INTRODUCTION TO
HEALTH SCIENCE
TECHNOLOGY

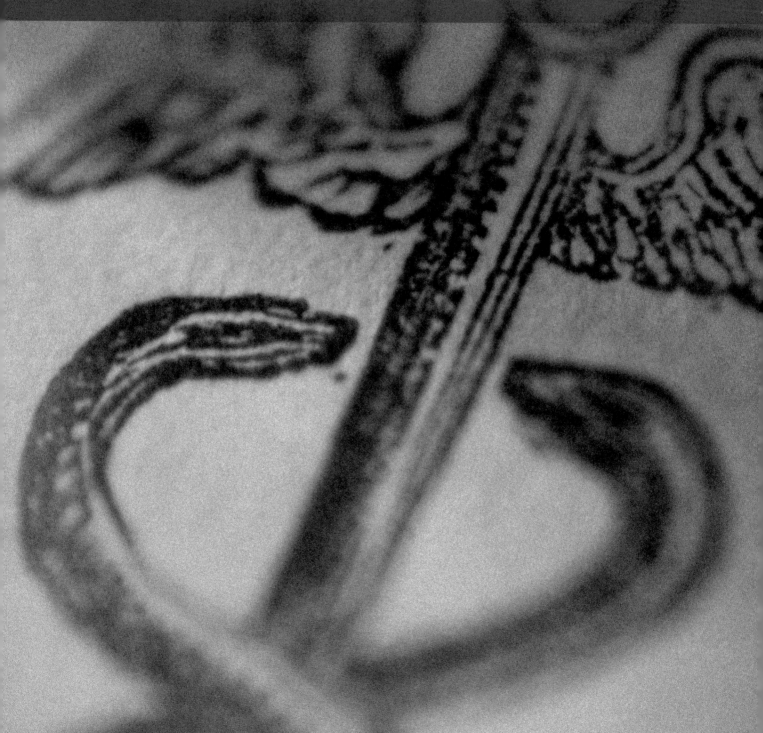

INTRODUCTION TO HEALTH SCIENCE TECHNOLOGY

Second Edition

Louise Simmers, MEd, RN
Karen Simmers-Nartker, BSN, RN
Sharon Simmers-Kobelak, BBA

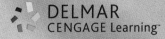

DELMAR
CENGAGE Learning

Australia • Brazil • Japan • Korea • Mexico • Singapore • Spain • United Kingdom • United States

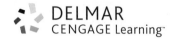
DELMAR
CENGAGE Learning

Introduction to Health Science Technology, Second Edition
Louise Simmers, MEd, RN
Karen Simmers-Nartker, BSN, RN
Sharon Simmers-Kobelak, BBA

Vice President, Career and Professional Editorial: Dave Garza

Director of Learning Solutions: Matthew Kane

Managing Editor: Marah Bellegarde

Acquisitions Editor: Matthew Seeley

Senior Product Manager: Juliet Steiner

Editorial Assistant: Megan Tarquinio

Vice President, Marketing, Career and Professional: Jennifer McAvey

Marketing Manager: Michele McTighe

Marketing Coordinator: Vanessa Carlson

Technology Product Manager: Mary Colleen Liburdi

Technology Project Manager: Carolyn Fox

Production Director: Carolyn Miller

Senior Art Director: Jack Pendleton

Content Project Manager: Anne Sherman

For product information and technology assistance, contact us at
Professional & Career Group Customer Support, 1-800-648-7450
For permission to use material from this text or product, submit all requests online at **www.cengage.com/permissions**
Further permissions questions can be emailed to
permissionrequest@cengage.com

Library of Congress Control Number: 2007941693

ISBN-13: 978-1-4180-2122-1
ISBN-10: 1-4180-2122-9

Delmar Cengage Learning   40761000673353
5 Maxwell Drive
Clifton Park, NY 12065-2919
USA

Cengage Learning products are represented in Canada by Nelson Education, Ltd.

For your lifelong learning solutions, visit **delmar.cengage.com**

Visit our corporate website at **www.cengage.com**

Notice to the Reader

4 5 6 7 12 11 10

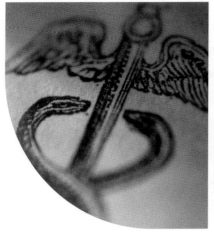

CONTENTS

CHAPTER 4   Personal and Professional Qualities of a Health Care Worker   81

CHAPTER 5   Legal and Ethical Responsibilities   103

PART 2
The Human Body   119

CHAPTER 6   Medical Terminology   121

CHAPTER 7   Anatomy and Physiology   142

PART 3
Special Considerations in Health Care   279

PART 4
Basics of Health Care   319

CHAPTER 15 First Aid 436

PART 5
Working in Health Care 517

CHAPTER 16 Preparing for the World of Work 518

CHAPTER 17 Computer Technology in Health Care 540

CHAPTER 18 Medical Math   562

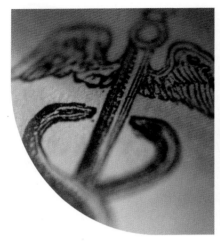

PREFACE

Introduction to Health Science Technology, second edition, was written to provide the beginning student with an overview of the health care field. The basic entry-level information that is covered serves as a solid foundation for all students in health sciences or health occupations, regardless of the particular health care profession they are interested in pursuing.

Content includes coverage of:

♦ Standard precautions, OBRA requirements, and isolation techniques

♦ Cultural diversity

♦ Medical math

♦ Principles of teamwork

♦ Professional leadership

♦ Time management

♦ Computer technology and how it influences the health care worker

♦ Industry efforts on cost containment, energy conservation, and accountability practices

♦ Health care career opportunities

♦ Growth and development

♦ Anatomy, physiology, and pathophysiology

♦ Medical terminology

♦ Vital signs

♦ First aid and CPR

ORGANIZATION OF TEXT

This book is divided into 18 chapters. Each chapter covers several topics. The topics presented are designed to provide the student with the basic knowledge and skills required for many different health careers.

Introduction to Health Science Technology, second edition, comprises both a textbook and a workbook. Each chapter in the textbook is subdivided into information sections. At the end of most of these sections, the student is told to go to the workbook to complete an assignment sheet on the information covered. Some chapters also include procedure sections, each of which refers the student to an evaluation sheet in the workbook. Following are brief explanations of these main components.

Information Sections (Textbook): The information sections provide the basic knowledge the student must acquire. These sections explain why the knowledge is important, the basic facts regarding the particular topic, and how this information is applied in various health careers. Most information sections refer the student to the assignment sheets found in the student workbook.

Assignment Sheets (Workbook): After students have read an information section, they are instructed to go to the corresponding assignment sheet. The assignment sheets allow them to test their comprehension and to return to the information section to check their answers. This enables them to reinforce their understanding of the information presented before moving on to another information section.

Procedure Sections (Textbook): The procedure sections provide step-by-step instructions on how to perform specific procedures. The student follows the steps while practicing the procedures. Each procedure begins with a list of the necessary equipment and supplies. **Note, Caution,** and **Checkpoint** may appear within the procedure. **Note** urges careful reading of the comments that follow. These comments usually stress points of knowledge or explain why certain techniques are used. **Caution** indicates that a safety factor is involved and that students should proceed carefully while doing the step in order to avoid injuring themselves or patients. **Checkpoint** alerts students to ask the instructor to check their work at that point in the procedure. Checkpoints are usually located at a critical stage. Each procedure section refers the student to a specific evaluation sheet in the workbook.

Evaluation Sheets (Workbook): Each evaluation sheet contains a list of criteria by which the students' performance will be tested after they have mastered a particular procedure. When a student feels he or she has mastered a particular procedure, he or she signs the evaluation sheet and gives it to the instructor. The instructor can grade the student's performance by using the listed criteria and checking each step against actual performance.

Because regulations vary from state to state regarding which procedures may be performed by a student in health science technology education (HSTE), it is important to check the specific regulations for your state. A health care worker should never perform any procedure without checking legal responsibilities. In addition, a student should perform no procedure unless the student has been properly taught the procedure and has been authorized to perform it.

Features

♦ More than 400 photos and illustrations are included to enhance learning and clarify technical content.

♦ The text material covers the *National Health Skill Standards,* helping instructors implement the curriculum elements of this important document. A new appendix provides a table showing the correlation of chapters in the book to the National Health Care Skill Standards.

♦ Mandates of the Health Insurance Portability and Accountability Act (HIPAA) have been incorporated throughout the textbook to emphasize the student's responsibilities with regard to this act and to stress how this act affects insurance portability and confidentiality of patient information.

♦ *Chapter objectives,* included in every chapter, help focus the student on the content discussed in the chapter.

♦ A list of *key terms* is included in the beginning of every chapter. These terms are defined within the chapter and in the glossary at the back of the book.

♦ The Anatomy and Physiology chapter has a listing of Related Health Careers as they pertain to specific body systems. This feature allows the student to associate a potential career with a specific body system.

♦ Internet search topics are included at the end of each chapter to encourage the student to explore the Internet to obtain current information on the many aspects of health care.

- A new chapter on Internet safety and security explains ways to protect computer hardware and software, methods used to maintain confidentiality of information, and safeguards that must be taken to protect computer security.

- Review questions at the end of each chapter enable the student to test his or her knowledge of information provided in the chapter.

- Career information has been updated and is stressed throughout the textbook to provide current information on a wide variety of health care careers. Careers have been organized according to the National Career Clusters. In addition, careers in forensic medicine and biotechnology have been added.

- A new section on bioterrorism provides information to make students aware of this constant threat and describes methods used to prevent and/or deal with it.

- The information on viruses has been expanded to include new viruses that can become potential sources of epidemics and pandemics. New emphasis is placed on infection control methods to prevent epidemics and pandemics.

- The section on cardiopulmonary resuscitation (CPR) has been revised to meet the American Heart Association's new 2005 standards for CPR for health care professionals.

- New nutritional guidelines from the U.S. Department of Agriculture have been incorporated into the nutrition chapter. Instructions are provided for using *My Pyramid* to plan a healthy diet.

- A new section on weight management discusses how to calculate ideal weight, how to lose or gain weight, and how to make food choices that will maintain a healthy weight.

- Various icons are included throughout the textbook. These icons denote the integration of academics such as math, science, and communication; occupational safety issues such as standard precautions and OBRA requirements; and workplace readiness issues such as career, legal, and technology information. An icon key similar to the one that follows can be found on the opening page of every chapter.

Observe Standard Precautions

Safety—Proceed with Caution

Math Skill

Science Skill

Communications Skill

Instructor's Check—Call Instructor at This Point

OBRA Requirement—Based on Federal Law

Legal Responsibility

Career Information

Technology

Extensive Teaching and Learning Package

Introduction to Health Science Technology, second edition, has a complete and specially designed supplement package to enhance student learning and workplace preparation. It is also designed to assist instructors in planning and implementing their instructional programs for the most efficient use of time and resources. The package contains:

Introduction to Health Science Technology, Student Workbook

This workbook contains perforated, performance-based assignments and evaluation sheets. The assignment sheets help students review what they have learned. The evaluation sheets provide criteria or standards for judging student performance for each procedure in the text.

Introduction to Health Science Technology Electronic Classroom Manager

This comprehensive teacher resource CD-ROM provides a wealth of resources to support the text.

A computerized Test Bank contains more than 1,800 modifiable test questions with answers. The user can also add his or her own questions. This software allows the user to create tests in less than 5 minutes and print them out in a variety of layouts. The Electronic Classroom Manager also contains a PowerPoint presentation with approximately 500 slides that can be used in the classroom to support lectures and generate discussion. Finally, an electronic Instructor's Manual provides answers to the workbook questions, teaching strategies, lesson plans, and applied academics. Additionally, critical thinking questions and case studies are included. The Instructor's Manual is provided as an MS Word document so it can be downloaded and modified to meet individual teacher needs.

Health Science Technology, Second Edition, Online Companion

An online companion that includes valuable information for both the student and instructor is available to accompany the text.

For the Student:

♦ PowerPoint presentations of important concepts

♦ Evaluation checklists from the Student Workbook

♦ Link to audio podcasts of medical terminology

♦ 14 animations that make anatomy and physiology concepts come alive

♦ StudyWARE software that is designed to offer additional review of concepts

The Online Companion tools for the instructor are on a password-protected site. Tools include:

♦ Online Instructor's Manual

♦ PowerPoint presentation to help you manage your classroom presentation

♦ Computerized Test Bank with over 1,800 questions.

♦ Evaluation checklists from the Student Workbook

♦ Conversion Grids to help you move from the 1st edition to the 2nd edition

♦ Correlation Grids demonstrating how the text meets national standards

♦ 14 Animations that make anatomy and physiology concepts come alive

To access the companion go to: http://www.delmarlearning/companions.com.

Diversified Health Occupations Video Series

A set of four videos that correlate to the text. The videos present career- and workplace-readiness issues.

Complete Video Package

Video 1: Is a Career in Health Care for You? Order # 0827382766; Video 2: A Day in the Life of Health Care Services, Order # 0827382774; Video 3: Professional and Personal Standards for Health Care Careers, Order # 0827382782; Video 4: How to Succeed in Your Health Care Career, Order # 0827382790.

About the Author

Louise Simmers received a Bachelor of Science degree in nursing from the University of Maryland and an MEd in education from Kent State University. She has worked as a public health nurse, medical–surgical nurse, charge nurse in a coronary–intensive care unit, instructor of practical nursing, and health occupations teacher and school-to-work coordinator at the Madison Comprehensive High School in Mansfield, Ohio. She is a member of the University of Maryland Nursing Alumni Association, Sigma Theta Tau, Phi Kappa Phi, National Education Association, and Association for Career and Technical Education (ACTE), and is a volunteer worker for the Red Cross. Mrs. Simmers received the Vocational Educator of the Year Award for Health Occupations in the State of Ohio and the Diversified Health Occupations Instructor of the Year Award for the State of Ohio. Mrs. Simmers is retired and lives with her husband in Venice, Florida. The author is pleased to announce that her twin daughters will now be assisting with the revisions of this textbook.

Karen Simmers-Nartker graduated from Kent State University, Ohio, with a Bachelor of Science degree in Nursing. She has been employed as a telemetry step-down, medical intensive care, surgical intensive care, and neurological intensive care nurse. She is currently employed as a shift coordinator in an open-heart intensive care unit. She has obtained certification from the Emergency Nurses Association for the Trauma Nursing Core Course (TNCC) and from the American Heart Association for Advanced Cardiac Life Support (ACLS). In her current position as charge nurse in her ICU, she coordinates patient care and staff assignments; manages interpersonal conflicts among staff and/or patients and family members; is responsible for ensuring quality care to meet the diverse needs of patients and/or family; actively participates in inservices to evaluate new equipment, medications, hospital services and supplies; and teaches and mentors newly employed nurses.

Sharon Simmers-Kobelak graduated from Miami University, Ohio, with a Bachelor of Business Administration degree. She is currently employed by Cengage Learning as a Career Account Manager. In this position, she assists instructors at private career schools in finding appropriate materials for classroom instruction. Sharon also provides inservice training for instructors on how to use the instructor and student resources in the most productive manner. She achieved President's Club status for two years and has repeatedly achieved quota with Cengage Learning during her tenure with the company.

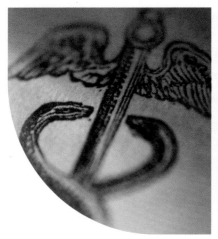

HOW TO USE

Objectives

Review this series of goals before you begin reading a chapter to help focus your study. When you have completed the chapter, go back and review these goals to see if you have grasped the key points of the chapter.

Icons

Icons are used throughout the text to highlight specific pieces of information. This icon key is presented to reinforce its meaning so when you see the icons used you will understand what they represent.

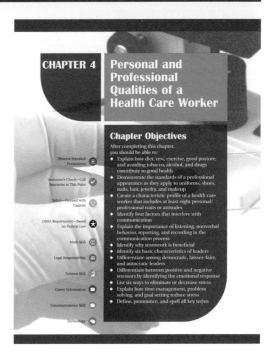

CHAPTER 4 — Personal and Professional Qualities of a Health Care Worker

Chapter Objectives

After completing this chapter, you should be able to:

- Explain how diet, rest, exercise, good posture, and avoiding tobacco, alcohol, and drugs contribute to good health
- Demonstrate the standards of a professional appearance as they apply to uniforms, shoes, nails, hair, jewelry, and makeup
- Create a characteristic profile of a health care worker that includes at least eight personal/professional traits or attitudes
- Identify four factors that interfere with communication
- Explain the importance of listening, nonverbal behavior, reporting, and recording in the communication process
- Identify why teamwork is beneficial
- Identify six basic characteristics of leaders
- Differentiate among democratic, laissez-faire, and autocratic leaders
- Differentiate between positive and negative stressors by identifying the emotional response
- List six ways to eliminate or decrease stress
- Explain how time management, problem solving, and goal setting reduce stress
- Define, pronounce, and spell all key terms

Icons (vertical list in image):
Observe Standard Precautions
Instructor's Check—Call Instructor at This Point
Safety—Proceed with Caution
OBRA Requirement—Based on Federal Law
Math Skill
Legal Responsibility
Science Skill
Career Information
Communications Skill
Technology

KEY TERMS

browser
central processing unit (CPU)
computer literacy *(come-pew'-tur lit'-er-ass-see)*
computer-assisted instruction (CAI)
computerized tomography (CT) *(com-pew'-tur-eyesd toe-mawg'-rah-fee)*
database
echocardiograph
electronic mail
file
fields

hardware
input
interactive video (computer-assisted video)
Internet
magnetic resonance imaging (MRI) *(mag-net'-ik rez'-oh-nance im'-adj-ing)*
mainframe computer
microcomputer
modem
networks
output
personal computer

positron emission tomography (PET) *(pos-ee'-tron ee-miss'-shun toe-mawg'-rah-fee)*
random access memory (RAM)
read only memory (ROM)
record
software
spreadsheet
stress test
telemedicine
telepharmacies
ultrasonography *(ul-trah-sawn-ahg'-rah-fee)*
virtual communities

Key Terms

Key Terms highlight the critical vocabulary words you will need to learn. Pronunciations are included for the harder to pronounce words. These terms are highlighted in color within the text where they are defined. You will also find most of these terms listed in the glossary section. Use this listing as part of your study and review of critical terms.

others, including family members. Information obtained from patients should not be repeated or used for personal gain. Gossiping about patients is ethically wrong.

♦ Refrain from immoral, unethical, and illegal practices. If you observe others taking part in illegal actions, report such actions to the proper authorities.

♦ Show loyalty to patients, co-workers, and employers. Avoid negative or derogatory statements, and always express a positive attitude.

♦ Be sincere, honest, and caring. Treat others as you want to be treated. Show respect and concern for the feelings, dignity, and rights of others.

When you enter a health occupation, learn the code of ethics for that occupation. Make every effort to abide by the code so as to become a competent and ethical health care worker. In doing so, you will earn the respect and confidence of patients, co-workers, and employers.

5:3 INFORMATION

Patients' Rights

Federal and state legislation requires health care agencies to have written policies concerning **patients' rights,** or the factors of care that patients can expect to receive. Agencies expect all personnel to respect and honor these rights.

The American Hospital Association has affirmed a **Patient's Bill of Rights** that is recognized and honored by many health care facilities. This bill of rights states, in part, that a patient has the right to:

♦ Considerate and respectful care

♦ Obtain complete, current information concerning diagnosis, treatment, and prognosis (expected outcome)

♦ Receive information necessary to give informed consent prior to the start of any procedure or treatment

♦ Have advance directives for health care and/or refuse treatment to the extent permitted under law (figure 5-7)

♦ Privacy concerning a medical care program

♦ Confidential treatment of all communications and records

FIGURE 5-7 Patients have the right to refuse treatment.

♦ Reasonable response to a request for services

♦ Obtain information regarding any relationship of the hospital to other health care and educational institutions

♦ Be advised of and have the right to refuse to participate in any research project

♦ Expect reasonable continuity of care

♦ Review medical records and examine bills and receive an explanation of all care and charges

♦ Be informed of any hospital rules, regulations, and/or policies and the resources available to resolve disputes or grievances

Residents in long-term care facilities are guaranteed certain rights under the Omnibus Budget Reconciliation Act (OBRA) of 1987. Every long-term care facility must inform residents or their guardians of these rights and a copy must be posted in each facility. This is often called a **Resident's Bill of Rights** and states, in part, that a resident has the right to:

♦ Free choice regarding physician, treatment, care, and participation in research

♦ Freedom from abuse and chemical or physical restraints

♦ Privacy and confidentiality of personal and clinical records

♦ Accommodation of needs and choice regarding activities, schedules, and health care

Information Sections

Information sections explain the basic facts of the topic, why you would need this information, and how the information is applied to various health care fields.

Related Health Careers

Related Health Careers appear in Chapter 7, *Anatomy and Physiology*. By reviewing the information presented in these boxes, you will relate specific health careers to specific body systems.

RELATED HEALTH CAREERS

NOTE: A basic knowledge of human anatomy and physiology is essential for almost every health care provider. However, some health careers are related to specific body systems. As each body system is discussed, examples of related health careers are listed. The following health career categories require knowledge of the structure and function of the entire human body and will not be listed in specific body system units.

♦ Athletic Trainer

♦ Emergency Medical Careers

♦ Medical Laboratory Careers

♦ Medical Assistant

♦ Medical Illustrator

♦ Nursing Careers

♦ Pharmacy Careers

♦ Physician Assistant

♦ Physician

♦ Surgical Technologist

Procedures Sections

Procedure sections provide step-by-step instructions on how to perform the procedure outlined in the Information section. Practice these procedures until you perform them correctly and proficiently.

PROCEDURE 14:2E

Measuring and Recording Tympanic (Aural) Temperature

Equipment and Supplies

Tympanic thermometer, probe cover, paper, pencil/pen, container for soiled probe cover

Procedure

1. Assemble equipment.

   NOTE: Read the operating instructions so you understand exactly how the thermometer must be used.

2. Wash hands. Put on gloves if needed.

   CAUTION: Follow standard precautions if contact with open sores or body fluids is possible.

3. Introduce yourself. Identify the patient. Explain the procedure.

4. Remove the thermometer from its base. Set the thermometer on the proper mode according to operating instructions. The equal mode is usually used for newborn infants, the rectal mode for children under 3 years of age, and the oral mode for children over 3 years of age and all adults. In areas where core body temperatures are recorded, such as critical care units, the core mode may be used.

5. Install a probe cover according to instructions. This will usually activate the thermometer, showing the mode selected and the word *ready*, indicating the thermometer is ready for use.

   CAUTION: Do not use the thermometer until *ready* is displayed because inaccurate readings will result.

6. Position the patient. Infants under 1 year of age should be positioned lying flat with the head turned for easy access to the ear. Small children can be held on the parent's lap, with the head held against the parent's chest for support. Adults who can cooperate and hold the head steady can either sit or lie flat. Patients in bed should have the head turned to the side, and stabilized against the pillow.

7. Hold the thermometer in your right hand to take a temperature in the right ear, and in your left hand to take a temperature in the left ear. With your other hand, pull the ear pinna (external lobe) up and back on any child over 1 year of age and on adults (figure 14-15A). Pull the ear pinna straight back for infants under 1 year of age.

   NOTE: Pulling the pinna correctly straightens the auditory canal so the probe tip will point directly at the tympanic membrane.

8. Insert the covered probe into the ear canal as far as possible to seal the canal (figure 14-15B). Do not apply pressure.

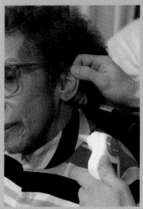

FIGURE 14-15A Before inserting the tympanic thermometer, pull the pinna up and back on adults and children older than 1 year.

Today's Research: Tomorrow's Health Care

Today's Research: Tomorrow's Health Care blocks are located in each chapter. These commentaries allow the student to learn about the many different types of research occurring today. If the research is successful, it may lead to possible cures and/or better methods of treatment in the future for a wide range of diseases and disorders. These blocks of information will also make the student aware of the fact that health care changes constantly because of new ideas and technology.

TODAY'S RESEARCH: TOMORROW'S HEALTH CARE

Draino for blood vessels?

Cardiovascular (heart and blood vessel) disease is the leading cause of death in the United States. Fatty plaques, caused mainly by an accumulation of LDL (low-density lipoprotein, or "bad" cholesterol), block the flow of blood in arterial walls, triggering a heart attack or stroke. HDL (high-density lipoprotein, or "good" cholesterol) helps protect the body from cardiovascular disease. HDL carries fats to the liver for disposal, helps prevent clots, and decreases inflammation in the blood vessels. For years, researchers have tried to find ways to increase the level of HDL while decreasing the level of LDL in the blood.

Scientists may have found the key to solve this problem in a small village in Italy. They discovered that residents of this village seemed to be immune to heart disease. Research showed that these individuals have a mutant gene that produces a powerful version of HDL. Scientists have produced a synthetic version of this HDL called *apo A-1 Milano*. When it was injected into a small group of volunteer heart patients, plaque in blood vessels was reduced by 4 percent and no new plaque buildup occurred. Scientists called it a miracle "blood vessel Draino." However, apo A-1 Milano is expensive to produce because it is a protein. It also must be injected into the body by an intravenous infusion, making it even more costly and inconvenient. Research is now directed toward gene therapy where the codes for the apo A-1 Milano protein are transferred into the body so the body can produce its own powerful version of HDL.

Scientists are also evaluating other methods to increase levels of HDL. They have discovered an enzyme called *cholesteryl ester transfer protein* that appears to reduce HDL levels and increase the levels of harmful LDL. Research is being conducted on new drugs that will block this enzyme. Who knows which approach will be most successful, but scientists will find the answer.

Full-Color Photos and Illustrations

Full-color photos are used through the text to illustrate important techniques you will be required to know and demonstrate when working within a health care field.

Illustrations are presented in full color and demonstrate important health care concepts, including the inner workings of the body. Use these illustrations for review while studying.

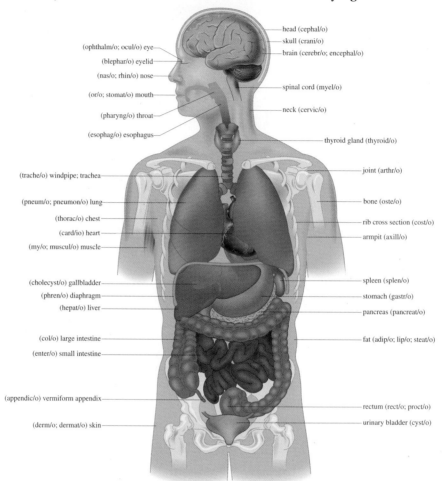

(ophthalm/o; ocul/o) eye
(blephar/o) eyelid
(nas/o; rhin/o) nose
(or/o; stomat/o) mouth
(pharyng/o) throat
(esophag/o) esophagus

(trache/o) windpipe; trachea
(pneum/o; pneumon/o) lung
(thorac/o) chest
(card/io) heart
(my/o; muscul/o) muscle

(cholecyst/o) gallbladder
(phren/o) diaphragm
(hepat/o) liver

(col/o) large intestine
(enter/o) small intestine

(appendic/o) vermiform appendix

(derm/o; dermat/o) skin

head (cephal/o)
skull (crani/o)
brain (cerebr/o; encephal/o)

spinal cord (myel/o)

neck (cervic/o)

thyroid gland (thyroid/o)

joint (arthr/o)

bone (oste/o)

rib cross section (cost/o)
armpit (axill/o)

spleen (splen/o)
stomach (gastr/o)
pancreas (pancreat/o)

fat (adip/o; lip/o; steat/o)

rectum (rect/o; proct/o)
urinary bladder (cyst/o)

FIGURE 6-3 The prefixes, suffixes, and word roots for parts of the human body.

Internet Searches

Internet Searches can enhance your comprehension of chapter information by offering the opportunity to read more information on the chapter topics.

Review Questions

Review Questions have been added to enhance your comprehension of chapter content. After you have completed reading the chapter, try to answer the review questions. If you find yourself unable to answer the questions, go back and review the chapter again.

INTERNET SEARCHES

Use the suggested search engines in the Using the Internet section in this chapter to search the Internet for additional information on the following topics:

1. *Computer hardware*: obtain information about different computer systems and compare and contrast the systems by searching the sites of computer manufacturers such as Gateway, Dell, Compaq, and IBM

2. *Computer software*: search for different types of software for health care providers

3. *Diagnostic devices*: search for additional information on blood analyzers, echocardiographs, computerized tomography, magnetic resonance imaging, positron emission tomography, and ultrasonography

REVIEW QUESTIONS

1. Define *computer literacy*.

2. Differentiate between hardware and software.

3. List five (5) examples of input devices and two (2) examples of output devices.

4. Identify ways confidentiality of patient information can be maintained while using computers.

5. Why is a contingency backup plan essential when computers are used to record information?

6. Briefly describe the main uses of the following imaging techniques:
   a. computerized tomography (CT)
   b. magnetic resonance imaging (MRI)
   c. positron emission tomography (PET)
   d. ultrasonography

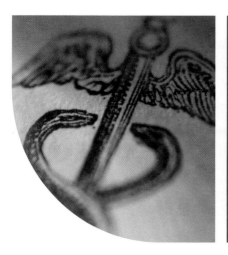

HOW TO USE INTRODUCTION TO HEALTH SCIENCE TECHNOLOGY, SECOND EDITION, STUDYWARE™

MINIMUM SYSTEM REQUIREMENTS

♦ Operating systems: Microsoft Windows 2000, Windows XP, Windows Vista
♦ Processor: Minimum required by operating system
♦ Memory: Minimum required by operating system
♦ Screen resolution: 800 × 600 pixels
♦ Color depth: 16-bit color (thousands of colors)
♦ Macromedia Flash Player 9. The Macromedia Flash Player is free and can be downloaded from **http://www.adobe.com/products/flashplayer/**

INSTALLATION INSTRUCTIONS

1. Insert disc into CD-ROM player. *Introduction to Health Science Technology*, Second Edition, StudyWARE™ installation program should start up automatically. If it does not, go to step 2.
2. From My Computer, double-click on the icon for the CD drive.
3. Double-click on the *setup.exe* file to start the program.

TECHNICAL SUPPORT

Telephone: 1-800-648-7450; 8:30 A.M.–5:30 P.M. Eastern Time
Fax: 1-518-881-1247
E-mail: delmar.help@cengage.com
StudyWARE™ is a trademark used herein under license.
Microsoft® and Windows® are registered trademarks of the Microsoft Corporation.
Pentium® is a registered trademark of the Intel Corporation.

GETTING STARTED

The StudyWARE™ software is designed to enhance your learning. As you study each chapter in the text, be sure to explore the activities in the corresponding chapter in the software. Use StudyWARE™ as your own private tutor to help you learn the material in the text.

Getting started is easy. Install the software by inserting the CD and following the on-screen instructions. Enter your first and last name so that the software can store you quiz results. Then choose a chapter from the menu and take a quiz or explore one of the activities.

Menus

You can access any of the menus from wherever you are within the program. The menus include Quizzes, Scores, Activities, and Animations.

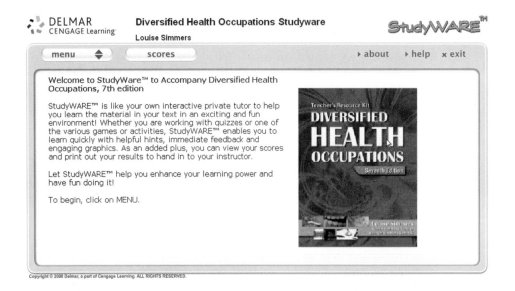

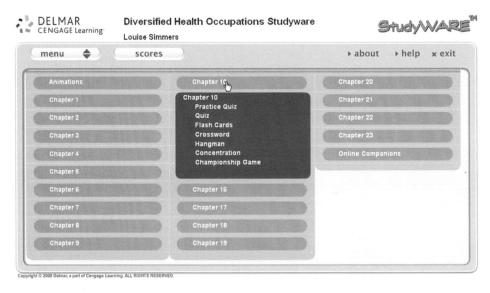

Quizzes

Quizzes include multiple choice and fill-in questions. You can take the quizzes in both Practice Mode and Quiz Mode. Use Practice Mode to improve your mastery of the material. You have multiple tries to get the answers correct. Instant feedback tells you whether you are right or wrong—and helps you learn quickly by explaining why an answer was correct or incorrect. Use Quiz Mode when you are ready to test yourself and keep a record of your scores. In Quiz Mode, you have one try to get the answers right, but you can take each Quiz as many times as you want.

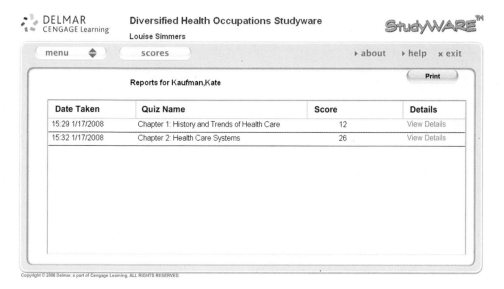

Scores

You can view your last scores for each quiz and print out your results to hand in to your instructor.

Activities

Activities include Flashcards, Crossword, Hangman, Ordering and Sorting, and a *Jeopardy!*-style Championship Game. Have fun while increasing your knowledge.

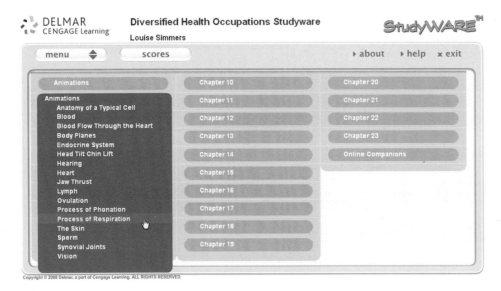

Animations

Animations help you visualize concepts related to pathological conditions and anatomy.

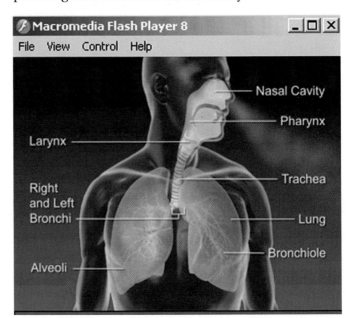

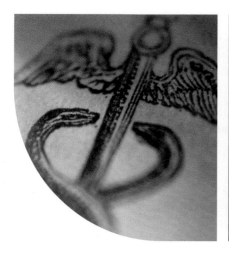

ACKNOWLEDGMENTS

Introduction to Health Science Technology, second edition, is dedicated to my grandchildren, Hayden Michael Kobelak, Kaleigh Ann Nartker, Kyla Ann Kobelak, Jesse Louise Nartker, and Brady Wayne Nartker. Our grandchildren help keep us young and bring so much joy and pleasure into our lives.

The author would like to thank everyone who participated in the development of this text, including

Nancy L. Raynor, former Chief Consultant, Health Occupations Education, State of North Carolina, who served as a consultant and major mentor in the development of this textbook

Dr. Charles Nichols, Department Head, and Ray Jacobs, Teacher Educator, Kent State University

Nancy Webber, RN, Diversified Health Occupations Instructor

Each person who consented to be a subject in the photographs

Administrative staff at Madison Comprehensive High School

Carolynn Townsend, Lisa Shearer Cooper, Donna Story, and Dorothy Fishman, who contributed chapter information

Kathryn G. Cutlip, Health and Safety Services Director at Richland County Red Cross, who reviewed and contributed information for the First Aid chapter

Sharon Logan, a true friend and health care professional, who never hesitated to review new material, research information, critique the manuscript, and offer encouragement

The author and Delmar Learning would like to thank those individuals who reviewed the manuscript and offered suggestions, feedback, and assistance. The text has been greatly improved as a result of the reviewers' helpful, insightful, and creative suggestions. Their work is greatly appreciated.

Becky Carter
Health Science Instructor
Charlotte, NC

Eleanore Cross
Health Science Instructor
Scotland High School
Laurinburg, NC

Beverly Fenley
Health Science Technology Instructor
Academy of Irving
Irving, TX

Christine Glass
ROP Instructor at Weber Institute
Stockton Unified School District
Lodi, CA

Natalie Kelly
Health Science Instructor
Hardaway High School
Columbus, GA

Julee T. Kristeller, RN
Health Occupations Instructor
Gray's Creek High School
Hope Mills, NC

Diane Sharp
Kentucky Department of Education
Career and Technical Education
Frankfort, KY

Lara Skaggs
State Program Manager
Health Careers Education
Oklahoma Department of CareerTech Education
Stillwater, OK

Linda Stanhope
Texas State Curriculum Writer
Health Science Instructor
Amarillo, TX

Kathy Turner
Health Occupations Consultant
North Carolina Department of Public Instruction
Cary, NC

Debra Ziegler, RN, BS
Health Sciences Instructor
Ralston High School
Ralston, NE

The author also wishes to thank the following companies, associations, and individuals for information and/or illustrations.

A-dec, Inc.

American Cancer Society

American Optometric Association

Becton Dickinson

Timothy Berger, MD

Bruce Black, MD

Boehringer Mannheim

Brevis Corporation

Briggs Corporation

Marcia Butterfield

Carson's Scholar Fund

Centers for Disease Control and Prevention

CIBA Pharmaceutical Company

Sandy Clark

The Clorox Company

Exergen Corporation

Food and Drug Administration (FDA)

Deborah Funk, MD

G.E. Medical Systems

Health Occupations Students of America

Hill-Rom

Kerr Corporation

Medline Industries

Michigan Pharmacists Association

Miltex Instrument Company

National Eye Institute

National Hospice and Palliative Care Organization

Omron Healthcare

Pfizer

Phoenix Society of Burn Survivors, Inc.

Photodisc

Poly-Medco

Professional Innovations

Sage Products, Inc.

Salk Institute

Skills USA

Robert A. Silverman

Smead Manufacturing

Spacelabs Medical, Inc.

Ron Stram, MD

Sunrise Medical

U.S. Army

U.S. Department of Agriculture

W.A. Foote Memorial Hospital

PART 1

Health Care Industry and Careers

CHAPTER 1

History and Trends of Health Care

Observe Standard Precautions

Instructor's Check—Call Instructor at This Point

Safety—Proceed with Caution

OBRA Requirement—Based on Federal Law

Math Skill

Legal Responsibility

Science Skill

Career Information

Communications Skill

Technology

Chapter Objectives

After completing this chapter,
you should be able to:

◆ Differentiate between early beliefs about the cause of disease and treatment and current beliefs about disease and treatment

◆ Identify at least 10 major events in the history of health care

◆ Name at least six historical individuals and explain how each one has helped to improve health care today

◆ Create a time line showing what you believe are the 20 most important discoveries in health care and explain why you believe they are important

◆ Identify at least five current trends or changes in health care

◆ Define, pronounce, and spell all key terms

KEY TERMS

alternative therapies
complementary therapies
cost containment
diagnostic related groups (DRGs)
energy conservation

geriatric care
holistic health care
home health care
integrative health care
Omnibus Budget Reconciliation Act (OBRA)

outpatient services
pandemic
telemedicine
wellness

NOTE: To further emphasize the Key Terms, they appear in color in the chapter copy. You will notice beginning in Chapter 3 on page 39 that pronunciations have been provided for the more difficult key terms. The single accent mark, _'_, shows where the main stress is placed when saying the word. The double accent, _"_, shows secondary stress (if present in the word).

1:1 INFORMATION

History of Health Care

Why is it important to understand the history of health care? Would you believe that some of the treatment methods in use today were also used in ancient times? In the days before drug stores, people used many herbs and plants as both food and medicine. Many of these herbs remain in use today. A common example is a medication called *morphine.* Morphine is made from a poppy plant and is used to manage pain. As you review each period of history, think about how the discoveries have helped to improve the health care you receive today.

ANCIENT TIMES

Table 1-1 lists many of the historical events of health care in ancient times. In primitive times, the common belief was that disease and illness were caused by evil spirits and demons. Treatment was directed toward eliminating the evil spirits. As civilizations developed, changes occurred as people began to study the human body and make observations about how it functions.

Religion played an important role in health care. A common belief was that illness and disease were punishments from the gods. Religious rites and ceremonies were frequently used to eliminate evil spirits and restore health. Explor-

ing the structure of the human body was limited because most religions did not allow dissection, or cutting apart of the body. For this reason, animals were frequently dissected to learn about different body parts.

The ancient Egyptians were the first people to record health records. It is important to remember that many people could not read; therefore, knowledge was limited to an educated few. Most of the records were recorded on stone and were created by priests, who also acted as physicians.

The ancient Chinese had a strong belief in the need to cure the spirit and nourish the entire body. This form of treatment remains important today, when holistic health methods stress treating the entire patient—mind, body, and soul.

Hippocrates (ca 460–377 BC), called the "Father of Medicine," was one of the most important physicians in ancient Greece (figure 1-1). The records that he and other physicians created helped establish that disease is caused by natural causes, not by supernatural spirits and demons. The ancient Greeks were also among the first to stress that a good diet and cleanliness would help to prevent disease.

With knowledge obtained from the Greeks, the Romans realized that some diseases were connected to filth, contaminated water, and poor sanitation. They began the development of sanitary systems by building sewers to carry away waste and aqueducts (waterways) to deliver clean water. They drained swamps and marshes to reduce the incidence of malaria. They created laws to keep streets clean and eliminate garbage.

TABLE 1-1 History of Health Care in Ancient Times

HISTORICAL EVENTS OF HEALTH CARE IN ANCIENT TIMES	
4000 BC–3000 BC **Primitive Times**	Believed that illness and disease were caused by supernatural spirits and demons Tribal witch doctors treated illness with ceremonies to drive out evil spirits Herbs and plants used as medicines, and some are still used today Trepanation or trephining (boring a hole in the skull) was used to treat insanity and epilepsy Average life span was 20 years
3000 BC–300 BC **Ancient Egyptians**	Earliest people known to maintain accurate health records Called upon the gods to heal them when disease occurred Physicians were priests who studied medicine and surgery in temple medical schools Imhotep (2635–2595? BC) may have been the first physician Believed the body was a system of channels for air, tears, blood, urine, sperm, and feces If channels became "clogged," bloodletting or leeches were used to "open" them Used magic and medicinal plants to treat disease Average life span was 20 to 30 years
1700 BC–220 AD **Ancient Chinese**	Religious prohibitions against dissection resulted in inadequate knowledge of body structure Carefully monitored the pulse to determine the condition of the body Believed in the need to treat the whole body by curing the spirit and nourishing the body Recorded a pharmacopoeia of medications based mainly on the use of herbs Used acupuncture, or puncture of the skin by needles, to relieve pain and congestion Also used moxibustion (a powdered substance was placed on the skin and then burned to cause a blister) to treat disease Began the search for medical reasons for illness Average life span was 20 to 30 years
1200 BC–200 BC **Ancient Greeks**	Began modern medical science by observing the human body and effects of disease Biochemist Alcmaeon in 6th century BC identified the brain as the physiological site of the senses Hippocrates (460–377 BC) called the Father of Medicine: • Developed an organized method to observe the human body • Recorded signs and symptoms of many diseases • Created a high standard of ethics, the Oath of Hippocrates, used by physicians today Aristotle (384–322 BC) dissected animals and is called the founder of comparative anatomy Believed illness is a result of natural causes Used therapies such as massage, art therapy, and herbal treatment that are still used today Stressed diet and cleanliness as ways to prevent disease Average life span was 25 to 35 years
753 BC–410 AD **Ancient Romans**	First to organize medical care by providing care for injured soldiers Early hospitals developed when physicians cared for ill people in rooms in their homes Later hospitals were religious and charitable institutions housed in monasteries and convents Began public health and sanitation systems: • Created aqueducts to carry clean water to the cities • Built sewers to carry waste materials away from the cities • Used filtering systems in public baths to prevent disease • Drained marshes to reduce the incidence of malaria Claudius Galen (129–199? AD), a physician, established many medical beliefs: • Body regulated by four fluids or humors: blood, phlegm, black bile, and yellow bile • An imbalance in the humors resulted in illness • Described symptoms of inflammation and studied infectious diseases • Dissected animals and determined function of muscles, kidney, and bladder Diet, exercise, and medications were used to treat disease Average life span was 25 to 35 years

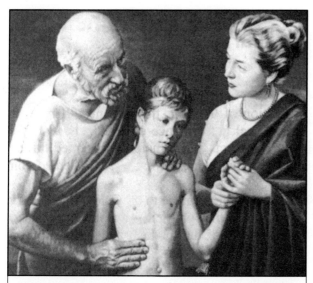

Hippocrates (ca 460–377 BC) was a Greek physician who is called the "Father of Medicine." He is best known for authoring a code of conduct for doctors, the "Hippocratic Oath." Today, physicians still recognize this oath and the guidelines it establishes for the practice of medicine.

The ancient Greeks thought that illness and disease were caused by the disfavor of the gods or evil spirits. Hippocrates' beliefs led medicine in a more accurate direction. He believed that illness and disease had rational and physical explanations.

Hippocrates stressed the importance of observation, diagnosis, and treatment. He was the first to accurately describe symptoms of pneumonia and epilepsy in children. He encouraged the use of a good diet, fresh air, cleanliness, and exercise to help the body heal itself.

Hippocrates founded a medical school in Cos, Greece, to teach his ideas on medicine. His students were held to a strict ethical code of behavior. This oath is the basis of medical practice today.

FIGURE 1-1 Hippocrates

The first hospitals were also established in ancient Rome when physicians began caring for injured soldiers or ill people in their homes.

Although many changes occurred in health care during ancient times, treatment was still limited. The average person had poor personal hygiene, drank contaminated water, and had unsanitary living conditions. Diseases such as typhoid, cholera, malaria, dysentery, leprosy, and smallpox infected many individuals. Because the causes of these diseases had not been discovered, the diseases were usually fatal. The average life span was 20 to 35 years. Today, individuals who die at this age are considered to be young people.

THE DARK AGES AND MIDDLE AGES

Table 1-2 lists many of the historical events of the Dark Ages and the Middle Ages. During the Dark Ages, after the fall of the Roman empire, the study of medicine stopped. Individuals again lived in unsanitary conditions with little or no personal hygiene. Epidemics of smallpox, dysentery, typhus, and the plague were rampant. Monks and priests stressed prayer to treat illness and disease.

The Middle Ages brought a renewed interest in the medical practices of the Romans and Greeks. Monks obtained and translated the writings of the Greek and Roman physicians, and recorded the knowledge in handwritten books. Medical universities were created in the 9th century to train physicians how to use this knowledge to treat illness. Later, Arabs began requiring that physicians pass examinations and obtain licenses.

In the 1300s, a major epidemic of bubonic plague killed almost 75 percent of the population of Europe and Asia. Other diseases such as smallpox, diphtheria, tuberculosis, typhoid, and malaria killed many others. The average life span of 20 to 35 years was often reduced even more by the presence of these diseases. Many infants died shortly after birth. Many children did not live into adulthood. Today, most of these diseases are almost nonexistent. They are prevented by vaccines or treated by medications.

THE RENAISSANCE

Table 1-3 lists many of the historical events that occurred between 1350 and 1650 AD, a period known as the Renaissance. This period often refers to the "rebirth of science of medicine." The major source of new information about the human body was a result of accepting and allowing human dissection. Doctors could now view body organs and see the connection between different systems in the body. Artists, such as Michelangelo and Leonardo da Vinci, were able to draw the body accurately. In addition, the development of the printing press resulted in the publication of medical books that were used by students at medical universities. Knowledge spread more rapidly. Physicians were more educated.

TABLE 1-2 History of Health Care in the Dark Ages and the Middle Ages

HISTORICAL EVENTS OF HEALTH CARE IN THE DARK AGES AND THE MIDDLE AGES	
400–800 AD **Dark Ages**	Emphasis was placed on saving the soul and the study of medicine was prohibited Prayer and divine intervention were used to treat illness and disease Monks and priests provided custodial care for sick people Medications were mainly herbal mixtures Average life span was 20 to 30 years
800–1400 AD **Middle Ages**	Renewed interest in the medical practice of Greeks and Romans Physicians began to obtain knowledge at medical universities in the 9th century A pandemic (worldwide epidemic) of the bubonic plague (black death) killed three quarters of the population of Europe and Asia Major diseases were smallpox, diphtheria, tuberculosis, typhoid, the plague, and malaria Arab physicians used their knowledge of chemistry to advance pharmacology Rhazes (al-Razi), an Arab physician, became known as the Arab Hippocrates: • Based diagnoses on observations of the signs and symptoms of disease • Developed criteria for distinguishing between smallpox and measles in 910 AD • Suggested blood was the cause of many infectious diseases • Began the use of animal gut for suture material Arabs began requiring that physicians pass examinations and obtain licenses Avenzoar, a physician, described the parasite causing scabies in the 12th century Average life span was 20 to 35 years

TABLE 1-3 History of Health Care in the Renaissance

HISTORICAL EVENTS OF HEALTH CARE IN THE RENAISSANCE	
1350–1650 AD **Renaissance**	Rebirth of science of medicine Dissection of the body began to allow a better understanding of anatomy and physiology Artists Michelangelo (1475–1564) and Leonardo da Vinci (1452–1519) used dissection to draw the human body more realistically First chairs (positions of authority) of medicine created at Oxford and Cambridge in England in 1440 Development of the printing press allowed knowledge to be spread to others First anatomy book was published by Andreas Vesalius (1514–1564) First book on dietetics written by Isaac Judaeus Michael Servetus (1511–1553): • Described the circulatory system in the lungs • Explained how digestion is a source of heat for the body Roger Bacon (1214?–1294): • Promoted chemical remedies to treat disease • Researched optics and refraction (bending of light rays) Average life span was 30 to 40 years

TABLE 1-4 History of Health Care in the 16th, 17th, and 18th Centuries

HISTORICAL EVENTS OF HEALTH CARE IN THE 16TH, 17TH, AND 18TH CENTURIES	
16th and 17th Centuries	Causes of disease were still not known and many people died from infections and puerperal (childbirth) fever Ambroise Paré (1510–1590), a French Surgeon, known as the Father of Modern Surgery: • Established use of ligatures to bind arteries and stop bleeding • Eliminated use of boiling oil to cauterize wounds • Improved treatment of fractures and promoted use of artificial limbs Gabriel Fallopius (1523–1562): • Identified the fallopian tubes in the female • Described the tympanic membrane in the ear William Harvey (1578–1657) described the circulation of blood to and from the heart in 1628 Anton van Leeuwenhoek (1632–1723) invented the microscope in 1666 First successful blood transfusion on animals performed in England in 1667 Bartolomeo Eustachio identified the eustachian tube leading from the ear to the throat Scientific societies, such as the Royal Society of London, were established Apothecaries (early pharmacists) made, prescribed, and sold medications Average life span was 35 to 45 years
18th Century	Gabriel Fahrenheit (1686–1736) created the first mercury thermometer in 1714 Joseph Priestley (1733–1804) discovered the element oxygen in 1774 John Hunter (1728–1793), an English surgeon: • Established scientific surgical procedures • Introduced tube feeding in 1778 Benjamin Franklin (1706–1790) invented bifocals for glasses Dr. Jessee Bennet performed the first successful Cesarean section operation to deliver an infant in 1794 James Lind prescribed lime juice containing vitamin C to prevent scurvy in 1795 Edward Jenner (1749–1823) developed a vaccination for smallpox in 1796 Average life span was 40 to 50 years

The life span increased to an average age of 30 to 40 years during the Renaissance, but common infections still claimed many lives. At this point in time, the actual causes of disease were still a mystery.

THE 16TH, 17TH, AND 18TH CENTURIES

Table 1-4 lists many of the historical events that occurred during the 16th, 17th, and 18th centuries. During this period, physicians gained an increased knowledge of the human body. William Harvey described the circulation of blood. Gabriel Fallopius described the tympanic membrane in the ear and the fallopian tubes of a female. Bartolomeo Eustachio identified the tube between the ear and throat. These discoveries allowed other physicians to see how the body functioned.

A major development was the invention of the microscope by Anton van Leeuwenhoek (figure 1-2). This allowed physicians to see organisms that are too small to be seen by the human eye. Even though they were not aware of it at the time, physicians were looking at many of the pathogenic organisms (germs) that cause disease. The microscope continues to be a major diagnostic tool.

This period also saw the start of drug stores, or pharmacies. Apothecaries (early pharmacists) made, prescribed, and sold medications. Many of the medications were made from plants and herbs similar to those used in ancient times. At the end of the 18th century, Edward Jenner developed a vaccine to prevent smallpox, a deadly disease.

During this time, the average life span increased to 40 to 50 years. However, the causes of many diseases were still unknown, and medical care remained limited.

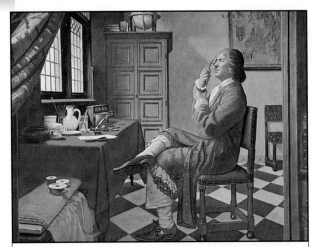

Anton van Leeuwenhoek (1632–1723) is one of several individuals who are called the "Father of Microbiology" because of his discovery of bacteria and other microscopic organisms. He was born in Delft, Holland, and worked as a tradesman and apprentice to a textile merchant. van Leeuwenhoek learned to grind lenses and make simple microscopes to use while examining the thread densities of materials.

In 1668, he visited London and saw a copy of Robert Hookes's *Micrographia,* a book depicting Hookes's own observations with the microscope. This stimulated van Leeuwenhoek's interest and he began to build microscopes that magnified more than 200 times, with clearer and brighter images than were available at the time. Using the improved microscope, van Leeuwenhoek began to observe bees, bugs, water, and other similar substances. He noticed tiny single-celled organisms that he called *animalcules,* now known as microorganisms. When van Leeuwenhoek reported his observations to the Royal Society of London, he was met with skepticism. However, other scientists researched his findings, and eventually his ideas were proved and accepted.

van Leeuwenhoek was the first individual to record microscopic observations on muscle fibers, blood vessels, and spermatozoa. He laid the foundations of plant anatomy and animal reproduction. He developed a method for grinding powerful lenses and made more than 400 different types of microscopes. Anton van Leeuwenhoek's discoveries are the basis for microbiology today.

FIGURE 1-2 Anton van Leeuwenhoek

THE 19TH CENTURY

Table 1-5 lists many of the historical events that occurred during the 19th century, a period also known as the Industrial Revolution. Major progress in medical science occurred because of the development of machines and ready access to books.

Early in the century, René Laënnec invented the stethoscope (figure 1-3). This invention

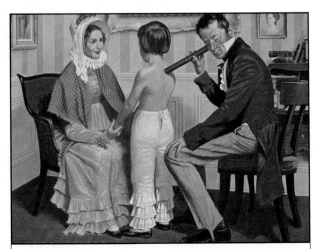

René-Théophile-Hyacinthe Laënnec (1781–1826) was a French physician who is frequently called the "Father of Pulmonary Diseases." In 1816, he invented the stethoscope, which began as a piece of rolled paper and evolved into a wooden tube that physicians inserted into their ears.

Laënnec used his stethoscope to listen to the various sounds made by the heart and lungs. For years he studied chest sounds and correlated them with diseases found on autopsy. In 1819, he published a book on his findings, *De l'auscultation mediate*, also known as *On Mediate Auscultation*. Laënnec's use of auscultation (listening to internal body sounds) and percussion (tapping body parts to listen to sounds) formed the basis of the diagnostic techniques used in medicine today.

Laënnec studied and diagnosed many medical conditions such as bronchiectasis, melanoma, cirrhosis, and tuberculosis. Cirrhosis of the liver is still called *Laënnec's cirrhosis* because Laënnec was the first physician to recognize this condition as a disease entity. Laënnec also conducted extensive studies on tuberculosis, but unfortunately he was not aware of the contagiousness of the disease and contracted tuberculosis himself. He died at the age of 45 of tuberculosis, leaving a legacy of knowledge that is still used by physicians today.

FIGURE 1-3 René Laënnec *(Courtesy of Parke-Davis and Company, copyright 1957)*

allowed physicians to listen to internal body sounds, which increased their knowledge of the human body. The original stethoscope, a rolled piece of paper, quickly evolved into a wooden tube that was inserted into the physician's ear.

Formal training for nurses began during this century. After training at a program in Germany, Florence Nightingale established sanitary nursing care units for injured soldiers during the Crimean War. She is known as the founder of modern nursing (figure 1-4).

TABLE 1-5 History of Health Care in the 19th Century

HISTORICAL EVENTS OF HEALTH CARE IN THE 19TH CENTURY	
19th Century	Royal College of Surgeons (medical school) founded in London in 1800
	French barbers acted as surgeons by extracting teeth, using leeches for treatment, and giving enemas
	First federal vaccination legislation enacted in 1813
	First successful blood transfusion was performed on humans in 1818 by James Blundell
	René Laënnec (1781–1826) invented the stethoscope in 1816
	Dr. Philippe Pinel (1755–1826) began humane treatment for mental illness
	Pandemic of cholera in 1832
	Theodor Fliedner started one of the first training programs for nurses in Germany in 1836, which provided Florence Nightingale with her formal training
	In the 1840s, Ignaz Semmelweis (1818–1865) encouraged physicians to wash their hands with lime after performing autopsies and before delivering babies to prevent puerperal (childbirth) fever, but the idea was resisted by hospital and medical personnel
	Dr. William Morton (1819–1868), an American dentist, began using ether as an anesthetic in 1846
	Dr. James Simpson (1811–1870) began using chloroform as an anesthetic in 1847
	American Medical Association was formed in Philadelphia in 1847
	Elizabeth Blackwell (1821–1910) became the first female physician in the United States in 1849; started the first Women's Medical College in New York in 1868
	American Pharmaceutical Association held its first convention in 1853
	Florence Nightingale (1820–1910) was the founder of modern nursing:
	• Established efficient and sanitary nursing units during Crimean War in 1854
	• Opened Nightingale School and Home for Nurses at St. Thomas' Hospital in London in 1860
	• Began the professional education of nurses
	Dorothea Dix (1802–1887) appointed Superintendent of Female Nurses of the Army in 1861
	International Red Cross was founded in 1863
	Joseph Lister (1827–1912) started using disinfectants and antiseptics during surgery to prevent infection in 1865
	Elizabeth Garrett Anderson (1836–1917) became the first female physician in Britain in 1870 and the first woman member of the British Medical Association in 1873
	Paul Ehrlich (1854–1915), a German bacteriologist, developed methods of detecting and differentiating between various diseases, developed the foundation for modern theories of immunity, and used chemicals to eliminate microorganisms
	Francis Clarke and M. G. Foster patented the first electrical hearing aid in 1880
	Clara Barton (1821–1912) founded the American Red Cross in 1881
	Robert Koch (1843–1910), another individual who is also called the "Father of Microbiology," developed the culture plate method to identify pathogens and in 1882 isolated the bacteria that causes tuberculosis
	Louis Pasteur (1822–1895) contributed many discoveries to the practice of medicine including:
	• Proving that microorganisms cause disease
	• Pasteurizing milk to kill bacteria
	• Creating a vaccine for rabies in 1885
	Gregory Mendel (1822–1884) established principles of heredity and dominant/recessive patterns
	Dimitri Ivanofski discovered viruses in 1892
	Lillian Wald (1867–1940) established the Henry Street Settlement in New York City in 1893 (the start of public health nursing)
	Dr. Emile Roux of Paris developed a vaccine for diphtheria in 1894
	Wilhelm Roentgen (1845–1923) discovered roentgenograms (X-rays) in 1895
	Almroth Wright developed a vaccine for typhoid fever in 1897
	Bayer introduced aspirin in powdered form in 1899
	Bacteria causing gonorrhea and leprosy were discovered and identified
	Average life span was 40 to 60 years

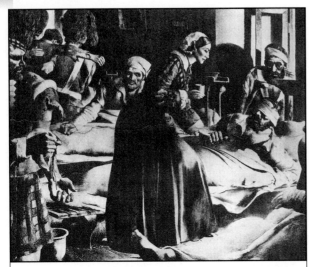

Florence Nightingale (1820–1910) is known as the founder of modern nursing. In 1854, Nightingale led 38 nurses to serve in the Crimean War. During the war, the medical services of the British army were horrifying and inadequate. Hundreds of soldiers died because of poor hygiene and unsanitary conditions. Nightingale fought for the reform of the military hospitals and for improved medical care.

Nightingale encouraged efficiency and cleanliness in the hospitals. Her efforts decreased the death rate of patients by two thirds. She used statistics to prove that the number of deaths decreased with improved sanitary conditions. Because of her statistics, sanitation reforms occurred and medical practice improved.

One of Nightingale's greatest accomplishments was starting the Nightingale Training School for nurses at St. Thomas' Hospital in London. Nurses attending her school received a year's training, which included lectures and practical ward work. Trained nurses were then sent to work in British hospitals and abroad. These trained nurses also established other nursing schools by using Nightingale's model. Nightingale published more than 200 books, pamphlets, and reports. Her writings on hospital organization had a lasting effect in England and throughout the world. Many of her principles are still used in health care today.

FIGURE 1-4 Florence Nightingale *(Courtesy of Parke-Davis, a division of Warner-Cambert Company)*

Infection control was another major development. Physicians began to associate the tiny microorganisms seen in the microscope with diseases. Methods to stop the spread of these organisms were developed by Theodor Fliedner, Joseph Lister, and Louis Pasteur (figure 1-5).

Women became active participants in medical care. Elizabeth Blackwell was the first female physician in the United States. Dorothea Dix was appointed superintendent of female nurses in

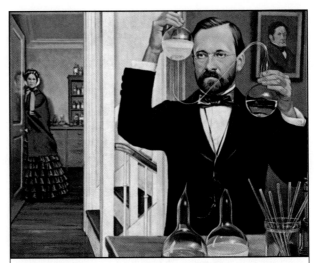

Louis Pasteur (1822–1895) was a French chemist and biologist. He is also called the "Father of Microbiological Sciences and Immunology" because of his work with the microorganisms that cause disease. Pasteur developed the germ theory and discovered the processes of pasteurization, vaccination, and fermentation. His germ theory proved that microorganisms cause most infectious diseases. He proved that heat can be used to destroy harmful germs in perishable food, a process now known as "pasteurization." Pasteur also discovered that weaker microorganisms could be used to immunize against more poisonous forms of a microorganism. He developed vaccines against anthrax, chicken cholera, rabies, and swine erysipelas. Through his studies of fermentation, he proved that each disease is caused by a specific microscopic organism.

Pasteur's principles for sanitation helped control the spread of disease and provided ideas on how to prevent disease. These discoveries reformed surgery and obstetrics. Pasteur is responsible for saving the lives of millions of people through vaccination and pasteurization. His accomplishments are the foundation of bacteriology, immunology, microbiology, molecular biology, and virology in today's health care.

FIGURE 1-5 Louis Pasteur *(Courtesy of Parke-Davis and Company, copyright 1957)*

the army. Clara Barton founded the American Red Cross (figure 1-6).

The average life span during this period increased to 40 to 65 years. Treatment for disease was more specific after the causes for diseases were identified. Many vaccines and medications were developed.

THE 20TH CENTURY

Table 1-6 lists many of the historical events that occurred during the 20th century. This period

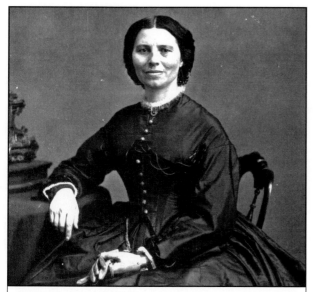

Clara Barton (1821–1912) is known as the founder of the American Red Cross. During the American Civil War, she served as a volunteer to provide aid to wounded soldiers. She appealed to the public to provide supplies and, after collecting the supplies, personally delivered them to soldiers of both the North and the South.

In 1869, Barton went to Geneva, Switzerland, to rest and improve her health. During her visit she learned about the Treaty of Geneva, which provided relief for sick and wounded soldiers. A dozen nations had signed the treaty, but the United States had refused. She also learned about the International Red Cross, which provided disaster relief during peacetime and war.

When Barton returned to the United States, she campaigned for the Treaty of Geneva until it was ratified. In 1881, the American Red Cross was formed. Barton served as its first president. She represented the American Red Cross by traveling all over the United States and the world to assist victims of natural disasters and war.

FIGURE 1-6 Clara Barton *(Courtesy of the National Archives, photo no. 111-B-4 246, Brady Collection)*

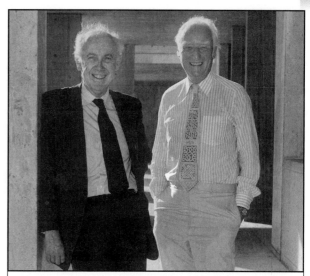

Francis Crick and James Watson shared the Nobel Prize in 1962 with Maurice Wilkins for discovering the structure of deoxyribonucleic acid (DNA). Crick is a biophysicist and chemist. Watson studied zoology. They met at the University of Cambridge and shared a desire to solve the mystery of the structure of DNA.

Crick and Watson built a three-dimensional model of the molecules of DNA to assist them in discovering the structure. In 1953, they discovered that the structure of DNA is a double helix, similar to a gently twisted ladder. It consists of pairs of bases, including adenine and thymine, and guanine and cytosine. The order in which these bases appear on the double helix determines the identity of a living organism. That is, DNA carries life's hereditary information.

Crick and Watson's model of the DNA double helix provided motivation for research in molecular genetics and biochemistry. Their work showed that understanding how a structure is arranged is critical to understanding how it functions. Crick and Watson's discovery is the foundation for most of the genetic research that is being conducted today.

FIGURE 1-7A Francis Crick and James Watson *(Courtesy of the Salk Institute)*

showed the most rapid growth in health care. Physicians were able to use new machines such as X-rays to view the body. Medicines, including insulin for diabetes, antibiotics to fight infections, and vaccines to prevent diseases, were developed. The causes for many diseases were identified. Physicians were now able to treat the cause of a disease to cure the patient.

A major development to understanding the human body occurred in the 1950s when Francis Crick and James Watson described the structure of DNA and how it carries genetic information

(figures 1-7A and B). Their studies began the search for gene therapy to cure inherited diseases. This research continues today.

Health care plans to help pay the costs of care also started in the 20th century. At the same time, standards were created to make sure that every individual had access to quality health care. This remains a major concern of health care in the United States today.

The first open-heart surgery in the 1950s has progressed to the heart transplants that occur today. Surgical techniques have provided cures for what were once fatal conditions. Infection

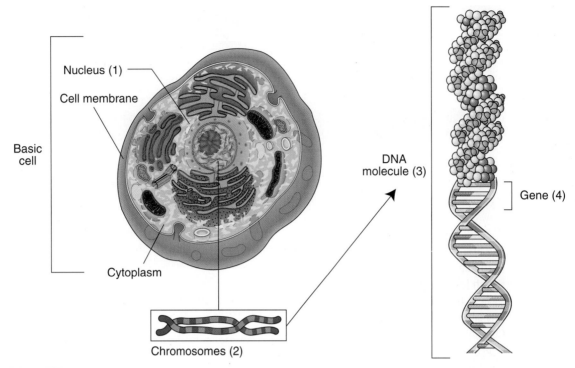

FIGURE 1-7B The discovery of the structure of DNA and how it carries genetic (inherited) information was the beginning of research on how to cure inherited diseases by gene therapy.

TABLE 1-6 History of Health Care in the 20th Century

HISTORICAL EVENTS OF HEALTH CARE IN THE 20TH CENTURY	
20th Century	Walter Reed demonstrated that mosquitoes carry yellow fever in 1900
	Carl Landsteiner classified the ABO blood groups in 1901
	Female Army Nurse Corps established as a permanent organization in 1901
	Miller Reese of New York patented the battery-driven hearing aid in 1901
	Dr. Harry Plotz developed a vaccine against typhoid in 1903
	Dr. Elie Metchnikoff (1845–1916) identified how white blood cells protect against disease
	Marie Curie (1867–1934) isolated radium in 1910
	Sigmund Freud's (1856–1939) studies formed the basis for psychology and psychiatry
	Influenza (flu) pandemic killed more than 21 million people in 1918
	Frederick Banting and Charles Best discovered and used insulin to treat diabetes in 1922
	Health insurance plans and social reforms were developed in the 1920s
	Mary Breckinridge (1881–1965) founded Frontier Nursing Service in 1925 to deliver health care to rural Kentuckians
	John Enders and Frederick Robbins developed methods to grow viruses in cultures in the 1930s
	Sir Alexander Fleming (1881–1955) discovered penicillin in 1928
	Buddy, a German shepherd, became the first guide dog for the blind in 1928
	Dr. Robert Smith (Dr. Bob) and William Wilson founded Alcoholics Anonymous in 1935
	President Franklin Roosevelt established the March of Dimes to fight poliomyelitis in 1937
	Gerhard Domagk (1895–1964) developed sulfa drugs to fight infections
	Dr. George Papanicolaou developed the Pap test to detect cervical cancer in females in 1941
	The first kidney dialysis machine was developed in 1944
	Jonas Salk (1914–1995) developed the polio vaccine using dead polio virus in 1952
	Francis Crick and James Watson described the structure of DNA and how it carries genetic information in 1953

(continues)

TABLE 1-6 History of Health Care in the 20th Century *(Continued)*

HISTORICAL EVENTS OF HEALTH CARE IN THE 20TH CENTURY

The first heart–lung machine was used for open-heart surgery in 1953

Conjoined (Siamese) twins were separated successfully for the first time in 1953

The first successful kidney transplant in humans was performed by Joseph Murray in 1954

Albert Sabin (1906–1993) developed an oral live-virus polio vaccine in the mid-1950s

Birth control pills approved by the U.S. Food and Drug Administration (FDA) in 1960

An arm severed at the shoulder was successfully reattached to body in 1962

The first liver transplant was performed by Thomas Starzl in 1963

The first lung transplant was performed by James Hardy in 1964

Medicare and Medicaid 1965 Amendment to Social Security Act marked the entry of the federal government into the health care arena as a major purchaser of health services

The first successful heart transplant was performed by Christian Barnard in 1967

The first hospice was founded in England in 1967

Hargobind Khorana synthesized a gene in 1970

Health Maintenance Organization Act of 1973 established standards for HMOs and provided an alternative to private health insurance

Physicians used amniocentesis to diagnose inherited diseases before birth in 1975

Computerized axial tomography (CAT) scan was developed in 1975

New Jersey Supreme Court ruled that parents of Karen Ann Quinlan, a comatose woman, had the power to remove life support systems in 1975

The first "test tube" baby, Louise Brown, was born in England in 1978

Genetic engineering led to development of vaccines against hepatitis, herpes simplex, and chicken pox in the 1980s

Acquired immune deficiency syndrome (AIDS) was identified as a disease in 1981

Dr. William DeVries implanted the first artificial heart, the Jarvik-7, in 1982

Cyclosporine, a drug to suppress the immune system after organ transplants, approved in 1983

The Human immunodeficiency virus (HIV) causing AIDS was identified in 1984

The Omnibus Budget Reconciliation Act (OBRA) of 1987 established regulations for the education and certification of nursing assistants

The Omnibus Budget Reconciliation Act of 1989 created an agency for health care policy and research to develop outcome measures of health care quality

The first gene therapy to treat disease occurred in 1990

President George H. Bush signed the Americans with Disabilities Act in 1990

The National Center for Complementary and Alternative Medicine (NCCAM) was established by the National Institutes of Health (NIH) to research and establish standards of quality care in 1992

A vaccine for chicken pox was approved in 1995

The British government admitted that an outbreak of "mad cow" disease was linked to Creutzfeldt–Jacob disease in humans in 1996

President Clinton signed the Health Insurance Portability and Accountability Act (HIPAA) of 1996 to protect patient privacy and to make it easier to obtain and keep health insurance

Identification of genes causing diseases increased rapidly in the 1990s

A sheep was cloned in 1997

The first successful larynx (voice box) transplant was performed in 1998

An international team of scientists sequenced the first human chromosome in 1999

Average life span was 60 to 80 years

control has helped decrease surgical infections that previously killed many patients.

The contribution of computer technology to medical science has helped medicine progress faster in the 20th century than in all previous periods combined. Today, computers are used in every aspect of health care. Their use will increase even more in the 21st century.

All of these developments have helped increase the average life span to 60 to 80 years. In

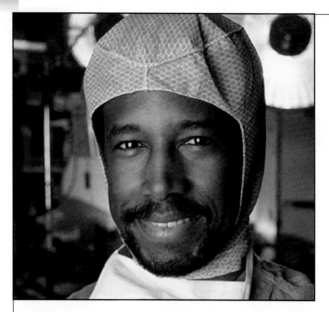

age system. After the operation, both boys were able to survive independently. This result was the first surgery to separate occipital craniopagus twins, meaning they were joined at the head near the occipital bone. In 1997, Dr. Carson was the lead surgeon in South Africa in another successful operation to separate 11-month-old boys who were vertical craniopagus twins, meaning they were joined at the top of the head looking in opposite directions.

Dr. Carson continues to perform landmark surgeries and conduct research for new techniques and procedures. He has refined hemispherectomy, a revolutionary surgical procedure performed on the brain to stop seizures that are difficult to treat or cure. He works with craniofacial (head or facial disfigurement) reconstructive surgery. Dr. Carson has developed an important craniofacial program that combines neurosurgery and plastic surgery for children with congenital (at birth) deformities. He is also known for his work in pediatric neurooncology (brain tumors).

Dr. Carson is the author of three best-selling books: *Gifted Hands,* the story of his life; *Think Big,* a story inspiring others to use their intelligence; and *The Big Picture,* a close-up look at the life of a professional surgeon. Dr. Carson is also cofounder and president of the Carson Scholar's Fund. This fund was established to recognize young people for superior academic performance and humanitarian achievement.

Benjamin Carson, MD, has become famous for his landmark surgeries to separate conjoined twins. Dr. Carson is one of the most skilled and accomplished neurosurgeons today.

In 1987, he was the primary surgeon of a 70-member surgical team that separated Siamese twins from West Germany. The 7-month-old boys were joined at the back of the head, sharing the major cerebral blood drain-

FIGURE 1-8 Benjamin Carson, MD *(Courtesy of Carson Scholar's Fund)*

fact, it is not unusual to see people live to be 100. With current pioneers such as Ben Carson (figure 1-8), as well as many other medical scientists and physicians, there is no limit to what future health care will bring.

THE 21ST CENTURY

The potential for major advances in health care in the 21st century is unlimited. Early in the century, the completion of the Human Genome Project by the U.S. Department of Energy and the National Institutes of Health (NIH) provided the basis for much of the current research on genetics. Research with embryonic stem cells and development of cloned cells could lead to treatments that will cure many diseases.

Some major threats to health care exist in this century. Bioterrorism, the use of microorganisms or biologic agents as weapons to infect humans, is a real and present threat. New viruses, such as the bird flu virus, could mutate and cause disease in humans. Pandemics, or worldwide epidemics, could occur quickly in our global society because people can travel easily from one country to another.

At the same time, however, scientists now have computers and rapid methods of communication to share new knowledge. Organizations such as the World Health Organization (WHO), an international agency sponsored by the United Nations, are constantly monitoring health problems throughout the world and taking steps to prevent pandemics. Health care has become a global concern and countries are working together to promote good health in all individuals.

Table 1-7 lists some of the events that have occurred so far in the 21st century and some possible advances that might occur soon. The potential for the future of health care has unlimited possibilities.

1:2 INFORMATION

Trends in Health Care

Health care has seen many changes during the past several decades, and many additional changes will occur in the years to come. An awareness of such changes and trends is important for any health care worker.

TABLE 1-7 History of Health Care in the 21st Century

HISTORICAL EVENTS OF HEALTH CARE IN THE 21ST CENTURY	
21st Century	Adult stem cells were used in the treatment of disease early in the 2000s
	The U.S. Food and Drug Administration (FDA) approved the use of the abortion pill RU-486 in 2000
	President George W. Bush approved federal funding for research using only existing lines of embryonic stem cells in 2001
	Advanced Cell Technology announced it cloned a human embryo in 2001 but the embryo did not survive
	The first totally implantable artificial heart was placed in a patient in Louisville, Kentucky, in 2001
	Smallpox vaccinations were given to military personnel and first responders to limit the effects of a potential bioterrorist attack in 2002
	The Netherlands became the first country in the world to legalize euthanasia in 2002
	The Human Genome Project to identify all of the approximately 20,000 to 25,000 genes in human DNA was completed in 2003
	The Standards for Privacy of Individually Identifiable Health Information, required under the Health Insurance Portability and Accountability Act (HIPAA) of 1996, went into effect in 2003
	The Medicare Prescription Drug Improvement and Modernization Act was passed in 2003
	The virus that causes severe acute respiratory syndrome (SARS) was identified in 2003 as a new coronavirus, never seen in humans previously
	National Institutes of Health (NIH) researchers discover that primary teeth can be a source of stem cells in 2003
	First face transplant was performed in France in 2005 on a woman whose lower face was destroyed by a dog attack
	Stem cell researchers at the University of Minnesota coaxed embryonic stem cells to produce cancer-killing cells in 2005
	The National Cancer Institute (NCI) and the National Human Genome Research Institute started a project to map genes associated with cancer so mutations that occur with specific cancers can be identified in 2006
	The FDA approved the use of the AbioCor totally implantable artificial heart in 2006
	The first inhalable insulin product, Exubera, was approved by the FDA in 2006
	Researchers propose a new method to generate embryonic stem cells from a blastocyst without destroying embryos in 2006
	Gardasil, a vaccine to prevent cervical cancer, was approved by the FDA in 2006
	Zostavax, a vaccine to prevent herpes zoster (shingles), was approved by the FDA in 2006
Potential for the 21st Century	Cures for AIDS, cancer, and heart disease are found
	Genetic manipulation to prevent inherited diseases is a common practice
	Development of methods to slow the aging process or stop aging are created
	Nerves in the brain and spinal cord are regenerated to eliminate paralysis
	Transplants of every organ in the body, including the brain, are possible
	Antibiotics are developed that do not allow pathogens to develop resistance
	Average life span is increased to 90 to 100 years and beyond

COST CONTAINMENT

Cost containment, a term heard frequently in health care circles, means trying to control the rising cost of health care and achieving the maximum benefit for every dollar spent. Some reasons for high health care costs include:

♦ *Technological advances*: highly technical procedures such as heart, lung, liver, or kidney transplants can cost hundreds of thousands of dollars. Even so, many of these procedures are performed daily throughout the United States. Artificial hearts are another new technology being used. Computers that can be used to examine internal body parts are valuable diagnostic tools, but these devices can cost millions of dollars. Advanced technology does allow people to survive illnesses that used to be fatal, but these individuals may require expensive and lifelong care.

♦ *The aging population*: older individuals use more pharmaceutical products (medications), have more chronic diseases, and often need frequent health care services.

♦ *Health-related lawsuits*: lawsuits force health care providers to obtain expensive malpractice insurance, order diagnostic tests even though they might not be necessary, and make every effort to avoid lawsuits by practicing defensive health care.

Because these expenses must be paid, a major concern is that health care costs could rise to levels that could prohibit providing services to all individuals. However, everyone should have equal access to care regardless of their ability to pay. Because of this, all aspects of health care are directed toward cost containment. Although there is no firm answer to controlling health costs, most agencies that deliver health care are trying to provide quality care at the lowest possible price. Some methods of cost containment that are used include:

♦ ***Diagnostic related groups (DRGs)***: one way Congress is trying to control costs for government insurance plans such as Medicare and Medicaid. Under this plan, patients with certain diagnoses who are admitted to hospitals are classified in one payment group. A limit is placed on the cost of care, and the agency providing care receives this set amount. This encourages the agency to make every effort to provide care within the expense limit allowed. If the cost of care is less than the amount paid, the agency keeps the extra money. If the cost of care is more than the amount paid, the agency must accept the loss.

♦ *Combination of services*: done to eliminate duplication of services. Clinics, laboratories shared by different agencies, health maintenance organizations (HMOs), preferred provider organizations (PPOs), and other similar agencies all represent attempts to control the rising cost of health care. When health care agencies join together or share specific services, care can be provided to a larger number of people at a decreased cost per person. For example, a large medical laboratory with expensive computerized equipment performing thousands of tests per day can provide quality service at a much lower price than smaller laboratories with less expensive equipment capable of performing only a limited numbers of tests per day.

♦ ***Outpatient services***: patients receive care without being admitted to hospitals or other care facilities. Hospital care is expensive. Reducing the length of hospital stays or decreasing the need for hospital admissions lowers the cost of health care. For example, patients who had open-heart surgery used to spend several weeks in a hospital. Today, the average length of stay is 5 to 7 days. Less expensive home care or transfer to a skilled-care facility can be used for individuals who require additional assistance. Surgery, radiographs, diagnostic tests, and many other procedures that once required admission to a hospital are now done on an outpatient basis.

♦ *Mass or bulk purchasing*: buying equipment and supplies in larger quantities at reduced prices. This can be done by combining the purchases of different departments in a single agency, or by combining the purchases of several different agencies. A major health care system purchasing medical supplies for hundreds or thousands of health care agencies can obtain much lower prices than an individual agency. Computerized inventory can be used to determine when supplies are needed and to prevent overstocks and waste.

♦ *Early intervention and preventive services*: providing care before acute or chronic disease occurs. Preventing illness is always more cost-effective than treating illness. Methods used to prevent illness include patient education, immunizations, regular physical examinations to detect problems early, incentives for individuals to participate in preventive activities, and easy access for all individuals to preventive health care services. Studies have shown that individuals with limited access to health services and restricted finances use expensive emergency rooms and acute care facilities much more frequently. Providing early intervention and care to these individuals is much more cost-efficient.

♦ ***Energy conservation***: monitoring the use of energy to control costs and conserve resources.

Major expenses for every health care industry/ agency are electricity, water, and/or gas. Most large health care facilities perform energy audits to determine how resources are being used and to calculate ways to conserve energy. Methods that can be used for energy conservation include designing and building new energy-efficient facilities; constantly monitoring and maintaining heating/cooling systems; using insulation and thermopane windows to prevent hot/cool air loss; repairing plumbing fixtures immediately to stop water loss; replacing energy-consuming lightbulbs with fluorescent or energy-efficient bulbs; installing infrared sensors to turn water faucets on and off; and using alternative forms of energy such as solar power. Recycling is also a form of energy conservation, and most health care facilities recycle many different materials.

The preceding are just a few examples of cost containment. Many other methods will undoubtedly be applied in the years ahead. It is important to note that the quality of health care should not be lowered simply to control costs. To prevent this from happening, the Agency for Health Care Policy and Research (AHCPR) researches the quality of health care delivery and identifies the standards of treatment that should be provided. In addition, every health care worker must make every effort to provide quality care while doing everything possible to avoid waste and keep expenditures down. Health care consumers must assume more responsibility for their own care, become better informed of all options for health care services, and follow preventive measures to avoid or limit illness and disease. Everyone working together can help control the rising cost of health care.

HOME HEALTH CARE

Home health care is a rapidly growing field. Diagnostic related groups and shorter hospital stays have created a need for providing care in the home. Years ago, home care was the usual method of treatment. Doctors made house calls, private duty nurses cared for patients in the patients' homes, babies were delivered at home, and patients died at home. Current trends show a return to some of these practices. Home care is also another form of cost containment because it is usually less expensive to provide this type of care. All aspects of health care can be involved. Nursing care, physical and occupational therapy,

respiratory therapy, social services, nutritional and food services, and other types of care can be provided in the home environment.

GERIATRIC CARE

Geriatric care, or care for the elderly, is another field that will continue to experience rapid growth in the future (figure 1-9). This is caused in part by the large number of individuals who are experiencing longer life spans because of advances in health care. Many people now enjoy life spans of 80 years or more. Years ago, very few people lived to be 100 years old. This is becoming more and more common. Also, the "baby boom" generation—the large number of people born after World War II—is now reaching the geriatric age classification. Projections from the U.S. Census Bureau indicate that the rate of population growth during the next 50 years will be slower for all age groups, but the number of people in older age groups will continue to grow more than twice as rapidly as the total population. Many different facilities will be involved in providing care and resources for this age group. Adult day care centers, retirement communities, assisted/independent living facilities, long-term care facilities, and other organizations will all see increased demand for the services they provide.

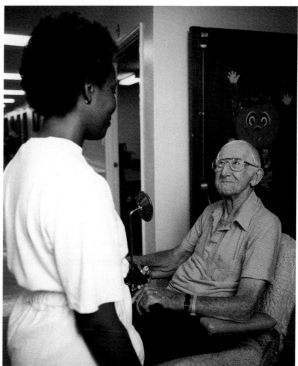

FIGURE 1-9 Geriatric care is a field that will continue to experience rapid growth.

✪ **OBRA** the **Omnibus Budget Reconciliation Act (OBRA)** of 1987 has led to the development of many regulations regarding long-term care and home health care. This act requires states to establish training and competency evaluation programs for nursing and geriatric assistants. Each assistant working in a long-term care facility or home health care is now required under federal law to complete a mandatory, state-approved training program and pass a written and/or competency examination to obtain certification or registration. OBRA also requires continuing education, periodic evaluation of performance, and retraining and/or testing if a nursing assistant does not work in a health care facility for more than 2 years. Each state then maintains a registry of qualified individuals.

The minimum skills required are specified in the Nurse Aide Competency Evaluation Program (NACEP) developed by the National Council of State Boards of Nursing. Programs that prepare nursing and geriatric assistants use NACEP as a guideline to ensure that the minimum requirements of OBRA are met. Many programs expand these requirements. OBRA also requires compliance with patients'/residents' rights, and forces states to establish guidelines to ensure that such rights are observed and enforced. These regulations serve to ensure certain standards of care. As the need for geriatric care increases, additional regulations may be created. It is important that every health care worker be informed about all OBRA regulations to comply with these regulations.

TELEMEDICINE

Telemedicine involves the use of video, audio, and computer systems to provide medical and/or health care services. New technology now allows interactive services between health care providers even though they are in different locations. For example, emergency medical technicians (EMTs), at the scene of an accident or illness, can use technology to transmit medical data such as an electrocardiogram to an emergency department physician. The physician can then monitor the data and direct the care of the patient. Surgeons using a computer can guide a remote-controlled arm (robotic) to perform surgery on a patient many miles away. In other instances, a surgeon can direct the work of another surgeon by watching the procedure on video beamed by a satellite system.

As consumers become computer literate, more health care services will be provided electronically. Telemedicine machines, operating over telephone lines, are "user-friendly," compact, and less expensive than when they were developed. They are already allowing individuals with chronic illnesses or disabilities to receive care in the comfort of their homes. This decreases the need for trips to medical care facilities. Patients can test blood sugar levels, oxygen levels, blood pressure measurements, and other vital signs, and send the results to a physician/nurse; monitor pacemakers; use online courses to learn how to manage their condition; schedule an "appointment" to talk with a health care provider "face to face" through video monitors; receive electronic reminders to take medications or perform diagnostic tests; and receive answers to specific health questions. In rural areas, where specialty care is often limited, telemedicine can provide a patient with access to specialists thousands of miles away. Telemedicine will become an important way of delivering health care in future years.

WELLNESS

⬛ **Wellness,** or the state of being in optimum health with a balanced relationship between physical, mental, and social health, is another major trend in health care. People are more aware of the need to maintain health and prevent disease because disease prevention improves the quality of life and saves costs. More individuals are recognizing the importance of exercise, good nutrition, weight control, and healthy living habits (figure 1-10). This has led to the establishment of wellness centers, weight-control facilities, health food stores, nutrition services, stress reduction counseling, and habit cessation management.

Wellness is determined by the lifestyle choices made by an individual and involves many factors. Some of the factors and ways to promote wellness include:

◆ *Physical wellness*: promoted by a well-balanced diet; regular exercise; routine physical examinations and immunizations; regular dental and vision examinations; and avoidance of alcohol, tobacco, caffeine, drugs, environmental contaminants, and risky sexual behavior

◆ *Emotional wellness*: promoted by understanding personal feelings and expressing them

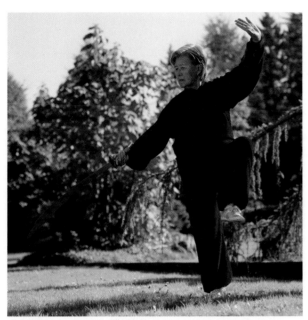

FIGURE 1-10 Individuals are recognizing the importance of exercise and healthy living habits. *(Courtesy of Photodisc)*

appropriately, accepting one's limitations, adjusting to change, coping with stress, enjoying life, and maintaining an optimistic outlook

♦ *Social wellness*: promoted by showing concern, fairness, affection, tolerance, and respect for others; communicating and interacting well with others; sharing ideas and thoughts; and practicing honesty and loyalty

♦ *Mental and intellectual wellness*: promoted by being creative, logical, curious, and open-minded; using common sense; obtaining continual learning; questioning and evaluating information and situations; learning from life experiences; and using flexibility and creativity to solve problems

♦ *Spiritual wellness*: promoted by using values, ethics, and morals to find meaning, direction, and purpose to life; often includes believing in a higher authority and observing religious practices

The trend toward wellness has led to **holistic health care,** or care that promotes physical, emotional, social, intellectual, and spiritual well-being by treating the whole body, mind, and spirit. Each patient is recognized as a unique person with different needs. Holistic health care uses many methods of diagnosis and treatment in addition to traditional Western medical practice. Treatment is directed toward protection and res-

toration. It is based on the body's natural healing powers, the various ways different tissues and systems in the body influence each other, and the effect of the external environment. It is essential to remember that the patient is responsible for choosing his or her own care. Health care workers must respect the patient's choices and provide care that promotes the well-being of the whole person.

COMPLEMENTARY AND ALTERNATIVE METHODS OF HEALTH CARE

The most common health care system in the United States is the biomedical or "Western" system. It is based on evaluating the physical signs and symptoms of a patient, determining the cause of disease, and treating the cause. A major trend, however, is an increase in the use of complementary or alternative (CAM) health care therapies. **Complementary therapies** are methods of treatment that are used in conjunction with conventional medical therapies. **Alternative therapies** can be defined as methods of treatment that are used in place of biomedical therapies. Even though the two terms are different, the term *alternative* is usually applied whether or not the therapy is used in place of, or in conjunction with, conventional medical therapies.

Many health care facilities now offer **integrative (integrated) health care,** which uses both mainstream medical treatments and CAM therapies to treat a patient. For example, chronic pain is treated with both medications and CAM therapies that encourage stress reduction and relaxation. Integrative health care is based on the principle that individuals have the ability to bring greater wellness and healing into their own lives and that the mind affects the healing process. In addition, integrative care recognizes that each person is unique and may require different medical treatments and a variety of CAM therapies. For this reason, an integrative treatment plan must be individualized to meet the patient's own special needs and circumstances.

The interest in holistic health care has increased the use of CAM therapies. Common threads in these therapies are that they consider the whole individual and recognize that the health of each part has an effect on the person's total health status; that each person has a life force or special type of energy that can be used in the healing process; and that skilled practitioners, rituals, and specialized practices are a part of the therapy. Many of these therapies are based on cultural values and beliefs. A few examples of CAM practitioners include:

♦ *Ayurvedic practitioners*: use an ancient philosophy, ayurveda, developed in India to determine a person's predominant dosha (body type) and prescribe diet, herbal treatment, exercise, yoga, massage, minerals, and living practices to restore and maintain harmony in the body

♦ *Chinese medicine practitioners*: use an ancient holistic-based healing practice based on the belief that a life energy (Chi) flows through every living person in an invisible system of meridians (pathways) to link the organs together and connect them to the external environment or universe; use acupuncture (figure 1-11), acupressure, tai chi, and herbal remedies to maintain the proper flow of energy and promote health

♦ *Chiropractors*: believe that the brain sends vital energy to all body parts through nerves in the spinal cord; when there is a misalignment of the vertebrae (bones), pressure is placed on spinal nerves that results in disease and pain; use spinal manipulation, massage, and exercise to adjust the position of the vertebrae and restore the flow of energy

♦ *Homeopaths*: believe in the ability of the body to heal itself through the actions of the immune system; use minute diluted doses of drugs made from plant, animal, and mineral substances to cause symptoms similar to the disease and activate the immune system

♦ *Hypnotists*: help an individual obtain a trance-like state with the belief that the person will be receptive to verbal suggestions and able to make a desired behavior change

♦ *Naturopaths*: use only natural therapies such as fasting, special diets, lifestyle changes, and supportive approaches to promote healing; avoid the use of surgery or medicinal agents to treat disease

Many different therapies are used in CAM medicine. Some of these therapies are discussed in Table 1-8. Most of the therapies are noninvasive and holistic. In many instances, they are less

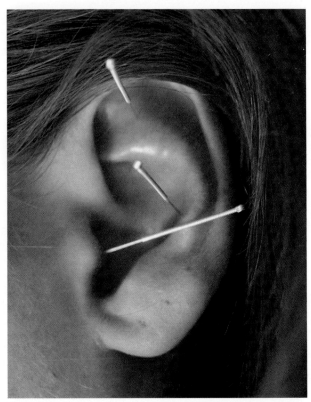

FIGURE 1-11 Acupuncture therapists insert very thin needles into specific points along the meridians (pathways) in the body to stimulate and balance the flow of energy.

expensive than other traditional treatments. Many insurance programs now cover a wide variety of CAM therapies.

Because of the increased use of CAM therapies, the federal government established the National Center for Complementary and Alternative Medicine (NCCAM) at the National Institutes of Health in 1992. Its purpose is to research the various therapies and determine standards of quality care. In addition, many states have passed laws to govern the use of various therapies. Some states have established standards for some therapies, forbidden the use of others, labeled specific therapies experimental, and require a license or certain educational requirements before a practitioner can administer a particular therapy. It is essential for health care workers to learn the legal requirements of their states regarding the different CAM therapies. Health care workers must also remember that patients have the right to choose their own type of care. A nonjudgmental attitude is essential.

TABLE 1-8 Complementary and Alternative Therapies

THERAPY	BASIC DESCRIPTION
Acupressure (Shiatsu)	Pressure is applied with fingers, palms, thumbs, or elbows to specific pressure points of the body to stimulate and regulate the flow of energy; based on the belief that Chi (life energy) flows through meridians (pathways) in the body, and illness and pain occur when the flow is blocked; used to treat muscular–joint pain, depression, digestive problems, and respiratory disorders; *Shiatsu* is the Japanese form of acupressure
Acupuncture	Ancient Chinese therapy that involves the insertion of very thin needles into specific points along the meridians (pathways) in the body to stimulate and balance the flow of energy; at times, heat (moxibustion) or electrical stimulation is applied to the needles; based on the belief that Chi (life energy) flows through the meridians, and illness and pain occur when the flow is blocked; used to relieve pain, especially headache and back pain, reduce stress-related illnesses, and treat drug dependency and obesity
Antioxidants (Free Radicals)	Nutritional therapy that encourages the use of substances called *antioxidants* to prevent or inhibit oxidation (chemical process in which a substance is joined to oxygen) and neutralize free radicals (molecules that can damage body cells by altering the genetic code); examples of antioxidants are vitamins A, C, and E, and selenium; may prevent heart disease, cataracts, and some types of cancer
Aromatherapy	Therapeutic use of selected fragrances (concentrated essences or essential oils that have been extracted from roots, bark, plants, and/or flowers) to alter mood and restore the body, mind, and spirit; fragrances may be diluted in oils for massages or placed in warm water or candles for inhalation; used to relieve tense muscles and tension headaches or backaches, lower blood pressure, and cause a stimulating, uplifting, relaxing, or soothing effect
Biofeedback	Relaxation therapy that uses monitoring devices to provide a patient with information about his/her reaction to stress by showing the effect of stress on heart rate, respirations, blood pressure, muscle tension, and skin temperature; patient is then taught relaxation methods to gain "mind" or voluntary control over the physical responses; used to treat hypertension (high blood pressure), migraine headaches, and stress-related illnesses, and to enhance relaxation
Healing Touch (Reiki)	Ancient Japanese/Tibetan healing art based on the idea that disease causes an imbalance in the body's energy field; begins with centering (inward focus of total serenity) before gentle hand pressure is applied to the body's chakras (energy centers) to harness and balance the life energy force, help clear blockages, and stimulate healing; at times, hands are positioned slightly above the energy centers; used to promote relaxation, reduce pain, and promote wound healing
Herbal or Botanical Medicine	Herbal medicine treatments that have been used in almost all cultures since primitive times; based on the belief that herbs and plant extracts, from roots, stems, seeds, flowers, and leaves, contain compounds that alter blood chemistry, remove impurities, strengthen the immune system, and protect against disease
Homeopathy	Treatment based on using very minute, dilute doses of drugs made from natural substances to produce symptoms of the disease being treated; based on the belief that these substances stimulate the immune system to remove toxins and heal the body; very controversial form of treatment
Hydrotherapy	Type of treatment that uses water in any form, internally and externally, for healing purposes; common external examples include water aerobics and exercises, massage in or under water, soaking in hot springs or tubs, and steam vapors; a common internal example is a diet that encourages drinking large amounts of water to help cleanse the body and stimulate the digestive tract

(continues)

TABLE 1-8 Complementary and Alternative Therapies *(Continued)*

THERAPY	BASIC DESCRIPTION
Hypnotherapy (Hypnosis)	Technique used to induce a trancelike state so a person is more receptive to suggestion; enhances a person's ability to form images; used to encourage desired behavior changes such as helping people lose weight, stop smoking, reduce stress, and/or relieve pain
Imagery	Technique of using imagination and as many senses as possible to visualize a pleasant and soothing image; used to decrease tension, anxiety, and adverse effects of chemotherapy
Ionization Therapy	Special machines called *air ionizers* are used to produce negatively charged air particles or ions; used to treat common respiratory disorders
Macrobiotic Diet	Macrobiotic (meaning "long life") is a nutrition therapy based on the Taoist concept of the balance between yin (cold, death, and darkness) and yang (heat, life, and light) and the belief that different foods represent yin (sweet foods) and yang (meat and eggs); diet encourages balanced foods such as brown rice, whole grains, nuts, vegetables, fruits, and fish; discourages overindulgence of yin or yang foods; processed and treated foods, red meat, sugar, dairy products, eggs, and caffeine should be avoided; similar to the American Dietary Association's low-fat, low-cholesterol, and high-fiber diet
Meditation	Therapy that teaches breathing and muscle relaxation techniques to quiet the mind by focusing attention on obtaining a sense of oneness within oneself; used to reduce stress and pain, slow heart rate, lower blood pressure, and stimulate relaxation
Pet Therapy	Therapy that uses pets, such as dogs, cats, and birds, to enhance health and stimulate an interest in life; helps individuals overcome physical limitations, decrease depression, increase self-esteem, socialize, and lower stress levels and blood pressure
Phytochemicals	Nutritional therapy that recommends foods containing phytochemicals (nonnutritive plant chemicals that store nutrients and provide aroma and color in plants) with the belief that the chemicals help prevent disease; found mainly in a wide variety of fruits and vegetables, so these are recommended for daily consumption; used to prevent heart disease, stroke, cancer, and cataracts
Play Therapy	Therapy that uses toys to allow children to learn about situations, share experiences, and express their emotions; important aspect of psychotherapy for children with limited language ability
Positive Thought	Therapy that involves developing self-awareness, self-esteem, and love for oneself to allow the body to heal itself and eliminate disease; based on the belief that disease is a negative process that can be reversed by an individual's mental processes
Reflexology	Ancient healing art based on the concept that the body is divided into ten equal zones that run from the head to the toes; illness or disease of a body part causes deposits of calcium or acids in the corresponding part of the foot; therapy involves applying pressure on specific points on the foot so energy movement is directed toward the affected body part; used to promote healing and relaxation, reduce stress, improve circulation, and treat asthma, sinus infections, irritable bowel syndrome, kidney stones, and constipation
Spiritual Therapies	Therapies based on the belief that a state of wholeness or health depends not only on physical health, but the spiritual aspects of an individual; uses prayer, meditation, self-evaluation, and spiritual guidance to allow an individual to use the powers within to increase the sense of well-being and promote healing
Tai Chi	Therapies based on the ancient theory that health is harmony with nature and the universe and a balanced state of yin (cold) and yang (heat); uses a series of sequential, slow, graceful, and precise body movements combined with breathing techniques to improve energy flow (Chi) within the body; improves stamina, balance, and coordination and leads to a sense of well-being; used to treat digestive disorders, stress, depression, and arthritis

TABLE 1-8 Complementary and Alternative Therapies *(Continued)*

THERAPY	BASIC DESCRIPTION
Therapeutic (Swedish) Massage	Treatment that uses kneeling, gliding, friction, tapping, and vibration motions by the hands to increase circulation of the blood and lymph, relieve musculoskeletal stiffness, pain, and spasm, increase range-of-motion, and induce relaxation
Therapeutic Touch	Therapy based on an ancient healing practice with the belief that illness is an imbalance in an individual's energy field; the practitioner assesses alterations or changes in a patient's energy fields, places his/her hands on or slightly above the patient's body, and balances the energy flow to stimulate self-healing; used to encourage relaxation, stimulate wound healing, increase the energy level, and decrease anxiety
Yoga	Hindu discipline that uses concentration, specific positions, and ancient ritual movements to maintain the balance and flow of life energy; encourages the use of both the body and mind to achieve a state of perfect spiritual insight and tranquility; used to increase spiritual enlightenment and well-being, develop an awareness of the body to improve coordination, relieve stress and anxiety, and increase muscle tone

NATIONAL HEALTH CARE PLAN

The high cost of health care and large number of uninsured individuals have created a demand for a national health care plan. Many different types of plans have been proposed. One plan involves nationalized medicine, where the federal government would pay for all health services and levy taxes to pay for those services. Another plan involves the creation of health care cooperatives, which would allow consumers to purchase health care at lower costs. A third plan is based on managed care and requires employers to provide coverage and the federal government to subsidize insurance for the poor. Still another plan would allow each state to establish its own health care plan paid for by employers, individuals, and/or government subsidies.

The main goal in health care reform is to ensure that all Americans can get health coverage. Related problems include the cost of creating such a system, the fact that those with insurance may pay more to cover uninsured individuals, the lack of freedom in choosing health care providers, and the regulations that will have to be created to establish a national health care system.

PANDEMIC

A **pandemic** exists when the outbreak of a disease occurs over a wide geographic area and affects a high proportion of the population. A major concern today is that worldwide pandemics will become more and more frequent. Because society is global and individuals can travel readily throughout the world, disease can spread much more rapidly from individual to individual.

The World Health Organization (WHO) is concerned about influenza pandemics occurring in the near future. Throughout history, influenza pandemics have killed large numbers of people. For example, the 1918 Spanish flu pandemic killed approximately 2.6 percent of individuals who contracted it, or about 40 million people. Recently, researchers identified the virus that caused this epidemic as an avian (bird) flu virus that jumped directly to humans. This caused a major alarm throughout the world because of the avian flu viruses, called *H5N1* viruses, which are present in countries in Asia and some other countries. These viruses pass readily from birds to birds and have devastated bird flocks in more than 11 countries. The infection has appeared in humans, but most cases have resulted from contact with infected poultry or contaminated surfaces. The spread from one person to another has been reported only rarely. However, because the death rate for this bird flu in humans is between 50 and 60 percent, a major concern is that the *H5N1* viruses will mutate and begin to spread from birds to humans more readily. Even if the *H5N1* viruses do not mutate and spread to humans, WHO is still concerned about many other viruses. Examples include the hantavirus spread by rodents, severe acute respiratory syndrome (SARS), monkeypox, and filoviruses such as the Ebola virus and the Marburg virus that cause hemorrhagic fever. Because viruses are prone to mutation and exchanging genetic information, the creation of a new lethal virus can occur at any time. WHO estimates that 2 to 7 million people worldwide could die from infections by this type of virus. Other estimates are that tens of millions of people could die.

Many governments are creating pandemic influenza plans to protect their populations. Components of most plans include the following:

◆ *Education*: information about the pandemic and ways to avoid its spread must be given to the entire population

◆ *Vaccine production*: more research must be directed toward producing effective vaccines in larger quantities and in a shorter period of time

◆ *Antiviral drugs*: drugs that are currently available must be stockpiled so they will be ready for immediate use, and more research must be done to develop and produce effective antiviral drugs

◆ *Development of protective public health measures*: influenza must be diagnosed rapidly and accurately, strict infection control methods must be implemented to limit the spread of the virus, first responders and health care personnel must be immunized so they will be able to care for infected individuals, and quarantine measures must be used if necessary to control the spread of the disease

◆ *International cooperation*: countries must be willing to work with each other to create an international plan that will limit the spread of lethal viruses and decrease the severity of a pandemic

In the near future, much effort will be directed toward identifying and limiting the effect of any organism that could lead to a pandemic. Health

TODAY'S RESEARCH: TOMORROW'S HEALTH CARE

The Food and Drug Administration regulating maggots and leeches as medical devices?

Throughout the history of health care, maggots and leeches have been used to treat infection and encourage blood flow. Maggots clean festering, gangrenous wounds that fail to heal. They eat the dead tissue and discharges to clean the wound and promote the growth of new tissue. Leeches drain excess blood from tissue and encourage new circulation.

Microsurgeons, doctors who specialize in reattaching fingers, hands, and other body appendages, have come to rely on the assistance of leeches. When microsurgeons reattach or transplant a body part, they can usually connect arteries that bring blood to the appendage. They find it more difficult to attach veins, which carry blood away from the appendage, because veins are smaller and are fragile. Without a good venous supply, blood tends to collect in the new attachment, clot, and in some cases, kill the tissue. To allow time for the body to create its own veins to the new appendage, doctors apply leeches. The leeches naturally inject the area with a chemical that includes an anticoagulant (a substance that prevents clotting), an anesthetic, an antibiotic, and a vasodilator (a substance that dilates or enlarges blood vessels). This chemical encourages the blood to flow quickly. The leeches drain this blood to reduce pressure and allow veins to form.

Even though many individuals are squeamish about the use of maggots and leeches, they have proved to be an effective method of treatment for chronic infections and microsurgery. The problem arises because the sources for maggots and leeches are not reliable. For this reason, the FDA has classified maggots and leeches as medical devices. Medical advisers have been asked to create basic guidelines to regulate how maggots and leeches are grown, transported, sold, and disposed of after use. This will provide a safe source for this unique method of treatment and encourage future research on the use of maggots and leeches as methods of treatment. It may also lead to a future in which every microsurgery has an excellent chance of success.

care workers must stay informed and be prepared to deal with the consequences of a pandemic.

CONCLUSION

Although the preceding are just several of the many trends in health care, they do illustrate how health care has changed and how it will continue to change. Every health care worker must stay abreast of such changes and make every attempt to learn about them.

STUDENT: *Go to the workbook and complete the assignment sheet for Chapter 1, History and Trends of Health Care.*

CHAPTER 1 SUMMARY

The history of health care shows that treating illness and disease has been an important part of every civilization. Even in ancient times, people were searching for ways to eliminate illness and disease. Some of the early plants and herbs that were used to treat disease are still in use today. Computers and modern technology have caused major changes in health care in the past century. Many more changes are expected in the future as scientists continue to study the human body and discover the causes of illness and disease.

As health care continues to grow as an industry, changes and trends will occur. Issues of primary importance are cost containment to control the high cost of health care, home health care, care for the elderly, telemedicine, wellness to prevent disease, complementary and alternative methods (CAM) of health care, a national health care plan, and pandemic preparation.

INTERNET SEARCHES

Use the suggested search engines in Chapter 17:4 of this textbook to search the Internet for additional information on the following topics:

1. *History of health care*: research individual names or discoveries such as the polio vaccine to gain more insight into how major developments in health care occurred.

2. *Trends in health care*: research topics such as home health care, the Omnibus Budget Reconciliation Act of 1987, telemedicine, holistic health care, cost containment, geriatric care, and wellness to obtain additional information on the present effect on health care.

3. *Complementary/alternative methods of health care*: search the Internet for additional information on specific therapies such as acupuncture. Refer to table 1–8 for a list of many different therapies.

4. *Pandemics*: search the Internet to obtain information on at least four (4) pandemics. Compare and contrast the cause of each pandemic, the number of people infected, and the death rate.

REVIEW QUESTIONS

1. Name the person responsible for each of the following events in the history of health care. Briefly state how their accomplishments contributed to the current state of health care.
   a. The ancient Greek who is known as the Father of Medicine
   b. An artist who drew the human body during the Renaissance
   c. The inventor of the microscope
   d. The individual who discovered roentgenograms (X-rays)
   e. The person who discovered penicillin

2. Create a time line for the history of health care showing the twenty (20) events you believe had the most impact on modern-day care. State why you believe these events are the most important.

3. List six (6) specific ways to control the rising cost of health care.

4. You are employed in a medical office with four doctors. Identify four (4) specific ways to conserve energy in the office.

5. Write a brief essay describing how you maintain physical, emotional, social, mental, and spiritual wellness. Be sure to include specific examples for each type of wellness.

6. Review all the CAM therapies shown in table 1-8. Identify two therapies that you believe would be beneficial. Explain why you think the therapies might be effective.

CHAPTER 2

Health Care Systems

Observe Standard
Precautions

Instructor's Check—Call
Instructor at This Point

Safety—Proceed with
Caution

OBRA Requirement—Based
on Federal Law

Math Skill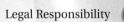

Legal Responsibility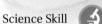

Science Skill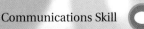

Career Information

Communications Skill

Technology

Chapter Objectives

After completing this chapter,
you should be able to:

◆ Describe at least eight types of private health
care facilities

◆ Analyze at least three government agencies
and the services offered by each

◆ Describe at least three services offered by
voluntary or nonprofit agencies

◆ Compare the basic principles of at least four
different health insurance plans

◆ Explain the purpose of organizational
structures in health care facilities

◆ Define, pronounce, and spell all key terms

KEY TERMS

Agency for Health Care
    Policy and Research
    (AHCPR)
assisted living facilities
Centers for Disease Control
    and Prevention (CDC)
clinics
dental offices
emergency care services
Food and Drug
    Administration (FDA)
genetic counseling centers
health departments
health insurance plans
Health Insurance Portability
    and Accountability Act
    (HIPAA)
health maintenance
    organizations (HMOs)

home health care
hospice
hospitals
independent living facilities
industrial health care
    centers
laboratories
long-term care facilities
    (LTCs or LTCFs)
managed care
Medicaid
medical offices
Medicare
Medigap
mental health
National Institutes of Health
    (NIH)
nonprofit agencies

Occupational Safety and
    Health Administration
    (OSHA)
optical centers
organizational structure
preferred provider
    organizations (PPOs)
rehabilitation
school health services
TRICARE
U.S. Department of Health
    and Human Services
    (USDHHS)
voluntary agencies
Workers' Compensation
World Health Organization
    (WHO)

2:1 INFORMATION

Private Health Care Facilities

Today, health care systems include the many agencies, facilities, and personnel involved in the delivery of health care. According to U.S. government statistics, health care is one of the largest and fastest-growing industries in the United States. This industry employs over 13 million workers in more than 200 different health careers. It attracts people with a wide range of educational backgrounds because it offers multiple career options. By the year 2012, employment is expected to increase to over 15 million workers. Health care has become a 4-billion-dollar-per-day business.

Many different health care facilities provide services that are a part of the industry called *health care* (figure 2-1). Most private health care facilities require a fee for services. In some cases, grants and contributions help provide financial support for these facilities. A basic description of the various facilities will help provide an understanding of the many different types of services included under the umbrella of the health care industry.

HOSPITALS

Hospitals are one of the major types of health care facilities. They vary in size and types of service provided. Some hospitals are small and serve the basic needs of a community; others are large, complex centers offering a wide range of services including diagnosis, treatment, education, and research. Hospitals are also classified as private or proprietary (operated for profit), religious, nonprofit or voluntary, and government, depending on the sources of income received by the hospital.

There are many different types of hospitals. Some of the more common ones include:

♦ *General hospitals*: treat a wide range of conditions and age groups; usually provide diagnostic, medical, surgical, and emergency care services

♦ *Specialty hospitals*: provide care for special conditions or age groups; examples include burn hospitals, oncology (cancer) hospitals, pediatric (or children's) hospitals, psychiatric hospitals (dealing with mental diseases and

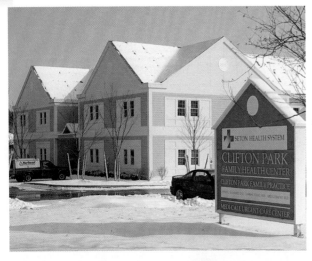

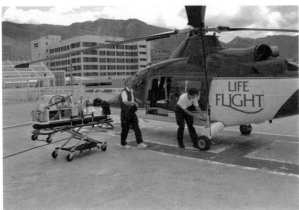

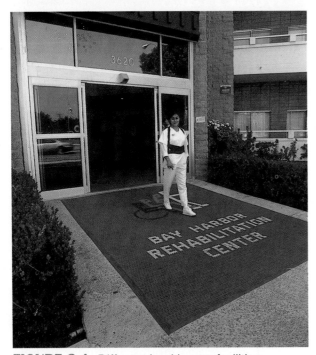

FIGURE 2-1 Different health care facilities.

disorders), orthopedic hospitals (dealing with bone, joint, or muscle disease), and rehabilitative hospitals (offering services such as physical and occupational therapy)

◆ *Government hospitals*: operated by federal, state, and local government agencies; include the many facilities located throughout the world that provide care for government service personnel and their dependents; examples are Veterans Administration hospitals (which provide care for veterans), state psychiatric hospitals, and state rehabilitation centers

◆ *University or college medical centers*: provide hospital services along with research and education; can be funded by private and/or governmental sources

In any type of hospital facility, a wide range of trained health workers is needed at all levels.

LONG-TERM CARE FACILITIES

Long-term care facilities (LTCs or LTCFs) mainly provide assistance and care for elderly patients, usually called *residents.* However, they also provide care for individuals with disabilities or handicaps and individuals with chronic or long-term illness.

There are many different types of long-term care facilities. Some of the more common ones include:

◆ *Residential care facilities* (*nursing homes or geriatric homes*): designed to provide basic physical and emotional care to individuals who can no longer care for themselves; help individuals with activities of daily living (ADLs), provide a safe and secure environment, and promote opportunities for social interactions

◆ *Extended care facilities or skilled care facilities*: designed to provide skilled nursing care and rehabilitative care to prepare patients* or residents for return to home environments or other long-term care facilities; some have *subacute units* designed to provide services to

*In some health care facilities, patients are referred to as *clients*. For the purposes of this text, *patient* will be used.

patients who need rehabilitation to recover from a major illness or surgery, treatment for cancer, or treatments such as dialysis for kidney disease or heart monitoring

♦ **Independent living** *and* **assisted living** *facilities*: allow individuals who can care for themselves to rent or purchase an apartment in the facility; provide services such as meals, housekeeping, laundry, transportation, social events, and basic medical care (such as assisting with medications)

Most assisted or independent living facilities are associated with nursing homes, extended care facilities, and/or skilled care facilities. This allows an individual to move readily from one level of care to the next when health needs change. Many long-term care facilities also offer special services such as the delivery of meals to the homes of the elderly, chronically ill, or people with disabilities. Some facilities offer senior citizen or adult day care centers, which provide social activities and other services for the elderly. The need for long-term care facilities has increased dramatically because of the large increase in the number of elderly people. Many health career opportunities are available in these facilities, and there is a shortage of nurses and other personnel.

MEDICAL OFFICES

Medical offices vary from offices that are privately owned by one doctor to large complexes that operate as corporations and employ many doctors and other health care professionals. Medical services obtained in these facilities can include diagnosis (determining the nature of an illness), treatment, examination, basic laboratory testing, minor surgery, and other similar care. Some medical doctors treat a wide variety of illnesses and age groups, but others specialize in and handle only certain age groups or conditions. Examples of specialities include pediatrics (infants and children), cardiology (diseases and disorders of the heart), and obstetrics (care of the pregnant female).

DENTAL OFFICES

Dental offices vary in size from offices that are privately owned by one or more dentists to dental clinics that employ a group of dentists. In some

areas, major retail or department stores operate dental clinics. Dental services can include general care provided to all age groups or specialized care offered to certain age groups or for certain dental conditions.

CLINICS OR SATELLITE CENTERS

Clinics, also called *satellite clinics* or *satellite centers,* are health care facilities found in many types of health care. Some clinics are composed of a group of medical or dental doctors who share a facility and other personnel. Other clinics are operated by private groups who provide special care. Examples include:

♦ *Surgical clinics* or *surgicenters*: perform minor surgical procedures; frequently called "one-day" surgical centers because patients are sent home immediately after they recover from their operation

♦ *Urgent* or *emergency care clinics*: provide first aid or emergency care to ill or injured patients

♦ *Rehabilitation clinics*: offer physical, occupational, speech, and other similar therapies

♦ *Specialty clinics*: provide care for specific diseases; examples include diabetic clinics, kidney dialysis centers, and oncology (cancer) clinics

♦ *Outpatient clinics*: usually operated by hospitals or large medical groups; provide care for outpatients (patients who are not admitted to the hospital)

♦ *Health department clinics*: may offer clinics for pediatric health care, treatment of sexually transmitted diseases and respiratory disease, immunizations, and other special services

♦ *Medical center clinics*: usually located in colleges or universities; offer clinics for various health conditions; offer care and treatment and provide learning experiences for medical students

OPTICAL CENTERS

Optical centers can be individually owned by an ophthalmologist or optometrist or they can be part of a large chain of stores. They provide vision examinations, prescribe eyeglasses or contact lenses, and check for the presence of eye diseases.

EMERGENCY CARE SERVICES

Emergency care services provide special care for victims of accidents or sudden illness. Facilities providing these services include ambulance services, both private and governmental; rescue squads, frequently operated by fire departments; emergency care clinics and centers; emergency departments operated by hospitals; and helicopter or airplane emergency services that rapidly transport patients to medical facilities for special care.

LABORATORIES

Laboratories are often a part of other facilities but can operate as separate health care services. Medical laboratories can perform special diagnostic tests such as blood or urine tests. Dental laboratories can prepare dentures (false teeth) and many other devices used to repair or replace teeth. Medical and dental offices, small hospitals, clinics, and many other health care facilities frequently use the services provided by laboratories.

HOME HEALTH CARE

Home health care agencies are designed to provide care in a patient's home (figure 2-2). The services of these agencies are frequently used by the elderly and disabled. Examples of such services include nursing care, personal care, therapy (physical, occupational, speech, respiratory), and homemaking (food preparation, cleaning, and other household tasks). Health departments, hospitals, private agencies, government agencies, and nonprofit or volunteer groups can offer home care services.

HOSPICE

Hospice agencies provide care for terminally ill persons who usually have life expectancies of 6 months or less. Care can be provided in the person's home or in a hospice facility. Hospice offers

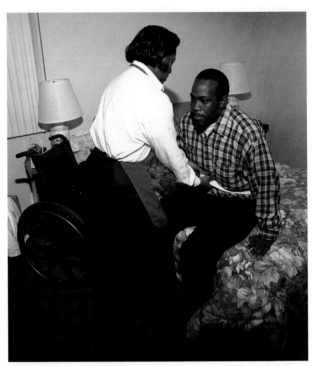

FIGURE 2-2 Many types of health care can be provided in a patient's home.

palliative care, or care that provides support and comfort, that is directed toward allowing the person to die with dignity. Psychological, social, spiritual, and financial counseling are provided for both the patient and the family. Hospice also provides support to the family following a patient's death.

MENTAL HEALTH FACILITIES

Mental health facilities treat patients with mental disorders and diseases. Examples of these facilities include guidance and counseling centers, psychiatric clinics and hospitals, chemical abuse treatment centers (dealing with alcohol and drug abuse), and physical abuse treatment centers (dealing with child abuse, spousal abuse, and geriatric [elderly] abuse).

GENETIC COUNSELING CENTERS

Genetic counseling centers can be an independent facility or located in another facility such as a hospital, clinic, or physician's office. Genetic counselors work with couples or individuals who are pregnant or considering a pregnancy. They perform prenatal (before birth) screening tests, check for genetic abnormalities and birth defects, explain the results of the tests, identify medical options when a birth defect is present, and help the individuals cope with the psychological issues caused by a genetic disorder. Examples of genetic disorders include Down's syndrome and cystic fibrosis. Counselors frequently consult with couples prior to a pregnancy if the woman is in her late childbearing years, has a family history of genetic disease, or is of a specific race or nationality with a high risk for genetic disease.

REHABILITATION FACILITIES

Rehabilitation facilities are located in hospitals, clinics, and/or private centers. They provide care to help patients with physical or mental disabilities obtain maximum self-care and function. Services may include physical, occupational, recreational, speech, and hearing therapy.

HEALTH MAINTENANCE ORGANIZATIONS

Health maintenance organizations (HMOs) are both health care delivery systems and types of health insurance. They provide total health care directed toward preventive health care for a fee that is usually fixed and prepaid. Services include examinations, basic medical services, health education, and hospitalization or rehabilitation services as needed. Some HMOs are operated by large industries or corporations; others are operated by private agencies. They often use the services of other health care facilities including medical and dental offices, hospitals, rehabilitative centers, home health care agencies, clinics, and laboratories.

INDUSTRIAL HEALTH CARE CENTERS

Industrial health care centers or *occupational health clinics* are found in large companies or industries. Such centers provide health care for employees of the industry or business by performing basic examinations, teaching accident prevention and safety, and providing emergency care.

SCHOOL HEALTH SERVICES

School health services are found in schools and colleges. These services provide emergency care for victims of accidents and sudden illness; perform tests to check for health conditions such as speech, vision, and hearing problems; promote health education; and maintain a safe and sanitary school environment. Many school health services also provide counseling.

2:2 INFORMATION

Government Agencies

In addition to the government health care facilities mentioned previously, other health services are offered at international, national, state, and local levels. Government services are tax supported. Examples of government agencies include:

- ◆ *World Health Organization (WHO):* an international agency sponsored by the United Nations; compiles statistics and information on disease, publishes health information, and investigates and addresses serious health problems throughout the world

- ◆ **U.S. Department of Health and Human Services (USDHHS):** a national agency that deals with the health problems in the United States

- ◆ *National Institutes of Health (NIH):* a division of the USDHHS; involved in research on disease

- ◆ *Centers for Disease Control and Prevention (CDC):* another division of the USDHHS; concerned with causes, spread, and control of diseases in populations

- ◆ *Food and Drug Administration (FDA):* a federal agency responsible for regulating food and drug products sold to the public

- ◆ *Agency for Health Care Policy and Research (AHCPR):* a federal agency established in 1990 to research the quality of health care delivery and identify the standards of treatment that should be provided by health care facilities

♦ *Occupational Safety and Health Administration (OSHA)*: establishes and enforces standards that protect workers from job-related injuries and illnesses

♦ *Health departments*: provide health services as directed by the U.S. Department of Health and Human Services (USDHHS); also provide specific services needed by the state or local community; examples of services include immunization for disease control, inspections for environmental health and sanitation, communicable disease control, collection of statistics and records related to health, health education, clinics for health care and prevention, and other services needed in a community

2:3 INFORMATION

Voluntary or Nonprofit Agencies

Voluntary agencies, frequently called **nonprofit agencies**, are supported by donations, membership fees, fund-raisers, and federal or state grants. They provide health services at national, state, and local levels.

Examples of nonprofit agencies include the American Cancer Society, American Heart Association, American Respiratory Disease Association, American Diabetes Association, National Mental Health Association, Alzheimer's Association, National Kidney Foundation, Leukemia and Lymphoma Society, National Foundation of the March of Dimes, and American Red Cross. Many of these organizations have national offices as well as branch offices in states and/or local communities.

As indicated by their names, many such organizations focus on one specific disease or group of diseases. Each organization typically studies the disease, provides funding to encourage research directed at curing or treating the disease, and promotes public education regarding information obtained through research. These organizations also provide special services to victims of disease, such as purchasing medical equipment and supplies, providing treatment centers, and supplying information regarding other community agencies that offer assistance.

Nonprofit agencies employ many health care workers in addition to using volunteer workers to provide services.

2:4 INFORMATION

Health Insurance Plans

The cost of health care is a major concern of everyone who needs health services. Statistics show that the cost of health care is more than 15 percent of the gross national product (the total amount of money spent on all goods and services). Also, health care costs are increasing much faster than other costs of living. To pay for the costs of health care, most people rely on **health insurance plans**. Without insurance, the cost of an illness can mean financial disaster for an individual or family.

Health insurance plans are offered by several thousand insurance agencies. A common example is Blue Cross/Blue Shield (figure 2-3). In this type of plan, a *premium*, or a fee the individual pays for insurance coverage, is made to the insurance company. When the insured individual incurs health care expenses covered by the insurance plan, the insurance company pays for the services. The amount of payment and the type of services covered vary from plan to plan. Common insurance terms include:

♦ *Deductibles*: amounts that must be paid by the patient for medical services before the policy begins to pay

♦ *Co-insurance*: requires that specific percentages of expenses are shared by the patient and insurance company; for example, in an 80–20 percent co-insurance, the company pays 80

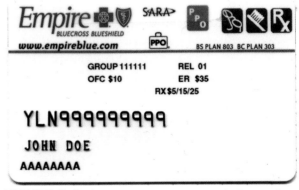

FIGURE 2-3 Health insurance plans help pay for the costs of health care. *(Courtesy of Empire Blue Cross/Blue Shield)*

percent of covered expenses, and the patient pays the remaining 20 percent

♦ *Co-payment:* a specific amount of money a patient pays for a particular service, for example, $10 for each physician visit regardless of the total cost of the visit

Many individuals have insurance coverage through their places of employment (called employer-sponsored health insurance or group insurance), where the premiums are paid by the employer. In most cases, the individual also pays a percentage of the premium. Private policies are also available for purchase by individuals.

A health maintenance organization (HMO) is another type of health insurance plan that provides a managed care plan for the delivery of health care services. A monthly fee or premium is paid for membership, and the fee stays the same regardless of the amount of health care used. The premium can be paid by an employer and/or an individual. Total care provided is directed toward preventive type health care. An individual insured under this type of plan has ready access to health examinations and early treatment and detection of disease. Because most other types of insurance plans do not cover routine examinations and preventive care, the individual insured by an HMO can therefore theoretically maintain a better state of health. The disadvantage of an HMO is that the insured is required to use only HMO-affiliated health care providers (doctors, laboratories, hospitals) for health care. If a nonaffiliated health care provider is used instead, the insured usually must pay for the care.

A **preferred provider organization (PPO)** is another type of managed care health insurance plan usually provided by large industries or companies to their employees. The PPO forms a contract with certain health care agencies, such as a large hospital and/or specific doctors and dentists, to provide certain types of health care at reduced rates. Employees are restricted to using the specific hospital and/or doctors, but the industry or company using the PPO can provide health care at lower rates. PPOs usually require a deductible and a co-payment. If an enrollee uses a nonaffiliated provider, the PPO may require co-payments of 40–60 percent.

The government also provides health insurance plans for certain groups of people. Two of the main plans are Medicare and Medicaid.

Medicare is a federal government program that provides health care for almost all individuals over the age of 65, for any person with a disability who has received Social Security benefits for at least 2 years, and for any person with end-stage renal (kidney) disease. Medicare consists of three kinds of coverage: type A for hospital insurance, type B for medical insurance, and type D for pharmaceutical (medication) expenses. Type A covers hospital services, care provided by an extended care facility or home-health care agency after hospitalization, and hospice care for people with a terminal illness. Type B offers additional coverage for doctors' services, outpatient treatments, therapy, clinical laboratory services, and other health care. The individual does pay a premium for type B coverage and also must pay an initial deductible for services. In addition, Medicare pays for only 80 percent of the services; the individual must either pay the balance or have another insurance policy to cover the expenses.

Medigap policies are health insurance plans that help pay expenses not covered by Medicare. These policies are offered by private insurance companies and require the payment of a premium by the enrollee. Medigap policies must meet specific federal guidelines. They provide options that allow enrollees to choose how much coverage they want to purchase.

Medicaid is a medical assistance program that is jointly funded by the federal government and state governments but operated by individual states. Benefits and individuals covered under this program vary slightly from state to state because each state has the right to establish its own eligibility standards, determine the type and scope of services, set the rate of payment for services, and administer its own program. In most states, Medicaid pays for the health care of individuals with low incomes, children who qualify for public assistance, and individuals who are physically disabled or blind. Generally, all state Medicaid programs provide hospital services, physician's care, long-term care services, and some therapies. In some states, Medicaid offers dental care, eye care, and other specialized services.

The *State Children's Health Insurance Program (SCHIP)* was established in 1997 to provide health care to uninsured children of working families who earn too little to afford private insurance but too much to be eligible for Medicaid. It provides inpatient and outpatient hospital services, physician's surgical and medical care, laboratory and X-ray tests, and well-baby and well-child care, including immunizations.

Workers' Compensation is a health insurance plan providing treatment for workers injured on the job. It is administered by the state, and payments are made by employers and the state. In addition to providing payment for needed health care, this plan also reimburses the worker for wages lost because of on-the-job injury.

TRICARE, formerly called CHAMPUS (the Civilian Health and Medical Programs for the Uniform Services) is a U.S. government health insurance plan for all military personnel. It provides care for all active duty members and their families, survivors of military personnel, and retired members of the Armed Forces. The Veterans Administration provides for military veterans.

Managed care is an approach that has developed in response to rising health care costs. Employers, as well as insurance companies who pay large medical bills, want to ensure that such money is spent efficiently rather than wastefully. The principle behind managed care is that all health care provided to a patient must have a purpose. A second opinion or verification of need is frequently required before care can be provided. Every effort is made to provide preventive care and early diagnosis of disease to avoid the high cost of treating disease. For example, routine physical examinations, well-baby care, immunizations, and wellness education to promote good nutrition, exercise, weight control, and healthy living practices are usually provided under managed care. Employers and insurance companies create a network of doctors, specialists, therapists, and health care facilities that provide care at the most reasonable cost. HMOs and PPOs are the main providers of managed care, but many private insurance companies are establishing health care networks to provide care to their subscribers. As these health care networks compete for the consumer dollar, they are required to provide quality care at the lowest possible cost. The health care consumer who is enrolled in a managed care plan receives quality care at the most reasonable cost but is restricted in choice of health care providers.

Health insurance plans do not solve all the problems of health care costs, but they do help many people by paying for all or part of the cost of health services. However, as the cost of insurance increases, many employers are less willing to offer health care insurance. Individuals with chronic illnesses often find they cannot obtain insurance coverage if their place of employment changes. This is one reason the federal government passed the **Health Insurance Portability and Accountability Act (HIPAA)** in 1996. This act has five main components:

♦ *Health Care Access, Portability, and Renewability*: limits exclusions on preexisting conditions to allow for the continuance of insurance even with job changes, prohibits discrimination against an enrollee or beneficiary based on health status, guarantees renewability in multiemployer plans, and provides special enrollment rights for individuals who lose insurance coverage in certain situations such as divorce or termination of employment

♦ *Preventing Health Care Fraud and Abuse; Administrative Simplification, and Medical Liability Reform*: establishes methods for preventing fraud and abuse and imposes sanctions or penalties if fraud or abuse does occur, reduces the costs and administration of health care by adopting a single set of electronic standards to replace the wide variety of formats used in health care, provides strict guidelines for maintaining the confidentiality of health care information and the security of health care records, and recommends limits for medical liability

♦ *Tax-Related Health Provisions*: promotes the use of medical savings accounts (MSAs) by allowing tax deductions for monies placed in the accounts, establishes standards for long-term care insurance, allows for the creation of state insurance pools, and provides tax benefits for some health care expenses

♦ *Application and Enforcement of Group Health Plan Requirements*: establishes standards that require group health care plans to offer portability, access, and renewability to all members of the group

♦ *Revenue Offsets*: provides changes to the Internal Revenue Code for HIPAA expenses

Compliance with all HIPAA regulations was required by April 2004 for all health care agencies. These regulations have not solved all of the problems of health care insurance, but they have provided consumers with more access to insurance and greater confidentiality in regard to medical records. In addition, standardization of electronic health care records, reductions in administrative costs, increased tax benefits, and decreasing fraud and abuse in health care have reduced health care costs for everyone.

2:5 INFORMATION

Organizational Structure

All health care facilities must have some type of **organizational structure.** The structure may be complex, as in larger facilities, or simple, as in smaller facilities. Organizational structure always, however, encompasses a line of authority or chain of command. The organizational structure should indicate areas of responsibility and lead to the most efficient operation of the facility.

A sample organizational chart for a large general hospital is shown in figure 2-4. This chart shows organization by department. Each department, in turn, can have an organizational chart similar to the one shown for the nursing department in figure 2-4. A sample organizational chart for a small medical office is shown in figure 2-5. The organizational structure will vary with the size of the office and the number of people employed.

In both organizational charts illustrated, the lines of authority are clearly indicated. It is important for health care workers to identify and understand their respective positions in a given facility's organizational structure. By doing this, they will know their lines of authority and understand who are the immediate supervisors in charge of their work. Health care workers must always take questions, reports, and problems to their immediate

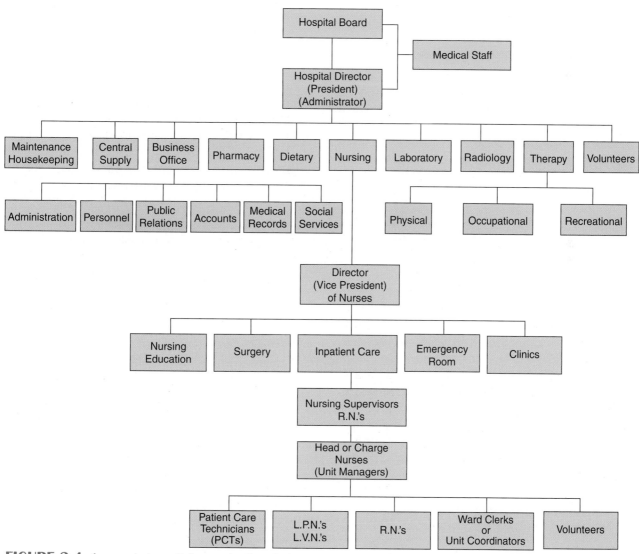

FIGURE 2-4 A sample hospital organizational chart.

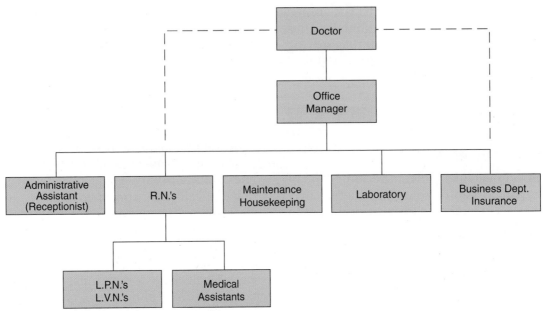

FIGURE 2-5 A sample medical office organizational chart.

TODAY'S RESEARCH: TOMORROW'S HEALTH CARE

Nature as a pharmacy?

Throughout history, many medicines have been derived from natural resources. Examples include aspirin, which comes from willow bark; penicillin, which comes from fungus; and the cancer drug Taxol, which comes from the Pacific yew tree. Recognizing this, many scientists believe that nature is a pharmaceutical gold mine and are exploring the vast supply of materials present in the oceans and in the earth.

The National Cancer Institute (NCI) has more than 100,000 samples of plants and marine life stored in Frederick, Maryland. Every sample is crushed into a powder and made into extracts that can be tested against human cancer cells. In addition, small quantities of the extracts are made available to other scientists who evaluate their effectiveness against other conditions, such as viral diseases and infections. To date, more than 4,000 extracts have shown promise and are being used in more advanced studies. One compound, Halichondrin B, labeled "yellow slimy" by researchers, appears to be effective at eliminating human tumors. Halichondrin B is an extract taken from a deep-sea sponge found in New Zealand. Scientists have created a synthetic version of the active component in Halichondrin B. This component, called E7389, is currently being tested in patients with a variety of tumors. By creating synthetic versions of the compounds, scientists are preserving natural resources while also benefiting from them.

Other natural products are now being tested and modified. Bristol-Myers is testing Ixabepilone, extracted from garden soil bacteria, in patients with advanced breast cancer. Wyeth isolated Rapamune from soil on Easter Island and proved it is effective in preventing kidney rejection after transplants. NCI developed a compound called prostratin from tree bark in Samoa. Healers in Samoa used the bark to treat hepatitis. The NCI has found that it is effective against the human immunodeficiency virus (HIV) that causes acquired immune deficiency syndrome (AIDS). As scientists continue to explore all that nature has to offer, it is possible they will find cures for many cancers, diseases, and infections.

supervisors, who are responsible for providing necessary assistance. If immediate supervisors cannot answer the question or solve the problem, it is their responsibility to take the situation to the next level in the organizational chart. It is also important for health care workers to understand the functions and goals of the organization.

STUDENT: *Go to the workbook and complete the assignment sheet for Chapter 2, Health Care Systems.*

CHAPTER 2 SUMMARY

Health care, one of the largest and fastest growing industries in the United States, encompasses many different types of facilities that provide health-related services. These include hospitals, long-term care facilities, medical and dental offices, clinics, laboratories, industrial and school health services, and many others. Government and nonprofit or voluntary agencies also provide health care services. All health care facilities require different health care workers at all levels of training.

Many types of health insurance plans are available to help pay the costs of health care. Insurance does not usually cover the entire cost of care, however. It is important for consumers to be aware of the types of coverage provided by their respective insurance plans.

Organizational structure is important in all health care facilities. The structure can be complex or simple, but it should show a line of authority or chain of command within the facility and indicate areas of responsibility.

INTERNET SEARCHES

Use the suggested search engines in Chapter 17:4 of this textbook to search the Internet for additional information on the following topics:

1. *Private health care facilities*: search for information on each of the specific types of facilities; for example, hospitals, hospice care, or emergency care services.

2. *Government agencies*: search for more detailed information about the activities of the World Health Organization, U.S. Department of Health and Human Services, National Insti-

tutes of Health, Centers for Disease Control and Prevention, Food and Drug Administration, and Occupational Safety and Health Administration.

3. *Voluntary or nonprofit agencies*: search for information on the purposes and activities of organizations such as the American Cancer Society, American Heart Association, American Respiratory Disease Association, American Diabetes Association, National Mental Health Association, National Foundation of the March of Dimes, and the American Red Cross.

4. *Health insurance*: search the Internet to find specific names of companies that are health maintenance organizations or preferred provider organizations. Check to see how their coverage for individuals is the same or how it is different.

5. *Government health care insurance*: search the Internet to learn about benefits provided under Medicare, Medicaid, and the State Children's Health Insurance Program.

REVIEW QUESTIONS

1. Differentiate between a private or proprietary, religious, nonprofit or voluntary, and government type of hospital.

2. Identify at least six (6) different types of private health care facilities by stating the functions of the facility. Provide specific examples of the care received at each facility.

3. Name each of the following federal agencies and briefly describe its function:
   a. CDC
   b. FDA
   c. NIH
   d. OSHA
   e. USDHHS
   f. WHO

4. What does the term *deductible* mean on health insurance policies? *co-insurance? co-payment? premium?*

5. An insurance policy has a co-payment of 70–30 percent. If an emergency department bill is $660.00, what amount will the patient have to pay?

6. Why is it important for every health care worker to know the organizational structure for his/her place of employment?

CHAPTER 3

Careers in Health Care

Observe Standard Precautions

Instructor's Check—Call Instructor at This Point

Safety—Proceed with Caution

OBRA Requirement—Based on Federal Law

Math Skill

Legal Responsibility

Science Skill

Career Information

Communications Skill

Technology

Chapter Objectives

After completing this chapter, you should be able to:

◆ Compare the educational requirements for associate's, bachelor's, and master's degrees

◆ Contrast certification, registration, and licensure

◆ Describe at least 10 different health careers by including a definition of the career, three duties, educational requirements, and employment opportunities

◆ Investigate at least one health career by writing to listed sources or using the Internet to request additional information on the career

◆ Interpret at least 10 abbreviations used to identify health care career workers

◆ Define, pronounce, and spell all key terms (see page 3 for explanation of accent mark use)

KEY TERMS

admitting officers/clerks

art, music, dance therapists

associate's degree

athletic trainers (ATs)

audiologists

bachelor's degree

biological or medical scientists

biological technician

biomedical (clinical) engineer

biotechnological engineer (bioengineer)

biomedical equipment technicians (BETs)

cardiovascular technologist

central/sterile supply workers

certification

continuing education units (CEUs)

dental assistants (DAs)

dental hygienists *(den'-tall hi-geen'-ists)*

dental laboratory technicians (DLTs)

dentists (DMDs or DDSs)

dialysis technicians *(die-ahl'-ih-sis tek-nish'ins)*

dietetic assistants

dietetic technicians (DTs)

dietitians (RDs)

Doctor of Chiropractic (DC) *(Ky-row-prak'-tik)*

Doctor of Medicine (MD)

Doctor of Osteopathic Medicine (DO) *(Oss-tee-ohp'-ath-ik)*

Doctor of Podiatric Medicine (DPM) *(Poh"-dee'-ah-trik)*

doctorate/doctoral/doctor's degree

electrocardiograph (ECG) technicians *(ee-lek"-trow-car'-dee-oh-graf tek-nish'-ins)*

electroencephalographic (EEG) technologist *(ee-lek"-troh-en-sef-ahl-oh-graf-ik tek-nahl'-oh-jist)*

electroneurodiagnostic technologist (END) *(ee-lek"-troh-new-roh-die-ag-nah'-stik)*

embalmers *(em-bahl'-mers)*

emergency medical technician (EMT)

endodontics *(en'-doe-don'-tiks)*

entrepreneur *(on"trah-peh-nor')*

epidemiologists

first responder

forensic science technician

funeral directors

genetic counselors

geriatric aides/assistants *(jerry-at'-rik)*

health care administrators

health information (medical records) administrators (RAs)

health information (medical records) technicians

health science technology education (HSTE)

home health care assistants

housekeeping workers/ sanitary managers

licensed practical/vocational nurses (LPNs/LVNs)

licensure *(ly'-sehn-shur)*

massage therapists

master's degree

medical assistants (MAs)

medical illustrators

medical interpreters/ translators

medical (clinical) laboratory assistants

medical (clinical) laboratory technicians (MLTs)

medical (clinical) laboratory technologists (MTs)

medical librarians

medical transcriptionists

medication aides/assistants

mortuary assistants

multicompetent/ multiskilled worker

nurse assistants

occupational therapists (OTs)

occupational therapy assistants (OTAs)

ophthalmic assistants (OAs)

ophthalmic laboratory technicians

ophthalmic medical technologists (OMTs)

ophthalmic technicians (OTs)

ophthalmologists

opticians *(ahp-tish'-ins)*

optometrists (ODs) *(ah'-tom'-eh-trists)*

oral surgery

orthodontics *(or"-thow-don'-tiks)*

paramedic (EMT-P)

patient care technicians (PCTs)

pedodontics *(peh"-doe-don'-tiks)*

perfusionists *(purr-few'-shun-ists)*

KEY TERMS

periodontics
  (peh″-ree-oh-don′-tiks)
pharmacists (PharmDs)
  (far′-mah-sists)
pharmacy technicians
phlebotomists
physical therapists (PTs)
physical therapist assistants
  (PTAs)
physicians
physician assistants (PAs)
process technician
prosthodontics
  (pross″-thow-don′-tiks)

psychiatric/mental health
  technicians
psychiatrists
psychologists
  (sy-koll″-oh-jists)
radiologic technologists
  (RTs) (ray′-dee-oh-loge′-ik
  tek-nahl′-oh-jists)
recreational therapists (TRs)
recreational therapy
  assistants
registered nurses (RNs)
registration
respiratory therapists (RTs)

respiratory therapy
  technicians (RTTs)
social workers (SWs)
speech–language
  pathologists
surgical technologists/
  technicians (STs)
unit secretaries/ward clerks/
  unit coordinators
veterinarians (DVMs or
  VMDs)
  (vet″-eh-ran-air′-e-ans)
veterinary assistants
veterinary technologists/
  technicians (VTs)

3:1 INFORMATION

Introduction to Health Careers

There are more than 250 different health care careers, so it would be impossible to discuss all of them in this chapter. A broad overview of a variety of careers is presented, however.

 Educational requirements for health careers depend on many factors and can vary from state to state. Basic preparation begins in high school (secondary education) and should include the sciences, social studies, English, and mathematics. Keyboarding, computer applications, and accounting skills are also utilized in most health occupations. Secondary **health science technology education (HSTE)** programs can prepare a student for immediate employment in many health careers or for additional education after graduation. Post-secondary education (after high school) can include training in a career/technical school, community college, or university. Some careers require an **associate's degree,** which is awarded by a career/technical school or a community college after completion of a prescribed two-year course of study. Other careers require a **bachelor's degree,** which is awarded by a college or university after a prescribed course of study that usually lasts for four or more years. In some cases, a **master's degree** is required. This is awarded by a college or university after completion of one or more years of work beyond a bachelor's degree. Other careers require a **doctorate, doctoral,** or **doctor's degree,** which is awarded by a college or university after completion of two or more years of work beyond a bachelor's or master's degree. Some doctorates can require four to six years of additional study.

A health science career cluster has been developed by the National Consortium on Health Science and Technology Education (NCHSTE) (figure 3-1). This cluster allows a student to see how early career awareness and exploration provide the foundation for making informed choices to prepare for a career in health care. Students who take required courses in middle school and high school have the foundation for success at the post-secondary level.

CERTIFICATION, REGISTRATION, AND LICENSURE

Three other terms associated with health careers are *certification, registration,* and *licensure.* These are methods used to ensure the skill and competency of health care personnel and to protect the consumer or patient.

Certification means that a person has fulfilled requirements of education and performance and meets the standards and qualifications estab-

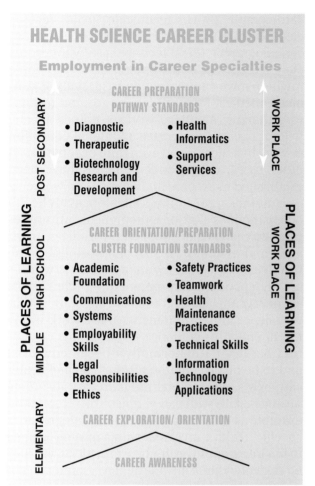

HEALTH SCIENCE CAREER CLUSTER

Employment in Career Specialties

CAREER PREPARATION
PATHWAY STANDARDS

POST SECONDARY

- Diagnostic
- Therapeutic
- Biotechnology Research and Development
- Health Informatics
- Support Services

WORK PLACE

CAREER ORIENTATION/PREPARATION
CLUSTER FOUNDATION STANDARDS

HIGH SCHOOL

- Academic Foundation
- Communications
- Systems
- Employability Skills
- Legal Responsibilities
- Ethics
- Safety Practices
- Teamwork
- Health Maintenance Practices
- Technical Skills
- Information Technology Applications

WORK PLACE

PLACES OF LEARNING

PLACES OF LEARNING

MIDDLE

ELEMENTARY

CAREER EXPLORATION/ ORIENTATION

CAREER AWARENESS

FIGURE 3-1 This cluster shows how early career awareness and exploration can provide a foundation for making informed choices to prepare for a career in health care.

lished by the professional association or government agency that regulates a particular career. A certificate or statement is issued by the association. Examples of certified positions include certified dental assistant, certified laboratory technician, and certified medical assistant.

Registration is required in some health care careers. This is performed by a regulatory body (professional association or state board) that administers examinations and maintains a current list ("registry") of qualified personnel in a given health care area. Examples of registered positions include registered dietitian, registered respiratory therapist, and registered radiologic technologist.

Licensure is a process whereby a government agency authorizes individuals to work in a given occupation. Health care careers requiring licensure can vary from state to state. Obtaining

and retaining licensure usually requires that a person complete an approved educational program, pass a state board test, and maintain certain standards. Examples of licensed positions include physician, dentist, physical therapist, registered nurse, and licensed practical/vocational nurse.

ACCREDITATION

For most health careers, graduation from an accredited program is required before certification, registration, and/or licensure will be granted. Accreditation ensures that the program of study meets the established quality competency standards and prepares students for employment in the health career. It is important for a student to make sure that a technical school, college, or university offers accredited programs of study before enrolling. Two major accrediting agencies for health care programs are the Commission on Accreditation of Allied Health Education Programs (CAAHEP) and the Accrediting Bureau of Health Education Schools (ABHES). A student can contact these agencies to determine whether an HSTE program at a specific school is accredited.

CONTINUING EDUCATION UNITS

Continuing education units (CEUs) are required to renew licenses or maintain certification or registration in many states (figure 3-2). An individual must obtain additional hours of education in the specific health career area during a specified period. For example, many states require registered nurses to obtain 24 to 48 CEUs every 1 to 2 years to renew licenses. Health care workers should be aware of the state requirements regarding CEUs for their given careers.

EDUCATION LEVELS, TRENDS, AND OPPORTUNITIES

Generally speaking, training for most health care careers can be categorized into four levels: professional, technologist or therapist, technician, and aide or assistant, as shown in table 3-1.

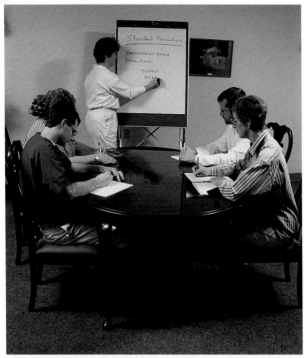

FIGURE 3-2 Continuing education units (CEUs) are required to renew licenses or maintain certification or registration in many states.

A common trend in health care is the **multicompetent or multiskilled worker.** Because of high health care costs, smaller facilities and rural areas often cannot afford to hire a specialist for every aspect of care. Therefore, workers are hired who can perform a variety of health care skills. For example, a health care worker may be hired to perform the skills of both an electrocardiograph (ECG) technician (who records electrical activity of the heart) and an electroencephalographic (EEG) technologist (who records electrical activity of the brain). Another example might involve combining the basic skills of radiology, medical (clinical) laboratory, and respiratory therapy. At times, workers trained in one field or occupation receive additional education to work in a second and even third occupation. In other cases, educational programs have been established to prepare multicompetent workers.

Another opportunity available in many health occupations is that of entrepreneur. An **entrepreneur** is an individual who organizes, manages, and assumes the risk of a business. Some health care careers allow an individual to work as an independent entrepreneur, while others encourage the use of groups of cooperating individuals. Many entrepreneurs must work under the direction or guidance of physicians or dentists. Because the opportunity to be self-employed and to be involved in the business area of health care exists, educational programs are including business skills with career objectives. A common example is combining a bachelor's degree in a specific health care career with a master's degree in business. Some health care providers who may be entrepreneurial include dental laboratory technicians, dental hygienists, nurse practitioners, physical therapists, physician assistants, respiratory therapists, recreational therapists, physicians, dentists, chiropractors, and optometrists. Although entrepreneurship involves many risks and requires a certain level of education and ability, it can be an

TABLE 3-1 Education and Levels of Training

CAREER LEVEL	EDUCATIONAL REQUIREMENT	EXAMPLES
Professional	Four or more years of college with bachelor's, master's, or doctoral degree	Medical doctor Dentist
Technologist or Therapist	Three to four years of college plus work experience, usually bachelor's degree and, at times, master's degree	Medical (clinical) laboratory technologist Physical therapist Speech therapist Respiratory therapist
Technician	Two-year associate's degree, special health science technology education, or three to four years of on-the-job training	Dental laboratory technician Medical (clinical) laboratory technician Surgical technician
Aide or Assistant	Specific number of hours of specialized education or one or more years of training combining classroom and/or on-the-job training	Dental assistant Medical assistant Nurse assistant

extremely satisfying choice for the individual who is well motivated, self-confident, responsible, creative, and independent.

NATIONAL HEALTH CARE SKILL STANDARDS

The National Health Care Skill Standards (NHCSS) were developed to indicate the knowledge and skills that are expected of health care workers primarily at entry and technical levels. The seven groups of standards include the following:

♦ *Health Care Core Standards*: specify the knowledge and skills that most health care workers should have; discuss an academic foundation, communication skills, employability skills, legal responsibilities, ethics, safety practices, teamwork, information technology applications, technical skills, health maintenance practices, and knowledge about the systems in the health care environment

♦ *Therapeutic/Diagnostic Core Standards*: specify the knowledge and skills required to focus on direct patient care in both the therapeutic and diagnostic health care careers; include health maintenance practices, patient interaction, intrateam communication, monitoring patient status, and patient movement

♦ *Therapeutic Cluster Standards (Therapeutic Services)*: specify the knowledge and skills required of workers in health care careers that are involved in changing the health status of the patient over time; include interacting with patients, communicating with team members, collecting information, planning treatment, implementing procedures, monitoring patient status, and evaluating patient response to treatment

♦ *Diagnostic Cluster Standards (Diagnostic Services)*: specify the knowledge and skills required of workers in health care careers that are involved in creating a picture of the health status of the patient at a single point in time; include communicating oral and written information, assessing patient's health status, moving and positioning patients safely and efficiently, explaining procedures and goals, preparing for procedures, performing diagnostic procedures, evaluating test results, and reporting required information

♦ *Health Informatics Services Cluster Standards*: specify the knowledge and skills required of workers in health care careers that are involved with the documentation of patient care; includes communicating information accurately within legal boundaries, analyzing information, abstracting and coding medical records and documents, designing and/or implementing effective information systems, documenting information, and understanding operations to enter, retrieve, and maintain information

♦ *Support (Environmental) Services Cluster Standards*: specify the knowledge and skills required of workers in health care careers that are involved with creating a therapeutic environment to provide direct or indirect patient care; include developing and implementing the administration, quality control, and compliance regulations of a health care facility; maintaining a clean and safe environment through aseptic techniques; managing resources; and maintaining an aesthetically appealing environment

♦ *Biotechnology Research and Development Standards*: specify the knowledge and skills required of workers in health care careers that are involved in bioscience research and development; include comprehending how biotechnology contributes to health and the quality of life, developing a strong foundation in math and science principles, performing biotechnology techniques, understanding and following laboratory protocols and principles, working with product design and development, and complying with bioethical policies

Examples of some of the health careers included in the NHCSS Clusters are shown in table 3-2. The careers listed are discussed in detail in this chapter.

INTRODUCTION TO HEALTH CAREERS

In the following discussion of health careers, a basic description of the job duties for each career is provided. The various levels in each health care career are also given. In addition, tables for each career group show educational requirements, job outlook, and average yearly earnings.

TABLE 3-2 Health Science Center Pathways

Planning, managing, and providing therapeutic services, diagnostic services, health informatics, support services, and biotechnology research and development

		Pathways		
Therapeutic Services	**Diagnostics Services**	**Health Informatics**	**Support Services**	**Biotechnology Research and Development**
Sample Career Specialties/Occupations				
Acupuncturist	Cardiovascular technologist	Admitting clerk	Biomedical/clinical engineer	Biochemist
Anesthesiologist assistant	Clinical lab technician	Applied researcher	Biomedical/clinical technician	Bioinformatics associate
Art/music/dance therapist	Computer tomography (CT) technologist	Community services specialist	Central services	Bioinformatics specialist
Athletic trainer	Cytogenetic technologist	Data analyst	Environmental health and safety	Biomedical chemist
Audiologist	Cytotechnologist	Epidemiologist	Environmental services	Biostatistician
Certified nursing assistant	Diagnostic medical sonographer	Ethicist	Facilities manager	Cell biologist
Chiropractor	Electrocardiographic (ECG) technician	Health educator	Food service	Clinical trials research associate
Dental assistant/hygienist	Electronic diagnostic (EEG) technologist	Health information coder	Hospital maintenance engineer	Clinical trials research coordinator
Dental lab technician	Exercise physiologist	Health information services	Industrial hygienist	Geneticist
Dentist	Geneticist	Health care administrator	Materials management	Lab assistant—genetics
Dietician	Histotechnologist	Medical assistant	Transport technician	Lab technician
Dosimetrist	Magnetic resonance (MR) technologist	Medical biller/patient financial services		Microbiologist
EMT	Mammographer	Medical information technologist		Molecular biologist
Exercise physiologist	Medical technologist/clinical laboratory scientist	Medical librarian/cybrarian		Pharmaceutical scientist
Home health aide		Patient advocate		Quality assurance technician
Kinesiotherapist		Public health educator		Quality control technician
Licensed practical nurse				Regulatory affairs specialist
Massage therapist				Research assistant
Medical assistant				
Mortician				

Research associate
Research scientist
Toxicologist

Reimbursement specialist
  (HFMA)
Risk management
Social worker
Transcriptionist
Unit coordinator
Utilization manager

Nuclear medicine technologist
Nutritionist
Pathologist
Pathology assistant
Phlebotomist
Positron emission tomography
  (PET) technologist
Radiologic technologist/
  radiographer

Occupational therapist/assistant
Ophthalmic medical personnel
Optometrist
Orthotist/prosthetist
Paramedic
Pharmacist/pharmacy technician
Physical therapist/assistant
Physician (MD/DO)
Physician's assistant
Psychologist
Recreation therapist
Registered nurse
Respiratory therapist
Social worker
Speech language pathologist
Surgical technician
Veterinarian/veterinary technician

Pathway Knowledge and Skills Clusters

• Academics foundation • Communications • Systems • Employability skills • Legal responsibilities • Ethics

• Safety practices Teamwork • Health maintenance practices • Technical skills • Information technology application

From National Consortium of Health Science and Technology Education, 2005.

To simplify the information presented in these tables, the highest level of education for each career group is listed. The designations used are as follows:

- *On-the-job*: training while working at a job
- *HSTE program*: health science technology education program
- *Associate's degree*: two-year associate's degree
- *Bachelor's degree*: four-year bachelor's degree
- *Master's degree*: one or more years beyond a bachelor's degree to obtain a master's degree
- *Doctoral (Doctor's) degree*: doctorate with four or more years beyond a bachelor's degree

It is important to note that although many health careers begin with HSTE programs, obtaining additional education after graduation from HSTE programs allows health care workers to progress in career level to higher-paying positions.

The job outlook or expected job growth through the year 2012 is stated in the tables as "below average," "average," or "above average."

Average yearly earning is presented as a range of income, because earnings will vary according to geographical location, specialty area, level of education, and work experience.

All career information presented includes a basic introduction. *Because requirements for various health care careers can vary from state to state, it is important for students to obtain information pertinent to their respective states.* More detailed information on any given career discussed can be obtained from the sources listed for that occupation's career cluster.

 3:2 INFORMATION

Therapeutic Services Careers

Therapeutic careers in health care are directed toward changing the health status of the patient over time.

Workers in the therapeutic services use a variety of treatments to help patients who are injured, physically or mentally disabled, or emotionally disturbed. All treatment is directed toward allowing patients to function at maximum capacity.

Places of employment include rehabilitation facilities, hospitals, clinics, mental health facilities, daycare facilities, long-term care facilities, home health care agencies, schools, and government agencies.

There are many health care careers in the therapeutic services cluster. Some of these careers are discussed in the following information sections.

 3:2A INFORMATION

Dental Careers

Dental workers focus on the health of the teeth and the soft tissues of the mouth. Care is directed toward preventing dental disease, repairing or replacing diseased or damaged teeth, and treating the gingiva (gums) and other supporting structures of the teeth.

Places of employment include private dental offices, laboratories, and clinics; or dental departments in hospitals, schools, health departments, or government agencies.

Most dental professionals work in general dentistry practices where all types of dental conditions are treated in people of all ages. Some, however, work in specialty areas such as the following:

- **Endodontics:** treatment of diseases of the pulp, nerves, blood vessels, and roots of the teeth; often called root canal treatment
- **Orthodontics:** alignment or straightening of the teeth
- **Oral Surgery:** surgery on the teeth, mouth, jaw and facial bones; often called *maxillofacial surgery*
- **Pedodontics:** dental treatment of children and adolescents
- **Periodontics:** treatment and prevention of diseases of the gums, bone, and structures supporting the teeth
- **Prosthodontics:** replacement of natural teeth with artificial teeth or dentures

Levels of workers in dentistry include dentist, dental hygienist, dental laboratory technician, and dental assistant (see table 3-3).

Dentists (DMD or DDS) are doctors who examine teeth and mouth tissues to diagnose and treat disease and abnormalities; perform corrective surgery on the teeth, gums, tissues, and supporting bones; and work to prevent dental disease. They also supervise the work of other dental workers. Most are entrepreneurs.

Dental hygienists (DHs) work under the supervision of dentists. They perform prelimi-

TABLE 3-3 Dental Careers

OCCUPATION	EDUCATION REQUIRED	JOB OUTLOOK TO YEAR 2012	AVERAGE YEARLY EARNINGS
Dentist (DMD or DDS)	• Doctor of Dental Medicine (DMD) or Doctor of Dental Surgery (DDS) • 2 or more years additional education for specialization • Licensure in state of practice	Below average growth	$84,000–$200,000
Dental Hygienist (DH) Licensed Dental Hygienist (LDH)	• Associate's, bachelor's, or master's degree • Licensure in state of practice	Above average growth	$39,300–$83,200
Dental Laboratory Technician (DLT) Certified Dental Laboratory Technician (CDLT)	• 3–4 years on-the-job or 1–2 years HSTE program or associate's or bachelor's degree • Certification can be obtained from National Board for Certification in Dental Technology	Average growth	$23,200–$53,600
Dental Assistant (DA) and Certified Dental Assistant (CDA)	• 1–3 years on-the-job or 1–2 years in HSTE program or associate's degree • Licensure or registration required in most states • Certification can be obtained from Dental Assisting National Board	Above average growth	$19,900–$38,700

nary examinations of the teeth and mouth, remove stains and deposits from teeth, expose and develop radiographs, apply cavity-preventing agents such as fluorides or pit and fissure sealants to the teeth, and perform other preventive or therapeutic (treatment) services to help the patient develop and maintain good dental health. In some states, dental hygienists are authorized to place and carve restorative materials, polish restorations, remove sutures, and/or administer anesthesia. Dental hygienists can be entrepreneurs.

Dental laboratory technicians (DLTs) make and repair a variety of dental prostheses (artificial devices) such as dentures, crowns, bridges, and orthodontic appliances according to the specifications of dentists. Specialities include dental ceramist and orthodontic technician. Some dental laboratory technicians are entrepreneurs.

Dental assistants (DAs), working under the supervision of dentists, prepare patients for examinations, pass instruments, prepare dental materials for impressions and restorations, take

and develop radiographs, teach preventive dental care, sterilize instruments, and/or perform dental receptionist duties such as scheduling appointments and handling accounts. Their duties may be limited by the dental practice laws of the state in which they work.

ADDITIONAL SOURCES OF INFORMATION

◆ American Dental Education Association
1400 K Street, NW
Washington, DC 20005
Internet address: *www.adea.org*

◆ American Dental Assistants Association
35 East Wacker Drive, Suite 1730
Chicago, IL 60601-2211
Internet address: *www.dentalassistant.org*

◆ American Dental Association
211 E. Chicago Avenue
Chicago, IL 60611-2678
Internet address: *www.ada.org*

♦ American Dental Hygienists' Association
444 N. Michigan Avenue, Suite 3400
Chicago, IL 60611
Internet address: *www.adha.org*

♦ Dental Assisting National Board, Inc.
676 North Saint Clair, Suite 1880
Chicago, IL 60611
Internet address: *www.danb.org*

♦ National Association of Dental Laboratories
325 John Knox Road
Tallahassee, FL 32303
Internet address: *www.nadl.org*

♦ National Association of Advisors for the Health
Professions, Inc.
P.O. Box 1518
Champaign, IL 61824-1518
Internet address: *www.naahp.org*

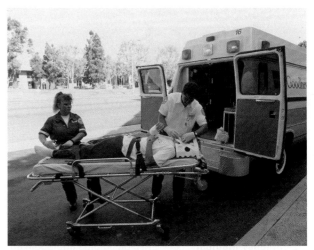

FIGURE 3-3 Emergency medical technicians (EMTs) provide emergency, prehospital care to victims of accidents, injuries, or sudden illness.

3:2B INFORMATION

Emergency Medical Services Careers

Emergency medical services personnel (figure 3-3) provide emergency, prehospital care to victims of accidents, injuries, or sudden illnesses. Although individuals with only basic training in first aid do sometimes work in this field, **emergency medical technician (EMT)** training is required for most jobs. Formal EMT training is available in all states and is offered by fire, police, and health departments, hospitals, career/technical schools, and as a nondegree course in technical/community colleges and universities.

Places of employment include fire and police departments, rescue squads, ambulance services, hospital or private emergency rooms, urgent care centers, industry, emergency helicopter services, and the military. Some EMTs are entrepreneurs. Emergency medical technicians sometimes serve as volunteers in fire and rescue departments.

Levels of EMT include the EMT basic, EMT intermediate, and EMT paramedic (see table 3-4). Another emergency medical person is a first responder.

A **first responder** is the first person to arrive at the scene of an illness or injury. Common examples include police officers, security guards, fire department personnel, and immediate family members. The first responder interviews and examines the victim to identify the illness or cause of injury, calls for emergency medical assistance as needed, maintains safety and infection control at the scene, and provides basic emergency medical care. A certified first responder (CFR) course prepares individuals by teaching airway management, oxygen administration, bleeding control, and cardiopulmonary resuscitation (CPR).

Emergency medical technicians basic (EMT-B) provide care for a wide range of illnesses and injuries including medical emergencies, bleeding, fractures, airway obstruction, basic life support (BLS), oxygen administration, emergency childbirth, rescue of trapped persons, and transporting of victims.

Emergency medical technician defibrillator (EMT-D) is a new level of EMT-B. It allows EMT-Bs with additional training and competency in basic life support to administer electrical defibrillation to certain heart attack victims.

Emergency medical technicians intermediate (EMT-I) perform the same tasks as do EMT-Bs together with assessing patients, interpreting electrocardiograms (ECGs), administering defibrillation as needed, managing shock, using intravenous equipment, and inserting esophageal airways.

TABLE 3-4 Emergency Medical Services Careers

OCCUPATION	EDUCATION REQUIRED	JOB OUTLOOK TO YEAR 2012	AVERAGE YEARLY EARNINGS
Emergency Medical Technician Paramedic (EMT-P)(EMT-4)	• EMT-Intermediate plus additional 6–9 months to 2 years (over 1,000 hours) approved paramedic training or associate's degree • 6 months experience as paramedic • State certification • Registration by the National Registry of EMTs (NREMT) required in most states • Other states identify as EMT-4 and administer their own certification examination	Above average growth	$28,400–$52,600
Emergency Medical Technician Intermediate (EMT-I) (EMT-2 and EMT-3)	• EMT-Basic plus additional approved training of at least 35–55 hours with clinical experience • State certification • Registration by the NREMT required in some states • Other states identify as EMT-2 and EMT-3 and administer their own certification examination	Above average growth	$21,200–$44,300
Emergency Medical Technician Basic (EMT-B)(EMT-1)	• Usually minimum 110 hours approved EMT program with 10 hours of internship in emergency room • State certification • Registration by National Registry of EMTs (NREMT) required in some states • Other states identify as EMT-1 and administer their own certification examination	Above average growth	$19,200–$35,700
First Responder	• Minimum 40 hours of approved training program • Certification can be obtained from the NREMT	Above average growth	Salary depends on individual's regular job

Emergency medical technicians **paramedic (EMT-P)** perform all the basic EMT duties plus in-depth patient assessment, provision of advanced cardiac life support (ACLS), ECG interpretation, endotracheal intubation, drug administration, and operation of complex equipment.

ADDITIONAL SOURCES OF INFORMATION

◆ National Association of Emergency Medical Technicians
132-A East Northside Drive
P.O. Box 1400
Clinton, MS 39060-1400
Internet address: *www.naemt.org*

◆ National Highway Transportation Safety Administration (NHTSA)
EMS Division
400 7th Street SW
Washington, DC 20590
Internet address: *www.nhtsa.dot.gov*

◆ National Registry of Emergency Medical Technicians
6610 Busch Boulevard
P.O. Box 29233
Columbus, OH 43229
Internet address: *www.nremt.org*

3:2C INFORMATION

Medical Careers

Medical careers is a broad category encompassing physicians (doctors) and other individuals who work in any of the varied careers under the supervision of physicians. All such careers focus on diagnosing, treating, or preventing diseases and disorders of the human body.

Places of employment include private practices, clinics, hospitals, public health agencies, research facilities, health maintenance organizations (HMOs), government agencies, and colleges or universities.

Levels include physician, physician assistant, and medical assistant (see table 3-5).

Physicians examine patients, obtain medical histories, order tests, make diagnoses, perform surgery, treat diseases/disorders, and teach preventive health. Several classifications are as follows:

♦ **Doctor of Medicine (MD):** Diagnoses, treats, and prevents diseases or disorders; may specialize as noted in table 3-6

♦ **Doctor of Osteopathic Medicine (DO):** Treats diseases/disorders, placing special emphasis on the nervous, muscular, and skeletal systems, and the relationship between the body, mind, and emotions; may also specialize

♦ **Doctor of Podiatric Medicine (DPM):** Examines, diagnoses, and treats diseases/disorders of the feet or of the leg below the knee

♦ **Doctor of Chiropractic (DC):** Focuses on ensuring proper alignment of the spine and optimal operation of the nervous and muscular systems to maintain health

Physician assistants (PAs), working under the supervision of physicians, take medical histories; perform routine physical examinations and basic diagnostic tests; make preliminary diagno-

TABLE 3-5 Medical Careers

OCCUPATION	EDUCATION REQUIRED	JOB OUTLOOK TO YEAR 2012	AVERAGE YEARLY EARNINGS
Physician	• Doctoral degree • 3–8 years additional postgraduate training of internship and residency depending on specialty selected • State licensure • Board certification in specialty area	Above average growth	$120,000–$425,500
Physician Assistant (PA), PAC (certified)	• 2 or more years of college and usually a bachelor's degree • 2 or more years accredited physician assistant program with certificate, associate's, or bachelor's degree • Registration, certification, or licensure required in all states • Certification can be obtained from National Commission on Certification of Physician's Assistants	Above average growth	$49,800–$104,600
Medical Assistant (MA), CMA (certified), RMA (registered)	• 1–2-year HSTE program or associate's degree • Certification can be obtained from American Association of Medical Assistants (AAMA) after graduation from CAAHEP or ABHES accredited medical assistant program • Registered credentials can be obtained from American Medical Technologists (AMT)	Above average growth	$18,400–$46,700

TABLE 3-6 Medical Specialties

PHYSICIAN'S TITLE	SPECIALTY
Anesthesiologist	Administration of medications to cause loss of sensation or feeling during surgery or treatments
Cardiologist	Diseases of the heart and blood vessels
Dermatologist	Diseases of the skin
Emergency Physician	Acute illness or injury
Endocrinologist	Diseases of the endocrine glands
Family Physician/Practice	Promote wellness, treat illness or injury in all age groups
Gastroenterologist	Diseases and disorders of the stomach and intestine
Gerontologist	Diseases of elderly individuals
Gynecologist	Diseases of the female reproductive organs
Internist	Diseases of the internal organs (lungs, heart, glands, intestines, kidneys)
Neurologist	Disorders of the brain and nervous system
Obstetrician	Pregnancy and childbirth
Oncologist	Diagnosis and treatment of tumors (cancer)
Ophthalmologist	Diseases and disorders of the eye
Orthopedist	Diseases and disorders of muscles and bones
Otolaryngologist	Diseases of the ear, nose, and throat
Pathologist	Diagnose disease by studying changes in organs, tissues, and cells
Pediatrician	Diseases and disorders of children
Physiatrist	Physical medicine and rehabilitation
Plastic Surgeon	Corrective surgery to repair injured or malformed body parts
Proctologist	Diseases of the lower part of the large intestine
Psychiatrist	Diseases and disorders of the mind
Radiologist	Use of X-rays and radiation to diagnose and treat disease
Sports Medicine	Prevention and treatment of injuries sustained in athletic events
Surgeon	Surgery to correct deformities or treat injuries or disease
Thoracic Surgeon	Surgery of the lungs, heart, or chest cavity
Urologist	Diseases of the kidney, bladder, or urinary system

ses; treat minor injuries; and prescribe and administer appropriate treatments. *Pathology assistants*, working under the supervision of pathologists, perform both gross and microscopic autopsy examinations.

Medical assistants (MAs), working under the supervision of physicians, prepare patients for examinations; take vital signs and medical histories; assist with procedures and treatments; perform basic laboratory tests; prepare and maintain equipment and supplies; and/or perform secretarial–receptionist duties (figure 3-4). The type of facility and physician determines the kinds of duties. The range of duties is determined by state law. Assistants working for physicians who specialize are called *specialty assistants*. For example, an assistant working for a pediatrician is called a *pediatric assistant.*

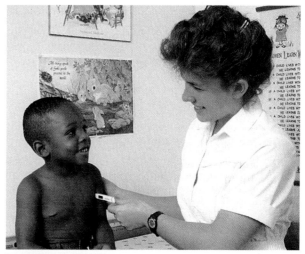

FIGURE 3-4 Medical assistants take vital signs and prepare patients for examinations.

ADDITIONAL SOURCES OF INFORMATION

- ◆ American Academy of Physician Assistants
  950 N. Washington Street
  Alexandria, VA 22314–1552
  Internet address: *www.aapa.org*

- ◆ American Association of Medical Assistants
  20 N. Wacker Drive, Suite 1575
  Chicago, IL 60606–2963
  Internet address: *www.aama-ntl.org*

- ◆ American Chiropractic Association
  1701 Clarendon Boulevard
  Arlington, VA 22209
  Internet address: *www.amerchiro.org*

- ◆ American Medical Association
  515 North State Street
  Chicago, IL 60610
  Internet address: *www.ama-assn.org*

- ◆ American Osteopathic Association
  142 East Ontario Street
  Chicago, IL 60611
  Internet address: *www.osteopathic.org*

- ◆ American Podiatric Medical Association
  9312 Old Georgetown Road
  Bethesda, MD 20814–1621
  Internet address: *www.apma.org*

- ◆ American Society of Podiatric Medical Assistants
  2124 S. Austin Boulevard
  Cicero, IL 60804
  Internet address: *www.aspma.org*

- ◆ Registered Medical Assistants of the American Medical Technologists
  710 Higgins Road
  Park Ridge, IL 60068
  Internet address: *www.amt1.org*

3:2D INFORMATION

Mental and Social Services Careers

Mental services professionals focus on helping people with mental or emotional disorders or those who are developmentally delayed or mentally impaired. Social workers help people deal with illnesses, employment, or community problems. Workers in both fields try to help individuals function to their maximum capacities.

Places of employment include hospitals; psychiatric hospitals or clinics; home health care agencies; public health departments; government agencies; crisis or counseling centers; drug and alcohol treatment facilities; prisons; educational institutions; and long-term care facilities.

Levels of employment range from psychiatrist (a physician), who diagnoses and treats mental illness, to psychologist and psychiatric technician. There are also various levels (including assistant) employed in the field of social work (see table 3-7).

Psychiatrists are physicians who specialize in diagnosing and treating mental illness. Some specialties include child or adolescent psychiatry, geriatric psychiatry, and drug/chemical abuse.

Psychologists study human behavior and use this knowledge to help individuals deal with problems of everyday living. Many specialize in specific aspects of psychology, which include child psychology, adolescent psychology, geriatric psychology, behavior modification, drug/chemical abuse, and physical/sexual abuse.

Psychiatric/mental health technicians, working under the supervision of psychiatrists or psychologists, help patients and their families follow treatment and rehabilitation plans. They provide understanding and encouragement, assist with physical care, observe and report behavior, and help teach patients constructive social behavior. Assistants or aides who have completed one or more years in an HSTE program are also employed in this field.

Social workers, also called *sociologists*, case managers, or counselors (figure 3-5), aid people

TABLE 3-7 Mental and Social Services Careers

OCCUPATION	EDUCATION REQUIRED	JOB OUTLOOK TO YEAR 2012	AVERAGE YEARLY EARNINGS
Psychiatrist	• Doctoral degree • 2–7 years postgraduate specialty training • State licensure • Certification in psychiatry	Average growth	$95,500–$297,000
Psychologist PsyD (Doctor of Psychology)	• Bachelor's or master's degree • Doctor of psychology required for many positions • Licensure or certification required in all states • Certification for specialty areas available from American Board of Professional Psychology	Above average growth	$34,900–$97,800 or $45,900–$136,500 with doctorate
Psychiatric/Mental Health Technicians	• Associate's degree • Licensure required in some states • A few states require a nursing degree	Average growth	$28,500–$52,600
Social Workers/ Sociologists	• Bachelor's or master's degree or Doctor of Philosophy or Social Work (DSW) • Licensure, certification or registration required in all states • Credentials available from National Association of Social Workers	Above average growth	$33,500–$76,800
Genetic Counselor (GC)	• Master's degree • Certification can be obtained from the American Board on Genetic Counseling	Above average growth	$38,900–$97,600

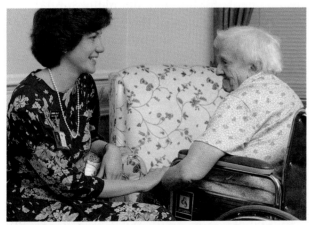

FIGURE 3-5 Social workers help people make life adjustments and refer patients to community resources for assistance.

who have difficulty coping with various problems by helping them make adjustments in their lives and/or by referring them to community resources for assistance. Specialties include child welfare, geriatrics, family, correctional (jail), and occupational social work. Many areas employ assistants or technicians who have one or more years of an HSTE program.

Genetic counselors provide information to individuals and families on genetic diseases or inherited conditions. They research the risk for occurrence of the disease or birth defect, analyze inheritance patterns, perform screening tests for potential genetic defects, identify medical options when a genetic disease or birth defect is present, and help individuals cope with the psychological issues caused by genetic diseases. Genetic counselors may specialize in prenatal (before birth) counseling, pediatric (child) counseling, neurogenetics (brain and nerves), cardiogenetics (heart and blood vessels), or genetic influences on cancer.

ADDITIONAL SOURCES OF INFORMATION

♦ American Board of Genetic Counseling
9650 Rockville Pike
Bethesda, MD 20814
Internet address: *www.abgc.net*

♦ American Psychiatric Association
1000 Wilson Boulevard, Suite 1825
Arlington, VA 22209-3901
Internet address: *www.psych.org*

♦ American Psychological Association
750 1st Street NE
Washington, DC 20002-4242
Internet address: *www.apa.org*

♦ American Sociological Association
1307 New York Avenue NW, Suite 700
Washington, DC 20005
Internet address: *www.asanet.org*

♦ National Mental Health Information Center
P.O. Box 42557
Washington, DC 20015
Internet address: *www.mentalhealth.org*

♦ National Association of Social Workers
750 First Street NE, Suite 700
Washington, DC 20002-4241
Internet address: *www.naswdc.org*

♦ National Mental Health Association
2001 N. Beauregard Street
Alexandria, VA 22311
Internet address: *www.nmha.org*

3:2E INFORMATION

Mortuary Careers

Workers in mortuary careers provide a service that is needed by everyone. Even though funeral practices and rites vary because of cultural diversity and religion, most services involve preparation of the body, performance of a ceremony that honors the deceased and meets the spiritual needs of the living, and cremation or burial of the remains.

Places of employment are funeral homes or mortuaries, crematoriums, or cemetery associations.

Levels include funeral director, embalmer, and mortuary assistant (see table 3-8).

Funeral directors, also called *morticians* or *undertakers,* provide support to the survivors; interview the family of the deceased to establish details of the funeral ceremonies or review arrangements the deceased person requested prior to death; prepare the body following legal requirements; secure information for legal documents; file death certificates; arrange and direct all the details of the wake and services; make arrangements for burial or cremation; and direct all business activities of the funeral home. Frequently, funeral directors help surviving individuals adapt to the death by providing post-death counseling and support group activities. Most funeral directors are also licensed embalmers.

TABLE 3-8 Mortuary Careers

OCCUPATION	EDUCATION REQUIRED	JOB OUTLOOK TO YEAR 2012	AVERAGE YEARLY EARNINGS
Funeral Director (Mortician)	• 2–4 years in a mortuary science college or associate's or bachelor's degree • Licensure required in all states except Colorado	Average growth	$28,600–$94,700
Embalmer	• 2–4 years in a mortuary science college or associate's or bachelor's degree • Licensure required in all states except Colorado	Average growth	$22,600–$71,500
Mortuary Assistant	• 1–2 years on-the-job training or 1-year HSTE program	Average growth	$14,500–$26,800

Embalmers prepare the body for interment by washing the body with germicidal soap, replacing the blood with embalming fluid to preserve the body, reshaping and restructuring disfigured bodies, applying cosmetics to create a natural appearance, dressing the body, and placing it in a casket. They are also responsible for maintaining embalming reports and itemized lists of clothing or valuables.

Mortuary assistants work under the supervision of the funeral director and/or embalmer. They may assist with preparation of the body, drive the hearse to pick up the body after death or to take it to the burial site, arrange flowers for the viewing, assist with preparations for the funeral service, help with filing and maintenance of records, clean the funeral home, and other similar duties.

ADDITIONAL SOURCES OF INFORMATION

♦ American Board of Funeral Service Education
38 Florida Avenue
Portland, ME 04103
Internet address: *www.abfse.org*

♦ International Conference of Funeral Service Examining Boards
1885 Shelby Lane
Fayetteville, AR 72704
Internet address: *www.cfseb.org*

♦ National Funeral Directors Association
13625 Bishop's Drive
Brookfield, WI 53005
Internet address: *www.nfda.org*

3:2F INFORMATION

Nursing Careers

Those in the nursing careers provide care for patients as directed by physicians. Care focuses on the mental, emotional, and physical needs of the patient.

Hospitals are the major places of employment, but nursing workers are also employed in long-term care facilities, rehabilitation centers, physicians' offices, clinics, public health agencies, home health care agencies, health maintenance organizations (HMOs), schools, government agencies, and industry.

Levels include registered nurse, licensed practical/vocational nurse, and nurse assistant/technician (see table 3-9).

TABLE 3-9 Nursing Careers

OCCUPATION	EDUCATION REQUIRED	JOB OUTLOOK TO YEAR 2012	AVERAGE YEARLY EARNINGS
Registered Nurse (RN)	• 2–3-year diploma program in hospital school of nursing, or associate's degree or bachelor's degree	Above average growth	$36,500–$84,600
	• Master's or doctoral for some administrative/educational positions and for some advanced practice nursing positions • Licensure in state of practice		$60,300–$108,900 with advanced specialities
Licensed Practical/ Vocational Nurse (LPN/LVN)	• 1–2-year state-approved HSTE practical/vocational nurse program • Licensure in state of practice	Above average growth	$25,800–$52,600
Nurse Assistant Geriatric Aide Home Health Care Assistant Medication Aide Certified Nurse Technician Patient Care Technician (PCT)	• HSTE program • Certification or registration required in all states for long-term care facilities— obtained by completing 75–120-hour state-approved program	Above average growth especially in geriatric or home care	$14,900–$29,200

Registered nurses (RNs) (figure 3-6), work under the direction of physicians and provide total care to patients. The RN observes patients, assesses patients' needs, reports to other health care personnel, administers prescribed medications and treatments, teaches health care, and supervises other nursing personnel. The type of facility determines specific job duties. Registered nurses with an advanced education can specialize. Examples of advanced practice nurses include:

♦ *Nurse practitioners (CRNPs)*: take health histories, perform basic physical examinations, order laboratory tests and other procedures, refer patients to physicians, help establish treatment plans, treat common illnesses such as colds or sore throats, and teach and promote optimal health

♦ *Nurse midwives (CNMs)*: provide total care for normal pregnancies, examine the pregnant woman at regular intervals, perform routine tests, teach childbirth and childcare classes, monitor the infant and mother during childbirth, deliver the infant, and refer any problems to a physician

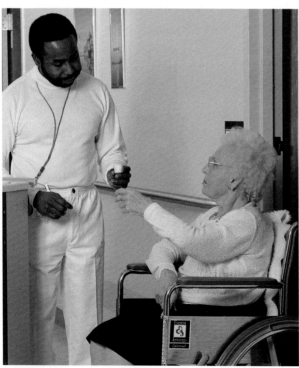

FIGURE 3-6 Registered nurses (RNs) administer prescribed medications to patients.

♦ *Nurse educators*: teach in HSTE programs, schools of nursing, colleges and universities, wellness centers, and health care facilities

♦ *Nurse anesthetists*: administer anesthesia, monitor patients during surgery, and assist anesthesiologists (who are physicians)

♦ *Clinical nurse specialists (CNSs)*: use advanced degree to specialize in specific nursing areas such as intensive care, trauma or emergency care, psychiatry, pediatrics (infants and children), neonatology (premature infants), and gerontology (elderly individuals)

Licensed practical/vocational nurses (LPNs/LVNs), working under the supervision of physicians or RNs, provide patient care requiring technical knowledge but not the level of education required of RNs. The type of care is determined by the work environment, which can include the home, hospital, long-term care facility, adult daycare center, physician's office, clinic, wellness center, and health maintenance organization. Care provided by LPN/LVNs is also determined by state laws regulating the extent of duties.

Nurse assistants (also called nurse aides, nurse technicians, **patient care technicians (PCTs)**, or orderlies) work under the supervision of RNs or LPNs/LVNs. They provide patient care such as baths, bedmaking, and feeding; assist in transfer and ambulation; and administer basic treatments. **Geriatric aides/assistants** acquire additional education to provide care for the elderly in work environments such as extended care facilities, nursing homes, retirement centers, adult daycare agencies, and other similar agencies. **Home health care assistants** are trained to work in the patient's home and may perform additional duties such as meal preparation or cleaning. **Medication aides/assistants** receive special training such as a 40-hour or more state-approved medication aide course to administer medications to patients or residents in long-term care facilities or patients receiving home health care. Most states that have the medication aide program require that the aide be on the state-approved list for nurse or geriatric assistants before taking the medication aide course. In addition, many states require a competency test.

✸ Each nursing assistant working in a long-term care facility or home health care is now required under federal law to complete a mandatory, state-approved training program and pass a written and/or competency examination to obtain certification or registration. Health workers in these environments should check the requirements of their respective states.

ADDITIONAL SOURCES OF INFORMATION

♦ American College of Nurse Practitioners
1111 19th Street NW, Suite 404
Washington, DC 20036
Internet address: *www.acnpweb.org*

♦ American Health Care Association
1201 L Street NW
Washington, DC 20005
Internet address: *www.ahca.org*

♦ American Nurses' Association
8515 Georgia Avenue, Suite 400
Silver Spring, MD 20910
Internet address: *www.nursingworld.org*

♦ National Association for Home Care and Hospice
228 Seventh Street SE
Washington, DC 20003
Internet address: *www.nahc.org*

♦ National Association for Practical Nurse Education and Service
P.O. Box 25647
Alexandria, VA 22313
Internet address: *www.napnes.org*

♦ National Federation of Licensed Practical Nurses
605 Poole Drive
Garner, NC 27529
Internet address: *www.nflpn.org*

♦ National League for Nursing
61 Broadway
New York, NY 10006
Internet address: *www.nln.org*

3:2G INFORMATION

Nutrition and Dietary Services Careers

Health, nutrition, and physical fitness have become a way of life. Workers employed in the nutrition and dietary services recognize the importance of proper nutrition to good health. Using knowledge of nutrition, they promote wellness and optimum health by providing dietary guidelines used to treat various diseases, teaching proper nutrition, and preparing foods for health care facilities.

Places of employment include hospitals, long-term care facilities, child and adult daycare facilities, wellness centers, schools, home health care agencies, public health agencies, clinics, industry, and offices.

Levels include dietitian, dietetic technician, and dietetic assistant (see table 3-10).

Dietitians (RDs) or *nutritionists* (figure 3-7) manage food service systems, assess patients'/residents' nutritional needs, plan menus, teach others proper nutrition and special diets, research nutrition needs and develop recommendations based on the research, purchase food and equip-

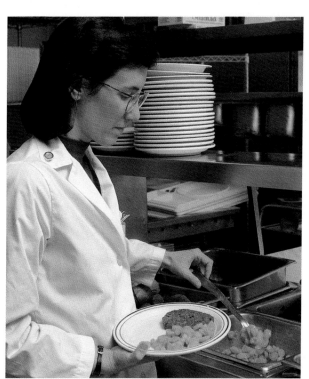

FIGURE 3-7 Dietitians manage food service systems, assess nutritional needs, and plan menus according to prescribed diets.

TABLE 3-10 Nutrition and Dietary Services Careers

OCCUPATION	EDUCATION REQUIRED	JOB OUTLOOK TO YEAR 2012	AVERAGE YEARLY EARNINGS
Dietitian, RD (registered)	• Bachelor's or master's degree • Registration can be obtained from Commission on Dietetic Registration of the American Dietetic Association • Licensure, certification, or registration required in many states	Average growth	$32,700–$68,300
Dietetic Technician, DTR (registered)	• Associate's degree • Licensure, certification, or registration required in some states • Registration can be obtained from the Commission on Dietetic Registration	Average growth	$24,200–$49,200
Dietetic Assistant	• 6–12 months on the job • One or more years HSTE or food service career/technical program	Average growth	$13,600–$24,900

ment, enforce sanitary and safety rules, and supervise and/or train other personnel. Some dietitians specialize in the care of pediatric (child), renal (kidney), or diabetic patients, or in weight management.

Dietetic technicians (DTs), working under the supervision of dietitians, plan menus, order foods, standardize and test recipes, assist with food preparation, provide basic dietary instruction, and teach classes on proper nutrition.

Dietetic assistants, also called *food service workers*, work under the supervision of dietitians and assist with food preparation and service, help patients select menus, clean work areas, and assist other dietary workers.

ADDITIONAL SOURCES OF INFORMATION

♦ American Dietetic Association
120 South Riverside Plaza, Suite 2000
Chicago, IL 60606-6995
Internet address: *www.eatright.org*

♦ Dietary Managers Association
406 Surrey Woods Drive
St. Charles, IL 60174
Internet address: *www.dmaonline.org*

♦ Institute of Food Technologists
525 West Van Buren, Suite 1000
Chicago, IL 60607
Internet address: *www.ift.org*

3:2H INFORMATION

Veterinary Careers

Veterinary careers focus on providing care to all types of animals—from house pets to livestock to wildlife.

Places of employment include animal hospitals, veterinarian offices, laboratories, zoos, farms, animal shelters, aquariums, drug or animal food companies; and fish and wildlife services.

Levels of employment include veterinarian, animal health technician, and assistant (see table 3-11).

Veterinarians (DVMs or VMDs) (figure 3-8) work to prevent, diagnose, and treat diseases and injuries in animals. Specialties include surgery, small-animal care, livestock, fish and wildlife, and research.

Veterinary technologists/technicians (VTs), also called *animal health technicians,* working under the supervision of veterinarians, assist with the handling and care of animals, collect specimens, assist with surgery, perform laboratory tests, take and develop radiographs, administer prescribed treatments, and maintain records.

TABLE 3-11 Veterinary Careers

OCCUPATION	EDUCATION REQUIRED	JOB OUTLOOK TO YEAR 2012	AVERAGE YEARLY EARNINGS
Veterinarian (DVM or VMD)	• 3–4 years preveterinary college • 4 years veterinary college and Doctor of Veterinary Medicine degree • State licensure required in all states	Above average growth	$45,300–$125,900
Veterinary (Animal Health) Technologist/Technician VTR (registered)	• Associate's degree for veterinary technician • Bachelor's degree for veterinary technologist • Registration, certification, or licensure required in most states • Certification for technologists/technicians employed in animal laboratory research facilities can be obtained from the American Association for Laboratory Animal Science (AALAS)	Above average growth	$20,200–$61,800
Veterinary Assistant (Animal Caretakers)	• 1–2 years on the job or 1–2-year HSTE program	Above average growth	$15,200–$35,300

Veterinary assistants, also called *animal caretakers,* feed, bathe, and groom animals; exercise animals; prepare animals for treatment; assist with examinations; clean and sanitize cages, examination tables, and surgical areas; and maintain records.

ADDITIONAL SOURCES OF INFORMATION

♦ American Association for Laboratory Animal Science
9190 Crestwyn Hills Drive
Memphis, TN 38125
Internet address: *www.aalas.org*

♦ American Veterinary Medical Association
1931 N. Meacham Road, Suite 100
Schaumburg, IL 60173-4360
Internet address: *www.avma.org*

♦ Animal Caretakers Information
The Humane Society of the United States
2100 L Street NW
Washington, DC 20037
Internet address: *www.hsus.org*

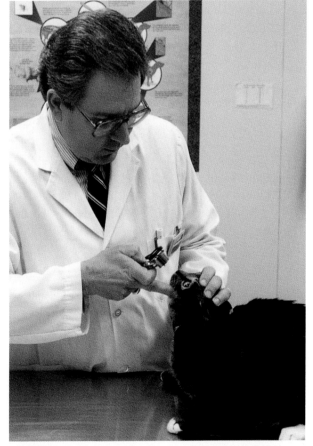

FIGURE 3-8 Veterinarians work to prevent, diagnose, and treat diseases and injuries in animals. (*Courtesy Warren, Small Animal Care and Management, 1995, Delmar Learning*)

♦ North America Veterinary Technician Association (NAVTA)
P. O. Box 224
Battle Ground, IN 47920
Internet address: *www.navta.net*

♦ For information about specific tasks of a veterinary assistant, ask your instructor for the Guideline for Clinical Rotations in the *Diversified Health Occupations Teacher's Resource Kit.*

3:21 INFORMATION

Vision Services Careers

Workers in the vision services provide care to prevent and treat vision disorders. Places of employment include offices, optical shops, department stores, hospitals, schools, health maintenance organizations (HMOs), government agencies, and clinics.

Levels include ophthalmologist, optometrist, ophthalmic medical technologist, ophthalmic technician, opthalmic assistant, optician, and ophthalmic laboratory technician (see table 3-12). Many individuals in this field are entrepreneurs.

Ophthalmologists are medical doctors specializing in diseases, disorders, and injuries of the eyes. They diagnose and treat disease, perform surgery, and correct vision problems or defects.

Optometrists (ODs), doctors of optometry, examine eyes for vision problems and defects, prescribe corrective lenses or eye exercises, and in some states, use drugs for diagnosis and/or treatment. If eye disease is present or if eye sur-

TABLE 3-12 Vision Services Careers

OCCUPATION	EDUCATION REQUIRED	JOB OUTLOOK TO YEAR 2012	AVERAGE YEARLY EARNINGS
Opthalmologist (MD)	• Doctoral degree • 2–7 years postgraduate specialty training • State licensure • Certification in ophthalmology	Average growth	$108,000–$248,500
Optometrist (OD)	• 3–4 years preoptometric college • Four years at college of optometry for doctor of optometry degree • State licensure	Average growth	$62,300–$125,300
Ophthalmic Medical Technologist COMT (certified)	• Associate's or bachelor's degree • Certification can be obtained from the Joint Commission on Allied Health Personnel in Ophthalmology (JCAHPO)	Average growth	$28,600–$68,500
Ophthalmic Technician COT (certified)	• Associate's degree • Certification can be obtained from JCAHPO	Average growth	$27,500–50,200
Ophthalmic Assistant COA (certified)	• Some on-the-job training • One month to 1-year HSTE program • Certification can be obtained from the JCAHPO	Average growth	$14,900–31,500
Optician	• 2–4 years on the job or 2–4-year apprenticeship or HSTE program or associate's degree • Licensure or certification required in some states • Certification can be obtained from Amercian Board of Opticianry and National Contact Lens Examiners	Average growth	$19,400–$46,500
Ophthalmic Laboratory Technician	• 2–3 years on the job or 1-year HSTE certificate program	Below average growth	$15,400–$35,600

gery is needed, the optometrist refers the patient to an ophthalmologist.

Ophthalmic medical technologists (OMTs), working under the supervision of opthalmologists, obtain patient histories, perform routine eye tests and measurements, fit patients for contacts, administer prescribed treatments, assist with eye surgery, perform advanced diagnostic tests such as ocular motility and biocular function tests, administer prescribed medications, and perform advanced microbiological procedures. In addition, they may perform any tasks that ophthalmic technicians or assistants perform.

Ophthalmic technicians (OTs) (figure 3-9) work under the supervision of ophthalmologists and optometrists. Technicians prepare patients for examinations, obtain medical histories, take ocular measurements, administer basic vision tests, maintain ophthalmic and surgical instruments, adjust glasses, teach eye exercises, measure for contacts, instruct patients on the care and use of contacts, and perform receptionist duties.

Ophthalmic assistants (OAs) work under the supervision of ophthalmologists, optometrists, and/or ophthalmic medical technologists or technicians. Assistants prepare patients for examinations, measure visual acuity, perform receptionist duties, help patients with frame selections and fittings, order lenses, perform minor adjustments and repairs of glasses, and teach proper care and use of contact lenses.

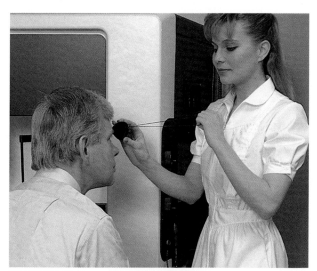

FIGURE 3-9 Ophthalmic technicians perform basic vision tests and teach eye exercises. *(Courtesy of the American Optometric Association, St. Louis, MO)*

Opticians make and fit the eyeglasses or lenses prescribed by ophthalmologists and optometrists. Some specialize in contact lenses.

Ophthalmic laboratory technicians cut, grind, finish, polish, and mount the lenses used in eyeglasses, contact lenses, and other optical instruments such as telescopes and binoculars.

ADDITIONAL SOURCES OF INFORMATION

◆ American Optometric Association
243 N. Lindbergh Boulevard
St. Louis, MO 63141
Internet address: *www.aoanet.org*

◆ Association of Schools and Colleges of Optometry
6110 Executive Boulevard, Suite 510
Rockville, MD 20852
Internet address: *www.opted.org*

◆ Commission on Opticianry Accreditation
8665 Sudley Road, Suite 341
Manassas, VA 20110
Internet address: *www.coaccreditation.com*

◆ Joint Commission on Allied Health Personnel in Ophthalmology
2025 Woodlane Drive
St. Paul, MN 55125-2995
Internet address: *www.jcahpo.org*

◆ National Federation of Opticianry Schools
1238 Robinson Point Road
Mountain Home, AR 72653
Internet address: *ww.nfos.org*

◆ Opticians Association of America
441 Carlisle Drive
Herndon, VA 20170
Internet address: *www.oaa.org*

3:2J INFORMATION

Other Therapeutic Services Careers

There are many other therapeutic service careers. Some are discussed in this section. Most therapeutic occupations include levels of therapist, technician, and assistant/aide (see table 3-13).

Occupational therapists (OTs) (figure 3-10) often work under the direction of a physia-

TABLE 3-13 Other Therapeutic Services Careers

OCCUPATION	EDUCATION REQUIRED	JOB OUTLOOK TO YEAR 2012	AVERAGE YEARLY EARNINGS
Occupational Therapist (OT) OTR (registered)	• Master's degree and internship • Licensure required in all states • Certification can be obtained from American Occupational Therapy Association	Above average growth	$43,900–$93,600
Occupational Therapy Assistant COTA (certified)	• Associate's degree or certificate and internship • Licensure or certification required by most states • Certification can be obtained from American Occupational Therapy Association	Above average growth	$32,500–$56,600
Pharmacist (PharmD)	• 5–6-year college program with Doctor of Pharmacy degree plus internship • Licensure required in all states	Above average growth	$56,800–$103,500
Pharmacy Technician	• 1 or more years on the job or 1–2-year HSTE program or associate's degree • Licensure required in many states • Certification can be obtained from the Pharmacy Technician Certification Board	Above average growth	$17,300–$36,400
Physical Therapist (PT)	• Master's or doctoral degree • Licensure required in all states	Above average growth	$48,400–$108,300
Physical Therapist Assistant (PTA)	• Associate's degree plus internship • Licensure required in most states	Above average growth	$23,500–$54,900
Massage Therapist	• 3-month to 1-year accredited Massage Therapy Program • Certification, registration, or licensure required in many states • Certification can be obtained from the National Certification Board for Therapeutic Massage and Bodywork (NCBTMB)	Above average growth	$22,400–$46,500
Recreational Therapist (TR) Certified Therapeutic Recreation Specialist (CTRS)	• Possibly associate's but usually bachelor's degree plus internship • Licensure or certification required in a few states • Certification can be obtained from National Council for Therapeutic Recreation Certification (NCTRC) • Registration can be obtained from Association for Rehabilitation Therapy	Average growth	$26,800–$54,500
Recreational Therapist Assistant (Activity Director)	• 1–2-year HSTE certificate program or associate's degree • Certification can be obtained from National Council for Therapeutic Recreation Certification	Average growth	$14,700–$32,800
Respiratory Therapist, RTRRT (registered)	• Associate's or bachelor's degree • Licensure required in most states • Registration can be obtained from National Board for Respiratory Care	Above average growth	$32,800–$66,300
Respiratory Therapy Technician (RTT) CRTT (certified)	• 1–2-year HSTE program or associate's degree • Licensure or certification required in most states • Certification can be obtained from National Board for Respiratory Care	Above average growth	$23,400–$49,800

TABLE 3-13 Other Therapeutic Services Careers *(Continued)*

OCCUPATION	EDUCATION REQUIRED	JOB OUTLOOK TO YEAR 2012	AVERAGE YEARLY EARNINGS
Speech–Language Therapist/Pathologist and/or Audiologist	• Master's degree and 9 months postgraduate clinical experience • Licensure required in most states • Clinical doctoral degree common for audiologists • Audiologists may obtain certification from the American Board of Audiology • Certificate of Clinical Competence in Speech–Language Pathology (CCC–SLP) or Audiology (CCC–A) can be obtained from American Speech-Language-Hearing Association (ASHA)	Above average growth	$40,100–$82,500
Surgical Technician/ Technologist CST (certified)	• 1–2-year HSTE program • Certificate, diploma, or associate's degree • Certification can be obtained from Liaison Council on Certification for Surgical Technologists	Above average growth	$24,800–$48,500
Art, Music, Dance Therapist	• Bachelor's or master's degree • Certification for art therapist can be obtained from American Art Therapy Association • Registration for music therapist can be obtained from National Association of Music Therapy and American Association for Music Therapy • Registration for dance therapist (DTR) can be obtained from American Dance Therapy Association • Registration for art therapist (ATR) can be obtained from the Art Therapy Credentials Board	Average growth	$25,700–$64,500
Athletic Trainer ATC (certified)	• Bachelor's or master's degree • Licensure required in some states • Most states require certification • Certification can be obtained from National Athletic Trainers Association	Above average growth	$35,000–$73,800
Dialysis Technician	• Varies with states • Some states require RN or LPN license and state-approved dialysis training • Other states require 1–2-year HSTE state-approved dialysis program or associate's degree • Certification can be obtained from National Association of Nephrology Technicians/ Technologists	Average growth	$18,700–$56,800
Perfusionist Certified Clinical Perfusionist (CCP) Extracorporeal Circulation Technologist	• Bachelor's degree • Specialized extracorporeal circulation training and supervised clinical experience • Licensure required in some states • Certification can be obtained from American Board of Cardiovascular Perfusion	Above average growth	$51,600–$112,800

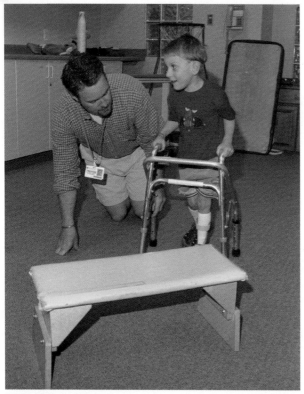

FIGURE 3-10 Occupational therapists (OTs) help patients with disabilities to overcome, correct, or adjust to the disabilities.

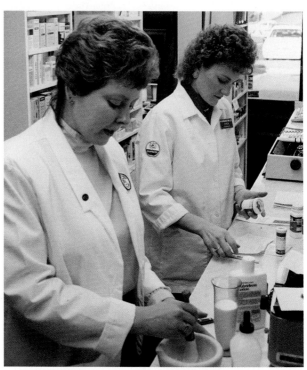

FIGURE 3-11 Pharmacists dispense medications and provide information on drugs. *(Courtesy of the Michigan Pharmacists Association and the Michigan Society of Pharmacy Technicians)*

trist, a physician specializing in physical medicine and rehabilitation. OTs help people with physical, developmental, mental, or emotional disabilities to overcome, correct, or adjust to their particular problems. The occupational therapist uses various activities to assist the patient in learning skills or activities of daily living (ADL), adapting job skills, or preparing for return to work. Treatment is directed toward helping patients acquire independence, regain lost functions, adapt to disabilities, and lead productive and satisfying lives.

Occupational therapy assistants (OTAs), working under the guidance of occupational therapists, help patients carry out programs of prescribed treatment. They direct patients in arts and crafts projects, recreation, or social events; teach and help patients carry out rehabilitation activities and exercises; use games to develop balance and coordination; assist patients trying to master the activities of daily living; and inform therapists of patients' responses and progress.

Pharmacists (PharmDs) (figure 3-11) dispense medications per written orders from physicians, dentists, and other health care pro-

fessionals authorized to prescribe medications. They provide information on drugs and correct ways to use them; order and dispense other health care items such as surgical and sickroom supplies; recommend nonprescription items to customers/patients; ensure drug compatibility; maintain records on medications dispensed; and assess, plan, and monitor drug usage. Pharmacists can also either be entrepreneurs or work for one of the many drug manufacturers involved in researching, manufacturing, and selling drugs.

Pharmacy technicians, working under the supervision of pharmacists, help prepare medications for dispensing to patients, label medications, perform inventories and order supplies, prepare intravenous solutions, help maintain records, and perform other duties as directed by pharmacists.

Physical therapists (PTs) (figure 3-12) often work under the direction of a physiatrist, a physician specializing in physical medicine and rehabilitation. PTs provide treatment to improve mobility and prevent or limit permanent disability of patients with disabling joint, bone, muscle, and/or nerve injuries or diseases. Treatment may

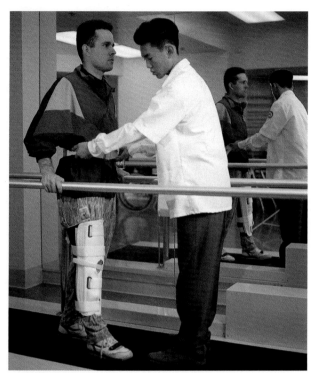

FIGURE 3-12 Physical therapists (PTs) provide treatment to improve mobility of patients with disabling injuries or diseases.

include exercise, massage, and/or applications of heat, cold, water, light, electricity, or ultrasound. Therapists assess the functional abilities of patients and use this information to plan treatment programs. They also promote health and prevent injuries by developing proper exercise programs and teaching patients correct use of muscles. Some physical therapists are entrepreneurs.

Physical therapist assistants (PTAs), working under the supervision of physical therapists, help carry out prescribed plans of treatment. They perform exercises and massages; administer applications of heat, cold, and/or water; assist patients to ambulate with canes, crutches, or braces; provide ultrasound or electrical stimulation treatments; inform therapists of patients' responses and progress; and perform other duties, as directed by therapists.

Massage therapists usually work under the supervision of physicians or physical therapists. They use many variations of massage, bodywork (manipulation or application of pressure to the muscular or skeletal structure of the body), and therapeutic touch to muscles to provide pain relief for chronic conditions (such as back pain)

or inflammatory diseases, improve lymphatic circulation to decrease edema (swelling), and relieve stress and tension. Some massage therapists are entrepreneurs.

Recreational therapists (TRs), or *therapeutic recreation specialists,* use recreational and leisure activities as forms of treatment to minimize patients' symptoms and improve physical, emotional, and mental well-being. Activities might include organized athletic events, dances, arts and crafts, musical activities, drama, field trips to shopping centers or other places of interest, movies, or poetry or book readings. All activities are directed toward allowing the patient to gain independence, build self-confidence, and relieve anxiety. Some recreational therapists are entrepreneurs.

Recreational therapy assistants, also called *activity directors,* work under the supervision of recreational therapists or other health care professionals. They assist in carrying out the activities planned by therapists and, at times, arrange activities or events. They note and inform therapists of patients' responses and progress.

Respiratory therapists (RTs), under physicians' orders, treat patients with heart and lung diseases by administering oxygen, gases, or medications; using exercise to improve breathing; monitoring ventilators; and performing diagnostic respiratory function tests (figure 3-13). Some respiratory therapists are entrepreneurs.

Respiratory therapy technicians (RTTs) work under the supervision of respiratory therapists and administer respiratory treatments, perform basic diagnostic tests, clean and maintain

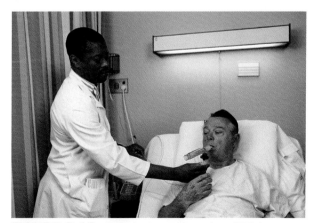

FIGURE 3-13 Respiratory therapists (RTs) provide treatments to patients with heart and lung diseases.

equipment, and note and inform therapists of patients' responses and progress.

Surgical technologists/technicians (STs), also called *operating room technicians* (figure 3-14), working under the supervision of RNs or physicians, prepare patients for surgery; set up instruments, equipment, and sterile supplies in the operating room; and assist during surgery by passing instruments and supplies to the surgeon. Although most surgical technologists/technicians work in hospital operating rooms, some are employed in outpatient surgical centers, emergency departments, urgent care centers, physicians' offices, and other facilities.

Speech–language pathologists, also called *speech therapists* or *speech scientists*, identify, evaluate, and treat patients with speech and language disorders. They help patients communicate as effectively as possible, and also teach patients to cope with the problems created by speech impairments.

Audiologists provide care to individuals who have hearing impairments. They test hearing, diagnose problems, and prescribe treatment, which may include hearing aids, auditory training, or instruction in speech or lip reading. They also test noise levels in workplaces and develop hearing protection programs.

Art, music, and **dance therapists** use the arts to help patients deal with social, physical, or emotional problems. Therapists usually work with individuals who are emotionally disturbed, mentally retarded, or physically disabled, but they may also work with adults and children who have no disabilities in an effort to promote physical and mental wellness.

Athletic trainers (ATCs) prevent and treat athletic injuries and provide rehabilitative services to athletes. The athletic trainer frequently works with a physician who specializes in sports medicine. Athletic trainers teach proper nutrition, assess the physical condition of athletes, give advice regarding a physical conditioning program to increase strength and flexibility or correct weaknesses, put tape or padding on players to protect body parts, treat minor injuries, administer first aid for serious injuries, and help carry out any rehabilitation treatment prescribed by sports medicine physicians or other therapists.

Dialysis technicians, also called *renal dialysis technicians*, *hemodialysis technicians*, or *nephrology technicians*, operate the kidney hemodialysis machines used to treat patients with limited or no kidney function. Careful patient monitoring is critical during the dialysis process. The dialysis technician must also provide emotional support for the patient and teach proper nutrition (because many patients must follow restricted diets).

Perfusionists, also called *extracorporeal circulation technologists,* are members of open-heart surgical teams and operate the heart–lung machines used in coronary bypass surgery (surgery on the coronary arteries in the heart). This field is expanding to include new advances such as artificial hearts. Monitoring and operating these machines correctly is critical because the patient's life depends on the machines. During surgery, the perfusionist monitors blood gases and vital signs; administers blood products, anesthetic agents, and/or drugs as needed; and induces hypothermia (low body temperature) to decrease the body's need for oxygen. After the surgery, the perfusionist must restore normal body circulation when the heart starts beating and wean the patient from the extracorporeal machine.

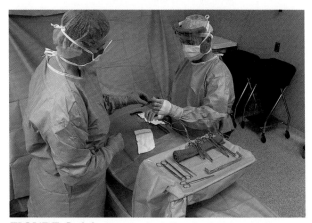

FIGURE 3-14 Surgical technologists assist by passing instruments and supplies to the surgeon.

ADDITIONAL SOURCES OF INFORMATION

♦ American Alliance for Health, Physical Education, Recreation, and Dance
1900 Association Drive
Reston, VA 22091-1598
Internet address: *www.aahperd.org*

♦ American Art Therapy Association
1202 Allanson Road
Mundelheim, IL 60060-3808
Internet address: *www.arttherapy.org*

♦ American Academy of Audiology
11730 Plaza America Drive, Suite 300
Reston, VA 20190
Internet address: *www.audiology.org*

♦ American Association for Respiratory Care
9425 N. MacArthur Boulevard, Suite 100
Irving, TX 75063-48706
Internet address: *www.aarc.org*

♦ American Association of Colleges of Pharmacy
1426 Prince Street
Alexandria, VA 22314
Internet address: *www.aacp.org*

♦ American Dance Therapy Association
10632 Little Patuxent Parkway
Columbia, MD 21044
Internet address: *www.adta.org*

♦ American Massage Therapy Association
820 Davis Street, Suite 100
Evanston, IL 60201-4444
Internet address: *www.amtamassage.org*

♦ American Music Therapy Association
8455 Colesville Road
Silver Spring, MD 20910
Internet address: *www.musictherapy.org*

♦ American Pharmacists Association
2215 Constitution Avenue NW
Washington, DC 20037-2985
Internet address: *www.aphanet.org*

♦ American Physical Therapy Association
1111 N. Fairfax Street
Alexandria, VA 22314-1488
Internet address: *www.apta.org*

♦ American Occupational Therapy Association
4720 Montgomery Lane, P. O. Box 31220
Bethesda, MD 20824-1220
Internet address: *www.aota.org*

♦ American Society of Extracorporeal Technologists
2209 Dickens Road
P.O. Box 11086
Richmond, VA 23230-1086
Internet address: *www.amsect.org*

♦ American Speech-Language-Hearing Association
10801 Rockville Pike
Rockville, MD 20852
Internet address: *www.asha.org*

♦ American Therapeutic Recreation Association
1414 Prince Street, Suite 204
Alexandria, VA 22314
Internet address: *www.atra-tr.org*

♦ Associated Bodywork and Massage Professionals
1271 Sugarbush Drive
Evergreen, CO 80439-9766
Internet address: *www.abmp.com*

♦ Association of Surgical Technologists
6 W. Dry Creek Circle
Littleton, CO 80120
Internet address: *www.ast.org*

♦ Massage and Bodywork Resource Center
Internet address: *www.massageresource.com*

♦ National Athletic Trainers Association
2952 Stemmons Freeway
Dallas, TX 75247
Internet address: *www.nata.org*

♦ National Therapeutic Recreation Society
22377 Belmont Ridge Road
Ashburn, VA 20148
Internet address: *www.nrpa.org*

♦ Pharmacy Technician Certification Board
2215 Constitution Avenue NW
Washington, DC 20037-2985
Internet address: *www.ptcb.org*

3:3 INFORMATION

Diagnostic Services Careers

Diagnostic service workers are involved with creating a picture of the health status of a patient at a single point in time. They perform tests or evaluations that aid in the detection, diagnosis, and treatment of disease, injury, or other physical conditions.

Many workers are employed in hospital laboratories, but others work in private laboratories, outpatient centers, doctors' offices, clinics, public health agencies, pharmaceutical (drug) firms, and research or government agencies. In some occupations, individuals are entrepreneurs, owning and operating their own businesses.

Many careers fall under the designation of diagnostic services. Some of the more common ones are discussed in this chapter. There are various levels of workers in most fields (table 3-14).

Electrocardiograph (ECG) technicians operate electrocardiograph machines, which record electrical impulses that originate in the heart. Physicians (especially cardiologists) use the electrocardiogram (ECG) to help diagnose

TABLE 3-14 Diagnostic Services Careers

OCCUPATION	EDUCATION REQUIRED	JOB OUTLOOK TO YEAR 2012	AVERAGE YEARLY EARNINGS
Cardiovascular Technologist Registered Diagnostic Vascular Technologist (RDVT)	• Associate's or bachelor's degree • Certification or registration can be obtained from Cardiovascular Credentialing International • Registration can be obtained from the American Registry of Diagnostic Medical Sonographers	Above average growth	$27,500–$58,600
Electrocardiograph (ECG Technician) Certified Cardiographic Technician (CCT)	• 1–12 months on-the-job or 6–12-month-HSTE program • Certification can be obtained from Cardiovascular Credentialing International	Below average growth	$17,300–$32,800
Electroencephalographic (EEG) Technologist	• Few have 1–2-years on-the-job • Most have 1–2-year HSTE certification program or associate's degree • Registration can be obtained from American Board of Registration of Electroencephalographic and Evoked Potential Technologists	Below average growth	$22,300–$46,200
Electroneurodiagnostic Technologist	• 1–2-year program usually leading to associate's degree • Registration can be obtained from the American Board of Electroencephalographic and Evoked Potential Technologists • Polysomnographic technologists can obtain registration from the Association of Polysomnographic Technologists	Above average growth	$35,800–$56,200
Medical (Clinical) Laboratory Technologist (MT) Certified Medical (Clinical) Laboratory Technologist (CMT) Registered Medical (Clinical) Laboratory Technologist (RMT)	• Bachelor's or master's degree • Licensure or registration required in some states • Certification can be obtained from the American Medical Technologists Association and the National Credentialing Agency for Laboratory Personnel	Average growth	$35,800–$66,900

(continued)

TABLE 3-14 Diagnostic Services Careers *(Continued)*

OCCUPATION	EDUCATION REQUIRED	JOB OUTLOOK TO YEAR 2012	AVERAGE YEARLY EARNINGS
Medical (Clinical) Laboratory Technician (MLT) Certified Laboratory Technician (CLT)	• 2-year HSTE certification program or associate's degree • Licensure or registration required in some states • Certification can be obtained from the American Medical Technologists Association and the National Credentialing Agency for Laboratory Personnel	Average growth	$26,300–$48,900
Medical (Clinical) Laboratory Assistant	• 1–2-year HSTE program or on-the-job training • Certification can be obtained from the Board of Certified Laboratory Assistants	Below average growth	$14,500–$26,300
Phlebotomist	• 1–2 years on the job or HSTE program or 100–300 hour certification program • Certification can be obtained from the National Credentialing Agency for Laboratory Personnel and the American Society of Phlebotomy Technicians	Average growth	$14,600–$28,300
Radiologic Technologist ARRT (Registered)	• Associate's or bachelor's degree • Licensure required in most states • Registration can be obtained from American Registry of Radiologic Technologies (ARRT)	Above average growth	$28,900–$68,600

heart disease and to note changes in the condition of a patient's heart. ECG or *cardiographic technicians* with more advanced training perform stress tests (which record the action of the heart during physical activity), Holter monitorings (ECGs lasting 24–48 hours, figure 3-15), thallium scans (a nuclear scan after thallium is injected), and other specialized cardiac tests that frequently involve the use of computers. An associate's or bachelor's degree leads to a position as a **cardiovascular technologist.** These individuals assist with cardiac catheterization procedures and angioplasty (a procedure to remove blockages in blood vessels), monitor patients during open-heart surgery and the implantation of pacemakers, and perform tests to check circulation in blood vessels. Some specialize in using ultrasound (high-frequency sound waves) to assess heart function and diagnose heart conditions and are called *echocardiographers* or *cardiac sonographers*. Others use ultrasound to diagnose disorders of blood vessels by checking blood pressure, oxygen saturation, and circulation of blood throughout the body. They are called *vascular technologists* or *vascular sonographers*.

An **electroencephalographic (EEG) technologist** operates an instrument called an *electroencephalograph,* which records the electrical activity of the brain. The record produced, called an *electroencephalogram,* is used by a variety of physicians, especially neurologists (doctors specializing in nerve and brain diseases), to diagnose and evaluate diseases and disorders of the brain, such as brain tumors, strokes, toxic/metabolic disorders, epilepsy, and sleep disorders. Advanced training leads to a position as an **electroneurodiagnostic technologist (END).** In addition to performing EEGs, these individuals perform nerve conduction tests, measure sensory and physical responses to specific stimuli, perform evoked potential (EP) tests that measure brain response when specific nerves are stimulated, and operate other monitoring devices. Technologists who specialize in administering sleep disorder evaluations are called *polysomnographic technologists.*

Medical (clinical) laboratory technologists (MTs) work under the supervision of doctors called *pathologists*. They study tissues, fluids, and cells of the human body to help determine

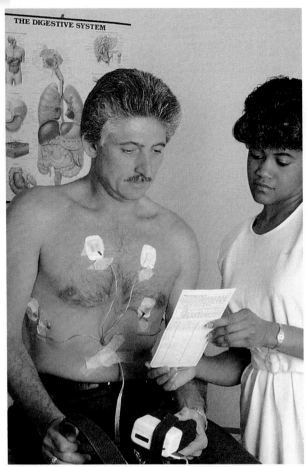

FIGURE 3-15 Cardiographic technicians assist with Holter monitorings of the heart.

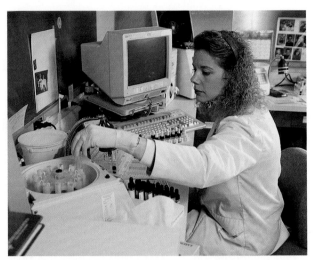

FIGURE 3-16 Medical laboratory technologists perform computerized blood analysis tests. *(Photo by Marcia Butterfield, courtesy of W. A. Foote Memorial Hospital, Jackson, MI)*

the presence and/or cause of disease. They perform complicated chemical, microscopic, and automated analyzer/computer tests (figure 3-16). In small laboratories, technologists perform many types of tests. In larger laboratories, they may specialize. Examples of specialization include:

♦ *Biochemistry*: chemical analysis of body fluids

♦ *Blood bank technology*: collection and preparation of blood and blood products for transfusions

♦ *Cytotechnology*: study of human body cells and cellular abnormalities

♦ *Hematology*: study of blood cells

♦ *Histology*: study of human body tissue

♦ *Molecular biology*: complex protein and nucleic acid testing on cell samples

♦ *Microbiology*: study of bacteria and other microorganisms

Medical (clinical) laboratory technicians (MLTs), working under the supervision of medical technologists or pathologists, perform many of the routine tests that do not require the advanced knowledge held by a medical technologist. Like the technologist, the technician can specialize in a particular field or perform a variety of tests.

Medical (clinical) laboratory assistants, working under the supervision of medical technologists, technicians, or pathologists, perform basic laboratory tests; prepare specimens for examination or testing; and perform other laboratory duties such as cleaning and helping to maintain equipment.

Phlebotomists (figure 3-17), or venipuncture technicians, collect blood and prepare it for testing. In some states, they perform blood tests under the supervision of medical technologists or pathologists.

Radiologic technologists (RTs), working under the supervision of doctors called radiologists, use X-rays, radiation, nuclear medicine, ultrasound, and magnetic resonance to diagnose and treat disease. Most techniques are noninvasive, which means examining or treating the internal organs of patients without entering the body. In many cases, recent advances in this field have eliminated the need for surgery and, therefore, offer less risk to patients. Radiologic tech-

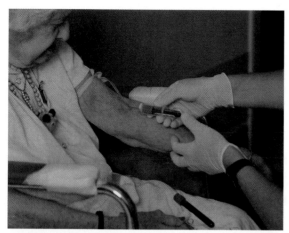

FIGURE 3-17 Phlebotomists collect blood and prepare it for testing.

nologists use different types of scanners to produce images of body parts. Examples include X-ray machines, fluoroscopes, ultrasonic scanners, computerized tomography (CT) scanners (formerly known as computerized axial tomography [CAT] scanners), magnetic resonance imagers (MRI), and positron emission tomography (PET) scanners. Many radiologic technologists also provide radiation treatment. Specific job titles exist for technologists who specialize:

♦ *Radiographers*: (figure 3-18) take X-rays of the body for diagnostic purposes.

♦ *Radiation therapists*: administer prescribed doses of radiation to treat disease (usually cancer).

♦ *Nuclear medicine technologists*: prepare radioactive substances for administration to patients. Once administered, these professionals use films, images on a screen, or body specimens such as blood or urine to determine how the radioactive substances pass through or localize in different parts of the body. This information is used by physicians to detect abnormalities or diagnose disease.

♦ *Ultrasound technologists* or *diagnostic medical sonographers*: use equipment that sends high-frequency sound waves into the body. As the sound waves bounce back from the part being examined, an image of the part is viewed on a screen. This can be recorded on a printout strip or be photographed. Ultrasound is frequently used to examine the fetus (developing infant) in a pregnant woman and can reveal the sex of the unborn child. Ultrasound is also used for neurosonography (the brain),

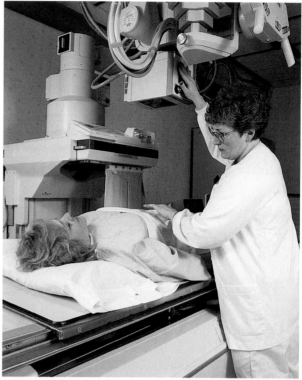

FIGURE 3-18 Radiologic technologists take X-rays used in the diagnosis of disease. *(Photo by Marcia Butterfield, courtesy of W. A. Foote Memorial Hospital, Jackson, MI)*

vascular (blood vessels and blood flow), and echocardiography (the heart) examinations.

♦ *Mammographer*: uses a special mammography machine to produce images of the breast. The mammograms are used to assist in the early detection and treatment of breast cancer.

♦ *Computer tomography technologists*: use a special X-ray machine called a computerized axial tomography (CT or CAT) scanner to obtain cross-sectional images of body tissues, bones, and organs. CT scans help locate tumors and other abnormalities.

♦ *Magnetic resonance imaging (MRI) technologists*: use superconductive magnets and radiowaves to produce detailed images of internal anatomy. The information is processed by a computer and displayed on a videoscreen. Examples of MRI use include identifying multiple sclerosis and detecting hemorrhaging (bleeding) in the brain.

♦ *Positron emission tomography (PET) technologists*: inject a slightly radioactive substance into the patient and then operate the PET scanner, which uses electrons to create a three-dimensional image of body parts and scan the body for disease processes. This allows physicians to see an organ or bone from all sides, similar to a model.

ADDITIONAL SOURCES OF INFORMATION

♦ Alliance of Cardiovascular Professionals
4356 Bonney Road, Suite 103
Virginia Beach, VA 23452-1200
Internet address: *www.acp-online.org*

♦ American College of Radiology
1891 Preston White Drive
Reston, VA 22091
Internet address: *www.acr.org*

♦ American Medical Technologists
710 Higgins Road
Park Ridge, IL 60068
Internet address: *www.amt1.com*

♦ American Registry of Radiologic Technologists
1255 Northland Drive
St. Paul, MN 55120-1155
Internet address: *www.arrt.org*

♦ American Society for Clinical Laboratory Science
6701 Democracy Boulevard, Suite 300
Bethesda, MD 20814
Internet address: *www.ascls.org*

♦ American Society of Electroneurodiagnostic Technologists
426 W. 42nd Street
Kansas City, MO 64111
Internet address: *www.aset.org*

♦ American Society of Radiologic Technologists
15000 Central Avenue SE
Albuquerque, NM 87123-3917
Internet address: *www.asrt.org*

♦ Association of Schools of Allied Health Professions
1730 M Street, Suite 500
Washington, DC 20036
Internet address: *www.asahp.org.*

♦ Cardiovascular Credentialing International (CCI)
1500 Sunday Drive, Suite 102
Raleigh, NC 27607
Internet address: *www.cci-online.org*

♦ International Society for Clinical Laboratory Technology
917 Locust Street, Suite 1100
St. Louis, MO 63101

♦ National Accrediting Agency for Clinical Laboratory Sciences
8410 West Bryn Mawr Avenue, Suite 670
Chicago, IL 60631-3415
Internet address: *www.naacls.org*

♦ National Credentialing Agency for Laboratory Personnel
P.O. Box 15945-289
Lenexa, KS 66285
Internet address: *www.nca-info.org*

♦ Society of Diagnostic Medical Sonography
2745 Dallas Parkway, Suite 350
Dallas, TX 75093-8730
Internet address: *www.sdms.org*

3:4 INFORMATION

Health Informatics Careers

Health informatics workers are involved with documentation of patient records and health information. There are many different types of health workers at all levels. Some examples of careers in health informatics include health information administrators or technicians, health educators, medical transcriptionists, admitting office personnel, epidemiologists, medical illustrators, photographers, writers, and librarians (see table 3-15). Computer technology is used in almost all the careers.

Places of employment include hospitals, clinics, research centers, health departments, long-term care facilities, colleges, law firms, health maintenance organizations (HMOs), and insurance companies.

Health information (medical records) administrators (RAs) develop and manage the systems for storing and obtaining information

TABLE 3-15 Health Informatics Careers

OCCUPATION	EDUCATION REQUIRED	JOB OUTLOOK TO YEAR 2012	AVERAGE YEARLY EARNINGS
Health Information (Medical Records) Administrator Registered (RRA)	• Bachelor's or master's degree • Registration can be obtained from American Health Information Management Association (AHIMA)	Above average growth	$41,400–$88,700
Health Information (Medical Records) Technician Registered (RHIT)	• Associate's degree • Registration can be obtained from the American Health Information Management Association (AHIMA) after passing a written examination	Above average growth	$22,700–$52,300
Medical Transcriptionist Certified Medical Transcriptionist (CMT)	• 1 or more years career or technical education program, on-the-job training, or associate's degree • Certification can be obtained from American Association for Medical Transcription	Above average growth	$18,700–$37,400
Admitting Officer or Clerk	• 1–2 year HSTE or business/office career/technical education • Admitting manager may require bachelor's degree • Few have on-the-job training	Average growth	$15,300–$36,800
Unit Secretary Ward Clerk Health Unit Coordinator Medical Records Clerk	• 1 or more years career or technical education program • Some have on-the-job training	Average growth	$14,200–$34,300
Epidemiologist	• Master's or doctoral degree in environmental health, public health, or health management sciences	Above average growth	$55,000–$96,500
Medical Interpreter/ Translator	• Associate's, bachelor's, or master's degree • Certification for translators can be obtained from the American Translators Association • Certification for sign language interpreters can be obtained from the National Association of the Deaf and the Registry of Interpreters for the Deaf	Above average growth	$31,800–$76,300
Medical Illustrator	• Bachelor's or master's degree • Certification can be obtained from Association of Medical Illustrators	Average growth	$43,700–$132,500
Medical Librarian	• Master's degree in library science	Average growth	$41,600–$136,300

from records, prepare information for legal actions and insurance claims, compile statistics for organizations and government agencies, manage medical records departments, ensure the confidentiality of patient information, and supervise and train other personnel. Because computers are used in almost all aspects of the job, it is essential for the medical records admin-istrator to be able to operate and use a variety of computer programs.

Health information (medical records) technicians, (figure 3-19), organize and code patient records, gather statistical or research data, record information on patient records, monitor electronic and paper-based information to ensure confidentiality, and calculate bills using

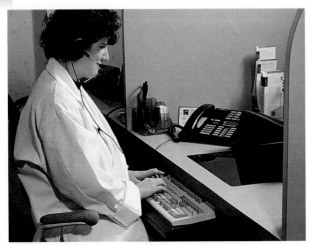

FIGURE 3-19 Health information (medical records) technicians organize and code patients' records.

health care data. Computers have simplified many of the duties and are used to organize records, compile and report statistical data, and perform similar tasks. Computer operation is an important part of the education program for health information technicians. Medical records departments also employ clerks, who organize records. Clerks typically complete a 1- or 2-year career/technical program, or are trained on the job.

Medical transcriptionists use a computer and word processing software to enter data that has been dictated on recorder by physicians or other health care professionals. Examples of data include physical examination reports, surgical reports, consultation findings, progress notes, and radiology reports.

Admitting officers/clerks work in the admissions department of a health care facility. They are responsible for obtaining all necessary information when a patient is admitted to the facility, assigning rooms, maintaining records, and processing information when the patient is discharged. An *admitting manager* is a higher level of worker in this field, usually having an associate's or bachelor's degree. The admitting manager is responsible for supervising staff, developing and implementing policies and procedures for the department, monitoring performance standards, and coordinating the operation of the department with other departments in the health care facility.

Unit secretaries, ward clerks, or health unit coordinators are employed in hospitals, extended care facilities, clinics, and other health facilities to record information on records; schedule procedures or tests; answer telephones; order supplies; and work with computers to record or obtain information.

Epidemiologists identify and track diseases as they occur in a group of people. They determine risk factors that make a disease more likely to occur, evaluate situations that may cause occupational exposure to toxic substances, develop methods to prevent or control the spread of new diseases, and evaluate statistics and data to help governments, health agencies, and communities deal with epidemics and other health issues. Some may specialize in areas such as cancer, cardiovascular (heart and blood vessels) diseases, occupational diseases, infectious or communicable (spread rapidly from person to person) diseases, and/or health care research.

Medical interpreters/translators assist cross-cultural communication processes by converting one language to another. Interpreters convert the spoken word while translators convert written material. Medical interpreters/translators must be proficient at translating words, relaying concepts and ideas between languages, practicing cultural sensitivity, editing written language, and determining that the communication has been comprehended. *Sign language interpreters* facilitate communication for individuals who are deaf or hard of hearing.

Medical illustrators use their artistic and creative talents to produce illustrations, charts, graphs, and diagrams for health textbooks, journals, magazines, and exhibits. Another related field is a *medical photographer*, who takes photographs or records videotapes of surgical procedures, health education information, documentation of conditions before and after reconstructive surgery, and legal information such as injuries received in an accident.

Medical librarians, also called *health sciences librarians*, organize books, journals, and other print materials to provide health information to other health care professionals. They use computer technology to create information centers for large health care facilities or to provide information to health care providers. Some librarians specialize in researching information for large pharmaceutical companies, insurance agencies, lawyers, industry, and/or government agencies.

ADDITIONAL SOURCES OF INFORMATION

♦ American Association for Medical Transcription
100 Sycamore Avenue
Modesto, CA 95354–0550
Internet address: *www.aamt.org*

♦ American Health Information Management Association
233 N. Michigan Avenue, Suite 2150
Chicago, IL 60601–5800
Internet address: *www.ahima.org*

♦ American Medical Association Commission on Accreditation of Allied Health Education Programs
515 N. State Street
Chicago, IL 60610
Internet address: *www.ama-assn.org*

♦ American Translators Association
225 Reinekers Lane, Suite 590
Alexandria, VA 22314
Internet address: *www.atanet.org*

♦ Association for Professionals in Infection Control and Epidemiology
1275 K Street NW, Suite 1000
Washington, DC 20005
Internet address: *www.apic.org*

♦ Association of Medical Illustrators
P.O. Box 1897
Lawrence, KS 66044
Internet address: *www.ami.org*

♦ Medical Library Association
65 East Wacker Plaza, Suite 1900
Chicago, IL 60602
Internet address: *www.mlanet.org*

♦ Registry of Interpreters for the Deaf
333 Commerce Street
Alexandria, VA 22314
Internet address: *www.rid.org*

TABLE 3-16 Support Services Careers

OCCUPATION	EDUCATION REQUIRED	JOB OUTLOOK TO YEAR 2012	AVERAGE YEARLY EARNINGS
Health Care Administrator Health Services Manager	• Usually master's or doctoral, but smaller facilities may accept a bachelor's degree • Licensure required for long-term care facilities • Certification can be obtained from American College of Health Care Executives	Above average growth	$48,500–$196,000
Biomedical (Clinical) Engineer	• Bachelor's or master's degree • Licensure required in some states • Certification available from the International Certification Commission for Clinical Engineering and Biomedical Technology	Above average growth	$48,500–$108,600
Biomedical Equipment Technician (CBET-Certified)	• Associate's or bachelor's degree • Certification can be obtained from the International Certification Commission for Clinical Engineering and Biomedical Technology of the Association for the Advancement of Medical Instrumentation	Above average growth	$26,300–$58,600
Central/Sterile Supply Technician	• On-the-job training or 1–2-year HSTE program	Average growth	$12,200–$23,500
Housekeeping Worker Sanitary Manager	• On-the-job training or 1-year career/technical program	Above average growth	$12,200–$24,700

3:5 INFORMATION

Support Services Careers

Support services workers are involved with creating a therapeutic environment to provide direct or indirect patient care. Any hospital or health care facility requires workers to operate the support departments such as administration, the business office, the admissions office, central/sterile supply, plant operations, equipment maintenance, and housekeeping. Each department has workers at all levels and with varying levels of education (see table 3-16).

Places of employment include hospitals, clinics, long-term care facilities, HMOs, and public health or governmental agencies.

Health care administrators, also called *health care executives* or *health services managers* plan, direct, coordinate, and supervise delivery of health care and manage the operation of health care facilities. They are frequently called chief executive officers (CEOs). A health care administrator may be responsible for personnel, supervise department heads, determine budget and finance, establish policies and procedures, perform public relations duties, and coordinate all activities in the facility. Duties depend on the size of the facility.

Biomedical (clinical) engineers combine knowledge of engineering with knowledge of biology and biomechanical principles to assist in the operation of health care facilities. They design and build sensor systems that can be used for diagnostic tests, such as the computers used to analyze blood; develop computer systems that can be used to monitor patients; design and produce monitors, imaging machines, surgical instruments, lasers, and other similar medical equipment; design clinical laboratories and other units in a health care facility that uses advanced technology; and monitor and maintain the operation of the technologic systems. They frequently work with other health team members such as physicians or nurses to adapt instrumentation or computer technology to meet the specific needs of the patients and health care team.

Biomedical equipment technicians (BETs) work with the many different machines used to diagnose, treat, and monitor patients. They install, test, service, and repair equipment such as patient monitors, kidney hemodialysis units, diagnostic imaging scanners, incubators,

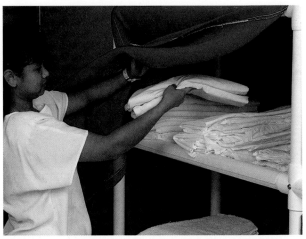

FIGURE 3-20 Central/sterile supply workers prepare all the equipment and supplies used by other departments in a health care facility.

electrocardiographs, X-ray units, pacemakers, sterilizers, blood-gas analyzers, heart–lung machines, respirators, and other similar devices. Lives depend on the accuracy and proper operation of many of these machines, so constant maintenance and testing for defects is critical. Some biomedical equipment technicians also teach other staff members how to use biomedical equipment.

Central/sterile supply workers (figure 3-20) are involved in ordering, maintaining, and supplying all the equipment and supplies used by other departments in a health care facility. They sterilize instruments or supplies, maintain equipment, inventory materials, and fill requisitions from other departments.

Housekeeping workers/sanitary managers, also called *environmental service workers,* help maintain the cleanliness of the health care facility to provide a pleasant, sanitary environment. They observe all principles of infection control to prevent the spread of disease.

ADDITIONAL SOURCES OF INFORMATION

◆ American College of Health Care Administrators
300 N. Lee Street Suite 301
Alexandria, VA 22314
Internet address: *www.achca.org*

◆ American College of Healthcare Executives
One North Franklin Street, Suite 1700

Chicago, IL 60606-4425
Internet address: *www.ache.org*

♦ American Health Care Association
1201 L Street NW
Washington, DC 20005
Internet address: *www.ahca.org*

♦ American Hospital Association
1 North Franklin Street
Chicago, IL 60606-3421
Internet address: *www.aha.org*

♦ Association for the Advancement of Medical
Instrumentation
3330 Washington Boulevard, Suite 400
Arlington, VA 22201-4598
Internet address: *www.aami.org*

♦ Biomedical Engineering Society
8401 Corporate Drive, Suite 110
Landover, MD 20785
Internet address: *www.bmes.org*

3:6 INFORMATION

Biotechnology Research and Development Careers

Biotechnology career workers are involved with using living cells and their molecules to make useful products. They work with cells and cell products from humans, animals, plants, and microorganisms. Through research and development, they help produce new diagnostic tests, forms of treatment, medications, vaccines to prevent disease, methods to detect and clean up environmental contamination, and food products. The potential for the use of biotechnology is unlimited.

Places of employment include pharmaceutical companies, chemical companies, agricultural facilities, research laboratories, colleges or universities, government facilities, forensic laboratories, hospitals, and industry. There are many career opportunities at all levels (table 3-17).

TABLE 3-17 Biotechnology Research and Development Careers

OCCUPATION	EDUCATION REQUIRED	JOB OUTLOOK TO YEAR 2012	AVERAGE YEARLY EARNINGS
Biological or Medical Scientists	• Bachelor's, master's, or doctoral degree • Licensure required in some states	Average growth	$52,600–$110,500
Biotechnological Engineers (Bioengineers)	• Bachelor's or master's degree • Licensure required in some states	Average growth	$48,600–$82,700
Biological Technicians	• Associate's or bachelor's degree • Certification can be obtained from the National Credentialing Agency for Laboratory Personnel	Average growth	$32,300–$62,500
Process Technicians	• Associate's degree • Some have bachelor's degree	Average growth	$32,300–$59,400
Forensic Science Technicians	• Associate's, bachelor's, or master's degree • Most states do not have licensing or certification requirements • Must meet proficiency levels established by national accreditation associations for criminal laboratories • Certification can be obtained from the American Society for Clinical Pathology	Above average growth	$38,600–$67,300

Biological or medical scientists study living organisms such as viruses, bacteria, protozoa, and other infectious substances. They assist in the development of vaccines, medicines, and treatments for diseases; evaluate the relationships between organisms and the environment; and administer programs for testing food and drugs. Some work on isolating and identifying genes associated with specific diseases or inherited traits, and perform research to correct genetic defects. Some specialties include:

♦ *Biochemists*: study the chemical composition of living things

♦ *Microbiologists*: investigate the growth and characteristics of microscopic organisms

♦ *Physiologists*: study the life functions of plants and animals

♦ *Forensic scientists*: study cells, fibers, and other evidence to obtain information about a crime

♦ *Biophysicists*: study the response and interrelationship of living cells and organisms to the principles of physics, such as electrical or mechanical energy

Most biological or medical scientists use research associates and assistants. These associates or assistants must have high-level math and science skills, computer technology proficiency, effective written and oral communication skills, knowledge of aseptic techniques, and laboratory skills.

Biotechnological engineers (bioengineers) use engineering knowledge to develop solutions to complex medical problems. They develop devices such as cardiac pacemakers, blood oxygenators, and defibrillators that aid in the diagnosis and treatment of disease; research various metals and other biomaterials to determine which can be used as implants in the human body; design and construct artificial organs, such as hip replacements, kidneys, heart valves, and artificial hearts; and research the biomechanics of injury and wound healing.

Biological technicians, working under the supervision of biological scientists or biotechnological engineers, assist in the study of living organisms. They perform many of the laboratory experiments used in medical research on diseases such as cancer and acquired immune deficiency syndrome (AIDS). They also assist in the development, testing, and manufacturing of pharmaceuticals or medications (figure 3-21).

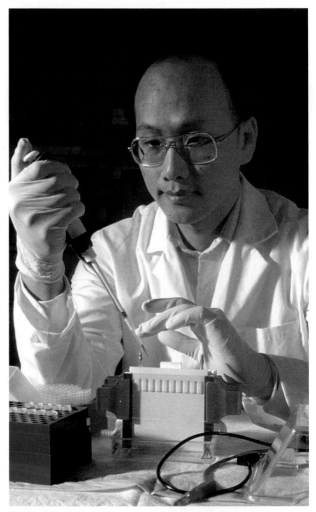

FIGURE 3-21 Biological technicians perform many of the laboratory experiments used for medical research. (*Courtesy of CDC Public Health Image Library/James Gathany*)

Biological technicians must be proficient in the use of clinical laboratory equipment and computers. They must also be adept at compiling statistics and preparing research reports to document experiments.

Process technicians, working under the supervision of biological scientists or research physicians, operate and monitor the machinery that is used to produce biotechnology products. They may install new equipment, monitor the operation process of the equipment, assess quality control of the finished product, and enforce environmental and safety regulations. For example, a process technician manufacturing drugs for a pharmaceutical company may prepare and measure raw materials, load the raw materials into the machinery, set the controls, operate the machinery, take test samples for quality control,

TODAY'S RESEARCH: TOMORROW'S HEALTH CARE

A robot that performs heart surgery?

Open-heart surgery is a major surgery. To correct heart defects or blocked blood vessels in the heart, surgeons must saw the breastbone in two, pull back the ribs, and open the thoracic (chest) cavity with an incision that is usually about 1 foot long. In addition, open-heart surgery requires a team of surgeons and other personnel.

Researchers have developed surgical robots that can perform this surgery with less trauma to the patient. A physician makes just three small incisions, called *ports,* into the chest. A tiny video camera is attached to one arm of a robot and inserted into one port. Surgical instruments, such as a scalpel (knife) or forceps, are attached to other arms on the robot and inserted into the other two ports as needed. The physician sits in front of a computer screen showing the images from the camera inside the patient. The physician then uses joystick-like controls to direct the actions of the robotic arms that hold the instruments. The robot never gets tired as physicians do during long and delicate surgeries. Its hands never "tremble" and its movements are exact. It simply follows the physician's instructions to perform the surgery. The patient recovers quickly and is usually sent home in one or two days.

Currently, robotic heart surgery is still being researched. Different types of robots are being evaluated. Researchers are trying to instill more artificial "intelligence" in the robots being used. However, the future of robotic surgery is promising. Patients with heart defects or disease may no longer have to dread open-heart surgery. A few small incisions in the chest will allow a blocked blood vessel to be replaced and a heart condition cured.

and record required information. Process technicians must use aseptic techniques and follow all safety and environmental regulations during the manufacturing process.

Forensic science technicians, also called *criminalists,* investigate crimes by collecting and analyzing physical evidence. Examples of physical evidence include weapons, clothing, shoes, fibers, hair, body tissues, blood, body fluids, fingerprints, chemicals, and even vapors in the air. After the physical evidence is analyzed and preserved, the forensic science technician works with other investigative officers such as police detectives to reconstruct a crime scene and find the individual who committed the crime. Forensic science technicians must be proficient in the use of laboratory equipment and computers. They must also be adept at preparing reports, compiling statistics, and testifying in trials or hearings.

ADDITIONAL SOURCES OF INFORMATION

♦ American Academy of Forensic Sciences
P.O. Box 669
Colorado Springs, CO 80901
Internet address: *www.aafs.org*

♦ American Institute of Biological Sciences
1444 I. Street NW, Suite 200
Washington, DC 20005
Internet address: *www.aibs.org*

♦ Biotechnology Industry Organization
1225 Eye Street, NW, Suite 400
Washington, DC 20005
Internet address: *www.bio.org*

♦ Biotechnology Institute
1840 Wilson Boulevard, Suite 202
Arlington, VA 22201
Internet address: *www.biotechinstitute.org*

♦ Pharmaceutical Research and Manufacturers of America
1100 Fifteenth Street, NW
Washington, DC 20005
Internet address: *www.phrma.org*

STUDENT: *Go to the workbook and complete the assignment sheet for Chapter 3, Careers in Health Care.*

CHAPTER 3 SUMMARY

More than 250 different careers in health care provide individuals with opportunities to find occupations they enjoy. Each health care career differs somewhat in the type of duties performed, the education required, the standards that must be met and maintained, and the salary earned.

This chapter has described some of the major health care careers. For each career group, levels of workers, basic job duties, educational requirements, anticipated need for workers through the year 2012, and average yearly salaries were provided. Use this chapter to evaluate the different health careers, and request additional information on specific careers from sources listed at the end of the respective career sections. In this way, you can research various occupational opportunities and determine which health care career is most appropriate for your interests and abilities.

INTERNET SEARCHES

Use the suggested search engines in Chapter 17:4 of this textbook to search the Internet for additional information on the following topics:

1. *National Health Care Skill Standards (NHCSS)*: review the history and development of health care skill standards, and search for additional information on the health science career cluster.

2. *Health care careers*: Search for information on specific careers by entering the name of the career.

3. *Career organizations*: Contact organizations at web addresses listed in each career cluster to determine the purpose of the organization, health careers it promotes, and advantages of membership.

4. *Accreditation Agencies*: Search the Commission on Accreditation of Allied Health Education Programs (CAAHEP) at www.caahep.org and the Accrediting Bureau of Health Education Schools (ABHES) at www.abhes.org to determine which health career programs are accredited by each agency. Research schools in your area that meet accreditation standards.

5. *Schools*: Search for technical schools, colleges, and universities that offer educational programs for a specific career. Evaluate entrance requirements, financial aid, and programs of study.

REVIEW QUESTIONS

1. Explain the differences and similarities between secondary and post-secondary health care education?

2. For each of the post-secondary degrees listed, state how many years of education are required to obtain the degree. For each degree, give three (3) examples of specific health care careers that require the degree for entry-level workers.
   a. Associate's degree
   b. Bachelor's degree
   c. Master's degree
   d. Doctorate

3. Differentiate between certification, registration, and licensure.

4. What are CEUs? Why are they required in many health care careers?

5. Name at least four (4) specific careers within each cluster of the National Health Care Skill Standards.

6. What is an entrepreneur? Identify five (5) examples of health care careers that may be an entrepreneur.

7. Choose one health care career in which you have an interest. Use references or search the Internet to list ten (10) specific tasks performed by personnel in the career.

8. Choose one health care career in which you have an interest. Use references or search the Internet to identify three (3) different schools that offer accredited programs in the career.

CHAPTER 4

Personal and Professional Qualities of a Health Care Worker

Observe Standard Precautions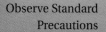

Instructor's Check—Call Instructor at This Point

Safety—Proceed with Caution

OBRA Requirement—Based on Federal Law

Math Skill

Legal Responsibility

Science Skill

Career Information

Communications Skill

Technology

Chapter Objectives

After completing this chapter, you should be able to:

◆ Explain how diet, rest, exercise, good posture, and avoiding tobacco, alcohol, and drugs contribute to good health

◆ Demonstrate the standards of a professional appearance as they apply to uniforms, shoes, nails, hair, jewelry, and makeup

◆ Create a characteristic profile of a health care worker that includes at least eight personal/professional traits or attitudes

◆ Identify four factors that interfere with communication

◆ Explain the importance of listening, nonverbal behavior, reporting, and recording in the communication process

◆ Identify why teamwork is beneficial

◆ Identify six basic characteristics of leaders

◆ Differentiate among democratic, laissez-faire, and autocratic leaders

◆ Differentiate between positive and negative stressors by identifying the emotional response

◆ List six ways to eliminate or decrease stress

◆ Explain how time management, problem solving, and goal setting reduce stress

◆ Define, pronounce, and spell all key terms

KEY TERMS

acceptance of criticism
autocratic leader
communication
competence
    (kom'-peh-tense)
cultural diversity
democratic leader
dependability
discretion
empathy *(em'-path-ee")*

enthusiasm
feedback
goal
honesty
laissez-faire leader
leader
leadership
listening
nonverbal communication
patience

personal hygiene
responsibility
self-motivation
stress
tact
team player
teamwork
time management
willingness to learn

INTRODUCTION

Although health care workers are employed in many different career areas and in a variety of facilities, certain personal/professional characteristics, attitudes, and rules of appearance apply to all health care professionals. This chapter discusses these basic requirements.

4:1 INFORMATION

Personal Appearance

As a worker in any health career, it is important to present an appearance that inspires confidence and a positive self-image. Research has shown that within 20 seconds to 4 minutes people form an impression about another person based mainly on appearance. Although the rules of suitable appearance may vary, certain professional standards apply to most health careers and should be observed to create a positive impression.

GOOD HEALTH

Health care involves promoting health and preventing disease. Therefore, a health care worker should present a healthy appearance. Five main factors contribute to good health:

♦ *Diet*: Eating well-balanced meals and nutritious foods provides the body with the materi-

als needed for optimum health. Foods from each of the five major food groups (milk; meat; vegetables; fruits; and bread, cereals, rice, and pasta) should be eaten daily. My Pyramid, discussed in Chapter 9:4, identifies the major food groups.

♦ *Rest*: Adequate rest and sleep help provide energy and the ability to deal with stress. The amount of sleep required varies from individual to individual.

♦ *Exercise*: Exercise maintains circulation, improves muscle tone, enhances mental attitude, aids in weight control, and contributes to more restful sleep. In addition, regular physical activity reduces the risk for coronary heart disease, diabetes, colon cancer, hypertension (high blood pressure), and osteoporosis. Individuals should choose the form of exercise best suited to their own needs, but should exercise daily.

♦ *Good posture*: Good posture helps prevent fatigue and puts less stress on muscles. Basic principles include standing straight with stomach muscles pulled in, shoulders relaxed, and weight balanced equally on each foot.

♦ *Avoid use of tobacco, alcohol, and drugs*: The use of tobacco, alcohol, and drugs can seriously affect good health. Tobacco affects the function of the heart, circulatory system, lungs, and digestive system. In addition, the odor of smoke is offensive to many individuals. For these reasons, most health care facilities are "smoke-free" environments. The use of alcohol and drugs impairs mental function, decreases ability to make decisions, and adversely affects many body systems. The use of alcohol or drugs can also result in job loss. Avoiding tobacco, alcohol, and drugs helps prevent damage to the body systems and contributes to good health.

PROFESSIONAL APPEARANCE

When you obtain a position in a health career, it is important to learn the rules or standards of dress and personal appearance that have been established by your place of employment. Abide by the rules and make every effort to maintain a neat, clean, and professional appearance.

Uniform

Many health occupations require uniforms. A uniform should always be neat, well fitting, clean, and free from wrinkles (figure 4-1). Some agencies require a white uniform, but others allow pastel colors. In some facilities, the colors identify groups of workers. If white uniforms are required, white or neutral undergarments should be worn. A large variety of uniform styles is available. Extreme styles in any type of uniform should be avoided. It is important that the health care worker learn what type and color uniform is required or permitted and follow the standards established by the place of employment.

Clothing

If regular clothing is worn in place of a uniform, the clothing must be clean, neat, and in good repair (figure 4-2). The style should allow for freedom of body movement and should be appropriate for the job. For example, while clean, neat jeans might be appropriate at times for a recreational therapist, they are not proper attire for most other health professionals. Washable fabrics are usually best because frequent laundering is necessary.

Name Badge

Most health care facilities require personnel to wear name badges or photo identification tags at all times. The badge usually states the name, title, and department of the health care worker. In some health care settings, such as long-term care facilities, workers are required by law to wear

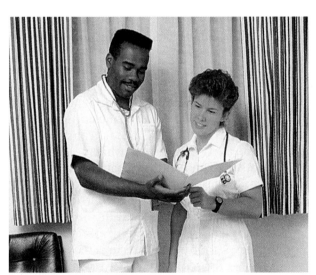

FIGURE 4-1 Uniform styles may vary, but a uniform should always be neat, well fitting, clean, and free from wrinkles.

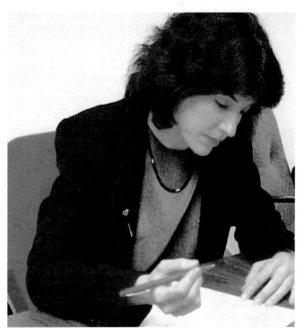

FIGURE 4-2 If regular clothing is worn in place of a uniform, the clothing should reflect a professional appearance.

identification badges. In addition, a health care facility's security regulations may require photo identification tags to gain access into the building or into certain areas inside the facility.

Shoes

Although white shoes are frequently required, many occupations allow other types of shoes. Any shoes should fit well and provide good support to prevent fatigue. Low heels are usually best because they help prevent fatigue and accidents. Avoid wearing sandals or open-toe shoes, unless they are standard dress for a particular occupation. Shoes should be cleaned daily. If shoelaces are part of the shoes, these must also be cleaned or replaced frequently. Women should wear white or beige stockings or pantyhose with dress uniforms; colored or patterned stockings should be avoided. White socks should be worn with white pants.

Personal Hygiene

Good **personal hygiene** is essential. Because health care workers typically work in close contact with others, body odor must be controlled. A daily bath or shower, use of deodorant or antiperspirant, good oral hygiene, and clean undergarments all help prevent body odor. Strong odors caused by tobacco, perfumes, scented hairsprays, and aftershave lotions can be offensive. In addition, certain scents can cause allergic reactions in some individuals. The use of these products should be avoided when working with patients and co-workers.

Nails

Nails should be kept short, clean, and natural. Many health care facilities prohibit the use of artificial nails. If fingernails are long and/or pointed, they can injure patients. They can also transmit germs, because dirt can collect under long nails and artificial nails. In addition, health care workers are now required to wear gloves for many procedures. Long nails can tear or puncture gloves. The use of colored nail polish is discouraged because the color can conceal any dirt that may collect under the nails. Further, because frequent handwashing causes polish to chip, germs can collect on the surfaces of nails.

Finally, the flash of bright colors may bother a person who does not feel well. If nail polish is worn, it should be clear or colorless, and the nails must be kept scrupulously clean. Hand cream or lotion should be used to keep the hands from becoming chapped and dry from frequent handwashing.

Hair

Hair should be kept clean and neat. It should be styled attractively and be easy to care for. Fancy or extreme hairstyles, hair ornaments, and/or unnatural hair colors should be avoided. If the job requires close contact with patients, long hair must be pinned back and kept off the collar. This prevents the hair from touching the patient/resident, falling on a tray or on equipment, or blocking necessary vision during procedures.

Jewelry

Jewelry is usually not permitted with a uniform because it can cause injury to the patient and transmit germs or pathogens. Exceptions sometimes include a watch, wedding ring, and small, pierced earrings. Earrings with hoops or dangling earrings should be avoided. Body jewelry, such as nose, eyebrow, or tongue-piercing jewelry, detracts from a professional appearance and is prohibited in many health care facilities. When a uniform is not required, jewelry should still be limited. Excessive jewelry can interfere with patient care and detracts from the professional appearance of the health care worker.

Makeup and Tattoos

Excessive makeup should be avoided. The purpose of makeup is to create a natural appearance and add to the attractiveness of a person.

Tattoos that are visible and/or offensive detract from a professional appearance and are prohibited in many health care facilities. An example is a tattoo on a hand or lower arm that promotes gang membership. Some health care facilities require that any tattoo be covered by clothing at all times. Learn and follow the policies established by your place of employment.

4:2 INFORMATION

Personal Characteristics

Many personal/professional characteristics and attitudes are required in the health occupations. As a health care worker, you should make every effort to develop the following characteristics and attitudes and to incorporate them into your personality.

♦ *Empathy:* Empathy means being able to identify with and understand another person's feelings, situation, and motives. As a health care worker, you may care for persons of all ages—from the newborn infant to the elderly adult. To be successful, you must be sincerely interested in working with people. You must care about others and be able to communicate and work with them. Understanding the needs of people and learning effective communication techniques is one way to develop empathy. This topic is covered in greater detail in Chapter 4:3 of this text.

♦ *Honesty:* Truthfulness and integrity are important in any career field. Others must be able to trust you at all times. You must be willing to admit mistakes so they can be corrected.

♦ *Dependability:* Employers and patients rely on you, so you must accept the responsibility required in your position. You must be prompt in reporting to work, and maintain a good attendance record (figure 4-3). You must perform assigned tasks on time and accurately.

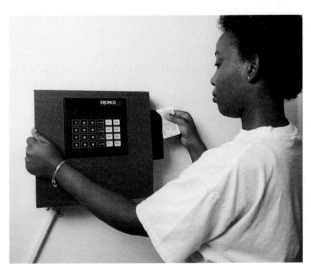

FIGURE 4-3 A health care worker must report to work on time and maintain a good attendance record.

♦ *Willingness to learn:* You must be willing to learn and to adapt to changes. The field of health care changes constantly because of research, new inventions, and technological advances. Change often requires learning new techniques or procedures. At times, additional education may be required to remain competent in a particular field. Be prepared for life-long learning to maintain a competent level of knowledge and skills.

♦ *Patience:* You must be tolerant and understanding. You must learn to control your temper and "count to ten" in difficult situations. Learning to deal with frustration and overcome obstacles is important.

♦ *Acceptance of criticism:* Patients, families, employers, co-workers, and others may criticize you. Some criticism will be constructive and allow you to improve your work. Remember that everyone has some areas where performance can be improved. Instead of becoming resentful, you must be willing to accept criticism and learn from it.

♦ *Enthusiasm:* You must enjoy your work and display a positive attitude. Enthusiasm is contagious; it helps you do your best and encourages others to do the same. If you do not like some aspects of your job, concentrating on the positive points can help diminish the importance of the negative points.

♦ *Self-motivation:* Self-motivation, or self-initiative, is the ability to begin or to follow through with a task. You should be able to determine things that need to be done and do them without constant direction. You set goals for yourself and work to reach the goals.

♦ *Tact:* Being tactful means having the ability to say or do the kindest or most fitting thing in a difficult situation. It requires constant practice. Tactfulness implies a consideration for the feelings of others. It is important to remember that all individuals have a right to their respective feelings, and that these feelings should not be judged as right or wrong.

♦ *Competence:* Being competent means that you are qualified and capable of performing a task. You follow instructions, use approved procedures, and strive for accuracy in all you do. You know your limits and ask for help or guidance if you do not know how to perform a procedure.

♦ **Responsibility:** Responsibility implies being willing to be held accountable for your actions. Others can rely on you and know that you will meet your obligations. Responsibility means that you do what you are supposed to do.

♦ **Discretion:** You must always use good judgment in what you say and do. In any health care career, you will have access to confidential information. This information should not be told to anyone without proper authorization. A patient is entitled to confidential care; you must be discreet and ensure that the patient's rights are not violated.

♦ **Team player:** In any health care field, you will become part of a team. It is essential that you become a team player and learn to work well with others. Each member of a health care team will have different responsibilities, but each member must do his or her part to provide the patient with quality care. By working together, a team can accomplish goals much faster than an individual.

Each of the preceding characteristics and attitudes must be practiced and learned. Some take more time to develop than do others. By being aware of these characteristics and striving constantly to improve, you will provide good patient/resident care and be a valuable asset to your employer and other members of the health care team.

4:3 INFORMATION

Effective Communications

 Communicating effectively with others is an important part of any health career. The health care worker must be able to relate to patients and their families, to co-workers, and to other professionals. An understanding of communication skills will assist the health care worker who is trying to relate effectively.

Communication is the exchange of information, thoughts, ideas, and feelings. It can occur through *verbal* means (spoken words), written communications, and *nonverbal* behavior such as facial expressions, body language, and touch.

COMMUNICATION PROCESS

The communication process involves three essential elements:

♦ *Sender*: an individual who creates a message to convey information or an idea to another person

♦ *Message*: information, ideas, or thoughts

♦ *Receiver*: an individual who receives the message from the sender

Without a sender, message, and receiver, communication cannot occur.

Feedback is a method that can be used to determine whether communication was successful. This occurs when the receiver responds to the message. Feedback allows the original sender to evaluate how the message was interpreted and to make any necessary adjustments or clarification. Feedback can be verbal or nonverbal.

Even though the communication process seems simple, many factors can interfere with the completion of the process. Important elements of effective communication include:

♦ *The message must be clear.* The message must be in terms that both the sender and receiver understand. Health care workers learn and use terminology that is frequently not understood by those people who are not employed in health care. Even though these terms are familiar to the health care worker, they must be modified, defined, or substituted with other words when messages are conveyed to people not employed in health care. For example, if a health care worker needs a urine specimen, some patients can be told to urinate in a container. Others, such as very small children or individuals with limited education, may have to be told to "pee" or "do number one." Even a term such as *apical pulse* is not understood by many individuals. Instead of telling a patient, "I am going to take your apical pulse," say, "I am going to listen to your heart." It requires experience and constant practice to learn to create a message that can be clearly understood.

♦ *The sender must deliver the message in a clear and concise manner.* Correct pronunciation and the use of good grammar are essential. The use of slang words or words with double meanings should be avoided. Meaningless phrases or terms such as "you know," "all that stuff," "um," and "OK," distract from the message and also must be avoided. In verbal communications, the tone and pitch of voice is important. A moderate level, neither too soft nor too loud, and good inflection, to avoid monotone, are essential. Think of the many different ways the sentence "I really like this job" can be said and the different meanings that can be interpreted depending on the tone and pitch of the voice. The proper rate, or speed, of delivering a message is also important. If a message is delivered too quickly, the receiver may not have enough time to hear all parts of the message. In written communications, the message should be spelled correctly, contain correct grammar and punctuation, and be concise but thorough.

♦ *The receiver must be able to hear and receive the message.* Patients who are heavily medicated or are weak may nod their heads as if messages are heard, when, in reality, the patients are not receiving the information. They may hear it, but it is not being interpreted and understood because of their physical states. Patients with hearing or visual impairments or patients with limited English-speaking abilities are other examples of individuals who may not be able to easily receive messages (figure 4-4). Repeating the message, changing the form of the message, and getting others to interpret or clarify the message are some ways to help the receiver receive and respond to the message.

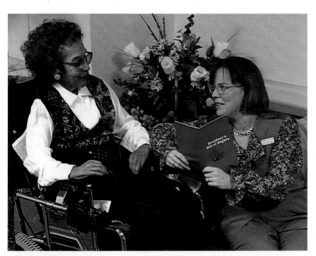

FIGURE 4-4 In communicating with a person who has a hearing impairment, face the individual and speak slowly and distinctly.

♦ *The receiver must be able to understand the message.* Using unfamiliar terminology can cause a breakdown in communication. Many people do not want to admit that they do not understand terms because they think others will think they are dumb. The health care worker should ask questions or repeat information in different terms if it appears that the patient does not understand the information. The receiver's attitude and prejudices can also interfere with understanding. If a patient feels that health care workers do not know what they are talking about, the patient will not accept the information presented. Receivers must have some confidence and belief in the sender before they will accept and understand a message. It is important that health care workers are willing to say, "I don't know, but I will try to find out that information for you," when they are asked a question about which they do not have correct knowledge. It is also important for health care workers to be aware of their own prejudices and attitudes when they are receiving messages from patients. If health care workers feel that certain patients are lazy, ignorant, or uncooperative, they will not respond correctly to messages sent by these patients. Health care workers must be aware of these feelings and work to overcome them so they can accept patients as they are.

♦ *Interruptions or distractions must be avoided.* Interruptions or distractions can interfere with any communication. Trying to talk with others while answering the phone or writing a message can decrease the effectiveness of spoken and/or written communication. Loud noises or distractions in the form of bright light or uncomfortable temperature can interrupt communication. When two people are talking outside in freezing temperatures, for example, the conversation will be limited because of the discomfort from the cold. A small child jumping around or climbing up and down off a mother's lap will distract the mother as she is getting instructions from a health care worker. A loud television or radio interferes with verbal messages, because receivers may pay more attention to the radio or television than to the person speaking to them. It is important to eliminate or at least limit distractions if meaningful communication is to take place.

LISTENING

Listening is another essential part of effective communication. Listening means paying attention to and making an effort to hear what the other person is saying. Good listening skills require constant practice. Techniques that can be used to learn good listening skills include:

♦ Show interest and concern for what the speaker is saying

♦ Be alert and maintain eye contact with the speaker

♦ Avoid interrupting the speaker

♦ Pay attention to what the speaker is saying

♦ Avoid thinking about how you are going to respond

♦ Try to eliminate your own prejudices and see the other person's point of view

♦ Eliminate distractions by moving to a quiet area for the conversation

♦ Watch the speaker closely to observe actions that may contradict what the person is saying

♦ Reflect statements back to the speaker to let the speaker know that statements are being heard

♦ Ask for clarification if you do not understand part of a message

♦ Keep your temper under control and maintain a positive attitude

Good listening skills will allow you to receive the entire message a person is trying to convey to you. For example, if a patient says, "I'm not worried about this surgery," but is very restless and seems nervous, the patient's body movements may indicate fear that is being denied by words. The health care worker could reflect the patient's statement by saying, "You're not at all worried about this surgery?" The patient may respond by saying, "Well, not really. It's just that I worry about my family if something should happen to me."

Good listening allowed the patient to express fears and opened the way to more effective communication. In this same case, the entire pattern of communication could have been blocked if the health care worker had instead responded, "That's good."

NONVERBAL COMMUNICATION

Nonverbal communication involves the use of facial expressions, body language, gestures, eye contact, and touch to convey messages or ideas (figure 4-5). If a person is smiling and sitting in a very relaxed position while saying, "I am very angry about this entire situation," two different messages are being conveyed. A smile, a frown, a wink, a shrug of the shoulders, a bored expression, a tapping of fingers or feet, and other similar body gestures or actions all convey messages to the receiver. It is important for health care workers to be aware of both their own and patients' nonverbal behaviors because these are an important part of any communication process. A touch of the hand, a pat on the back, a firm handshake, and a hug can convey more interest and caring than words could ever do. When verbal and nonverbal messages agree, the receiver is more likely to understand the message being sent.

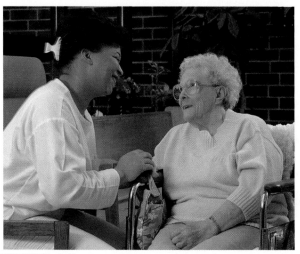

FIGURE 4-5 What aspects of listening and nonverbal behavior can you see in this picture?

BARRIERS TO COMMUNICATION

A communication barrier is something that gets in the way of clear communication. Three common barriers are physical disabilities, psychological attitudes and prejudice, and cultural diversity.

Physical Disabilities

♦ *Deafness or hearing loss*: People who are deaf or hearing impaired have difficulty receiving messages. To improve communication, it is essential to use body language such as gestures and signs, speak clearly in short sentences, face the individual to improve the potential for lip reading, write messages if necessary, and make sure that any hearing aids have good batteries and are inserted correctly (figure 4-6). At times, it may be neces-

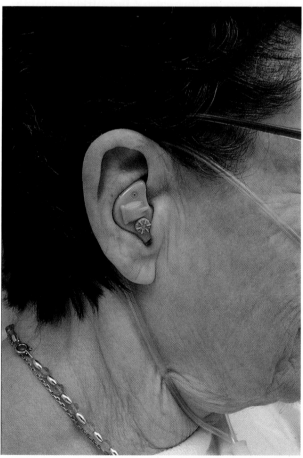

FIGURE 4-6 To be effective, hearing aids must be inserted correctly and have good batteries.

sary to obtain the assistance of a sign language interpreter to communicate with a deaf individual.

♦ *Blindness or impaired vision*: People who are blind or visually impaired may be able to hear what is being said, but they will not see body language, gestures, or facial expressions. To improve communication, use a soft tone of voice, describe events that are occurring, announce your presence as you enter a room, explain sounds or noises, and use touch when appropriate.

♦ *Aphasia or speech impairments*: Aphasia is the loss or impairment of the power to use or comprehend words, usually as a result of injury or damage to the brain. Individuals with aphasia or speech impairments can have difficulty with not only the spoken word but also written communications. They may know what they want to say but have difficulty remembering the correct words, may not be able to pronounce certain words, or may have slurred and distorted speech. Patience is essential while working with these individuals. Allow them to try to speak, encourage them to take their time, ask questions that require only short responses, speak slowly and clearly, pause between sentences to allow them to comprehend what has been said, repeat messages to be sure they are correct, encourage them to use gestures or point to objects, provide writing materials if they can write messages, or use pictures with key messages to communicate (figure 4-7).

Psychological Barriers

Psychological barriers to communication are often caused by prejudice, attitudes, and personality. Examples include closed-mindedness, judging, preaching, moralizing, lecturing, overreacting, arguing, advising, and prejudging. Our judgments of others are too often based on appearance, lifestyle, and social or economic status. Stereotypes such as "dumb blonde," "lazy bum," or "fat slob" cause us to make snap judgments about an individual and affect the communication process.

Health care workers must learn to put prejudice aside and show respect to all individuals. A homeless person deserves the same quality of health care

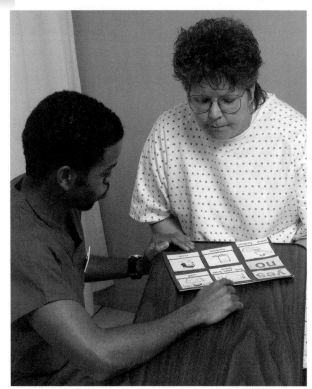

FIGURE 4-7 Picture cards make it easier to communicate with a patient who has aphasia or a speech impairment.

as the president of the United States. It is important to respect each person as an individual and to remember that each person has the right to good care and considerate treatment. At times, this can be extremely difficult, and patience and practice are essential. When individuals have negative attitudes or constantly complain or criticize your work, it can be difficult to show them respect. The health care worker must learn to see beyond the surface attitude to the human being underneath.

Frequently, fear is the cause of anger or a negative attitude. Allow patients to express their fears or anger, encourage them to talk about their feelings, avoid arguing, remain calm, talk in a soft and non-threatening tone of voice, and provide quality care. If other health care workers seem to be able to communicate more effectively with patients, watch these workers to learn how they handle difficult or angry patients. This is often the most effective means of learning good communication skills.

Cultural Diversity

Cultural diversity, discussed in detail in Chapter 10, is another possible communication barrier. Culture consists of the values, beliefs, attitudes, and customs shared by a group of people and passed from one generation to the next. It is often defined as a set of rules, because culture allows an individual to interpret the environment and actions of others and behave appropriately. The main barriers created by cultural diversity include:

♦ *Beliefs and practices regarding health and illness*: Individuals from different cultures may have their own beliefs about the cause of an illness and the type of treatment required. It is important to remember that they have the right to determine their treatment plans and even to refuse traditional treatments. At times, these individuals may accept traditional health care but add their own cultural remedies to the treatment plan.

♦ *Language differences*: Language differences can create major barriers. In the United States, English is a primary language used in health care. If a person has difficulty communicating in English, and a health care worker is not fluent in another language, a barrier exists. When providing care to people who have limited English-speaking abilities, speak slowly, use simple words, use gestures or pictures to clarify the meaning of words, and use nonverbal communication in the form of a smile or gentle touch. Avoid the tendency to speak louder because this does not improve comprehension. Whenever possible, try to find an interpreter who speaks the language of the patient. Frequently, another health care worker, a consultant, or a family member may be able to assist in the communication process. In addition, many health care facilities provide written instructions or explanations in several different languages to facilitate the communication process (figure 4-8).

♦ *Eye contact*: In some cultures, direct eye-to-eye contact while communicating is not acceptable. These cultures believe that looking down shows proper respect for another individual. A health care worker who feels that eye contact is important must learn to accept and respect this cultural difference and a person's inability to engage in eye contact while communicating.

♦ *Ways of dealing with terminal illness and/or severe disability*: In the United States, a traditional health care belief is that the patient

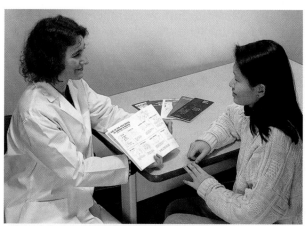

FIGURE 4-8 Many health care facilities provide written instructions or explanations in several different languages to facilitate communication with individuals who have limited English-speaking abilities.

should be told the truth about his or her diagnosis and informed about the expected outcome. Some cultural groups believe that a person should not be told of a fatal diagnosis or be burdened with making decisions about treatment. In these cultures, the family, the mother or father, or another designated individual is expected to make decisions about care, treatment, and information given to the patient. In such instances, it is important for health care workers to recognize and respect this and to involve these individuals in the patient's care. At times, it may be necessary for a patient to use legal means, such as power of attorney for health care, to designate responsibility for his or her care to another person.

♦ *Touch*: In some cultures, it is inappropriate to touch someone on the head. Other cultures have clearly defined areas of the body that can be touched or that should be avoided. Even a simple handshake can be regarded as showing a lack of respect. In some cultures, only family members provide personal care. For this reason, health care workers should always get permission from the patient before providing care and should avoid any use of touch that seems to be inappropriate for the individual.

Respect for and acceptance of cultural diversity is essential for any health care worker. When beliefs, ideas, concepts, and ways of life are different, communication barriers can result. By making every attempt to learn about cultural differences and by showing respect for an individu-

al's right to cultural beliefs, a health care worker can provide quality health care.

RECORDING AND REPORTING

In health care, an important part of effective communication is reporting or recording all observations while providing care. To do this, it is important to not only listen to what the patient is saying, but to make observations about the patient. All senses are used to make observations:

♦ *Sense of sight*: notes the color of skin, swelling or edema, the presence of a rash or sore, the color of urine or stool, the amount of food eaten, and other similar factors

♦ *Sense of smell*: alerts a health care worker to body odor or unusual odors of breath, wounds, urine, or stool

♦ *Sense of touch*: used to feel the pulse, dryness or temperature of the skin, perspiration, and swelling

♦ *Sense of hearing*: used while listening to respirations, abnormal body sounds, coughs, and speech

By using all senses, the health care worker can learn a great deal about a patient's condition and be able to report observations accurately.

Observations should be reported promptly to an immediate supervisor. There are two types of observations:

♦ *Subjective observations*: These cannot be seen or felt, and are commonly called *symptoms*. They are usually statements or complaints made by the patient. They should be reported in the exact words the patient used.

♦ *Objective observations*: These can be seen or measured, and are commonly called *signs*. A bruise, cut, rash, or swelling can be seen. Blood pressure and temperature are measurable.

For example, the health care worker should not state, "I think Mr. B. has a fever." The report should state, "Mr. B. is complaining of feeling hot. His skin is red and flushed, and his temperature is 102°."

In some health care facilities, observations are recorded on a patient's health care record. Effective communication requires these written observations to be accurate, concise, and complete (figure 4-9). The writing should be neat and legible, and spelling and grammar should be correct. Only objective observations should be noted. Subjective observations that the health care worker feels or thinks should be avoided. If a patient's statement is recorded, the statement should be written in the patient's own words and enclosed in quotation marks. All information should be signed with the name and title of the person recording the information. Errors should be crossed out neatly with a straight line, have "error" recorded by them, and show the initials of the person making the error. In this way, recorded communication will be effective communication.

The Health Insurance Portability and Accountability Act (HIPAA) has established strict standards for maintaining confidentiality of health care records. Under this act, patients have total control on how information in their medical records is used. Patients must be able to see and obtain copies of their records. They can set limits on who can obtain this information. They can even prevent other family members from seeing the information. If any health care provider allows information to be released from a medical record without the patient's permission, the patient can file a complaint that the privacy act has been violated. This act is discussed in more detail in Chapter 5:1. It is important for every health care provider to be aware of all parts of this act and to make every effort to protect the privacy and confidentiality of the patient's health care records.

SUMMARY

Good communication skills allow health care workers to develop good interpersonal relationships. Patients feel accepted, they feel that others have an interest and concern in them, they feel free to express their ideas and fears, they develop confidence in the health care workers, and they feel they are receiving quality health care. In addition, the health care worker will relate more effectively with co-workers and other individuals.

4:4 INFORMATION

Teamwork

In almost any health care career, you will be a part of an interdisciplinary health care team. The team concept was created to provide quality holistic health care to every patient. **Teamwork** consists of many professionals, with different levels of education, ideas, backgrounds, and interests, working together for the benefit of the patient. For example, a surgical team might include the following people:

♦ *Admitting clerk*: collects admission information

♦ *Insurance representative*: obtains approval for the surgery

♦ *Nurses or patient care technicians*: prepare the patient for surgery

♦ *Surgeons*: perform the operation

♦ *Anesthesiologist*: administer anesthetics, medications that decrease pain and/or consciousness

♦ *Operating room nurses*: assist the surgeon

♦ *Surgical technicians*: prepare and pass instruments

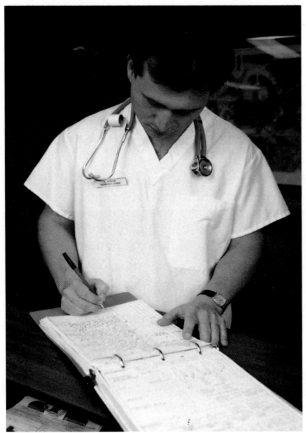

FIGURE 4-9 Information recorded on health care records must be accurate, concise, and complete.

- *Housekeepers*: clean and sanitize the area
- *Sterile supply personnel*: sterilize the instruments
- *Recovery room personnel*: care for the patient after surgery

After the surgery is complete, a dietitian, social worker, physical therapist, occupational therapist, home health personnel, and other team members might be needed to assist the patient as he/she recuperates. Each team member has an important job to do. When the team members work well together, the patient receives quality care.

Teamwork improves communication and continuity of care. When a team is assigned to a particular patient, the patient knows his/her caregivers and support staff. All the team members can help to identify the needs of the patient, offer opinions on the best type of care, participate as decisions are made on options of care, and suggest additional professionals who might be able to assist with specific needs. This allows a patient to become more educated about health care options and to make informed decisions regarding treatment and care.

For a team to function properly, every person on the team must understand the role of each team member. This knowledge provides a picture of the patient's total care plan. It also helps clarify each person's responsibility and establishes the goals that the team wants to achieve. Most teams have frequent patient care conferences, and in many instances, the patient is an active participant (figure 4-10). Opinions are shared, options are discussed, decisions are made, and goals are established. During the conference, each team member must listen, be honest, express his/her own opinion, and be willing to try different solutions.

A leader is an important part of any team. The leader is responsible for organizing and coordinating the team's activities, encouraging everyone to share ideas and give opinions, motivating all team members to work toward established goals, assisting with problems, monitoring the progress of the team, and providing reports and feedback to all team members on the effectiveness of the team. A good team leader will also allow others to assume the leadership role when circumstances indicate that another person can handle a particular situation more effectively.

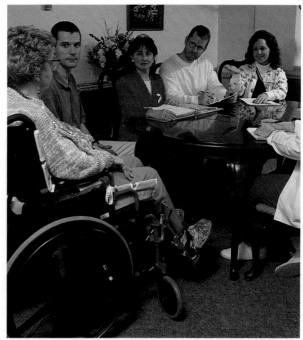

FIGURE 4-10 Most health care teams have frequent patient care conferences to establish team goals.

Leadership is discussed in more detail in Chapter 4:5.

Good interpersonal relationships are also essential. Poor interpersonal relationships among team members can harm the quality of care and prevent the team from meeting its goals. In the same way, good interpersonal relationships can improve the quality of care. Members of a team will have different cultural and ethnic backgrounds, sexes, ages, socioeconomic statuses, lifestyle preferences, beliefs, and levels of education. Each team member must understand that these differences affect the way a person thinks and acts. Each person must be sensitive to the hopes, feelings, and needs of other team members. The Golden Rule of "treat others as you would want to be treated" should be the main rule of teamwork. Some ways to develop good interpersonal relationships include:

- Maintain a positive attitude and learn to laugh at yourself
- Be friendly and cooperate with others
- Assist others when you see that they need help
- Listen carefully when another person is sharing ideas or beliefs

♦ Respect the opinions of others even though you may not agree with them

♦ Be open-minded and willing to compromise

♦ Avoid criticizing other team members

♦ Learn good communication skills so you can share ideas, concepts, and knowledge

♦ Support and encourage other team members

♦ Perform your duties to the best of your ability

Conflict among individuals with different personalities is a problem that can occur when a group of people is working as a team. When conflict occurs, it is essential for each person to deal with the conflict in a positive way. The people involved in the conflict should meet, talk with each other to identify the problem, listen to the other person's point of view, avoid accusations and hostility, try to determine a way to resolve the problem in a cooperative manner, and put the agreed-upon solution into action. If a situation occurs where two people do not feel comfortable talking privately with each other, a mediator may be able to assist with finding a solution to the problem. Some health care facilities have grievance committees to assist with conflicts that may occur. If a team is to meet its goals, conflict must be resolved.

 Legal responsibilities are another important aspect of teamwork. Each member of a team must be aware of the legal limitations on duties that can be performed. All members must function within legal boundaries. No team member should ever attempt to solve a problem or perform a duty that is beyond the range of duties legally permitted.

Effective teams are the result of hard work, patience, commitment, and practice. When each individual participates fully in the team and makes every effort to contribute to the team, the team achieves success.

4:5 INFORMATION
Professional Leadership

Leadership is an important concept in health occupations. **Leadership** is the skill or ability to encourage people to work together and do their best to achieve common goals. A **leader** is frequently defined as an individual who leads or guides others, or who is in charge or in command of others. A myth exists that leaders are born. In fact, leaders develop by their own efforts. Leaders combine visions of excellence with the ability to inspire others. They promote positive changes that benefit their professions and the people they serve. Anyone can learn to be a leader by making an effort to understand the principles of leadership. In a group, every member who makes a contribution to an idea can be considered a leader. The leadership in the group passes from person to person as each individual contributes to the achievement of the group's goals.

Many different characteristics are assigned to a leader. All the characteristics can be learned. In this way, leadership becomes a skill or function that can be learned, rather than an inherited set of characteristics.

Some common characteristics may include:

♦ Respects the rights, dignity, opinions, and abilities of others

♦ Understands the principles of democracy

♦ Works with a group and guides the group toward a goal

♦ Believes that changes and improvements can be accomplished

♦ Participates in continuing education and professional development, and understands the concept of lifelong learning

♦ Understands own strengths and weaknesses

♦ Displays self-confidence and willingness to take a stand

♦ Communicates effectively and verbalizes ideas clearly

♦ Shows self-initiative, a willingness to work, and completes tasks

♦ Shows optimism, is open-minded, and can compromise

♦ Praises others and gives credit to others

♦ Dedicated to meeting high standards

Leaders can often be classified into broad categories. Some of the categories include: religious, political, club or organizational, business, community, expertise in a particular area, and even informal or peer group. Leaders in these categories often develop based on their involvement with the particular category. An individual who joins a club or organization may become a leader when the group elects the individual to an office or position of leadership within the group.

Leaders are frequently classified as one of three types based on how they perform their leadership skills. The three main types of leader are *democratic, laissez-faire,* and *autocratic.*

♦ **Democratic leader:** encourages the participation of all individuals in decisions that have to be made or problems that have to be solved. This leader listens to the opinions of others, and then bases decisions on what is best for the group as a whole. By guiding the individuals to a solution, the leader allows the group to take responsibility for the decision.

♦ **Laissez-faire leader:** more of an informal type of leader. This leader believes in noninterference in the affairs of others. A laissez-faire leader will strive for only minimal rules or regulations, and allow the individuals in a group to function in an independent manner with little or no direction. This leader almost has a "hands-off" policy, and usually avoids making decisions until forced by circumstances to do so. The term *laissez-faire* comes from a French idiom meaning "to let alone" and can be translated to mean "allow to act"; therefore, it is an appropriate term to use for this type of leader.

♦ **Autocratic leader:** often called a "dictator." This individual maintains total rule, makes all of the decisions, and has difficulty delegating or sharing duties. This type of leader seldom asks for the opinions of others, emphasizes discipline, and expects others to follow directions at all times. Individuals usually follow this type of leader because of a fear of punishment or because of an extreme loyalty.

All types of leadership have advantages and disadvantages. In some rare situations, an autocratic leader may be beneficial. However, the democratic leader is the model frequently presented as most effective for group interactions. By allowing a group to share in deciding what, when, and how something is to be done, members of the group will usually do what has to be done because they want to do it. Respecting the rights and opinions of others becomes the most important guide for the leader.

4:6 INFORMATION

Stress

Stress can be defined as the body's reaction to any stimulus that requires a person to adjust to a changing environment. Change always initiates stress. The stimuli to change, alter behavior, or adapt to a situation are called *stressors*. Stressors can be situations, events, or concepts. Stressors can also be external or internal forces. For example, a heart attack is an internal stressor, and a new job is an external stressor.

No matter what the cause, a stressor will cause the body to go into an alarm or warning mode. This mode is frequently called the "fight or flight" reaction because of the physical changes that occur in the body. When the warning is received from a stressor, the sympathetic nervous system prepares the body for action. Adrenaline, a hormone from the adrenal glands, is released into the bloodstream. It dilates blood vessels to the heart and brain to increase blood circulation to these areas. At the same time, it constricts blood vessels to the skin and other internal organs, resulting in cool skin, decreased movement in the digestive tract, and decreased production of urine. The pupils in the eyes dilate to improve vision. Saliva production decreases and the mouth becomes dry. The heart beats more rapidly, blood pressure rises, and the respiratory rate increases. These actions by the sympathetic nervous system help provide the body with a burst of energy and the stamina needed to respond to the stressor.

After the individual responds to the stressor and adapts or changes as needed, the parasympathetic system slowly causes opposite reactions in the body. This results in fatigue or exhaustion while the body returns to normal and recuperates. If the body is subjected to continual stress with constant "up and down" nervous system reactions, the normal functions of the body will be disrupted. This can result in a serious illness or disease. Many diseases have stress-related origins. Examples include migraine headaches, anxiety reactions, depression, allergies, asthma, digestive disorders, hypertension (high blood pressure), insomnia (inability to sleep), and heart disease.

Everyone experiences a certain degree of stress on a daily basis. The amount of stress felt usually depends on the individual's reaction to and perception of the situation causing stress. For example, a blood test can be a routine event for some individuals, such as a diabetic who performs three or four blood tests on a daily basis. Another individual who is terrified of needles might feel extreme stress when a blood test is necessary. Many different things can cause stress. Examples include relationships with family, friends, and co-workers; job or school demands; foods such as caffeine, excessive sweets, and salt; illness; lifestyle; financial problems; family events such as birth, death, marriage, or divorce; overwork; boredom and negative feelings; time limitations (too much to do and not enough time to do it); and failure to achieve goals.

Not all stress is harmful. In fact, a small amount of stress is essential to an individual's well-being because it makes a person more alert and raises the energy level. The individual is able to make quick judgments and decisions, becomes more organized, and is motivated to accomplish tasks and achieve goals. The way in which an individual responds to stressors determines whether the situation is helpful or harmful. If stress causes positive feelings such as excitement, anticipation, self-confidence, and a sense of achievement, it is helpful. If stress causes negative feelings such as boredom, frustration, irritability, anger, depression, distrust of others, self-criticism, emotional and physical exhaustion, and emotional outbursts, it is harmful. Negative stress can also lead to substance abuse. An individual may smoke more, drink large amounts of alcohol, take drugs, or eat excessively to find comfort and escape from the negative feelings. Prolonged periods of harmful stress can lead to burnout or a mental breakdown. For this reason, an individual must become aware of the stressors in his/her life and learn methods to control them.

The first step in learning how to control stress is to identify stressors. Recognizing the symptoms of "fight or flight" can lead to an awareness of the factors that cause these symptoms. By keeping a list or diary of stressors, an individual can begin to evaluate ways to deal with the stressors and/or ways to eliminate them. When stressful events occur, note what the event was, why you feel stress, how much stress you experience, and how you deal with the stress. Do you tackle the cause of the stress or the symptom? This type of information allows you to understand the level

of stress you are comfortable with, the type of stress that motivates you effectively, and the type of stress that is unpleasant. If a chronic daily stressor is heavy traffic on the road to work, it may be time to evaluate the possibility of finding a new way to work, leaving earlier or later to avoid traffic, or finding a way to relax while stuck in traffic. Stressors are problems that must be solved or eliminated. One way to do this is to use the *problem-solving method.* It consists of the following steps:

- *Gather information or data.* Assess the situation to obtain all facts and opinions.
- *Identify the problem.* Try to identify the real stressor and why it is causing a reaction.
- *List possible solutions.* Look at all ways to eliminate or adapt to the stressor; include both good and bad ideas; then, evaluate each of the ideas and try to determine how effective it will be.
- *Make a plan.* After evaluating the solutions, choose one that you think will have the best outcome.
- *Act on your solution.* Use the solution to your problem to see if it has the expected outcome. Does it allow you to eliminate or adapt to the stressor?
- *Evaluate the results.* Determine whether the action was effective. Did it work or is another solution better?
- *Change the solution.* If necessary, use a different solution that might be more effective.

Learning to manage a stress reaction is another important way of dealing with stressors. When you become aware that a stressor is causing a physical reaction in your body, use the following four-step plan to gain control:

- *Stop*: immediately stop what you are doing to break out of the stress response
- *Breathe*: take a slow deep breath to relieve the physical tension you are feeling
- *Reflect*: think about the problem at hand and the cause of the stress
- *Choose*: determine how you want to deal with the stress

The brief pause that the four-step method requires allows an individual to become more aware of the stressor, the physical reaction to the stressor, and the actual cause of the stress. This awareness can then be used to determine whether a problem exists. If a problem does exist, a solution to the problem must be found.

Many other stress-reducing techniques can be used to manage stress. Some of the more common techniques include:

♦ *Live a healthy life*: eat balanced meals, get sufficient amounts of rest and sleep, and exercise on a regular basis

♦ *Take a break from stressors*: sit in a comfortable chair with your feet up

♦ *Relax*: take a warm bath

♦ *Escape*: listen to quiet, soothing music

♦ *Relieve tension*: shut your eyes, take slow deep breaths, and concentrate on relaxing each muscle that is tense

♦ *Rely on others*: talk with a friend and reach out to your support system (figure 4-11)

♦ *Meditate*: think about your values or beliefs in a higher power

♦ *Use imagery*: close your eyes and use all your senses to place yourself in a scene where you are at peace and relaxed

♦ *Enjoy yourself*: find an enjoyable leisure activity or hobby to provide "time outs"

♦ *Renew yourself*: learn new skills, take part in a professional organization, participate in community activities, and make every effort to continue growing as an individual

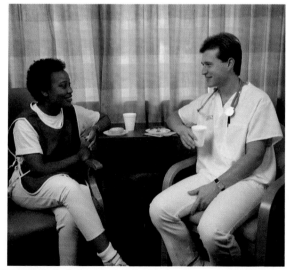

FIGURE 4-11 Relaxing and talking with a friend is one way to reduce stress.

♦ *Think positively*: reflect on your accomplishments and be proud of yourself

♦ *Develop outside interests*: provide time for yourself; do not allow a job to dominate your life

♦ *Seek assistance or delegate tasks*: ask others for help or delegate some tasks to others; remember that no one can do everything all of the time

♦ *Avoid too many commitments*: learn to say "no"

It is important to remember that stress is a constant presence in every individual's life and cannot be avoided. However, by being aware of the causes of stress, by learning how to respond when a stress reaction occurs, by solving problems effectively to eliminate stress, and by practicing techniques to reduce the effect of stress, an individual can deal with the daily stressors in his/her life and even benefit from them. It is also important for every health care worker to remember that patients also experience stress, especially when they are dealing with an illness and/or disability. The same techniques can be used by the health care worker to help patients learn to deal with stress.

4:7 INFORMATION

Time Management

One way to help prevent stress is to use time management. **Time management** is a system of practical skills that allows an individual to use time in the most effective and productive way possible. Time management helps prevent or reduce stress by putting the individual in charge, keeping things in perspective when events are overwhelming, increasing productivity, using time more effectively, improving enjoyment of activities, and providing time for relaxing and enjoying life.

The first step of time management is to keep an activity record for a period of several days. This allows an individual to determine how he/she actually uses the time available. By listing activities as they are performed, noting the amount of time each activity takes, and evaluating how effective the activity was, an individual can see patterns emerging. Certain periods of the day will show higher energy levels and an improved quality of work. Other periods may indicate that accomplishments are limited because of fatigue. Wasted time will also become apparent. Time spent looking for objects, talking on the telephone, playing games on a computer, and doing things that are not worthwhile is time that can be put to more constructive use. After this information has been obtained, an individual can begin to organize time. Important projects can be scheduled during the periods of the day when energy levels are high. Rest or relaxation periods can be scheduled when energy levels are low.

SETTING GOALS

Goal setting is another important factor of time management. A **goal** can be defined as a desired result or purpose toward which one is working. Goals can be compared with maps that help you find your direction and reach your destination. An old saying states, "If you don't know where you are going, you will never get there." Goals allow you to know where you are going and provide direction to your life.

Everyone should have both short- and long-term goals. Long-term goals are achievements that may take a period of years or even a lifetime to accomplish. Short-term goals usually take days, weeks, or months to accomplish. They are the smaller steps that are taken to reach the long-term goal. For example, a long-term goal might be to graduate from college with a health care degree.

If the person with this goal is starting high school, short-term goals might include:

♦ Research and learn about the wide variety of health careers.

♦ Job-shadow health careers that seem most interesting.

♦ Talk with people in different health care careers to find out about the careers.

♦ Complete job interest surveys to determine how your own skills and interests match requirements for different health careers.

♦ Discuss career opportunities with a guidance or career counselor.

♦ Attend job fairs or career planning days to obtain information on specific health careers.

♦ Use a computer to research health careers on the Internet.

♦ Narrow your career choices to the health care fields that you like best.

♦ Investigate which high-school courses you should take to meet college entry requirements for these health careers.

♦ Take the required courses in English, math, science, computer technology, and other specific academic areas.

♦ Explore the career and technology programs offered by your high school.

♦ Enroll in a health science technology education (HSTE) program if one is available.

♦ Join a student organization for HSTE students to network with other people who have similar interests.

♦ Obtain a job or work as a volunteer in health care areas to determine which career you like best.

♦ Research and visit different colleges or technical schools to learn about course offerings, financial aid, entry requirements, and other similar information.

When this person is in the junior or senior year of high school, short-term goals might include:

♦ Complete all required high-school courses and maintain a high grade point average.

♦ Confer with guidance or career counselors to obtain information on scholarships, financial help, career planning, college life, and other similar topics.

♦ Apply to several colleges or technical schools that have accredited programs in the chosen health field.

♦ Arrange for financial assistance and/or obtain a part-time job to save money for college.

♦ Check living arrangements at the college areas if living away from home will be necessary.

♦ After being accepted by colleges or technical schools, evaluate each individually to choose the school you will attend.

♦ Notify the school you have selected before the established deadline for enrollment.

These short-term goals are basic suggestions. Each individual has to establish his/her own goals. It is important to remember that short-term goals will change constantly as one set is completed and a new set is established. Completion of a goal, however, will lead to a sense of satisfaction and accomplishment, and provide motivation to attempt other goals. To set goals effectively, you must observe certain points. These points include:

♦ *State goals in a positive manner.* Use words such as "accomplish" rather than "avoid."

♦ *Define goals clearly and precisely.* If possible, set a time limit to accomplish the goal.

♦ *Prioritize multiple goals.* Determine which goals are the most important and complete them first.

♦ *Write goals down.* This makes the goal seem real and attainable.

♦ *Make sure each goal is at the right level.* Goals should present a challenge, but not be too difficult or impossible to complete.

After goals have been established, concentrate on ways to accomplish them. Review necessary skills, information that must be obtained, resources you can use, problems that may occur, and which goal should be completed first. Basically, this is just organizing the steps that will lead to achieving the goal. After the goal has been achieved, enjoy your sense of accomplishment and satisfaction for a job well done. If you fail in obtaining the goal, evaluate the situation and determine why you failed. Was the goal unrealistic? Did you lack the skills or knowledge to obtain the goal? Is there another way to achieve the goal? Remember that failure can be a positive learning experience.

TIME MANAGEMENT PLAN

Time management is used to ensure success in meeting established goals. A daily planner and calendar are essential tools. These tools allow an individual to write everything down, organize all information, become aware of conflicts (two things to do at the same time), and provide an organized schedule to follow. An effective time management plan involves the following seven steps:

♦ *Analyze and prioritize*: review and list established goals; determine what tasks must be completed to achieve goals; list tasks in order,

from the most important to the least important; decide if any tasks can be delegated to another person to complete and delegate whenever possible; eliminate unnecessary tasks

♦ *Identify habits and preferences*: know when you have the most energy to complete work and when it is best to schedule rest, exercise, or social activities

♦ *Schedule tasks*: use the daily planner and calendar to write down all events; be sure to include time for rest, exercise, meals, hobbies, and social activities; if a conflict arises with two things scheduled at the same time, prioritize and reschedule

♦ *Make a daily "to do" list*: list all tasks on a daily basis; as you complete each one, cross it off the list; enjoy the sense of satisfaction that occurs as you complete each job; if some things on the list are not completed at the end of the day, determine if they should be added to the next day's list or if they can be eliminated

♦ *Plan your work*: work at a comfortable pace; try to do the hardest tasks first; do one thing at a time whenever possible so you can complete it and cross it off the list; make sure you have everything you need to complete the task before you begin; ask for assistance when needed; work smarter, not harder

♦ *Avoid distractions*: make every effort to avoid interruptions; use a telephone answering system and screen calls; avoid procrastination; learn to say "no" when asked to interrupt your work for something that is not essential

♦ *Take credit for a job well done*: when a job is complete, recognize your achievement; cross the completed work off the list; if the task was a particularly hard one, reward yourself with a short break or other positive thing before going on to the next job on the list

These steps of time management provide for an organized and efficient use of time. However, even with careful planning, things do not always get done according to plan. Unexpected emergencies, a new assignment, a complication, and/or overscheduling are common events in the life of a health care worker. When a time management plan does not work, try to determine the reasons for failure. Reevaluate goals and revise the plan. Patience, practice, and an honest effort will eventually produce a plan that provides self-satisfaction for achieving goals, less stress, qual-

ity time for rest and relaxation, a sense of being in control, a healthier lifestyle, and increased productivity.

TODAY'S RESEARCH: TOMORROW'S HEALTH CARE

Melting fat to lose weight?

According to statistics from the National Health and Nutrition Examination Survey, nearly two-thirds of adults in the United States are overweight. In addition, more than one-third of these individuals are extremely overweight, or obese (20 percent or more above the recommended weight). Research has shown that obesity is a risk factor for the development of diabetes, heart disease, hypertension (high blood pressure), stroke, and even some forms of cancer.

Scientists are now researching a unique approach to treat obesity. They are trying to starve adipose (fatty) tissue by destroying the blood vessels that feed it. Fat cells grow and multiply quickly by creating tiny blood vessels called *capillaries*, which provide nourishment. Estimates are that 1 pound of fat contains a mile of blood vessels. A protein, prohibitin, located on the surface of fat-feeding blood vessels, seems to regulate cell growth. Scientists have developed a compound that attaches to prohibitin and selectively destroys the blood vessels. When the compound was injected into obese mice, the mice lost about 30 percent of their body weight within 4 weeks. Further research is now being conducted to determine the effect of this compound on baboons.

One obstacle to using this compound in humans is that prohibitin is found in cells throughout the body. Care will have to be taken to make sure that other tissues and blood vessels are not destroyed. If researchers are able to create a substance that destroys only the blood vessels to adipose tissue, they will be able to "melt" fat by literally starving it to death. If this occurs, obesity and many of the diseases caused by obesity will be eliminated.

STUDENT: *Go to the workbook and complete the assignment sheet for Chapter 4, Personal and Professional Qualities of a Health Care Worker.*

CHAPTER 4 SUMMARY

Certain personal characteristics, attitudes, and rules of appearance apply to health care workers in all health careers. Every health care worker must constantly strive to develop the necessary characteristics and to present a professional appearance.

A professional appearance helps inspire confidence and a positive self-image. Good health is an important part of appearance. By eating correctly, obtaining adequate rest, exercising daily, observing the rules of good posture, and avoiding the use of tobacco, alcohol, and drugs, a health care worker can strive to maintain good health. Wearing the appropriate uniform or appropriate clothing and shoes is essential to projecting the proper image. Proper hair and nail care, good personal hygiene, and limited makeup also help create a professional appearance.

Personal characteristics such as honesty, dependability, patience, enthusiasm, responsibility, discretion, and competence are essential. In addition, health care workers must be willing to learn and to accept criticism. These characteristics must be practiced and learned.

Effective communication is an important aspect of helping individuals through stages of growth and development and in meeting needs. A health care worker must have an understanding of the communication process, factors that interfere with communication, the importance of listening, and verbal and nonverbal communication. Another important aspect of communication is the proper reporting or recording of all observations noted while providing care.

Communication barriers such as physical disabilities, psychological attitudes, and cultural diversity can interfere with the communication process. Special consideration must be given to these barriers to improve communication. Some cultural groups have beliefs and practices that may relate to health and illness. Because individuals will respond to health care according to their cultural beliefs, a health care worker must be aware of and show respect for different cultural values in order to provide optimal patient care.

Teamwork is important in any health care career. Interdisciplinary health care teams provide quality holistic health care to every patient. Teamwork improves communication and continuity of care. A picture of the patient's total care plan is clear when the role of each team member is known. For a team to function effectively, it needs a qualified leader, good interpersonal relationships, ways to avoid or deal with conflict, positive attitudes, and respect for legal responsibilities. Effective teams are the result of hard work, patience, commitment, and practice.

Leadership is a skill that can be learned by mastering the characteristics of a leader. A leader may or may not be a supervisor; any member of a group that contributes to the group's goals can be considered a leader. Of the three types of leaders—democratic, laissez-faire, and autocratic—the democratic leader is the most effective for group interaction.

Stress is a component in every individual's life. Stress can be good or bad, depending on the person's perception of and reaction to the stress. By being aware of the causes of stress, learning how to respond when a stress reaction occurs, solving problems to eliminate stress, and practicing techniques to reduce the effect of stress, an individual can deal with stress and even benefit from it.

Time management is a system of practical skills that allow an individual to use time in the most effective and productive way possible. It involves analyzing how one actually uses the time available, establishing short- and long-term goals, prioritizing tasks that must be accomplished, identifying habits and preferences, preparing written "to do" lists and crossing off work that has been completed, planning work carefully, avoiding distractions, and taking credit for a job well done. An effective time management plan will reduce stress, help an individual attain goals, increase self-confidence, lead to a healthier lifestyle, and provide quality time for rest and relaxation.

Health care workers must learn and follow the standards and requirements established by the health care facility in which they are employed.

INTERNET SEARCHES

Use the suggested search engine in Chapter 17:4 of this textbook to search the Internet for additional information on the following topics:

1. *Uniform companies*: search "uniform suppliers" to locate companies that sell professional uniforms and compare styles, prices, and so forth.

2. *Professional characteristics*: choose a specific health care career and search for career descriptions; list the required personal qualities or characteristics necessary for the career you have chosen.

3. *Communication*: search for information on listening skills, nonverbal communication, and the communication process.

4. *Leadership*: search for information on types and characteristics of leaders; evaluate which types would be most effective in guiding a health care team.

5. *Stress*: search for information on stress and stress-reducing techniques.

6. *Time management*: search for information on time management.

REVIEW QUESTIONS

1. What five (5) main factors contribute to good health?

2. Identify eight (8) specific principles that must be followed for a professional appearance.

3. Create a personal description of yourself showing why you display at least six (6) of the

personal characteristics desired in a health care worker.

4. Why is it important to observe both verbal and nonverbal communication? Create a specific example of a situation showing how both verbal and nonverbal communication convey a message.

5. List five (5) factors that can interfere with the communication process. Give two (2) specific examples for each factor.

6. Differentiate between objective and subjective observations. List two (2) examples for each type of observation.

7. A patient is admitted to a hospital to give birth to her baby. Identify at least ten (10) health care professionals who may be on the team that provide her care. Review the many careers in Chapter 3 to prepare your list.

8. List six (6) characteristics of an effective leader.

9. Identify the three (3) types of leaders and describe their style of leadership.

10. Identify at least one major stress in your life. List the steps of the problem-solving method and then apply the stressor you have chosen to each of the steps. Identify at least three (3) courses of action that you can take.

11. List six (6) stress-reducing techniques that you find beneficial. State why they help you reduce stress.

12. Differentiate between short- and long-term goals. How are they related? How are they different?

13. What are the main goals of time management?

CHAPTER 5

Legal and Ethical Responsibilities

Chapter Objectives

After completing this chapter,
you should be able to:

◆ Provide one example of a situation that might result in legal action for each of the following: malpractice; negligence; assault and battery; invasion of privacy; false imprisonment; abuse; and defamation

◆ Describe how contract laws affect health care

◆ Define *privileged communications* and explain how they apply to health care

◆ State the legal regulations that apply to health care records

◆ Define HIPAA and explain how it provides confidentiality for health care information

◆ List at least six basic rules of ethics for health care personnel

◆ List at least six rights of the patient who is receiving health care

◆ Justify at least eight professional standards by explaining how they help meet legal/ethical requirements

◆ Define, pronounce, and spell all key terms

Observe Standard Precautions

Instructor's Check—Call Instructor at This Point

Safety—Proceed with Caution

OBRA Requirement—Based on Federal Law

Math Skill

Legal Responsibility

Science Skill

Career Information

Communications Skill

Technology

KEY TERMS

abuse
advance directives
agent
assault and battery
civil law
confidentiality *(con"-fih-den-chee"-ahl'-ih-tee)*
contract
criminal law
defamation *(deff"-ah-may'-shun)*
Designation of Health Care Surrogate

Durable Power of Attorney (POA)
ethics *(eth'-iks)*
expressed contracts
false imprisonment
health care records
implied contracts
informed consent
invasion of privacy
legal
legal disability
libel *(ly'-bull)*

living wills
malpractice
negligence *(neg'-lih-gents)*
Patient Self-Determination Act (PSDA)
Patient's Bill of Rights
patients' rights
privileged communications
Resident's Bill of Rights
slander
tort

5:1 INFORMATION
Legal Responsibilities

INTRODUCTION

In every aspect of life, there are certain laws and legal responsibilities formulated to protect you and society. An excellent example is the need to obey traffic laws when driving a motor vehicle. A worker in any health career also has certain responsibilities. Being aware of and following legal regulations is important for your own protection, the protection of your employer, and the safety and well-being of the patient.

Legal responsibilities are those that are authorized or based on law. A law is a rule that must be followed. Laws are created and enforced by the federal, state, or local government. Health care workers must follow any laws that affect health care. In addition, *health care professionals/ workers are also required to know and follow the state laws that regulate their respective licenses or registrations or set standards for their respective professions.* Failure to meet your legal responsibilities can result in legal action against you and your employer.

Two main types of laws affect health care workers: criminal laws and civil laws.

♦ *Criminal law:* focuses on behavior known as crime; deals with the wrongs against a person, property, or society; examples include practicing in a health profession without having the required license, illegal possession of drugs, misuse of narcotics, theft, sexual assault, and murder

♦ *Civil law:* focuses on the legal relationships between people and the protection of a person's rights; in health care, civil law usually involves torts and contracts

TORTS

A **tort** is a wrongful act that does not involve a contract. It is called a civil wrong instead of a crime. A tort occurs when a person is harmed or injured because a health care provider does not meet the established or expected standards of care. Many different types of torts can lead to legal action. These offenses may be quite complex and may be open to different legal interpretations. Some of the more common torts include the following:

♦ *Malpractice:* Malpractice can be interpreted as "bad practice" and is commonly called "professional negligence." It can be defined as the failure of a professional to use the degree of skill and learning commonly expected in that individual's profession, resulting in injury, loss, or damage to the person receiving care. Examples might include a physician not administering a tetanus injection when a patient has a puncture wound, or a nurse performing minor surgery without having any training.

♦ **Negligence:** Negligence can be described as failure to give care that is normally expected of a person in a particular position, resulting in injury to another person. Examples include falls and injuries that occur when siderails are left down (figure 5-1), using or not reporting defective equipment, infections caused by the use of nonsterile instruments and/or supplies, and burns caused by improper heat or radiation treatments.

♦ **Assault and battery:** Assault includes a threat or attempt to injure, and battery includes the unlawful touching of another person without consent. They are closely related and often used together. Examples of assault and battery include performing a procedure after a patient has refused to give permission, threatening a patient, and improper handling or rough treatment of a patient while providing care.

It is important to remember that patients must give consent for any care, and that they have the right to refuse care. Some procedures or practices require written consent from the patient. Examples can include surgery, certain diagnostic tests, experimental procedures, treatment of minors (individuals younger than legal age, which varies from state to state), and even simple things such as siderail releases for a patient who wants siderails left down when other factors indicate siderails should be up to protect the patient. Verbal consent is permitted in other cases, but the law states that this

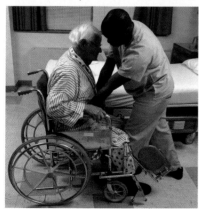

FIGURE 5-1 A nurse assistant could be charged with negligence if a patient is injured because the foot rests on a wheelchair are not moved up and out of the way before the patient is transferred to the chair.

must be "informed consent." **Informed consent** is permission granted voluntarily by a person who is of sound mind after the procedure and all risks involved have been explained in terms the person can understand. It is important to remember that a person has the right to withdraw consent at any time. Therefore, all procedures must be explained to the patient, and no procedure should be performed if the patient does not give consent.

♦ **Invasion of privacy:** Invasion of privacy includes unnecessarily exposing an individual or revealing personal information about an individual without that person's consent. Examples include improperly draping or covering a patient during a procedure so that other patients or personnel can see the patient exposed; sending information regarding a patient to an insurance company without the patient's written permission; or informing the news media of a patient's condition without the patient's permission.

♦ **False imprisonment:** False imprisonment refers to restraining an individual or restricting an individual's freedom. Examples include keeping patients hospitalized against their will, or applying physical restraints without proper authorization or with no justification.

It is important to remember that patients have the right to leave a hospital or health care facility without a physician's permission. If this occurs, the patient is usually asked to sign an AMA (Against Medical Advice) form. If the patient refuses to sign the form, this must be documented in the patient record and the physician must be notified.

Physical restraints are devices used to limit a patient's movements. They should be used *only* to protect patients from harming themselves or others and when all other measures to control the situation have failed. A physician's order must be obtained before they are used, and strict guidelines must be observed while they are in use.

♦ **Abuse:** Abuse includes any care that results in physical harm, pain, or mental anguish. Examples of types of abuse include:

♦ *Physical abuse:* hitting, forcing people against their will, restraining movement, depriving people of food or water, and/or not providing physical care

♦ *Verbal abuse*: speaking harshly, swearing or shouting, using inappropriate words to describe a person's race or nationality, and/or writing threats or abusive statements

♦ *Psychological abuse*: threatening harm; denying rights; belittling, intimidating, or ridiculing the person; and/or threatening to reveal information about the person

♦ *Sexual abuse*: any unwanted sexual touching or act, using sexual gestures, and/or suggesting sexual behavior

Patients may experience abuse before entering a health care facility. Domestic abuse occurs when an intimate partner uses threatening, manipulative, aggressive, or violent behavior to maintain power and control over another person. If abuse is directed toward a child, it is child abuse. If it is directed toward an older person, it is elder abuse. Health care providers must be alert to the signs and symptoms that may indicate patients in their care are victims of abuse. These may include:

♦ unexplained bruises, fractures, burns, or injuries

♦ signs of neglect such as poor personal hygiene

♦ irrational fears or a change in personality

♦ aggressive or withdrawn behavior

♦ patient statements that indicate abuse or neglect

Many of the other torts can lead to charges of abuse, or a charge of abuse can occur alone. Laws in all states require that any form of abuse be reported to the proper authorities. Even though the signs and symptoms do not always mean a person is being abused, their presence indicates a need for further investigation. Health care workers are required to report any signs or symptoms of abuse to their immediate supervisor or to the individual in the health care facility responsible for reporting the suspicions to the proper authorities.

Defamation: Defamation occurs when false statements either cause a person to be ridiculed or damage the person's reputation. Incorrect information given out in error can result in defamation. If the information is spoken, it is **slander;** if it is written, it is **libel.** Examples include reporting that a patient has an infectious disease to a gov-ernment agency when laboratory results are inaccurate, telling others that a person has a drug problem when another medical condition actually exists, or saying that a co-worker is incompetent.

CONTRACTS

In addition to tort laws, contract laws also affect health care. A **contract** is an agreement between two or more parties. Most contracts have three parts:

♦ *Offer*: a competent individual enters into a relationship with a health care provider and offers to be a patient

♦ *Acceptance*: the health care provider gives an appointment or examines or treats the patient

♦ *Consideration*: the payment made by the patient for the services provided

Contracts in health care are implied or expressed. **Implied contracts** are those obligations that are understood without verbally expressed terms. For example, when a qualified health worker prepares a medication and a patient takes the medication, it is implied that the patient accepts this treatment. **Expressed contracts** are stated in distinct and clear language, either orally or in writing. An example is a surgery permit. Promises of care must be kept. Therefore, all risks associated with treatment must be explained completely to the patient (figure 5-2).

All parties entering into a contract must be free of **legal disability.** A person who has a legal disability does not have the legal capacity to form a contract. Examples of people with legal disabilities are minors (individuals under legal age), mentally incompetent persons, individuals under the influence of drugs that alter the mental state, and semiconscious or unconscious people. In such cases, parents, guardians, or others permitted by law must form the contract for the individual.

A contract requires that certain standards of care be provided by competent, qualified individuals. If the contract is not performed according to agreement, the contract is breached. Failure to provide care and/or giving improper care on the part of the health provider, or failure on the part of the patient to pay according to the consid-

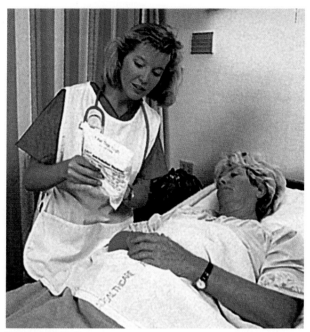

FIGURE 5-2 All risks of treatment must be explained to a patient before asking the patient for permission to administer treatment.

eration, can be considered breach of contract and cause for legal action.

To comply with legal mandates, an interpreter/translator must be used when a contract is explained to a non-English-speaking individual. In addition, many states require the use of interpreter services for individuals who are deaf or hard of hearing. Most health care agencies have a list of interpreters who can be used in these situations. At times, an English-speaking relative or friend of the patient can also serve as an interpreter.

A final important consideration in contract law is the role of the **agent.** When a person works under the direction or control of another person, the employer is called the *principal*, and the person working under the employer is called the *agent*. The principal is responsible for the actions of the agent and can be required to pay or otherwise compensate people who have been injured by the agent. For example, if a dental assistant tells a patient "your dentures will look better than your real teeth," the dentist may have to compensate the patient financially should this statement prove false. Health care workers should therefore be aware of their role as agents of their employers and work to protect the interests of their employers.

PRIVILEGED COMMUNICATIONS

Privileged communications are another important aspect of legal responsibility. Privileged communications comprise all information given to health care personnel by a patient; by law, this information must be kept confidential and shared only with other members of the patient's health care team. It cannot be told to anyone else without the written consent of the patient. The consent should state what information is to be released, to whom the information should be given, and any applicable time limits. Certain information is exempt by law and must be reported. Examples of exempt information are births and deaths; injuries caused by violence (such as assault and battery, abuse, stabbings) that may require police involvement; drug abuse; communicable diseases; and sexually transmitted diseases.

Health care records are also considered privileged communications. Such records contain information about the care provided to the patient. Although such records belong to the health care provider (for example, the physician, dentist, hospital, long-term care facility), the patient has a right to obtain a copy of any information in the record. Health care records can be used as legal records in a court of law. Erasures are therefore not allowed on such records. Errors should be crossed out with a single line so material is still readable. Correct information should then be inserted, initialed, and dated. If necessary, an explanation for the correction should also be provided. Health care records must be properly maintained, kept confidential, and retained for the amount of time required by state law (figure 5-3). When records are destroyed after the legal time for retention, they should be burned or shredded to maintain confidentiality.

The growing use of computerized records has created a dilemma in maintaining confidentiality (figure 5-4). In a large health care facility such as a hospital, many different individuals may have access to a patient's records. For this reason, health care providers are creating safeguards to maintain computer confidentiality. Some examples include limiting personnel who have access to such records, using codes to prevent access to certain information, requiring passwords to access specific information on records, and constantly monitoring and evaluating computer use.

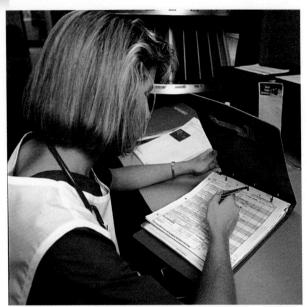

FIGURE 5-3 Confidentiality must be maintained with regard to health care records.

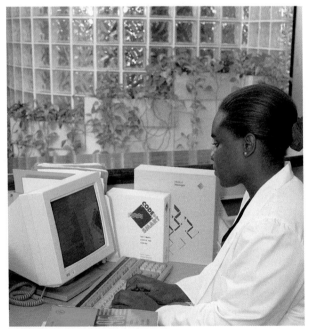

FIGURE 5-4 The growing use of computerized records has created the need for limiting access to computers to maintain confidentiality.

PRIVACY ACT

The federal government is concerned about protecting privileged communications and maintaining confidentiality of health care records. In the Health Insurance Portability and Account- ability Act (HIPAA) of 1996, Congress required the U.S. Department of Health and Human Services (USDHHS) to establish standards to protect health information. The USDHHS published the *Standards for Privacy of Individually Identifiable Health Information* (commonly called the Privacy Rule), which went into effect in 2003. These standards provide federal protection for privacy of health information in all states.

HIPAA regulations in the Privacy Rule require every health care provider to inform patients about how their health information is used. Patients must sign a consent form (figure 5-5) ascertaining that they have received the information before any health care provider can use the health information for diagnosis, treatment, billing, insurance claims, or quality care assessments.

In addition, before a health care provider can release information to anyone else, such as another health care provider, attorney, insurance company, federal or state agency, or even other members of the patient's family, a patient must sign an authorization form for the release of this information (figure 5-6). This authorization form must identify the purpose or need for the information, the extent of the information that may be released, any limits on the release of information, the date of authorization, and the signature of the person authorized to give consent. These requirements are used to ensure the privacy and confidentiality of a patient's health care information. The only exception to these regulations is for the release of information on diseases or injuries that must be reported by law to protect the safety and welfare of the public. Examples of exempt information include births, deaths, injuries caused by violence that require police involvement, communicable diseases, and sexually transmitted diseases.

Other requirements of the privacy standards are that patients must be:

♦ able to see and obtain copies of their medical records

♦ given information by health care providers about how they use medical information

♦ allowed to set limits on how personal health information is used

♦ permitted to request that health care providers take reasonable care to keep communications confidential

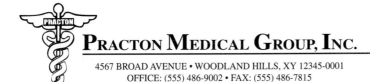

PRACTON MEDICAL GROUP, INC.

4567 BROAD AVENUE • WOODLAND HILLS, XY 12345-0001
OFFICE: (555) 486-9002 • FAX: (555) 486-7815

Fran Practon, M.D.
Gerald Practon, M.D.

CONSENT TO THE USE AND DISCLOSURE OF HEALTH INFORMATION

I understand that this organization originates and maintains health records which describe my health history, symptoms, examination, test results, diagnoses, treatment, and any plans for future care or treatment. I understand that this information is used to:

- plan my care and treatment
- communicate among health professionals who contribute to my care
- apply my diagnosis and services, procedures, and surgical information to my bill
- verify services billed by third-party payers
- assess quality of care and review the competence of health care professionals in routine health care operations

I further understand that:

- a complete description of information uses and disclosures is included in a *Notice of Information Practices* which has been provided to me
- I have a right to review the notice prior to signing this consent
- the organization reserves the right to change their notice and practices
- any revised notice will be mailed to the address I have provided prior to implementation
- I have the right to object to the use of my health information for directory purposes
- I have the right to request restrictions as to how my health information may be used or disclosed to carry out treatment, payment, or health care operations
- the organization is not required to agree to the restrictions requested
- I may revoke this consent in writing, except to the extent that the organization has already taken action in reliance thereon.

☐ I request the following restrictions to the use or disclosure of my health information.

June 29, 20XX
Date

June 29, 20XX
Notice Effective Date

Consuelo Hernandez
Signature of Patient or Legal Representative

Witness

Signature

Title

_____ Accepted _____ Rejected

Date

FIGURE 5-5 Example of a Health Insurance Portability and Accountability Act (HIPAA) required form providing consent to the use and disclosure of health information.

AUTHORIZATION FOR RELEASE OF INFORMATION

Section A: Must be completed for all authorizations.

I hereby authorize the use or disclosure of my individually identifiable health information as described below.
I understand that this authorization is voluntary. I understand that if the organization authorized to receive the information is not a health plan or health care provider, the released information may no longer be protected by federal privacy regulations.

Identity of person/organization disclosing protected health information

Patient name: _Hilda F. Goodman_   **ID Number:**   _4309_

Persons/organizations providing information: **Persons/organizations receiving information:**
Practon Medical Group, Inc   _Jennifer P. Lee, MD_
4567 Broad Avenue   _400 North M Street_
Woodland Hills, XY 12345-4700   _Anytown, XY 54098-1235_

Identity of those authorized to use protected health information

Specific description of information [including from and to date(s)]:
Complete medical records from 4-22-XX to 9-15-XX

Specific description of information to be used or disclosed with dates

Section B: Must be completed only if a health plan or a heath care provider has requested the authorization.

Purpose for disclosure

1. The health plan or health care provider must complete the following:
   a. What is the purpose of the use or disclosure?_____Patient relocating to another city_____

   b. Will the health plan or health care provider requesting the authorization receive financial or in-kind compensation in exchange for using or disclosing the health information described above? Yes___ No_X_

2. The patient or the patient's representative must read and initial the following statements:
   a. I understand that my health care and the payment for my health care will not be affected if I do not sign this form.
                                                         Initials: _hfg_

   b. I understand that I may see and copy the information described on this form if I ask for it, and that I get a copy of this form after I sign it.
                                                         Initials: _hfg_

Section C: Must be completed for all authorizations.

The patient or the patient's representative must read and initial the following statements:

Expiration date

1. I understand that this authorization will expire on _12_ / _31_ / _20XX_ (DD/MM/YR).
                                                         Initials: _hfg_

Individual's right to revoke this authorization in writing

2. I understand that I may revoke this authorization at any time by notifying the providing organization in writing, but if I do not it will not have any effect on any actions they took before they received the revocation.
                                                         Initials: _hfg_

Redisclosure conditions

3. I understand that any disclosure of information carries with it the potential for an unauthorized redisclosure and the information may not be protected by federal confidentiality rules.
                                                         Initials: _hfg_

Individual's signature

_____Hilda F. Goodman_____   _____September 15, 20XX_____
Signature of patient or patient's representative   **Date**
(Form MUST be completed before signing)

Date of signature

Printed name of patient's representative:_____

Relationship to the patient:_____

YOU MAY REFUSE TO SIGN THIS AUTHORIZATION
You may not use this form to release information for treatment or payment except
when the information to be released is psychotherapy notes or certain research information.

FIGURE 5-6 Example of an authorization to release health information form.

- given the right to state who has access to their information, and even limit providing information to their family
- provided with information on how to file a complaint against a health care provider who violates the privacy act

Health care providers must be aware of these standards and make every effort to protect the privacy and confidentiality of a patient's health care information.

SUMMARY

Legal responsibilities are important aspects of health care. All states have rules and regulations governing health care. In addition, most health care agencies have specific rules, regulations, and standards that determine activities performed by individuals holding different positions of employment. Standards can vary from state to state, and even from agency to agency. It is important to remember that you are liable, or legally responsible, for your own actions regardless of what anyone tells you or what position you hold. Therefore, when you undertake a particular position of employment in a health agency, *it is your responsibility to learn exactly what you are legally permitted to do, and to familiarize yourself with your exact responsibilities.*

5:2 INFORMATION

Ethics

Legal responsibilities are determined by law. **Ethics** are a set of principles relating to what is morally right or wrong. Ethics provide a standard of conduct or code of behavior. This allows a health care provider to analyze information and make decisions based on what people believe is right and good conduct. Modern health care advances, however, have created many ethical dilemmas for health care providers. Some of these dilemmas include:

♦ Is euthanasia (assisted death) justified in certain patients?

♦ Should a patient be told that a health care provider has AIDS?

♦ Should aborted fetuses be used for research?

♦ When should life support be discontinued?

♦ Do parents have a religious right to refuse a life-saving blood transfusion for their child?

♦ Can a health care facility refuse to provide expensive treatment such as a bone marrow transplant if a patient cannot pay for the treatment?

♦ Who decides whether a 75-year-old patient or a 56-year-old patient gets a single kidney available for transplant?

♦ Should people be allowed to sell organs for use in transplants?

♦ If a person can benefit from marijuana, should a physician be allowed to prescribe it as a treatment?

♦ Should animals be used in medical research even if it results in the death of the animal?

♦ Should genetic researchers be allowed to transplant specific genes to create the "perfect" human being?

♦ Should human beings be cloned?

♦ Should aborted embryos be used to obtain stem cells for research, especially since scientists may be able to use the stem cells to cure diseases such as diabetes, osteoporosis, and Parkinson's?

Although there are no easy answers to any of these questions, some guidelines are provided by an ethical code. Most of the national organizations affiliated with the different health care occupations have established ethical codes for personnel in their respective occupations. Although such codes differ slightly, most contain the same basic principles:

♦ Put the saving of life and the promotion of health above all else.

♦ Make every effort to keep the patient as comfortable as possible and to preserve life whenever possible.

♦ Respect the patient's choice to die peacefully and with dignity when all options have been discussed with the patient and family and/or predetermined by advance directives.

♦ Treat all patients equally, regardless of race, religion, social or economic status, sex, or nationality. Bias, prejudice, and discrimination have no place in health care.

♦ Provide care for *all* individuals to the best of your ability.

♦ Maintain a competent level of skill consistent with your particular occupation.

♦ Stay informed and up to date, and pursue continuing education as necessary.

♦ Maintain **confidentiality.** Confidentiality means that information about the patient must remain private and can be shared *only* with other members of the patient's health care team. A legal violation can occur if a patient suffers personal or financial damage when confidential information is shared with others, including family members. Information obtained from patients should not be repeated or used for personal gain. Gossiping about patients is ethically wrong.

♦ Refrain from immoral, unethical, and illegal practices. If you observe others taking part in illegal actions, report such actions to the proper authorities.

♦ Show loyalty to patients, co-workers, and employers. Avoid negative or derogatory statements, and always express a positive attitude.

♦ Be sincere, honest, and caring. Treat others as you want to be treated. Show respect and concern for the feelings, dignity, and rights of others.

When you enter a health occupation, learn the code of ethics for that occupation. Make every effort to abide by the code so as to become a competent and ethical health care worker. In doing so, you will earn the respect and confidence of patients, co-workers, and employers.

5:3 INFORMATION

Patients' Rights

 Federal and state legislation requires health care agencies to have written policies concerning **patients' rights,** or the factors of care that patients can expect to receive. Agencies expect all personnel to respect and honor these rights.

The American Hospital Association has affirmed a **Patient's Bill of Rights** that is recognized and honored by many health care facilities. This bill of rights states, in part, that a patient has the right to:

♦ Considerate and respectful care

♦ Obtain complete, current information concerning diagnosis, treatment, and prognosis (expected outcome)

♦ Receive information necessary to give informed consent prior to the start of any procedure or treatment

♦ Have advance directives for health care and/or refuse treatment to the extent permitted under law (figure 5-7)

♦ Privacy concerning a medical care program

♦ Confidential treatment of all communications and records

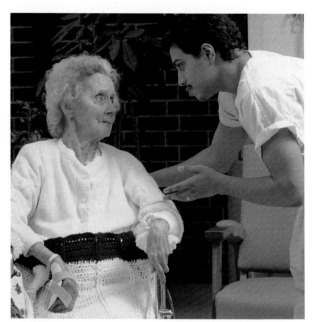

FIGURE 5-7 Patients have the right to refuse treatment.

♦ Reasonable response to a request for services

♦ Obtain information regarding any relationship of the hospital to other health care and educational institutions

♦ Be advised of and have the right to refuse to participate in any research project

♦ Expect reasonable continuity of care

♦ Review medical records and examine bills and receive an explanation of all care and charges

♦ Be informed of any hospital rules, regulations, and/or policies and the resources available to resolve disputes or grievances

Residents in long-term care facilities are guaranteed certain rights under the Omnibus Budget Reconciliation Act (OBRA) of 1987. Every long-term care facility must inform residents or their guardians of these rights and a copy must be posted in each facility. This is often called a **Resident's Bill of Rights** and states, in part, that a resident has the right to:

♦ Free choice regarding physician, treatment, care, and participation in research

♦ Freedom from abuse and chemical or physical restraints

♦ Privacy and confidentiality of personal and clinical records

♦ Accommodation of needs and choice regarding activities, schedules, and health care

♦ Voice grievances without fear of retaliation or discrimination

♦ Organize and participate in family/resident groups and in social, religious, and community activities

♦ Information on medical benefits, medical records, survey results, deficiencies of the facility, and advocacy groups including the ombudsman program (state representative who checks on resident care and violation of rights)

♦ Manage personal funds and use personal possessions

♦ Unlimited access to immediate family or relatives and to share a room with his or her spouse, if both are residents (figure 5-8)

♦ Remain in the facility and not be transferred or discharged except for medical reasons, the welfare of the resident or others, failure to pay, or if the facility either cannot meet the resident's needs or ceases to operate

All states have adopted these rights, and some have added additional rights. It is important to check state law and obtain a list of rights established in your state. Health care workers can face job loss, fines, and even imprisonment if they do not follow and grant established patients' or residents' rights. By observing these rights, the health care worker helps ensure the patient's safety, privacy, and well-being, and provides quality care at all times.

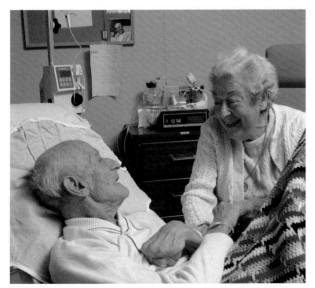

FIGURE 5-8 A married couple in a long-term care facility has the legal right to share a room if both members of the couple are residents in the facility.

5:4 INFORMATION

Advance Directives for Health Care

Advance directives for health care, also known as *legal directives,* are legal documents that allow individuals to state what medical treatment they want or do not want in the event that they become incapacitated and are unable to express their wishes regarding medical care. Two main directives are a living will and a Designation of Health Care Surrogate or a Durable Power of Attorney (POA) for Health Care.

Living wills (figure 5-9) are documents that allow individuals to state what measures should or should not be taken to prolong life when their conditions are terminal (death is expected). The document must be signed when the individual is competent and witnessed by two adults who cannot benefit from the death. Most states now have laws that allow the withholding of life-sustaining procedures and that honor living wills. A living will frequently results in a Do Not Resuscitate (DNR) order for a terminally ill individual. The DNR order means that cardiopulmonary resuscitation is not performed when the patient stops breathing. The patient is allowed to die with peace and dignity. At times this is extremely difficult for health care workers to honor. It is important to remember that many individuals believe that the quality of life is important and a life on support systems has no meaning or purpose for them.

A **Designation of Health Care Surrogate,** also called a **Durable Power of Attorney (POA)** for Health Care, is a document that permits an individual (known as a principal) to appoint another person (known as an agent) to make any decisions regarding health care if the principal should become unable to make decisions (figure 5-10). This includes providing or withholding specific medical or surgical procedures, hiring or dismissing health care providers, spending or withholding funds for health care, and having access to medical records. Although they are most frequently given to spouses or adult children, POAs can be given to any qualified adult. To meet legal requirements, the POA must be signed by the principal, agent, and one or two adult witnesses.

A federal law, called the **Patient Self-Determination Act (PSDA)** of 1990, mandates that all

FLORIDA LIVING WILL – PAGE 1 OF 2

INSTRUCTIONS

PRINT THE DATE

Declaration made this _____ day of _____, _____,
(day)   (month)   (year)

PRINT YOUR NAME

I, _____,
willfully and voluntarily make known my desire that my dying not be
artificially prolonged under the circumstances set forth below, and I do
hereby declare that :

PLEASE INITIAL
EACH THAT APPLIES

If at any time I am incapacitated and

_____ I have a terminal condition, or

_____ I have an end-stage condition, or

_____ I am in a persistent vegetative state

and if my attending or treating physician and another consulting physician
have determined that there is no reasonable medical probability of my
recovery from such condition, I direct that life-prolonging procedures be
withheld or withdrawn when the application of such procedures would
serve only to prolong artificially the process of dying, and that I be
permitted to die naturally with only the administration of medication or
the performance of any medical procedure deemed necessary to provide
me with comfort care or to alleviate pain.

It is my intention that this declaration be honored by my family and
physician as the final expression of my legal right to refuse medical or
surgical treatment and to accept the consequences for such refusal. In the
event that I have been determined to be unable to provide express and
informed consent regarding the withholding, withdrawal, or continuation
of life-prolonging procedures, I wish to designate, as my surrogate to
carry out the provision of this declaration:

PRINT THE NAME,
HOME ADDRESS
AND TELEPHONE
NUMBER OF YOUR
SURROGATE

Name: _____

Address: _____

_____ Zip Code: _____

Phone: _____

© 2005 National
Hospice and
Palliative Care
Organization
2006 Revised

FLORIDA LIVING WILL - PAGE 2 OF 2

PRINT NAME, HOME
ADDRESS
AND TELEPHONE
NUMBER OF YOUR
ALTERNATE
SURROGATE

I wish to designate the following person as my alternate surrogate, to carry
out the provisions of this declaration should my surrogate be unwilling or
unable to act on my behalf:

Name: _____

Address: _____

_____ Zip Code: _____

Phone: _____

ADD PERSONAL
INSTRUCTIONS
(IF ANY)

Additional instructions (optional):

SIGN THE
DOCUMENT

I understand the full import of this declaration, and I am emotionally and
mentally competent to make this declaration.

Signed: _____

WITNESSING
PROCEDURE

Witness 1:

Signed: _____

Address: _____

TWO WITNESSES
MUST SIGN AND
PRINT THEIR
ADDRESSES

Witness 2:

Signed: _____

Address: _____

© 2005 National
Hospice and
Palliative Care
Organization
2006 Revised

Courtesy of Caring Connections
1700 Diagonal Road, Suite 625, Alexandria, VA 22314
www.caringinfo. , 800/658-8898

FIGURE 5-9 A living will is a legal document that allows an individual to state what measures should or should not be taken to prolong life. *(Copyright © 2005 National Hospice and Palliative Care Organization. All rights reserved. Reproduction and distribution by an organization or organized group without the written permission of the National Hospice and Palliative Care Organization is expressly forbidden. For more information, please visit our Web site at www.caringinfo.org)*

FLORIDA DESIGNATION OF HEALTH CARE SURROGATE – PAGE 1 OF 2

INSTRUCTIONS

PRINT YOUR NAME

Name: _____

_____
(Last)   (First)   (Middle Initial)

In the event that I have been determined to be incapacitated to provide
informed consent for medical treatment and surgical and diagnostic
procedures, I wish to designate as my surrogate for health care decisions:

PRINT THE NAME,
HOME ADDRESS
AND TELEPHONE
NUMBER OF YOUR
SURROGATE

Name: _____

Address: _____

_____ Zip Code: _____

Phone: _____

If my surrogate is unwilling or unable to perform his or her duties, I wish
to designate as my alternate surrogate:

PRINT THE NAME,
HOME ADDRESS
AND TELEPHONE
NUMBER OF YOUR
ALTERNATE
SURROGATE

Name: _____

Address: _____

_____ Zip Code: _____

Phone: _____

ADD PERSONAL
INSTRUCTIONS
(IF ANY)

I fully understand that this designation will permit my designee to make
health care decisions, except for anatomical gifts, unless I have executed
an anatomical gift declaration pursuant to law, and to provide, withhold,
or withdraw consent on my behalf; to apply for public benefits to defray
the cost of health care; and to authorize my admission to or transfer from
a health care facility.

Additional instructions (optional):

© 2005 National
Hospice and
Palliative Care
Organization
2006 Revised

FLORIDA DESIGNATION OF HEALTH CARE SURROGATE PAGE 2 OF 2

I further affirm that this designation is not being made as a condition of
treatment or admission to a health care facility. I will notify and send a
copy of this document to the following persons other than my surrogate,
so they may know who my surrogate is:

Name: _____

PRINT THE NAMES
AND ADDRESSES OF
THOSE WHO YOU
WANT TO KEEP
COPIES OF THIS
DOCUMENT

Address: _____

Name: _____

Address: _____

Signed: _____

SIGN AND DATE
THE DOCUMENT

Date: _____

Witness 1:

WITNESSING
PROCEDURE

Signed: _____

Address: _____

TWO WITNESSES
MUST SIGN AND
PRINT THEIR
ADDRESSES

Witness 2:

Signed: _____

Address: _____

© 2005 National
Hospice and
Palliative Care
Organization
2006 Revised

Courtesy of Caring Connections
1700 Diagonal Road, Suite 625, Alexandria, VA 22314
www.caringinfo.org, 800/658-8898

FIGURE 5-10 A designation of health care surrogate is a legal document that allows an individual to appoint another person to make health care decisions if the individual is unable to make his or her own decisions. *(Copyright © 2005 National Hospice and Palliative Care Organization. All rights reserved. Reproduction and distribution by an organization or organized group without the written permission of the National Hospice and Palliative Care Organization is expressly forbidden. For more information, please visit our Web site at www.caringinfo.org)*

health care facilities receiving any type of federal aid comply with the following requirements:

◆ Inform every adult, both orally and in writing, of their right under state law to make decisions concerning medical care, including the right to refuse treatment and right-to-die options

◆ Provide information and assistance in preparing advance directives

◆ Document any advance directives on the patient's record

◆ Provide written statements to implement the patient's rights in the decision-making process

◆ Affirm that there will be no discrimination or effect on care because of advance directives

◆ Educate the staff on the medical and legal issues of advance directives

The PSDA ensures that patients are informed of their rights and have the opportunity to determine the care they will receive.

All health care workers must be aware of and honor advance or legal directives. In addition, health care workers should give serious consideration to preparing their own advance directives.

5:5 INFORMATION

Professional Standards

Legal responsibilities, ethics, patients' rights, and advance directives all help determine the type of care provided by health care workers. By following certain standards at all times, you can protect yourself, your employer, and the patient. Some of the basic standards are as follows:

◆ *Perform only those procedures for which you have been trained and are legally permitted to do.* Never perform any procedure unless you are qualified. The necessary training may be obtained from an educational facility, from your employer, or in special classes provided by an agency. If you are asked to perform any procedure for which you are not qualified, it is your responsibility to state that you have not been trained and to refuse to do it until you receive the required instruction. If you are not legally permitted to either perform a procedure or to sign documents, it is your responsibility to refuse to do so because of legal limitations.

◆ *Use approved, correct methods while performing any procedure.* Follow specific methods taught by qualified instructors in educational facilities, or observe and learn procedures from your employer or authorized personnel. Most health care agencies have an approved procedure manual that explains the step-by-step methods for performing tasks. Use this manual or read the manufacturer's instructions on specific equipment or supplies.

◆ *Obtain proper authorization before performing any procedure.* In some health careers, you will obtain authorization directly from the doctor, therapist, or individual in charge of a patient's care. In other careers, you will obtain authorization by checking written orders (figure 5-11). In careers where you have neither access to patients' records nor direct contact with the individuals in charge of care, an immediate supervisor will interpret orders and then direct you to perform procedures.

◆ *Identify the patient.* In some health care agencies, patients wear identification bands. If this is the case, check this name band (figure 5-12). In addition, state the patient's name clearly, repeating it if necessary. For example, say "Miss Jones?" followed by "Miss Sandra Jones?" to be sure you have the correct patient. Some health care facilities now use bar codes on patient identification bands. A scanner is

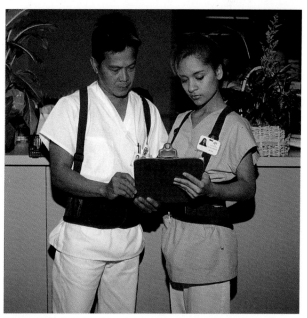

FIGURE 5-11 Obtain proper authorization before performing any procedure on a patient.

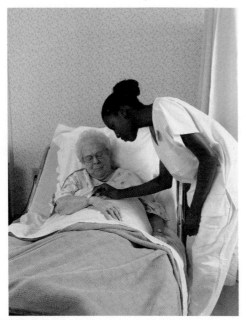

FIGURE 5-12 If a name band is present, use it to identify the patient.

used to check the bar code and verify the identification of the patient.

♦ *Obtain the patient's consent before performing any procedure.* Always explain a procedure briefly or state what you are going to do, and obtain the patient's consent. It is best to avoid statements such as "May I take your blood pressure?" because the patient can say "No." By stating, "The doctor would like me to check your blood pressure," you are identifying the procedure and obtaining consent by the patient's acceptance and/or lack of objection. If a patient refuses to allow you to perform a procedure, check with your immediate supervisor. Some procedures require written consent from the patient. Follow the agency policy with regard to such procedures. Never sign your name as a witness to any written consent or document unless you are authorized to do so.

♦ *Observe all safety precautions.* Handle equipment carefully. Be alert to all aspects of safety to protect the patient. Know and follow safety rules and regulations. Be alert to safety hazards in any area and make every effort to correct or eliminate such hazards as quickly as possible.

♦ *Keep all information confidential.* This includes oral and written information. Ensure that you do not place patient records in any area where they can be seen by unauthorized individuals. Do not reveal any information contained in the records without proper authorization and patient consent. If you are reporting specific information about a patient to your immediate supervisor, ensure that your conversation cannot be heard by others. Avoid discussing patients with others at home, in social situations, in public places, or anywhere outside the agency.

♦ *Think before you speak and carefully consider everything you say.* Do not reveal information, such as a blood pressure reading, to the patient unless you are specifically instructed to do so.

♦ *Treat all patients equally regardless of race, religion, social or economic status, sex, or nationality.* Provide care for *all* individuals to the best of your ability.

♦ *Accept no tips or bribes for the care you provide.* You receive a salary for your services, and the care you provide should not be influenced by the amount of money a patient can afford to pay. A polite refusal, such as "I'm sorry, I am not allowed to accept tips," is usually the best way to handle this situation.

♦ *If any error occurs or you make a mistake, report it immediately to your supervisor.* Never try to hide or ignore an error. Make every effort to correct the situation as soon as possible, and take responsibility for your actions.

♦ *Behave professionally in dress, language, manners, and actions.* Take pride in your occupation and in the work you do. Promote a positive attitude at all times.

Even when standards are followed, errors leading to legal action sometimes still occur. Liability insurance constitutes an additional form of protection in such cases. Many insurance companies offer policies at reasonable cost for health care workers and students. Some companies will even issue liability protection under a homeowner's policy or through a liability policy that protects the person against all liabilities, not just those related to occupation.

Again, remember that it is your responsibility to understand the legal and ethical implications of your particular health career. Never hesitate to ask specific questions or to request written policies from your employer. Contact your state board of health or state board of education to obtain information regarding regulations and guidelines for your occupation. By obtaining this information and by following the

TODAY'S RESEARCH: TOMORROW'S HEALTH CARE

Frozen stem cells that cure major diseases?

Stem cells are a major area of research today. Stem cells are important because they can become any of the specialized cell types needed in the human body. They can turn into muscle cells in the heart, nerve cells in the brain, or cells that secrete the insulin needed by a patient with diabetes. The major sources of stem cells are a developing embryo (infant); adult tissues such as bone marrow, brain, muscle, skin, and liver; and blood from the umbilical cord of a newborn infant.

Scientists the world over are finding ways to grow stem cells and force them to generate special cells that can be used to treat injury or disease. Early research has proved it is easier to work with embryonic cells, but this has created ethical dilemmas because it means embryos are destroyed. However, if adult cells can be harvested and grown, it would be easier to use an adult's own cells because they would not be rejected by the body.

Many scientists believe that, eventually, the study of stem cells will help explain how cells grow and develop. Conditions such as cancer and birth defects are caused by abnormal cell division. If scientists can learn how the abnormal development occurs, they could find ways to treat and even prevent the conditions. Major research is directed toward learning what makes the cells specialize to become a specific type of cell in the body.

Currently, parents have the option of preserving umbilical cord blood for its stem cells. When their baby is born, blood from the umbilical cord can be collected and stored in liquid nitrogen. If the child later develops a disease such as cancer and needs stem cells, the cells can be recovered and used for the transplant. The cost of this procedure still limits its widespread use, but hopefully less expensive methods will be found to maintain this source of stem cells. Many stem cell transplants have already been performed successfully, and lives have been saved.

basic standards listed, you will protect yourself, your employer, and the patient to whom you provide health care.

STUDENT: *Go to the workbook and complete the assignment sheet for Chapter 5, Legal and Ethical Responsibilities.*

CHAPTER 5 SUMMARY

All health care workers have legal and ethical responsibilities that exist to protect the health care worker and employer, and to provide for the safety and well-being of the patient.

Legal responsibilities in health care usually involve torts and contracts. Torts are wrongful acts that do not involve contracts. Examples of torts that can lead to legal action include malpractice, negligence, assault and battery, invasion of privacy, false imprisonment, abuse, and defamation. A contract is an agreement between two or more parties. Contracts create obligations that must be met by all involved individuals. If a contract is not performed according to agreement, the contract is breached, and legal action can occur.

Understanding privileged communications is another important aspect of legal responsibilities. A health care worker must be aware that all information given by a patient is confidential and should not be told to anyone other than members of the patient's health care team without the written consent of the patient. Health care records are also privileged communications and can be used as legal records in a court of law.

Ethical responsibilities are based not on law, but rather, on what is morally right or wrong. Most health care occupations each have an established code of ethics that provides a standard of conduct or code of behavior. Health care workers should make every effort to abide by the codes of ethics established for their given professions.

Health care workers must respect patients' rights. Health care agencies have written policies concerning the factors of care that patients can expect to receive. All personnel must respect and honor these rights.

Advance directives for health care are legal documents that allow individuals to state what medical treatment they want or do not want in the event that they become incapacitated. Two main examples are a living will and a Designation of Health Care Surrogate or Durable Power of Attorney for Health Care. As a result of a federal law called the Patient Self-Determination Act (PSDA), any health care facility receiving federal funds must provide patients with information regarding and assistance in preparing advance or legal directives.

Professional standards of care help provide guidelines for meeting legal responsibilities, ethics, and patients' rights. Every health care worker should follow these standards at all times. In addition, all health care workers should know and follow the state laws that regulate their respective occupations.

INTERNET SEARCHES

Use the suggested search engines in Chapter 17:4 of this textbook to search the Internet for additional information on the following topics:

1. *Torts*: search for additional information or actual legal cases involving malpractice, negligence, assault and battery, invasion of privacy, false imprisonment, and defamation.

2. *Abuse*: research domestic violence or abuse, child abuse, and elder abuse to determine how victims might react, signs and symptoms indicative of abuse, and information on how to help these victims.

3. *Contracts*: search for information on components of a contract and legal cases in health care caused by a breach of contract.

4. *Ethics*: use Internet addresses for professional organizations (see Chapter 3) to find two or three different codes of ethics; compare and contrast the codes of ethics.

5. *Patient's rights*: search for complete copies of a patient's or resident's bill of rights; compare and contrast the different bills of rights (*Hint:* check American Hospital Association Web site).

6. *Advance directives*: search for different examples of a living will and/or a designation of health

care surrogate or durable power of attorney for health care; compare the different forms.

7. *Patient Self Determination Act of 1990*: locate a copy of this act or information on the purposes of this act (*Hint:* check federal legislation Web sites).

8. *Insurance*: search for different types of liability insurance for health care providers; determine what different policies cover and their cost.

REVIEW QUESTIONS

1. Choose a specific health care profession (i.e., dental hygienist, physical therapist) and create a situation where this individual might be subject to legal action for each of the following torts: malpractice, negligence, assault, battery, invasion of privacy, false imprisonment, abuse, and defamation.

2. Differentiate between slander and libel.

3. What is the difference between an implied contract and an expressed contract?

4. You are employed as a geriatric assistant. A resident tells you that he is saving sleeping pills so he can commit suicide. He has terminal cancer and is in a great deal of pain. What should you do? Why?

5. What is HIPAA? Identify three (3) specific ways that HIPAA protects the privacy and confidentiality of health care information.

6. Obtain at least two different codes of ethics for health professions by contacting professional organizations or searching the Internet. Compare the codes of ethics.

7. Mr. Gonzales is a healthy 55-year-old man with a living will that contains a DNR (Do Not Resuscitate) order for terminal conditions. He goes into cardiac arrest as a result of an allergic reaction to an injection of dye for a laboratory test. Should cardiopulmonary resuscitation (CPR) be started? Why or why not?

8. How does a living will differ from a Designation of Health Care Surrogate?

9. List five (5) different patient or resident rights.

10. Identify six (6) professional standards by explaining why they are important to meet legal responsibilities, ethics, and/or patient's rights.

♦ @ symbol for at; mistaken for the number 2 if written poorly; write out "at"

♦ < or >: symbols for less than or greater than; can be misinterpreted as the number 7 or letter L; write greater than or less than

♦ *Apothecary unit symbols such as ʒ or ℥*: symbols for dram and ounce; easily mistaken for each other; write dram or ounce or use metric units

Health care workers must use only the abbreviations or symbols approved by the facility in which they are employed. In addition, extreme care must be used while writing abbreviations and symbols so they are legible and readily understood.

NOTE: In the lists that follow, these abbreviations and symbols are included because they are still used in some health facilities. However, an asterisk (*) has been placed in front of the abbreviation or symbol to alert the user that it is on the Do Not Use list.

NOTE: There is a growing trend toward eliminating periods from most abbreviations. Although the following list does not show periods, you may work in an agency that chooses to use them. When in doubt, follow the policy of your agency.

Learn the abbreviations in the following way:

♦ Use a set of index cards to make a set of flashcards of the abbreviations found on the abbreviation list. Print one abbreviation in big letters on each card. Put the abbreviation on the front of the card and the meaning on the back of the card.

♦ Use the flashcards to study the abbreviations. A realistic goal is to learn all abbreviations for one letter per week. For example, learn all of the *A*s the first week, all of the *B*s the second week, all of the *C*s the third week, and so on until all are learned.

♦ Follow your instructor's guidelines for tests on the abbreviations. Many instructors give weekly tests. The tests may be cumulative. They may cover the letter of the week plus any letters learned in previous weeks.

A

*@	at
ā	before
A&D	admission and discharge
A&P	anterior and posterior, anatomy and physiology

āā	of each
Ab	abortion
abd	abdomen, abdominal
ABG	arterial blood gas
ac	before meals
ACLS	advanced cardiac life support
ACTH	adrenocorticotrophic hormone
AD	right ear
ADH	antidiuretic hormone
ad lib	as desired
ADL	activities of daily living
adm	admission
AED	automated external defibrillation
AHA	American Hospital Association
AIDS	acquired immune deficiency syndrome
am, AM	morning, before noon
AMA	American Medical Association, against medical advice
amal	amalgam
amb	ambulate, walk
amt	amount
ANA	American Nurses' Association
ANS	autonomic nervous system
ant	anterior
AP	apical pulse
approx	approximately
aq, aqua	aqueous (water base)
ARC	AIDS-related complex
ART	accredited records technician
AS	left ear
as tol	as tolerated
ASA	aspirin (acetylsalicylic acid)
ASAP	as soon as possible
ASCVD	arteriosclerotic cardiovascular disease
ASHD	arteriosclerotic heart disease
AU	both ears
av	average
AV	arteriovenous, atrioventricular
A&W	alive and well
Ax	axilla, axillary, armpit

B

Ba	barium
bacti	bacteriology
B&B	bowel and bladder training
BBB	bundle branch block
B&C	biopsy and conization
BE	barium enema
bid	twice a day

bil	bilateral
Bl	blood
Bl Wk	blood work
BM	bowel movement
BMI	body mass index
BMR	basal metabolic rate
BP	blood pressure
BR	bed rest
BRP	bathroom privileges
BS	blood sugar
BSA	body surface area
BSC, bsc	bedside commode
BSE	breast self-examination
BUN	blood urea nitrogen
Bx, bx	biopsy

C

°C	degrees Celsius (Centigrade)
c̄, w/	with
Ca	calcium
CA	cancer
cal	calorie
Cap	capsule
CAT	computerized axial tomography
Cath	catheter, catheterize
CBC	complete blood count
CBET	certified biomedical equipment technician
CBR	complete bed rest
*cc	cubic centimeter
CC	chief complaint
CCU	coronary care unit, critical care unit
CDA	certified dental assistant
CDC	Centers for Disease Control and Prevention
CEO	chief executive officer
CF	cystic fibrosis
CHD	coronary heart disease
CHF	congestive heart failure
CHO	carbohydrate
chol	cholesterol
CICU	cardiac intensive care unit
ck	check
Cl	chloride or chlorine
cl liq	clear liquids
cm	centimeter
CMA	certified medical assistant
CNP	certified nurse practitioner
CNS	central nervous system

co, c/o	complains of
CO	carbon monoxide, coronary occlusion
CO_2	carbon dioxide
Comp	complete, compound
cont	continued
COPD	chronic obstructive pulmonary disease
COTA	certified occupational therapy assistant
CP	cerebral palsy
CPK	creatine phosphokinase (cardiac enzyme)
CPR	cardiopulmonary resuscitation
CPT	current procedure terminology
CRTT	certified respiratory therapy technician
CS	central supply or service
C&S	culture and sensitivity
CSF	cerebrospinal fluid
CSR	central supply room
CST	certified surgical technologist
CT	computerized tomography
Cu	copper
CVA	cerebral vascular accident (stroke)
CVD	cardiovascular disease
Cx	cervix, complication, complaint

D

d	day
D&C	dilatation and curettage
DA	dental assistant
DAT	diet as tolerated
DC	Doctor of Chiropractic
D/C, dc, disc	discontinue, discharge
DDS	Doctor of Dental Surgery
DEA	Drug Enforcement Agency
del	delivery
Dept	department
DH	dental hygienist
DHHS	Department of Health and Human Services
Diff	differential white blood cell count
dil	dilute, dissolve
DM	diabetes mellitus
DMD	Doctor of Dental Medicine
DMS	diagnostic medical sonography
DNA	deoxyribonucleic acid

DNR	do not resuscitate
DO	Doctor of Osteopathic Medicine
DOA	dead on arrival
DOB	date of birth
DOD	date of death
DON	director of nursing
DPM	Doctor of Podiatric Medicine
DPT	diphtheria, pertussis, tetanus
Dr	doctor
dr	dram, drainage
DRG	diagnostic related group
drg, drsg, dsg	dressing
D/S	dextrose in saline
DSD	dry sterile dressing
DTs	delirium tremors
DVM	Doctor of Veterinary Medicine
DW	distilled water
D/W	dextrose in water
Dx, dx	diagnosis

E

ea	each
EBL	estimated blood loss
ECG, EKG	electrocardiogram
ED	emergency department
EEG	electroencephalogram
EENT	ear, eye, nose, throat
elix	elixir
EMG	electromyogram
EMS	emergency medical services
EMT	emergency medical technician
ENT	ear, nose, throat
EPA	Environmental Protection Agency
ER	emergency room
ESR	erythrocyte sedimentation rate
et, etiol	etiology (cause of disease)
Ex, exam	examination
Exc	excision
Exp	exploratory, expiration
ext	extract, extraction, external

F

°F	degrees Fahrenheit
FAS	fetal alcohol syndrome
FBS	fasting blood sugar
FBW	fasting blood work
FC	Foley catheter

FDA	Food and Drug Administration
Fe	iron
FF, FFl	force fluids
FH	family history
FHR	fetal heart rate
Fl, fl	fluid
FSH	follicle-stimulating hormone
ft	foot
FUO	fever of unknown origin
Fx, Fr	fracture

G

GA	gastric analysis, general anesthesia
gal	gallon
GB	gallbladder
Gc	gonococcus, gonorrhea
GH	growth hormone
GI	gastrointestinal
Gm, g	gram
gr	grain
gt, gtt, gtts	drop, drops
GTT	glucose tolerance test
GU	genitourinary
Gyn	gynecology

H

H	hydrogen
H&H	hemoglobin and hematocrit
H_2O	water
H_2O_2	hydrogen peroxide
H, (h), hypo	hypodermic injection
HA	hearing aid, headache
HBP	high blood pressure
HBV	hepatitis B virus
HCG	human chorionic gonadotrophin hormone
HCl	hydrochloric acid
hct	hematocrit
HCV	hepatitis C virus
HDL	high-density lipoproteins (healthy type of cholesterol)
Hg	mercury
Hgb, Hb	hemoglobin
HHA	home health assistant/aide
HIPAA	Health Insurance Portability and Accountability Act

HIV	human immunodeficiency virus (AIDS virus)
HMO	health maintenance organization
HOB	head of bed
HOH	hard of hearing
H&P	history and physical
Hr, hr, H, h	hour, hours
HRT	hormone replacement therapy
HS	hour of sleep (bedtime)
Ht	height
Hx, hx	history
hypo	hypodermic injection
Hyst	hysterectomy

I

I&D	incision and drainage
I&O	intake and output
ICCU	intensive coronary care unit
ICD	international classification of diseases
ICU	intensive care unit
ID	intradermal, infectious disease
IDDM	insulin-dependent diabetes mellitus
IH	infectious hepatitis
IM	intramuscular
imp	impression
in	inch
inf	infusion, inferior, infection
ing	inguinal
inj	injection
int	internal, interior
IPPB	intermittent positive pressure breathing
irr, irrig	irrigation
Isol, isol	isolation
IT	inhalation therapy
IUD	intrauterine device
IV	intravenous
IVP	intravenous pyelogram

J

jt	joint

K

K	potassium
KCl	potassium chloride

Kg, kg	kilogram
KUB	kidney, ureter, bladder X-ray

L

L	lumbar
L&D	labor and delivery
L&W	living and well
(L), lt, lft	left
L, l	liter (1,000 cc)
Lab	laboratory
Lap	laparotomy
lat	lateral
lb	pound
LCT	long-term care
LDH	lactose dehydrogenase (cardiac enzyme)
LDL	low-density lipoprotein (unhealthy type of cholesterol)
lg	large
liq	liquid
LLQ	left lower quadrant
LMP	last menstrual period
LOC	laxative of choice, level of consciousness
LP	lumbar puncture
LPN	licensed practical nurse
LS	lumbar sacral
LTC	long-term care
LUQ	left upper quadrant
LVN	licensed vocational nurse

M

m	minim
MA	medical assistant
Mat	maternity
mcg	microgram
MD	Medical Doctor, muscular dystrophy, myocardial disease
Med	medical, medicine
mEq	milliequivalent
mg	milligram
Mg	magnesium
MI	myocardial infarction (heart attack)
MICU	medical intensive care unit
min	minute
mL, ml	milliliter
MLT	medical laboratory technician
mm	millimeter

MN	midnight
mod	moderate
MOM	milk of magnesia
MRI	magnetic resonance imaging
MS	multiple sclerosis, mitral stenosis, muscular–skeletal
MT	medical technologist

N

N	nitrogen
N/A	not applicable
Na	sodium
NA	nurse aide/assistant
NaCl	sodium chloride (salt)
NB	newborn
N/C	no complaints
neg	negative, none
Neur	neurology
NG, ng, N/G	nasogastric tube
NICU	neurological intensive care unit
NIDDM	non-insulin-dependent diabetes mellitus
NIH	National Institutes of Health
nil	none
NKA	no known allergies
NKDA	no known drug allergies
no	number
NO	nursing office
noc, noct	at night, night
NP	nurse practitioner
NPN	nonprotein nitrogen
NPO	nothing by mouth
N/S, NS	normal saline
Nsy	nursery
N/V, N&V	nausea and vomiting
NVD	nausea, vomiting, diarrhea
NVS	neurological vital signs

O

O_2	oxygen
O&P	ova and parasites
Ob, Obs	obstetrics
OBRA	Omnibus Budget Reconciliation Act
od	overdose
OD	right eye, occular dextra, Doctor of Optometry
oint	ointment
OJ	orange juice

OOB	out of bed
OP	outpatient
OPD, OPC	outpatient department or clinic
opp	opposite
OR	operating room
Ord	orderly
Orth	orthopedics
os	mouth
OS	left eye, occular sinistra
OSHA	Occupational Safety and Health Administration
OT	occupational therapy/therapist
OTC	over the counter
OU	each eye
OV	office visit
oz	ounce

P

$\overline{p}$	after
P	pulse, phosphorus
PA	physician's assistant
PAC	premature atrial contraction
PAP	Papanicolaou test (smear)
para	number of pregnancies
Path	pathology
Pb	lead
PBI	protein-bound iodine
pc	after meals
PCA	patient-controlled analgesia
PCC	poison control center
PCP	patient care plan
PCT	patient/personal care technician
PDR	*Physicians' Desk Reference*
PE	physical examination, pulmonary edema
Peds	pediatrics
per	by, through
PET	positron emission tomography
pH	measure of acidity/alkalinity
Pharm	pharmacy
PI	present illness
PID	pelvic inflammatory disease
PKU	phenylketonuria
PM, pm	after noon
PMC	postmortem (after death) care
PMS	premenstrual syndrome
PNS	peripheral nervous system
po	by mouth
PO	phone order
post	posterior, after
post-op	after an operation

PP	postpartum (after delivery)
PPE	personal protective equipment
PPO	preferred provider organization
pre-op	before an operation
prep	prepare
prn	whenever necessary, as needed
Psy	psychology, psychiatry
pt	patient, pint (500 mL or cc)
Pt	prothrombin time
PT	physical therapy/therapist
PTT	partial thromboplastin time
PVC	premature ventricular contraction
PVD	peripheral vascular disease
Px	prognosis, physical examination

Q

q, $\bar{q}$	every
*qd	every day
qh	every hour
q2h	every 2 hours
q3h	every 3 hours
q4h	every 4 hours
qhs	every night at bedtime
*qid	four times a day
qns	quantity not sufficient
*qod	every other day
qol	quality of life
qs	quantity sufficient
qt	quart

R

R	respiration, rectal
®, Rt	right
Ra	radium
RBC	red blood cell
RDA	recommended daily allowance
REM	rapid eye movement
RHD	rheumatic heart disease
RLQ	right lower quadrant
RN	registered nurse
RNA	ribonucleic acid
R/O	rule out
RO	reality orientation
ROM	range of motion
RR	recovery room
RRT	registered respiratory therapist, registered radiologic technologist

RT	respiratory therapy/therapist
RUQ	right upper quadrant
Rx	prescription, take, treatment

S

S	sacral
S&A	sugar and acetone
$\bar{s}$, w/o	without
SA	sinoatrial
sc, SC	subcutaneous
SGOT, SGPT	transaminase test
SICU	surgical intensive care unit
SIDS	sudden infant death syndrome
Sig	give the following directions
sm	small
SOB	short of breath
sol	solution
sos	if necessary
spec	specimen
SpGr, spgr	specific gravity
SPN	student practical nurse
spt	spirits, liquor
$\bar{\bar{s}}$	one half
S/S, S&S	signs and symptoms
SSE	soap solution enema
staph	staphylococcus infection
stat	immediately, at once
STD	sexually transmitted disease
STH	somatotropic hormone
strep	streptococcus infection
supp	suppository
Surg	surgery, surgical
susp	suspension
Sx	symptom, sign
syp	syrup

T

T&A	tonsillectomy and adenoidectomy
T, Temp	temperature
tab	tablet
TB	tuberculosis
tbsp	tablespoon
TCDB	turn, cough, deep breathe
TH	thyroid hormone
TIA	transient ischemic attack
tid	three times a day
TLC	tender loving care

TO	telephone order
tol	tolerated
TPN	total parenteral nutrition
TPR	temperature, pulse, respiration
tr, tinct	tincture
TSH	thyroid-stimulating hormone
tsp	teaspoon
TUR	transurethral resection
TWE	tap water enema
tx	traction, treatment, transplant

U

UA, U/A	urinalysis
ung	ointment
Ur, ur	urine
URI	upper respiratory infection
UTI	urinary tract infection
UV	ultraviolet

V

Vag	vaginal
VD	venereal disease
VDM	Veterinarian Degree of Medicine
VDRL	serology for syphilis, Venereal Disease Research Laboratory
VO	verbal order
Vol	volume
vp	venipuncture, venous pressure
VS	vital signs (TPR & BP)

W

WBC	white blood cell
WC	ward clerk/secretary
w/c	wheelchair
WHO	World Health Organization
WNL	within normal limits
w/o, wo	without
W/P	whirlpool
wt	weight

X

x	times (2x means do 2 times)
x-match	cross-match
XR	X-ray

Y

y/o	years old
YOB	year of birth
yr	year

Z

Zn	zinc

MISCELLANEOUS SYMBOLS

*>	greater than
*<	less than
↑	higher, elevate, or up
↓	lower or down
#	pound or number
*ʒ	dram
*ℨ	ounce
′	foot or minute
″	inch or second
°	degree
♀ or F	female
♂ or M	male
I or *i* or Ť	one
II or *ii* or ŤŤ	two
V	five
X	ten
L	fifty
C	one hundred
D	five hundred
M	one thousand

STUDENT: *Go to the workbook and complete the assignment and evaluation sheets for 6:1, Using Medical Abbreviations.*

6:2 INFORMATION

Interpreting Word Parts

Medical dictionaries have been written to include the many words used in health occupations. It would be impossible to memorize all such words. By breaking the words into parts, however, it is sometimes possible to figure out their meanings. This section provides basic information on doing just that.

A word is often a combination of different parts. The parts include prefixes, suffixes, and word roots (see figure 6-2).

A **prefix** can be defined as a syllable or word placed at the beginning of a word. A **suffix** can be defined as a syllable or word placed at the end of the word.

The meanings of prefixes and suffixes are set. For example, the suffix *itis* means "inflammation of." *Tonsillitis* means "an inflammation of the tonsils," and *appendicitis* means "an inflammation of the appendix." Note that the meaning of the suffix is usually placed first when the word is defined.

Word roots can be defined as main words or parts to which prefixes and suffixes can be added. In the example *appendicitis*, the word root is *appendix*. By adding the prefix *pseudo-*, which means "false," and the suffix *itis*, which means "inflammation of," the word becomes *pseudoappendicitis*. This is interpreted as a "false inflammation of the appendix."

The prefix usually serves to further define the word root. The suffix usually describes what is happening to the word root.

When prefixes, suffixes, and/or word roots are joined together, vowels are frequently added. Common examples include *a, e, i, ia, io, o,* and *u*. These are listed in parentheses in the lists that follow. The vowels are not used if the word root or suffix begins with a vowel. For example, *encephal (o)* means brain. When it is combined with *itis* meaning inflammation of, the vowel is not used for *encephalitis*. When it is combined with *gram*, meaning tracing or record, the vowel *o* is added for *encephalogram*. *Hepat (o)* means liver. When it is combined with *itis*, the vowel is not used for *hepatitis*. When it is combined with *megaly*, meaning enlarged, the vowel *o* is added for *hepatomegaly*.

By learning basic prefixes, suffixes, and word roots, you will frequently be able to interpret the meaning of a word even when you have never before encountered the word. A list of common prefixes, suffixes, and word roots follows. An example of a medical term using the word part and the meaning of the medical term is also provided. In addition, the prefixes, suffixes, and word roots for parts of the human body are shown in figure 6-3.

Learn the prefixes, suffixes, and word roots in the following way:

♦ Use a set of index cards to make flashcards of the word parts found on the prefix, suffix, and word root list. Place one prefix, suffix, or word root on each card. Put the word part on the front of the card and the meaning of the word part on the back of the card. Ensure that each is spelled correctly.

♦ Use the flashcards to learn the meanings of the word parts. A realistic goal is to learn one letter per week. For example, learn all word parts starting with the letter *A* the first week, all of those starting with *B* the second week, all of those starting with *C* the third week, and so on until all are learned. Practice correct spelling of all of the word parts.

♦ Follow your instructor's guidelines for tests on the word parts. Many instructors give weekly tests. The tests may be cumulative. They may cover the letter of the week plus any letters learned in previous weeks. Words may be presented that use the various word parts.

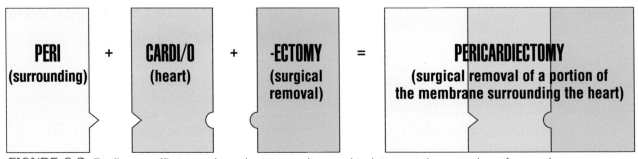

FIGURE 6-2 Prefixes, suffixes, and word roots can be used to interpret the meaning of a word.

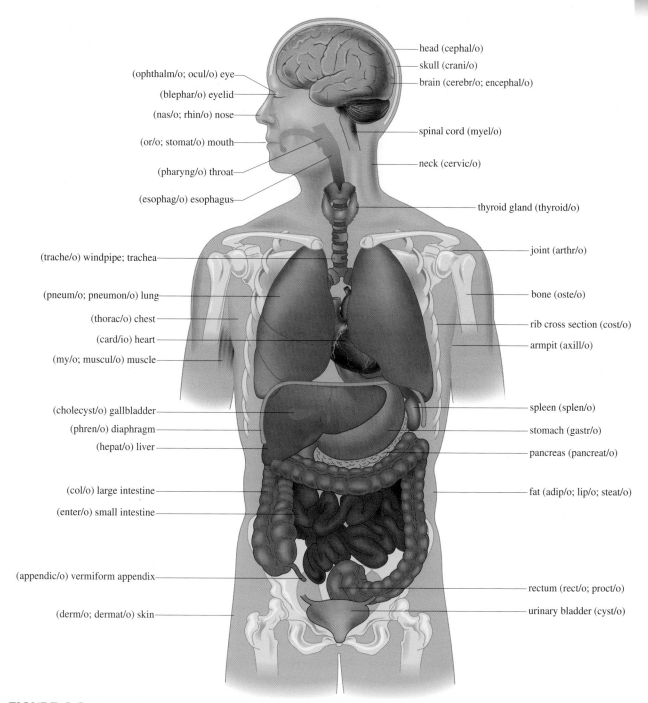

FIGURE 6-3 The prefixes, suffixes, and word roots for parts of the human body.

Word Part	Meaning	Medical Term	Meaning
A			
a-, an-	without, lack of	a/pnea	without or lack of breathing
ab-	from, away	ab/duct	to move away from the body
-ac, -ic	pertaining to	cardi/ac	pertaining to the heart
acr- (o)	extremities (arms and legs)	acro/cyan/osis	condition of blueness of the extremities
ad-	to, toward, near	ad/duct	to move toward the body
aden- (o)	gland, glandular	adeno/cele	a tumor of a gland
adren- (o)	adrenal gland	adreno/pathy	disease of the adrenal gland
aer- (o)	air	aero/cele	a cavity or pouch swollen with gas or air
-al	like, similar, pertaining to	neur/al	pertaining to a nerve
alba-, albi-	white	albi/no	an organism deficient in pigment, white
alges- (i, ia)	pain	algesi/meter	instrument for measuring pain
-algia	pain	my/algia	muscle pain
ambi-	both, both sides	ambi/lateral	both sides
an- (o, us)	anus (opening to rectum)	ano/scope	an instrument for examining the anus and rectum
angi- (o)	vessel	angio/pathy	disease of blood vessels
ankyl-	crooked, looped, immovable, fixed	ankyl/osis	stiffness or fixation of a joint
ante- (ro)	before, in front of, ahead of	ante/partum	before labor or childbirth
anti-	against	anti/bacterial	against bacteria
append- (i, o)	appendix	append/ectomy	surgical removal of the appendix
arter- (io)	artery	aterio/gram	tracing or picture of the arteries
arthr- (o)	joint	arthr/itis	inflammation of a joint
-ase	enzyme	peptid/ase	an enzyme that aids in the digestion of proteins
-asis	condition of	chole/lithi/asis	condition of stones in the gallbladder
-asthenia	weakness, lack of strength	my/asthenia	weakness in a muscle
ather- (o)	fatty, lipid	athero/sclerosis	a fatty hardening
audi- (o)	sound, hearing	audio/meter	an instrument to measure sound or hearing
aur-	ear	aur/al	pertaining to the ear
auto-	self	auto/phobia	a fear of being by oneself or alone
B			
bi- (s)	twice, double, both	bi/lateral	two sides
bio-	life	bio/logy	study of science of life
-blast	germ/embryonic cell	hemo/cyto/blast	an embryonic or stem cell for blood cells
blephar- (o)	eyelid	blepharo/plasty	plastic surgery on an eyelid
brachi-	arm	brachi/algia	arm pain
brachy-	short	brachy/dactyl/ic	condition of having short fingers
brady-	slow	brady/cardia	slow heart
bronch- (i, o)	air tubes in lungs	bronch/itis	inflammation of the air tubes in the lungs
bucc- (a, o)	cheek	bucco/lingu/al	pertaining to the cheek and tongue
C			
calc- (u, ulus)	stone	calcul/osis	condition of having a stone
carcin- (o)	cancer, malignancy	carcin/oma	cancerous tumor
cardi- (a, o)	pertaining to heart	cardi/ologist	physician who studies and treats heart disease
carp- (o)	wrist	carp/itis	inflammation of the wrist

Word Part	Meaning	Medical Term	Meaning
-cele, -coele	swelling, tumor, cavity, hernia	meningo/cele	swelling or tumor of the membranes of the brain and spinal cord
cent- (i)	one hundred	centi/meter	hundred part of a meter (unit of measurement)
-centesis	surgical puncture to remove fluid	thora/centesis	surgical puncture to remove fluid from the chest
cephal- (o)	head, pertaining to head	cephal/algia	pain in the head, headache
cerebro-	brain	cerebro/spin/al	pertaining to the brain and spinal cord
cerv- (ic, io)	neck, neck of uterus	cervio/facial	relating to the neck and face
cheil- (o)	lip	cheilo/plasty	plastic surgery to repair lip defects
chem- (o)	drug, chemical	chemo/therapy	treatment with drugs or chemicals
chlor- (o)	green	chlor/opsia	a visual defect in which all objects appear green
chol- (e, o)	bile, gallbladder	chole/cyst/ic	pertaining to the gallbladder or bag
chond- (i, r, ri)	cartilage	chondr/itis	inflammation of cartilage
chrom- (a, at, o)	color	chromato/meter	an instrument for measuring color perception
-cide	causing death	germi/cide	causing death to germs
circum-	around, about	circum/duction	movement in a circular motion
-cise	cut	ex/cise	cut out
co- (n)	with, together	co/chromato/graphy	identifying a substance by comparing color hues with a known substance
-coccus	round	strepto/coccus	round germ causing strep infection
col- (in, o)	colon, bowel, large intestine	col/ostomy	creating an opening into the colon or large intestine
colp- (i, o)	vagina	colp/orrhaphy	surgical repair of the vaginal wall
contra-	against, counter	contra/stimulant	against a stimulant
cost- (a, i, o)	rib	cost/ectomy	surgical removal of a rib
crani- (o)	pertaining to the skull	crani/otomy	cutting into the skull
-crine	secrete	exo/crine	secrete outside of
cryo-	cold	cryo/therapy	treatment with cold
crypt- (o)	hidden, obscure	crypto/genic	obscure or unknown origin
cut- (an)	skin	cutane/ous	pertaining to the skin
cyan- (o)	blue	cyan/osis	condition of blueness
cyst- (i, o)	bladder, bag, sac	cyst/itis	inflammation of the bladder
cyt- (e, o)	cell	cyt/ology	study of cells

D

Word Part	Meaning	Medical Term	Meaning
dacry- (o)	tear duct, tear	dacryo/cyst/itis	inflammation of the lacrimal (tear duct) sac
dactyl- (o)	finger, toe	dactyl/oscopy	the scientific study of fingerprints
dec- (a, i)	ten	deci/meter	tenth part of a meter (unit of measurement)
dent- (i, o)	tooth	dent/al	pertaining to teeth
derm- (a, at, o)	pertaining to skin	dermat/itis	inflammation of the skin
-desis	surgical union or fixation	arthro/desis	surgical immobilization of a joint to allow the bones to grow together
dextr- (i, o)	to the right	dextro/ocular	right eye
di- (plo)	double, twice	diplo/coccus	two round circles
dia-	through, between, part	dia/dermal	cutting through the skin
dis- (ti, to)	separation, away from	dis/infect	to separate or free from infection
dors- (i, o)	to the back, back	dors/al	pertaining to the back

Word Part	Meaning	Medical Term	Meaning
duoden- (o)	duodenum	duoden/ectomy	surgical removal of all or part of the duodenum
dys-	difficult, painful, bad	dys/uria	difficult or painful urination

E

Word Part	Meaning	Medical Term	Meaning
e- (c)	without	e/dentu/lous	condition of being without teeth
ec- (ti, to)	outside, external	ecto/genous	capable of developing away from the host
-ectasis	expansion, dilation, stretching	bronchi/ectasis	dilation or expansion of air tubes in lungs
-ectomy	surgical removal of	tonsil/ectomy	surgical removal of the tonsils
electr- (o)	electrical	electro/cardio/gram	recording of electrical activity in the heart
-emesis	vomit	hemat/emesis	vomiting blood
-emia	blood	glyc/emia	sugar in the blood
encephal- (o)	brain	encephal/itis	inflammation of the brain
endo-	within, innermost	endo/crine	secrete within
enter- (i, o)	intestine	enter/itis	inflammation of the intestine
epi-	upon, over, upper	epi/gastric	above the stomach
erythro-	red	erythro/cyte	red (blood) cell
-esis	condition of	par/esis	condition of paralysis
-esthesia	sensation, perception, feel	an/esthesia	without feeling
eu-	well, easy, normal	eu/pnea	normal respiration or breathing
ex- (o)	outside of, beyond	exo/path/ic	disease that originates outside the body

F

Word Part	Meaning	Medical Term	Meaning
faci-	face	facio/plegia	paralysis of the face
-fascia (l)	fibrous band	myo/fascial	muscle fiber
fibr- (a, i, o)	fiber, connective tissue	fibr/oma	tumor of fibrous tissue
fore-	in front of	fore/arm	the front part of the arm
-form	having the form of, shape	uni/form	one shape or form
-fuge	driving away, expelling	centri/fuge	driving away from the center

G

Word Part	Meaning	Medical Term	Meaning
galacto-	milk, galactose (milk sugar)	galact/orrhea	flow of milk
gast- (i, ro)	stomach	gastr/itis	inflammation of the stomach
-genesis	development, production, creation	fibro/genesis	the development of fibrous tissue
-genetic, -genic	origin, producing, causing	cyto/genic	origin of cells
genito-	organs of reproduction	genito/urinary	organs of reproductive and urinary systems
-genous	kind, type	exo/genous	outside kind or type
geront- (o)	old age, elderly	geront/ology	study of the elderly
gingiv-	gums, gingiva	gingiv/itis	inflammation of the gums
gloss- (o)	tongue	glosso/graph	instrument for recording movements of the tongue
gluc- (o)	sweetness, sugar, glucose	gluco/lipid	sugar fat
gly- (c, co)	sugar	glyc/emia	sugar in the blood
-gram	tracing, picture, record	electro/cardio/gram	tracing of the electrical activity in the heart
-graph	diagram, instrument for recording	electro/cardio/graph	instrument for recording electrical activity in the heart
gyn- (ec, o)	woman, female	gynec/ology	the study of women

Word Part	Meaning	Medical Term	Meaning
H			
hem- (a, ato, o)	blood	hemat/ology	study of the blood
hemi-	half	hemi/plegia	paralysis on half of the body
hepat- (o)	liver	hepat/itis	inflammation of the liver
herni-	rupture	hernio/plasty	surgical repair of a rupture
hetero-	other, unlike, different	hetero/genous	different kind or type
hist- (o)	tissue	hist/ologist	person who studies tissue
hom- (eo, o)	same, like	homeo/stasis	maintaining a constant level
hydro-	water	hydro/therapy	water treatment
hyper-	excessive, high, over, increased, more than normal	hyper/tension	high blood pressure
hypno-	sleep	hypno/sis	process of sleep
hypo-	decreased, deficient, low, under, less than normal	hypo/tension	low blood pressure
hyster- (o)	uterus	hyster/ectomy	surgical removal of the uterus
I			
-ia, -iasis	condition of, abnormal/pathological state	pneumon/ia	abnormal condition of the lung
-ic, -ac	pertaining to	thorac/ic	pertaining to the chest
idio-	peculiar to an individual, self-originating	idio/pathic	disease arising by itself or from an unknown cause
ile- (o, um)	ileum	ileo/stomy	creating an artificial opening into the ileum
infra-	beneath, below	infra/sonic	sound waves below the frequency of the human ear
inter-	between, among	inter/costal	between the ribs
intra-	within, into, inside	intra/ven/ous	into a vein
-ism	condition, theory, state of being	albin/ism	condition of being white
iso-	equal, alike, same	iso/chromatic	constant or same color
-itis	inflammation, inflammation of	pharyng/itis	inflammation of the throat
K			
kerat- (o)	cornea of eye	kerato/meter	instrument to measure the curvature of the cornea
-kinesis, -kinetic	motion	dys/kinetic	difficult movement
L			
labi- (a, o)	lip	labio/lingual	pertaining to the lips and tongue
lacrima-	tears	lacrima/tion	secretion of tears
lact- (o)	milk	lacto/genesis	production of milk
lapar- (o)	abdomen, abdominal wall	lapar/otomy	cutting into the abdomen
laryng- (o)	larynx (voicebox)	laryng/itis	inflammation of the voicebox
latero- (al)	side	ambi/lateral	both sides
-lepsy	seizure, convulsion	narco/lepsy	sleep seizure
leuco-, leuko-	white	leuko/cyte	white (blood) cell
lingu- (a, o)	tongue	lingu/al	pertaining to the tongue
lip- (o)	fat, lipids	lipo/cyte	fat cell
lith- (o)	stone, calculus	litho/tripsy	crushing a stone
-logy	study of, science of	bio/logy	study or science of life

Word Part	Meaning	Medical Term	Meaning
lymph- (o)	lymph tissue	lymph/oma	tumor of lymph tissue
-lys (is, o)	destruction, dissolving of	thrombo/lysis	destruction or dissolving of clots

M

Word Part	Meaning	Medical Term	Meaning
macro-	large	macro/cyte	large cell
mal-	bad, abnormal, disordered, poor	mal/nutrition	poor nutrition
malac- (ia)	softening of a tissue	malac/ia	tissue softening
mamm- (o)	breast, mammary glands	mammo/gram	radiographic (X-ray) image of the breast
-mania	insanity, mental disorder	pyro/mania	individual with the insane desire to start fires
mast- (o)	breast	masto/pathy	disorder of the breast
med- (i, io)	middle, midline	medio/carpal	in the middle of or between the two rows of carpals (wrist bones)
-megaly, mega-	large, enlarged	cardio/megaly	enlarged heart
melan- (o)	black	melan/oma	black cancer
mening- (o)	membranes covering the brain and spinal cord	mening/itis	inflammation of the membranes of the brain and spinal cord
meno-	monthly, menstruation	meno/rrhea	monthly flow or discharge
mes- (o)	middle, midline	meso/cephal/ic	condition of having a head of medium proportions
-meter	measuring instrument, measure	urino/meter	instrument to measure (specific gravity of) urine
-metry	measurement	audio/metry	measurement of hearing acuity
micro-	small	micro/scope	instrument to examine small things
mono-	one, single	mono/cyte	single cell
-mortem	death	post/mortem	after death
muc- (o, us)	mucus, secretion of mucous membrane	muco/static	stopping the secretion of mucus
multi-	many, much, a large amount	multi/para	woman who has borne more than one child
my- (o)	muscle	my/algia	muscle pain
myc- (o)	fungus	myco/cide	substance that kills fungus
myel- (o)	bone marrow, spinal cord	myelo/blast	bone marrow cell
myring- (o)	eardrum, tympanic membrane	myring/otomy	cutting into the eardrum

N

Word Part	Meaning	Medical Term	Meaning
narc- (o)	sleep, numb, stupor	narco/lepsy	sleep seizure
nas- (o)	nose	nas/al	pertaining to the nose
-natal	birth	pre/natal	before birth
necr- (o)	death	necr/osis	condition or process of death
neo-	new	neo/natal	newborn (infant)
neph- (r, ro)	kidney	nephro/lith	kidney stone
neur- (o)	nerve, nervous system	neur/algia	nerve pain
noct- (i)	night, at night	noct/uria	urination at night
non-	no, none	non/toxic	not poison

O

Word Part	Meaning	Medical Term	Meaning
ocul- (o)	eye	oculo/graph	machine to measure eye (movement)
odont- (o)	tooth	odont/algia	pain in a tooth, toothache
olig- (o)	few, less than normal, small	olig/uria	less than normal (amounts of) urine
-ologist	person who does/studies	radi/ologist	person who studies radiographs

Word Part	Meaning	Medical Term	Meaning
-ology	study of, science of	hemat/ology	study of blood
-oma	tumor, a swelling	carcin/oma	cancerous tumor
onco- (i)	mass, bulk, tumor	oncol/ogist	physician who studies cancer
oophor- (o)	ovary, female egg cell	oophor/ectomy	surgical removal of the ovaries
ophthalm- (o)	eye	ophthalmo/scope	instrument for examining the eye
-opia	vision	dipl/opia	double vision
-opsy	to view	aut/opsy	view internal organs of a dead person
opt- (ic)	vision, eye	optic/al	pertaining to the eye
or- (o)	mouth	or/al	pertaining to the mouth
orch- (ido)	testicle, testes	orch/itis	inflammation of a testis
-orrhea	flow, discharge	rhin/orrhea	flow or discharge from the nose
orth- (o)	normal, straight	ortho/dontics	branch of dentistry involved with aligning or straightening the teeth
ost- (e, eo)	bone	osteo/genesis	formation of bone
-oscopy	diagnostic examination	colon/oscopy	diagnostic examination of the colon or large intestine
-osis	condition, state, process	necr/osis	condition or process of death
ot- (o)	ear	oto/scope	instrument for examining the ear
-otic	pertaining to a condition	leuko/cyt/otic	condition of white blood cells
-otomy	cutting into	crani/otomy	cutting into the skull
-ous	full of, containing, pertaining to, condition	ven/ous	pertaining to a vein
ovi-, ovario-	egg, female sex gland, ovary	ovari/ectomy	surgical removal of an ovary

P

Word Part	Meaning	Medical Term	Meaning
pan-	all, complete, entire	pan/ater/itis	inflammation of all layers of an artery
pancreat- (o)	pancreas	pancreat/itis	inflammation of the pancreas
para-	near, beside, beyond, abnormal, lower half of the body	para/plegia	paralysis of the lower half of the body
-paresis	paralysis	hemi/paresis	paralysis on one side of the body
-partum	birth, labor	post/partum	after birth
path- (ia, o, y)	disease, abnormal condition	path/ology	study of disease
ped- (ia)	child	pedia/tric	pertaining to children
-penia	lack of, abnormal reduction in number, deficiency	erythro/cyto/penia	deficiency of red blood cells
pent- (a)	five	penta/dactyl	having five digits (fingers or toes)
-pepsia, -pepsis	digestion	dys/pepsia	difficult digestion (indigestion)
per-	through, by, excessive	per/axillary	through the axilla or armpit
peri-	around	peri/cardi/al	pertaining to area around the heart
-pexy	fixation	gastro/pexy	surgical operation in which the stomach is sutured or fixed to the abdominal wall
phag- (o)	eat, ingest	phago/cyt/osis	process of cells engulfing and destroying microorganisms
-phage, -phagia	to eat, consuming, swallow	dys/phagia	difficult or painful swallowing
pharyng- (o)	pharynx, throat	pharyng/itis	inflammation of the throat or pharynx
-phas, -phasia	speech	a/phasia	without speech
-philia, -philic	affinity for, attracted to	necro/philia	attracted to or unusual interest in death
phleb- (o)	vein	phleb/otomy	cutting into a vein
-phobia	fear	hydro/phobia	fear of water
phon- (o)	sound, voice	phon/asthenia	weakness or hoarseness of the voice
-phylaxis	protection, prevention	pro/phylaxis	for prevention

Word Part	Meaning	Medical Term	Meaning
-plasty	surgical correction or repair	chondro/plasty	surgical repair of cartilage
-plegia	paralysis	hemi/plegia	paralysis of half of the body
pleuro-	side, rib	pleur/itis	inflammation of the pleural membranes lining the side of the thorax
-pnea	breathing	a/pnea	without breathing
pneum- (o, on)	lung, pertaining to the lungs, air	pneumon/ectomy	surgical removal of a lung (or part of a lung)
pod- (e, o)	foot	pod/algia	foot pain
poly-	many, much	poly/uria	much urine (more than normal amounts)
post-	after, behind	post/operative	after an operation
pre-	before, in front of	pre/operative	before an operation
pro-	in front of, forward	pro/cephalic	in front of the head
proct- (o)	rectum, rectal, anus	procto/scope	instrument for examining the rectum
pseudo-	false	pseudo/appendic/itis	false inflammation of the appendix
psych- (i, o)	pertaining to the mind	psych/ology	study of the mind
-ptosis	drooping down, sagging, downward displacement	visero/ptosis	drooping down or displacement of internal organs
pulmon- (o)	lung	pulmon/ary	pertaining to the lung
py- (o)	pus	pyo/genic	producing pus
pyel- (o)	renal pelvis of kidney	pyelo/lith/otomy	surgical incision of the renal pelvis to remove a stone
pyr- (o)	heat, fever	pyro/genic	produced by a fever

Q

Word Part	Meaning	Medical Term	Meaning
quad- (ra, ri)	four	quadra/plegia	paralysis of four extremities (arms and legs)

R

Word Part	Meaning	Medical Term	Meaning
radi- (o)	radiographs (X-rays), radiation	radi/ologist	person who studies radiographs
rect- (o)	rectum	recto/cele	rupture of the rectum
ren- (o)	kidney	ren/al	pertaining to the kidney
retro-	backward, in back, behind	retro/lingual	occurring behind or near the base of the tongue
rhin- (o)	nose, pertaining to the nose	rhino/plasty	surgical correction of the nose
-rraphy	suture of, sewing up of a gap or defect	angio/rraphy	sewing (suturing) a gap or defect in a vessel
-rrhagia	sudden or excessive flow	rhino/rrhagia	sudden flow from the nose (nosebleed)
-rrhea	flow, discharge	meno/rrhea	monthly flow or discharge
-rrhexis	rupture of, bursting	hystero/rrhexis	rupture of the uterus

S

Word Part	Meaning	Medical Term	Meaning
salping- (i, o)	tube, fallopian tube	salping/ectomy	surgical removal of a fallopian tube
sanguin- (o)	blood	sanguino/purulant	containing blood and pus
sarc- (o)	malignant (cancer) connective tissue	sarc/oma	cancerous tumor of connective tissue
-sarcoma	tumor, cancer	adeno/sarcoma	cancerous tumor of a gland
scler- (o)	hardening	sclero/derma	thickening or hardening of the skin
-sclerosis	dryness or hardness	arterio/sclerosis	hardness of an artery
-scope	examining instrument	oto/scope	instrument for examining the ear
-scopy	observation	procto/scopy	examination of the rectum
-sect	cut	bi/sect	to cut into two parts

Word Part	Meaning	Medical Term	Meaning
semi-	half, part	semi/cartilagin/ous	partly of cartilage
sep- (ti, tic)	poison, rot, infection	septic/emia	blood infection
sinistr- (o)	left	sinistr/ocular	left eye
soma- (t, to)	body	somato/genic	originating in the body
son- (o)	sound	sono/gram	an image produced by sound waves
-spasm	involuntary contraction	myo/spasm	contraction of muscle
sperm- (ato)	spermatozoa, male germ (sex) cell	spermat/uria	discharge of sperm in the urine
splen- (o)	spleen	spleno/megaly	abnormal enlargement of the spleen
-stasis	stoppage, maintaining a constant level	homeo/stasis	maintaining the same constant level
steno-	contracted, narrow	steno/sis	condition of narrowing
stern- (o)	sternum, breast bone	sterno/cost/al	pertaining to the ribs and breastbone (sternum)
stoma- (t)	mouth	stomat/ology	scientific study of the mouth and its disorders
-stomy	artificial opening	colo/stomy	creating an opening into the colon or large intestines
sub-	less, under, below	sub/lingual	under the tongue
sup- (er, ra)	above, upon, over, higher in position	supra/thorac/ic	pertaining to the area in the upper part of the chest
sym-, syn-	joined, fused, together	syn/dactyl	two or more digits (fingers or toes) joined together

T

tach- (o, y)	rapid, fast	tachy/cardia	fast or rapid heart
ten- (do, don, o)	tendon	tendon/itis	inflammation of a tendon
tetra-	four	tetra/paresis	weakness or paralysis of all four limbs
-therapy	treatment	chemo/therapy	treatment with drugs or chemicals
therm- (o, y)	heat	therm/algesia	sensitive to heat
thorac- (o)	thorax, chest	thorac/otomy	cutting into the chest
thromb- (o)	clot, thrombus	thrombo/lysis	dissolving or destruction of clots
thym- (o)	thymus gland	thym/oma	tumor of the thymus gland
thyr- (o, oid)	thyroid gland	thyroid/ologist	individual who studies the thyroid gland
-tome	instrument that cuts	myo/tome	instrument for cutting muscle
-tox (ic)	poison	cyto/toxic	cell poison
trach- (e, i, o)	trachea, windpipe	trache/otomy	cutting into the trachea or windpipe
trans-	across, over, beyond	trans/neural	across a nerve
tri-	three	tri/angle	three angles
trich- (o)	hair	tricho/myo/sis	fungus disease of the hair
-trips (y)	crushing by rubbing or grinding	litho/tripsy	crushing of stone
-trophy	nutrition, growth, development	a/trophy	without nutrition (wasting away)
tympan- (o)	eardrum, tympanic membrane	tympan/itis	inflammation of the eardrum (tympanic membrane)

U

ultra-	beyond, excess	ultra/sonic	beyond sound waves
uni-	one	uni/ocular	one eye
ur- (in, o)	urine, urinary tract	urino/meter	instrument to measure (specific gravity) urine
ureter- (o)	ureter (tube from kidney to bladder)	uretero/cele	dilation of the ureter into the bladder

Word Part	Meaning	Medical Term	Meaning
urethr- (o)	urethra (tube from bladder to urinary meatus)	urethro/scope	instrument to view the urethra
-uria	urine	hemat/uria	blood in urine
uter- (o)	uterus, womb	utero/vaginal	pertaining to the uterus and vagina

V

Word Part	Meaning	Medical Term	Meaning
vas- (o)	vessel, duct	vaso/neur/otic	pertaining to blood vessels and nerves
ven- (a)	vein	ven/ous	pertaining to vein
ventro-	to the front, abdomen	ventr/al	pertaining to the front
vertebr- (o)	spine, vertebrae	vertebr/al	pertaining to the spine or vertebrae
vesic- (o)	urinary bladder	vesico/urethral	connecting the urinary bladder and urethra
viscer- (o)	internal organs	viscero/ptosis	drooping or displacement of internal organs
vit- (a)	necessary for life	vit/al	important to life

X

Word Part	Meaning	Medical Term	Meaning
xanth- (o)	yellow	xantho/derma	yellowish discoloration of the skin
-xen (ia, a)	strange, abnormal	xeno/genetic	derived or originating from a foreign species

Z

Word Part	Meaning	Medical Term	Meaning
zoo-	animal	zoo/ology	study of animals
zymo-	enzymes	zymo/gram	picture or tracing of enzymes

TODAY'S RESEARCH: TOMORROW'S HEALTH CARE

Artificial red blood cells that replace the need for blood transfusions?

Blood is needed for life. Erythrocytes (red blood cells) in the blood carry the oxygen that is needed by all body cells. The erythrocytes also carry carbon dioxide, a waste product of the cells, to the lungs so it can be expelled from the body. Without oxygen, body cells will die in 4 to 6 minutes.

When a person has a hemorrhage and loses a large amount of blood, an immediate blood transfusion is needed. The blood for the transfusion comes from other individuals who are willing to donate blood. However, the annual worldwide shortage of blood is estimated to be about 100 million units. Scientists are busy researching the development of "artificial" blood or some type of blood cell that will carry the oxygen needed by the body.

Already several products have been developed that meet this need. Dr. Thomas Chang is one researcher who has worked on this problem since the 1960s. He invented microencapsulation, a technique that allows a biochemical to be held inside an artificial membrane. His work has led to the development of a modified hemoglobin called *polyhemoglobin*. This substance carries oxygen in the same way hemoglobin on red blood cells carries oxygen. Clinical trials of the product are currently being conducted. Another product that has been developed by Alliance Pharmaceutical is *Oxygent*. *Oxygent* is a sterile perfluorochemical solution that can be used with all blood types, has a shelf life of about 2 years, and contains no human or animal blood. It carries oxygen in the bloodstream and is used in place of a blood transfusion. Studies on *Oxygent* are currently being conducted in Europe. There is little doubt that researchers will eventually find a substitute for blood transfusions.

cell, has 46 chromosomes: 23 from the ovum and 23 from the sperm. Thus, the zygote has 46, or 23 pairs, of chromosomes, the normal number for all body cells except the sex cells.

Immediately after the ovum and sperm join to form a zygote, the zygote begins a period of rapid mitotic division. Within 4–5 days, the zygote is a hollow ball-like mass of cells called a *blastocyst*. Within this blastocyst are embryonic **stem cells.** These stem cells have the ability to transform themselves into any of the body's specialized cells and perform many different functions. A controversial area of research is now concentrated on these stem cells. Scientists are attempting to determine whether stem cells can be transplanted into the body and used to cure diseases such as diabetes mellitus, Parkinson's, heart disease, osteoporosis, arthritis, and spinal cord injuries. The hope is that the stem cells can be programmed to produce new specialized cells that can replace a body's damaged cells and cure a disease. The controversy arises from the fact that a 4–5-day embryo, capable of creating a new life, is used to obtain the cells. Right-to-life advocates are strongly opposed to stem cell research if the cells are obtained from embryos. Another source of stem cells is the blood in the discarded umbilical cord and placenta of a newborn. Currently, parents have the option of preserving this blood for its stem cells. The blood is collected and frozen in liquid nitrogen. If the child later develops a disease for which a stem cell transplant can provide a cure, the cells can be harvested from the blood and used for the transplant. The cost of this procedure limits its use, however. Stem cells also exist in adult tissues, such as bone marrow and the liver. Adult stem cells, however, do not have the ability to evolve into every kind of cell; these stem cells evolve into more cells of their own kind. This controversy will continue as scientists expand stem cell research.

TISSUE

Although most cells contain the same basic parts, cells vary greatly in shape, size, and special function. When cells of the same type join together for a common purpose, they form a **tissue.** Tissues are 60–99 percent water with various dissolved substances. This water is slightly salty in nature and is called *tissue fluid*. If there is an insufficient amount (not enough tissue fluid), a condition

called **dehydration** occurs. When there is an excess amount (too much tissue fluid), a condition called **edema,** or swelling of the tissues, occurs.

There are four main groups of tissues: epithelial, connective, nerve, and muscle (figure 7-3).

Epithelial tissue covers the surface of the body and is the main tissue in the skin. It forms the lining of the intestinal, respiratory, circulatory, and urinary tracts, as well as that of other body cavities. Epithelial tissue also forms the body glands, where it specializes to produce specific secretions for the body, such as mucus and digestive juices.

Connective tissue is the supporting fabric of organs and other body parts. There are two main classes of connective tissue: soft and hard. One

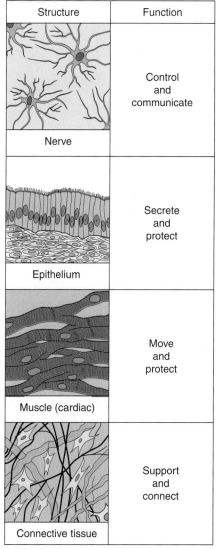

Structure	Function
Nerve	Control and communicate
Epithelium	Secrete and protect
Muscle (cardiac)	Move and protect
Connective tissue	Support and connect

FIGURE 7-3 Four main groups of tissues and their functions.

type of soft connective tissue is adipose, or fatty, tissue, which stores fat as a food reserve or source of energy, insulates the body, fills the area between tissue fibers, and acts as padding. A second type of soft connective tissue is fibrous connective tissue, such as ligaments and tendons, which help hold body structures together. Hard connective tissue includes cartilage and bone. Cartilage is a tough, elastic material that is found between the bones of the spine and at the end of long bones. It acts as a shock absorber and allows for flexibility. It is also found in the nose, ears, and larynx, or "voice box," to provide form or shaping. Bone is similar to cartilage but has calcium salts, nerves, and blood vessels; it is frequently called *osseous tissue*. Bone helps form the rigid structure of the human body. Blood and lymph are classified as liquid connective tissue, or *vascular tissue*. Blood carries nutrients and oxygen to the body cells and carries metabolic waste away from cells. Lymph transports tissue fluid, proteins, fats, and other materials from the tissues to the circulatory system.

Nerve tissue is made up of special cells called *neurons*. It controls and coordinates body activities by transmitting messages throughout the body. The nerves, brain, and spinal cord are composed of nerve tissue.

Muscle tissue produces power and movement by contraction of muscle fibers. There are three main kinds of muscle tissue: skeletal, cardiac,

TABLE 7-1 Systems of the Body

SYSTEM	FUNCTIONS	MAJOR ORGANS/STRUCTURES
Integumentary	Protects body from injury, infection, and dehydration; helps regulate body temperature; eliminates some wastes; produces vitamin D	Skin, sweat and oil glands, nails, and hair
Skeletal	Creates framework of body, protects internal organs, produces blood cells, acts as levers for muscles	Bones and cartilage
Muscular	Produces movement, protects internal organs, produces body heat, maintains posture	Skeletal, smooth, and cardiac muscles
Nervous	Coordinates and controls body activities	Nerves, brain, spinal cord
Special Senses	Allow body to react to environment by providing sight, hearing, taste, smell, and balance	Eye, ear, tongue, nose, general sense receptors
Circulatory	Carries oxygen and nutrients to body cells; carries waste products away from cells; helps produce cells to fight infection	Heart, blood vessels, blood, spleen
Lymphatic	Carries some tissue fluid and wastes to blood, assists with fighting infection	Lymph nodes, lymph vessels, spleen, tonsils, and thymus gland
Respiratory	Breathes in oxygen and eliminates carbon dioxide	Nose, pharynx, larynx, trachea, bronchi, lungs
Digestive	Digests food physically and chemically, transports food, absorbs nutrients, eliminates waste	Mouth, salivary glands, pharynx, esophagus, stomach, intestine, liver, gallbladder, pancreas
Urinary	Filters blood to maintain fluid and electrolyte balance in the body, produces and eliminates urine	Kidneys, ureters, urinary bladder, urethra
Endocrine	Produces and secretes hormones to regulate body processes	Pituitary, thyroid, parathyroid, adrenal, and thymus glands; pancreas, ovaries, testes
Reproductive	Provides for reproduction	Male: testes, epididymis, vas deferens, ejaculatory duct, seminal vesicles, prostate gland, penis, urethra Female: ovaries, fallopian tubes, uterus, vagina, breasts

and visceral (smooth). Skeletal muscle attaches to the bones and provides for movement of the body. Cardiac muscle causes the heart to beat. Visceral muscle is present in the walls of the respiratory, digestive, urinary tract, and blood vessels.

ORGANS AND SYSTEMS

Two or more tissues joined together to perform a specific function are called an **organ.** Examples of organs include the heart, stomach, and lungs.

Organs and other body parts joined together to perform a particular function are called a **system.** The basic systems (discussed in more detail in succeeding sections) are the integumentary, skeletal, muscular, circulatory, lymphatic, nervous, respiratory, digestive, urinary (or excretory), endocrine, and reproductive. Their functions and main organs are shown in table 7-1.

In summary, cells combine to form tissues, tissues combine to form organs, and organs and other body parts combine to form systems. These systems working together help create the miracle called the human body (figure 7-4).

STUDENT: *Go to the workbook and complete the assignment sheet for 7:1, Basic Structure of the Human Body.*

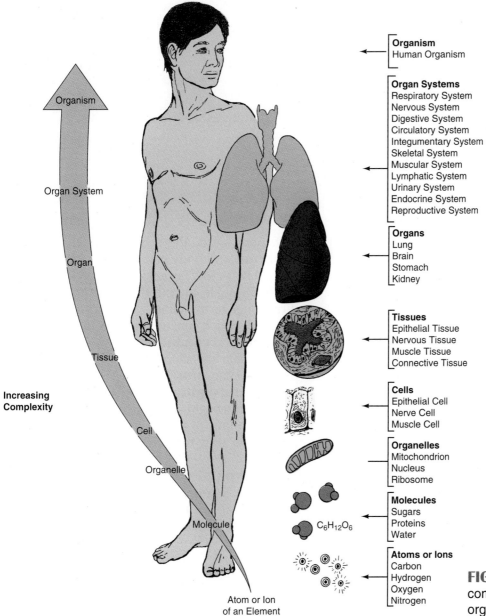

Organism
Human Organism

Organ Systems
Respiratory System
Nervous System
Digestive System
Circulatory System
Integumentary System
Skeletal System
Muscular System
Lymphatic System
Urinary System
Endocrine System
Reproductive System

Organs
Lung
Brain
Stomach
Kidney

Tissues
Epithelial Tissue
Nervous Tissue
Muscle Tissue
Connective Tissue

Cells
Epithelial Cell
Nerve Cell
Muscle Cell

Organelles
Mitochondrion
Nucleus
Ribosome

Molecules
Sugars
Proteins
Water

$C_6H_{12}O_6$

Atoms or Ions
Carbon
Hydrogen
Oxygen
Nitrogen

Organism

Organ System

Organ

Tissue

Increasing Complexity

Cell

Organelle

Molecule

Atom or Ion of an Element

FIGURE 7-4 The levels of complexity in the human organism.

7:2 Body Planes, Directions, and Cavities

Objectives

After completing this section, you should be able to:

♦ Label the names of the planes and the directional terms related to these planes on a diagram of the three planes of the body

♦ Label a diagram of the main body cavities

♦ Identify the main organs located in each body cavity

♦ Locate the nine abdominal regions

♦ Define, pronounce, and spell all key terms

KEY TERMS

abdominal cavity
abdominal regions
anterior
body cavities
body planes
buccal cavity
caudal *(kaw'-doll)*
cranial *(kray'-nee-al)*
cranial cavity
distal

dorsal
dorsal cavity
frontal (coronal) plane
inferior
lateral *(lat'-eh-ral)*
medial *(me'-dee-al)*
midsagittal (median) plane
    (mid-saj'-ih-tahl)
nasal cavity
orbital cavity

pelvic cavity
posterior
proximal *(prox'-ih-mahl)*
spinal cavity
superior
thoracic cavity *(tho-rass'-ik)*
transverse plane
ventral
ventral cavity

7:2 INFORMATION

Because terms such as *south* and *east* would be difficult to apply to the human body, other directional terms have been developed. These terms are used to describe the relationship of one part of the body to another part. The terms are used when the body is in anatomic position. This means the body is facing forward, standing erect, and holding the arms at the sides with the palms of the hands facing forward.

BODY PLANES

Body planes are imaginary lines drawn through the body at various parts to separate the body into sections. Directional terms are created by these planes. The three main body planes are the transverse, midsagittal, and frontal (figure 7-5).

The **transverse plane** is a horizontal plane that divides the body into a top half and a bottom half. Body parts above other parts are termed **superior,** and body parts below other parts are termed **inferior.** For instance, the knee is superior to the ankle, but inferior to the hip. Two other directional terms related to this plane include **cranial,** which means body parts located near the head, and **caudal,** which means body parts located near the sacral region of the spinal column (also known as the "tail").

The **midsagittal** or **median plane** divides the body into right and left sides. Body parts close to the midline, or plane, are called **medial,** and body parts away from the midline are called **lateral.**

The **frontal** or **coronal plane** divides the body into a front section and a back section. Body parts in front of the plane, or on the front of the body, are called **ventral** or **anterior.** Body parts on the back of the body are called **dorsal** or **posterior.**

Two other directional terms are **proximal** and **distal.** These are used to describe the loca-

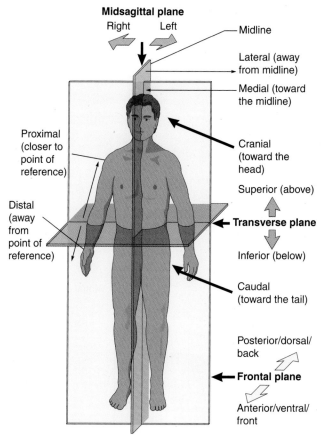

Midsagittal plane
Right — Left
— Midline
— Lateral (away from midline)
— Medial (toward the midline)
Proximal (closer to point of reference)
— Cranial (toward the head)
Superior (above)
Distal (away from point of reference)
◄ **Transverse plane**
Inferior (below)
Caudal (toward the tail)
Posterior/dorsal/back
◄ **Frontal plane**
Anterior/ventral/front

FIGURE 7-5 Body planes and directional terms.

tion of the extremities (arms and legs) in relation to the main trunk of the body, generally called the *point of reference.* Body parts close to the point of reference are called *proximal,* and body parts distant from the point of reference are called *distal.* For example, in describing the relationship of the wrist and elbow to the shoulder (or point of reference), the wrist is distal and the elbow is proximal to the shoulder.

BODY CAVITIES

Body cavities are spaces within the body that contain vital organs. There are two main body cavities: the dorsal, or posterior, cavity and the ventral, or anterior, cavity (figure 7-6).

The **dorsal cavity** is one long, continuous cavity located on the back of the body. It is divided into two sections: the **cranial cavity,** which contains the brain, and the **spinal cavity,** which contains the spinal cord.

The **ventral cavities** are larger than the dorsal cavities. The ventral cavity is separated into two distinct cavities by the dome-shaped muscle called the *diaphragm,* which is important for respiration (breathing). The **thoracic cavity** is located in the chest and contains the esophagus, trachea, bronchi, lungs, heart, and large blood vessels. The **abdominal cavity,** or abdomino-pelvic cavity, is divided into an upper part and a lower part. The upper abdominal cavity contains the stomach, small intestine, most of the large intestine, appendix, liver, gallbladder, pancreas, and spleen. The lower abdominal cavity, or **pelvic cavity,** contains the urinary bladder, the reproductive organs, and the last part of the large intestine. The kidneys and adrenal glands are technically located outside the abdominal cavity because they are behind the peritoneal membrane (peritoneum) that lines the abdominal cavity. This area is called the *retroperitoneal space.*

Three small cavities are the **orbital cavity** for the eyes, the **nasal cavity** for the nose structures, and the **buccal cavity,** or mouth, for the teeth and tongue.

ABDOMINAL REGIONS

The abdominal cavity is so large that it is divided into regions or sections. One method of division is into quadrants, or four sections. As shown in figure 7-7, this results in a right upper quadrant (RUQ), left upper quadrant (LUQ), right lower quadrant (RLQ), and left lower quadrant (LLQ). A more precise method of division is into nine **abdominal regions** (figure 7-8). The center regions are the epigastric (above the stomach), umbilical (near the umbilicus or belly button), and hypogastric, or pelvic (below the stomach). On either side of the center the regions are the hypochondriac (below the ribs), lumbar (near the large bones of the spinal cord), and iliac, or inguinal (near the groin).

The terms relating to body planes, directions, and cavities are used frequently in the study of human anatomy.

STUDENT: *Go to the workbook and complete the assignment sheet for 7:2, Body Planes, Directions, and Cavities.*

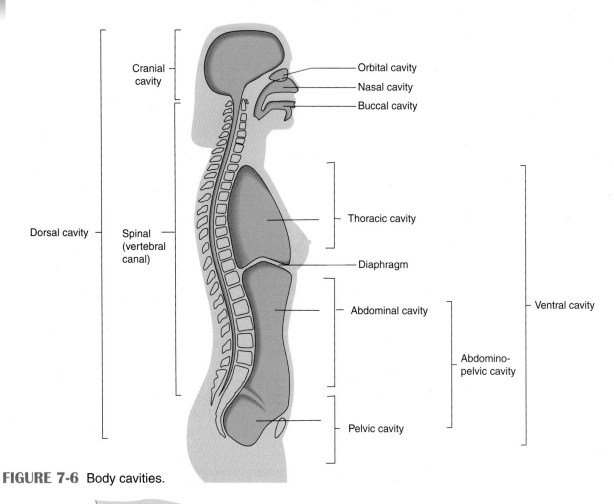

FIGURE 7-6 Body cavities.

Right upper quadrant (RUQ)

Left upper quadrant (LUQ)

Umbilicus

Right lower quadrant (RLQ)

Left lower quadrant (LLQ)

FIGURE 7-7 Abdominal quadrants.

Right hypo-chondriac region	Epigastric region	Left hypo-chondriac region
Right lumbar region	Umbilical region	Left lumbar region
Right iliac region	Hypogastric region	Left iliac region

FIGURE 7-8 Nine abdominal regions.

7:3 Integumentary System

Objectives

After completing this section, you should be able to:

◆ Label a diagram of a cross section of the skin

◆ Differentiate between the two types of skin glands

◆ List six functions of the skin

◆ Provide the correct names for three abnormal colors of the skin and identify the cause of each abnormal color

◆ Describe at least four skin eruptions

◆ Describe at least four diseases of the integumentary system

◆ Define, pronounce, and spell all key terms

KEY TERMS

albino	**integumentary system** *(in-teg-u-men'-tah-ree)*	**subcutaneous fascia (hypodermis)** *(sub-q-tay'-nee-us fash'-ee-ah)*
alopecia		
constrict *(kun-strict')*	**jaundice** *(jawn'-diss)*	
crusts	**macules** *(mack'-youlz)*	**sudoriferous glands** *(sue-de-rif'-eh-rus)*
cyanosis *(sy'-eh-noh'-sis)*	**melanin**	
dermis	**papules** *(pap'-youlz)*	**ulcer**
dilate *(die'-late)*	**pustules** *(pus'-tyoulz)*	**vesicles** *(ves'-i-kulz)*
epidermis *(eh-pih-der'-mis)*	**sebaceous glands** *(seh-bay'-shus)*	**wheals**
erythema *(err-ih-thee'-ma)*		

RELATED HEALTH CAREERS

◆ Allergist   ◆ Dermatologist   ◆ Plastic Surgeon

FIGURE

◆ *Body te* sels in heat. V larger), throug **strict** (body. T the boc tion.

◆ *Storage*: storage and salt taneous

◆ *Absorpti* absorbe tions for nicotine medicati applied mal med

◆ *Excretion* salt, a m water and

◆ *Productic* of vitami sun to fo that matu

7:3 INFORMATION

The **integumentary system,** or skin, has been called both a membrane, because it covers the body, and an organ, because it contains several kinds of tissues. Most anatomy courses, however, refer to it as a system because it has organs and other parts that work together to perform a particular function. On an average adult, the skin covers more than 3,000 square inches of surface area and accounts for about 15 percent of total body weight.

Three main layers of tissue make up the skin (figure 7-9):

◆ **Epidermis:** the outermost layer of skin. This layer is actually made of five smaller layers but no blood vessels or nerve cells. Two main layers are the *stratum corneum,* the outermost layer, and the *stratum germinativum,* the innermost layer. The cells of the stratum corneum are constantly shed and replaced by new cells from the stratum germinativum.

◆ **Dermis:** also called *corium,* or "true skin." This layer has a framework of elastic connective tissue and contains blood vessels, lymph vessels, nerves, involuntary muscle, sweat and oil glands, and hair follicles. The top of the dermis is covered with papillae, which fit into ridges on the stratum germinativum of the epidermis. These ridges form lines, or striations, on the skin. Because the pattern of ridges is unique to each individual, fingerprints and footprints are often used as methods of identification.

Cyanosis is a bluish discoloration of the skin caused by insufficient oxygen. It can be associated with heart, lung, and circulatory diseases or disorders. Chronic poisoning may cause a gray or brown skin discoloration.

SKIN ERUPTIONS

Skin eruptions can also indicate disease. The most common eruptions include:

♦ **Macules:** (macular rash) flat spots on the skin, such as freckles

♦ **Papules:** (papular rash) firm, raised areas such as pimples and the eruptions seen in some stages of chickenpox and syphilis

♦ **Vesicles:** blisters, or fluid-filled sacs, such as those seen in chickenpox

♦ **Pustules:** pus-filled sacs such as those seen in acne, or pimples

♦ **Crusts:** areas of dried pus and blood, commonly called *scabs*

♦ **Wheals:** itchy, elevated areas with an irregular shape; hives and insect bites are examples

♦ **Ulcer:** a deep loss of skin surface that may extend into the dermis; may cause periodic bleeding and the formation of scars

DISEASES AND ABNORMAL CONDITIONS

Acne Vulgaris

Acne vulgaris is an inflammation of the sebaceous glands. Although the cause is unknown, acne usually occurs at adolescence. Hormonal changes and increased secretion of sebum are probably underlying causes. Symptoms include papules, pustules, and blackheads. These occur when the hair follicles become blocked with dirt, cosmetics, excess oil, and/or bacteria. Treatment methods include frequent, thorough skin washing; avoidance of creams and heavy makeup; antibiotic or vitamin A ointments; oral antibiotics; and/or ultraviolet light treatments.

Athlete's Foot

Athlete's foot is a contagious fungal infection that usually affects the feet. The skin itches, blisters,

and cracks into open sores. Treatment involves applying an antifungal medication and keeping the area clean and dry.

Skin Cancer

Cancer of the skin is the most common type of cancer. There are three main types of skin cancer: basal cell carcinoma, squamous cell carcinoma, and melanoma. *Basal cell carcinoma* is cancer of the basal cells in the epidermis of the skin. It grows slowly and does not usually spread (figure 7-11). The lesions can be pink to yellow-white. They are usually smooth with a depressed center and an elevated, irregular-shaped border.

Squamous cell carcinoma affects the thin cells of the epithelium but can spread quickly to other areas of the body. The lesions start as small, firm, red, flat sores that later scale and crust (figure 7-12). Sores that do not heal are frequently squamous cell carcinomas.

Melanoma develops in the melanocytes of the epidermis and is the most dangerous type of

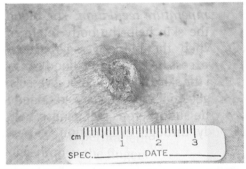

FIGURE 7-11 Basal cell carcinomas usually grow more slowly. *(Courtesy of Robert A. Silverman, MD, Clinical Associate Professor, Department of Pediatrics, Georgetown University)*

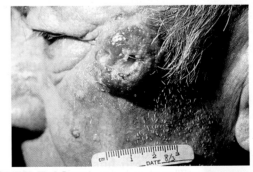

FIGURE 7-12 Squamous cell carcinomas resemble sores that scale and crust. *(Courtesy of Robert A. Silverman, MD, Clinical Associate Professor, Department of Pediatrics, Georgetown University)*

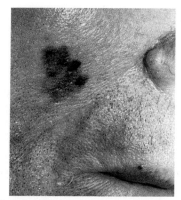

FIGURE 7-13 Melanoma is the most dangerous form of skin cancer. *(Courtesy of Robert A. Silverman, MD, Clinical Associate Professor, Department of Pediatrics, Georgetown University)*

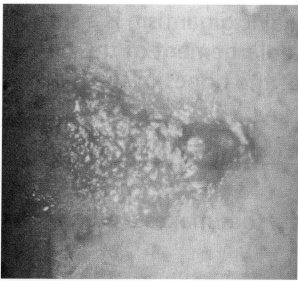

FIGURE 7-14 A contact dermatitis caused by contact with poison oak. *(Courtesy of Timothy Berger, MD, Clinical Professor, Department of Dermatology, University of California, San Francisco)*

skin cancer (figure 7-13). The lesions can be brown, black, pink, or multicolored. They are usually flat or raised slightly, asymmetric and irregular or notched on the edges.

Frequently, skin cancer develops from a mole or nevus that changes in color, shape, size, or texture. Bleeding or itching of a mole can also indicate cancer. Exposure to the sun, prolonged use of tanning beds, irritating chemicals, or radiation are the usual causes of skin cancer. Treatment involves surgical removal of the cancer, radiation, and/or chemotherapy.

Dermatitis

Dermatitis, an inflammation of the skin, can be caused by any substance that irritates the skin. It is frequently an allergic reaction to detergents, cosmetics, pollen, or certain foods. One example of contact dermatitis is the irritation caused by contact with poison ivy, poison sumac, or poison oak (figure 7-14). Symptoms include dry skin, erythema, itching, edema, macular-papular rashes, and scaling. Treatment is directed at eliminating the cause, especially in the case of allergens. Anti-inflammatory ointments, antihistamines, and/or steroids are also used in treatment.

Eczema

Eczema is a noncontagious, inflammatory skin disorder caused by an allergen or irritant. Diet, cosmetics, soaps, medications, and emotional stress can all cause eczema. Symptoms include dryness, erythema, edema, itching, vesicles, crusts, and scaling. Treatment involves removing the irritant and applying corticosteroids to reduce the inflammatory response.

Impetigo

Impetigo is a highly contagious skin infection usually caused by streptococci or staphylococci organisms. Symptoms include erythema, oozing vesicles, pustules, and the formation of a yellow crust. Lesions should be washed with soap and water and kept dry. Antibiotics, both topical and oral, are also used in treatment.

Psoriasis

Psoriasis is a chronic, noncontagious skin disease with periods of exacerbations (symptoms present) and remission (symptoms decrease or disappear). The cause is unknown, but there may be a hereditary link. Stress, cold weather, sunlight, pregnancy, and endocrine changes tend to cause an exacerbation of the disease. Symptoms include thick, red areas covered with white or silver scales, (figure 7-15). Although there is no cure, treatment methods include coal/tar or cortisone ointments, ultraviolet light, and/or scale removal.

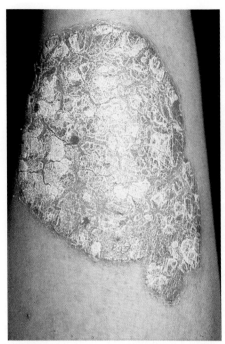

FIGURE 7-15 Psoriasis is characterized by white or silver scales. *(Courtesy of Robert A. Silverman, MD, Pediatric Dermatology, Georgetown University)*

Ringworm

Ringworm (tineas) is a highly contagious fungal infection of the skin or scalp. The characteristic symptom is the formation of a flat or raised circular area with a clear central area surrounded by an itchy, scaly, or crusty outer ring. Antifungal medications, both oral and topical, are used in treatment.

Verrucae

Verrucae, or warts, are caused by a viral infection of the skin. Plantar warts usually occur at pressure points on the sole of the foot. A rough, hard, elevated, rounded surface forms on the skin. Some warts disappear spontaneously, but others must be removed with electricity, liquid nitrogen, acid, chemicals, or laser.

STUDENT: *Go to the workbook and complete the assignment sheet for 7:3, Integumentary System.*

7:4 Skeletal System

Objectives

After completing this section, you should be able to:

♦ List five functions of bones

♦ Label the parts of a bone on a diagram of a long bone

♦ Name the two divisions of the skeletal system and the main groups of bones in each division

♦ Identify the main bones of the skeleton

♦ Compare the three classifications of joints by describing the type of motion allowed by each

♦ Give one example of each joint classification

♦ Describe at least four diseases of the skeletal system

♦ Define, pronounce, and spell all key terms

KEY TERMS

appendicular skeleton
    (ap-pen-dick'-u-lar)
axial skeleton
carpals
clavicles *(klav'-ih-kulz)*
cranium
diaphysis *(dy-af'-eh-sis)*
endosteum *(en-dos'-tee-um)*
epiphysis *(ih-pif'-eh-sis)*
femur *(fee'-mur)*

fibula *(fib'-you-la)*
fontanels
foramina *(for-ahm'-e-nah)*
humerus *(hue'-mer-us)*
joints
ligaments
medullary canal
    (med'-hue-lair-ee)
metacarpals
    (met-ah-car'-pulz)

metatarsals
    (met-ah-tar'-sulz)
os coxae *(ahs cock'-see)*
patella *(pa-tell'-ah)*
periosteum
    (per-ee-os'-tee-um)
phalanges *(fa-lan'-jeez)*
radius
red marrow
ribs

(continues)

KEY TERMS (continued)

scapula	sutures	ulna
sinuses *(sigh'-nuss-ez)*	tarsals	vertebrae *(vur'-teh-bray)*
skeletal system	tibia	yellow marrow
sternum		

RELATED HEALTH CAREERS

- ◆ Athletic Trainer
- ◆ Chiropractor
- ◆ Orthopedist
- ◆ Orthoptist
- ◆ Osteopathic Physician
- ◆ Physiatrist
- ◆ Physical Therapist
- ◆ Podiatrist
- ◆ Prosthetist
- ◆ Radiologic Technologist
- ◆ Sports Medicine Physician

7:4 INFORMATION

The **skeletal system** is made of organs called *bones*. An adult human has 206 bones. These bones work as a system to perform the following functions:

- ◆ *Framework*: bones form a framework to support the body's muscles, fat, and skin

- ◆ *Protection*: bones surround vital organs to protect them (for example the skull, which surrounds the brain, and the ribs, which protect the heart and lungs)

- ◆ *Levers*: muscles attach to bones to help provide movement

- ◆ *Production of blood cells*: bones help produce red and white blood cells and platelets, a process called *hemopoiesis* or *hematopoiesis*

- ◆ *Storage*: bones store most of the calcium supply of the body in addition to phosphorus and fats

Bones vary in shape and size depending on their locations within the body. Bones of the extremities (arms and legs) are called *long bones*. The basic parts of these bones are shown in figure 7-16. The long shaft is called the **diaphysis,** and the two extremities, or ends, are each called an **epiphysis.** The **medullary canal** is a cavity in the diaphysis. It is filled with **yellow marrow,** which is mainly a storage area for fat cells. Yellow marrow also contains cells that form leukocytes,

or white blood cells. The **endosteum** is a membrane that lines the medullary canal and keeps the yellow marrow intact. It also produces some bone growth. **Red marrow** is found in certain bones, such as the vertebrae, ribs, sternum, and cranium, and in the proximal ends of the humerus and femur. It produces red blood cells (erythrocytes), platelets (thrombocytes), and some white blood cells (leukocytes). Because bone marrow is important in the manufacture of blood cells and is involved with the body's immune response, the red marrow is used to diagnose blood diseases and is sometimes transplanted in people with defective immune systems. The outside of bone is covered with a tough membrane, called the **periosteum,** which contains blood vessels, lymph vessels, and *osteoblasts,* special cells that form new bone tissue. The periosteum is necessary for bone growth, repair, and nutrition. A thin layer of articular cartilage covers the epiphysis and acts as a shock absorber when two bones meet to form a joint.

The skeletal system is divided into two sections: the axial skeleton and the appendicular skeleton. The **axial skeleton** forms the main trunk of the body and is composed of the skull, spinal column, ribs, and breastbone. The **appendicular skeleton** forms the extremities and is composed of the shoulder girdle, arm bones, pelvic girdle, and leg bones.

The skull is composed of the cranial and facial bones (figure 7-17). The **cranium** is the spherical structure that surrounds and protects the

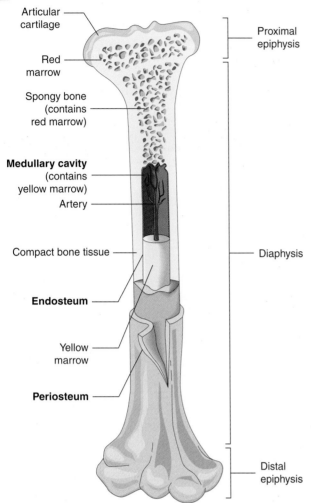

Articular cartilage

Red marrow

Spongy bone (contains red marrow)

Medullary cavity (contains yellow marrow)

Artery

Compact bone tissue

Endosteum

Yellow marrow

Periosteum

Proximal epiphysis

Diaphysis

Distal epiphysis

FIGURE 7-16 Anatomic parts of a long bone.

brain. It is made of eight bones: one frontal, two parietal, two temporal, one occipital, one ethmoid, and one sphenoid. At birth, the cranium is not solid bone. Spaces called **fontanels,** or "soft spots," allow for the enlargement of the skull as brain growth occurs. The fontanels are made of membrane and cartilage, and turn into solid bone by approximately 18 months of age. There are 14 facial bones: 1 mandible (lower jaw), 2 maxilla (upper jaw), 2 zygomatic (cheek), 2 lacrimal (inner aspect of eyes), 5 nasal, and 2 palatine (hard palate or roof of the mouth). **Sutures** are areas where the cranial bones have joined together. **Sinuses** are air spaces in the bones of the skull that act as resonating chambers for the voice. They are lined with mucous membranes. **Foramina** are openings in bones that allow nerves and blood vessels to enter or leave the bone.

The spinal column is composed of 26 bones called **vertebrae** (figure 7-18). These bones protect the spinal cord and provide support for the head and trunk. They include 7 cervical (neck), 12 thoracic (chest), 5 lumbar (waist), 1 sacrum (back of pelvic girdle), and 1 coccyx (tailbone). Pads of cartilage tissue, called *intervertebral disks,* separate the vertebrae. The disks act as shock absorbers and permit bending and twisting movements of the vertebral column.

There are 12 pairs of **ribs,** or costae. They attach to the thoracic vertebrae on the dorsal sur-

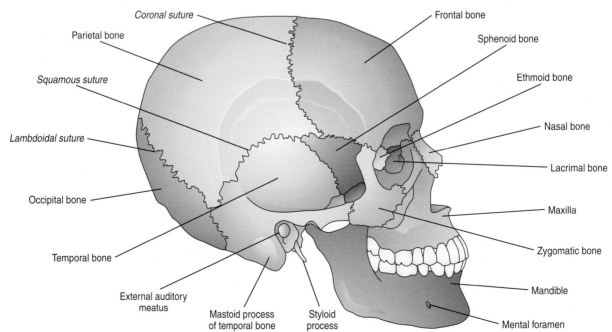

Coronal suture

Parietal bone

Squamous suture

Lambdoidal suture

Occipital bone

Temporal bone

External auditory meatus

Mastoid process of temporal bone

Styloid process

Frontal bone

Sphenoid bone

Ethmoid bone

Nasal bone

Lacrimal bone

Maxilla

Zygomatic bone

Mandible

Mental foramen

FIGURE 7-17 Bones of the skull.

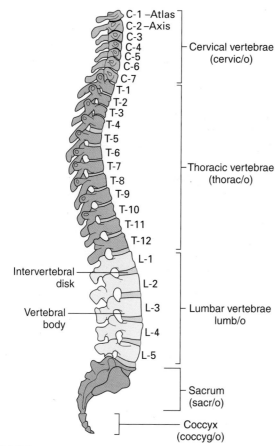

FIGURE 7-18 Lateral view of the vertebral, or spinal, column.

face of the body. The first seven pairs are called *true ribs* because they attach directly to the sternum, or breastbone, on the front of the body. The next five pairs are called *false ribs.* The first three pairs of false ribs attach to the cartilage of the rib above. The last two pairs of false ribs are called *floating ribs* because they have no attachment on the front of the body.

The **sternum,** or breastbone, is the last bone of the axial skeleton. It consists of three parts: the manubrium (upper region), the gladiolus (body), and the xiphoid process (a small piece of cartilage at the bottom). The two collarbones, or clavicles, are attached to the manubrium by ligaments. The ribs are attached to the sternum with costal cartilages to form a "cage" that protects the heart and lungs.

The shoulder, or pectoral, girdle is made of two **clavicles** (collarbones) and two **scapulas** (shoulder bones). The scapulas provide for attachment of the upper arm bones.

Bones of each arm include one **humerus** (upper arm), one **radius** (lower arm on thumb side that rotates around the ulna to allow the hand to turn freely), one **ulna** (larger bone of lower arm with a projection called the *olecranon process* at its upper end, forming the elbow), eight **carpals** (wrist), five **metacarpals** (palm of the hand), and fourteen **phalanges** (three on each finger and two on the thumb).

The pelvic girdle is made of two **os coxae** (coxal, or hip, bones), which join with the sacrum on the dorsal part of the body (figure 7-19). On the ventral part of the body, the os coxae join together at a joint called the *symphysis pubis.* Each os coxae is made of three fused sections: the ilium, the ischium, and the pubis. The pelvic girdle contains two recessed areas, or sockets. These sockets, called *acetabula,* provide for the attachment of the smooth rounded head of the femur (upper leg bone). An opening between the ischium and pubis, called the *obturator foramen,* allows for the passage of nerves and blood vessels to and from the legs.

Each leg consists of one **femur** (thigh), one **patella** (kneecap), one **tibia** (the larger weight-bearing bone of the lower leg commonly called the *shin bone*), and one **fibula** (the slender smaller bone of the lower leg that attaches to the proximal end of the tibia), seven **tarsals** (ankle), five **metatarsals** (instep of foot), and fourteen phalanges (two on the great toe and three on each of the other four toes). The heel is formed by the large tarsal bone called the *calcaneous.* The bones of the skeleton are shown in figure 7-20.

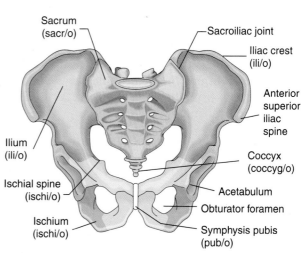

FIGURE 7-19 Anterior view of the pelvic girdle.

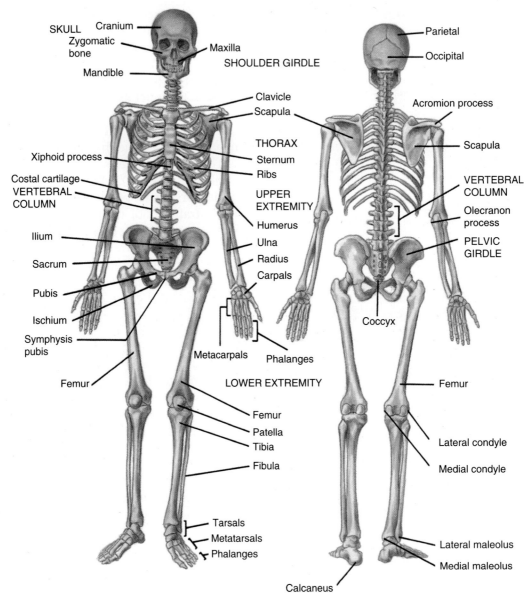

FIGURE 7-20 Bones of the skeleton.

Joints

Joints are areas where two or more bones join together. Connective tissue bands, called **ligaments,** help hold long bones together at joints. There are three main types of joints:

◆ *Diarthrosis* or *synovial*: freely movable; examples include the ball-and-socket joints of the shoulder and hip, or the hinge joints of the elbow and knee

◆ *Amphiarthrosis*: slightly movable; examples include the attachment of the ribs to the thoracic vertebrae and the symphysis pubis, or joint between the two pelvic bones

◆ *Synarthrosis*: immovable; examples are the suture joints of the cranium

DISEASES AND ABNORMAL CONDITIONS

Arthritis

Arthritis is actually a group of diseases involving inflammation of the joints. Two main types are osteoarthritis and rheumatoid arthritis. *Osteoarthritis,* the most common form, is a chronic disease that usually occurs as a result of aging. It frequently affects the hips and knees. Symptoms include joint pain, stiffness, aching, and limited range of motion. Although there is no cure, rest, applications of heat and cold, aspirin and anti-inflammatory medications, injection of steroids into the joints, and special exercises are used to relieve the symptoms. *Rheumatoid arthritis* is a chronic inflammatory disease that affects the connective tissues and joints. It is three times more common in women than in men, and onset often occurs between the ages of 35 and 45. Progressive attacks can cause scar tissue formation and atrophy of bone and muscle tissue, which result in permanent deformity and immobility (figure 7-21). Early treatment is important to reduce pain and limit damage to joints. Rest, prescribed exercise, anti-inflammatory medications such as aspirin, and careful use of steroids are the main forms of treatment. Surgery, or arthroplasty, to replace damaged joints, such as those in the hips and knees, is sometimes performed when severe joint damage has occurred.

Bursitis

Bursitis is an inflammation of the bursae, which are small, fluid-filled sacs surrounding the joints. It frequently affects the shoulders, elbows, hips, or knees. Symptoms include severe pain, limited movement, and fluid accumulation in the joint. Treatment consists of administering pain medications, injecting steroids and anesthetics into the affected joint, rest, aspirating (withdrawing fluid with a needle) the joint, and physical therapy to preserve joint motion.

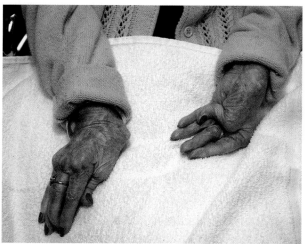

FIGURE 7-21 Rheumatoid arthritis can cause permanent deformity and immobility.

Fractures

A fracture is a crack or break in a bone. Types of fractures, shown in figure 7-22, include:

♦ *Greenstick*: bone is bent and splits, causing a crack or incomplete break; common in children

♦ *Simple* or *closed*: complete break of the bone with no damage to the skin

♦ *Compound* or *open*: bone breaks and ruptures through the skin; creates an increased chance of infection

♦ *Impacted*: broken bone ends jam into each other

♦ *Comminuted*: bone fragments or splinters into more than two pieces

♦ *Spiral*: bone twists, resulting in one or more breaks; common in skiing and skating accidents

♦ *Depressed*: a broken piece of skull bone moves inward; common with severe head injuries

♦ *Colles*: breaking and dislocation of the distal radius that causes a characteristic bulge at the wrist; caused by falling on an outstretched hand

Before a fracture can heal, the bone must be put back into its proper alignment. This process is called *reduction. Closed reduction* involves positioning the bone in correct alignment, usually with traction, and applying a cast or splint to maintain the position until the fracture heals. *Open reduction* involves surgical repair of the bone. In some cases, special pins, plates, or other devices are surgically implanted to maintain correct position of the bone.

Dislocation

A dislocation is when a bone is forcibly displaced from a joint. It frequently occurs in shoulders, fingers, knees, and hips. After the dislocation is reduced (the bone is replaced in the joint), the dislocation is immobilized with a splint, a cast, or traction.

Sprain

A sprain is when a twisting action tears the ligaments at a joint. The wrists and ankles are common sites for sprains. Symptoms include pain,

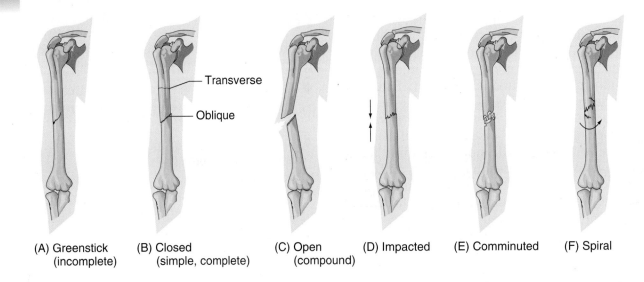

(A) Greenstick   (B) Closed   (C) Open   (D) Impacted   (E) Comminuted   (F) Spiral
     (incomplete)   (simple, complete)   (compound)

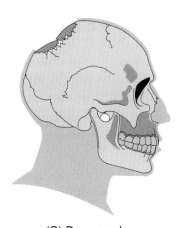

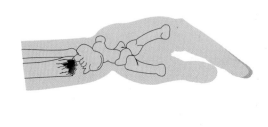

(G) Depressed   (H) Colles

FIGURE 7-22 Types of fractures.

swelling, discoloration, and limited movement. Treatment methods include rest, elevation, immobilization with an elastic bandage or splint, and/or cold applications.

Osteomyelitis

Osteomyelitis is a bone inflammation usually caused by a pathogenic organism. The infectious organisms cause the formation of an abscess within the bone and an accumulation of pus in the medullary canal. Symptoms include pain at the site, swelling, chills, and fever. Antibiotics are used to treat the infection.

Osteoporosis

Osteoporosis, or increased porosity or softening of the bones, is a metabolic disorder caused by a hormone deficiency (especially estrogen in women), prolonged lack of calcium in the diet, and a sedentary lifestyle. The loss of calcium and phosphate from the bones causes the bones to become porous, brittle, and prone to fracture. Bone density tests lead to early detection and preventative treatment for osteoporosis. Treatment methods include increased intake of calcium and vitamin D, medications such as Fosamax and Citracel to increase bone mass, exercise, and/or estrogen replacement.

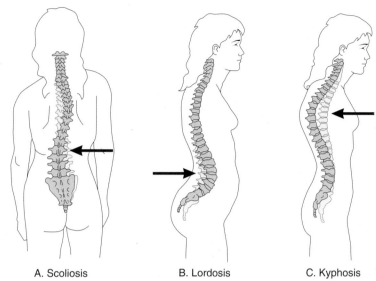

A. Scoliosis   B. Lordosis   C. Kyphosis

FIGURE 7-23 Abnormal curvatures of the spinal column.

Ruptured Disk

A ruptured disk, also called a *herniated* or *slipped disk*, occurs when an intervertebral disk (pad of cartilage separating the vertebrae) ruptures or protrudes out of place and causes pressure on the spinal nerve. The most common site is at the lumbar–sacral area, but a ruptured disk can occur anywhere on the spinal column. Symptoms include severe pain, muscle spasm, impaired movement, and/or numbness. Pain, anti-inflammatory, and muscle relaxant medications may be used as initial forms of treatment. Other treatments include rest, traction, physical therapy, massage therapy, chiropractic treatment, and/or heat or cold applications. A laminectomy, surgical removal of the protruding disk, may be necessary in severe cases that do not respond to conservative treatment. If pain persists, a spinal fusion may be performed to insert a screw/rod assembly into the spine to permanently immobilize the affected vertebrae.

Spinal Curvatures

Abnormal curvatures of the spinal column include kyphosis, scoliosis, and lordosis (figure 7-23). *Kyphosis*, or "hunchback," is a rounded bowing of the back at the thoracic area. *Scoliosis* is a side-to-side, or lateral, curvature of the spine. *Lordosis*, or "swayback," is an abnormal inward curvature of the lumbar region. Poor posture, congenital (at birth) defects, structural defects of the vertebrae, malnutrition, and degeneration of the vertebrae can all be causes of these defects. Therapeutic exercises, firm mattresses, and/or braces are the main forms of treatment. Severe deformities may require surgical repair.

STUDENT: *Go to the workbook and complete the assignment sheet for 7:4, Skeletal System.*

7:5 Muscular System

Objectives

After completing this section, you should be able to:

♦ Compare the three main kinds of muscle by describing the action of each

♦ Differentiate between voluntary muscle and involuntary muscle

♦ List at least three functions of muscles

♦ Describe the two main ways muscles attach to bones

♦ Demonstrate the five major movements performed by muscles

♦ Describe at least three diseases of the muscular system

♦ Define, pronounce, and spell all key terms

KEY TERMS

abduction *(ab-duck'-shun)*
adduction *(ad-duck'-shun)*
cardiac muscle
circumduction
contract *(con-trackt')*
contractibility
contracture *(con-track'-shur)*
elasticity

excitability
extensibility
extension
fascia *(fash'-ee''-ah)*
flexion *(flek'-shun)*
insertion
involuntary
muscle tone

muscular system
origin
rotation
skeletal muscle
tendons
visceral (smooth) muscle
voluntary

RELATED HEALTH CAREERS

◆ Athletic Trainer

◆ Chiropractor

◆ Doctor of Osteopathic Medicine

◆ Massage Therapist

◆ Myologist

◆ Neurologist

◆ Orthopedist

◆ Physiatrist

◆ Physical Therapist

◆ Podiatrist

◆ Prosthetist

◆ Rheumatologist

◆ Sports Medicine Physician

7:5 INFORMATION

More than 600 muscles make up the system known as the **muscular system.** Muscles are bundles of muscle fibers held together by connective tissue. All muscles have certain properties or characteristics:

◆ **Excitability:** irritability, the ability to respond to a stimulus such as a nerve impulse

◆ **Contractibility:** muscle fibers that are stimulated by nerves **contract,** or become short and thick, which causes movement

◆ **Extensibility:** the ability to be stretched

◆ **Elasticity:** allows the muscle to return to its original shape after it has contracted or stretched

There are three main kinds of muscle: cardiac, visceral, and skeletal (figure 7-24). **Cardiac muscle** forms the walls of the heart and contracts to circulate blood. **Visceral,** or **smooth, muscle** is found in the internal organs of the body, such as those of the digestive and respiratory systems, and

the blood vessels and eyes. Visceral muscle contracts to cause movement in these organs. Cardiac muscle and visceral muscle are **involuntary,** meaning they function without conscious thought or control. **Skeletal muscle** is attached to bones and causes body movement. Skeletal muscle is **voluntary** because a person has control over its action. Because cardiac muscle and visceral muscle are discussed in sections on other systems, the following concentrates on skeletal muscle.

Skeletal muscles perform four important functions:

◆ Attach to bones to provide voluntary movement

◆ Produce heat and energy for the body

◆ Help maintain posture by holding the body erect

◆ Protect internal organs

Skeletal muscles attach to bones in different ways. Some attach by **tendons,** which are strong, tough, fibrous connective-tissue cords. An example is the gastrocnemius muscle on the calf of the

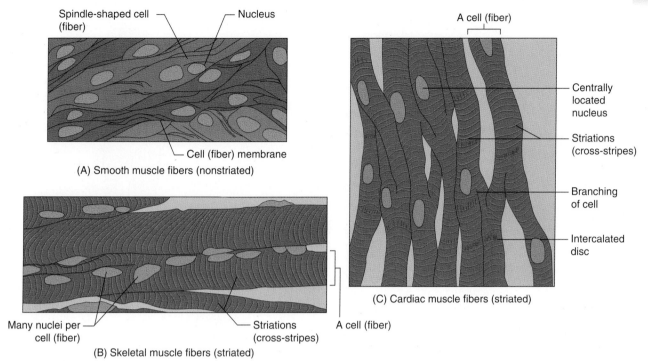

Spindle-shaped cell (fiber)

Nucleus

Cell (fiber) membrane

(A) Smooth muscle fibers (nonstriated)

A cell (fiber)

Centrally located nucleus

Striations (cross-stripes)

Branching of cell

Intercalated disc

(C) Cardiac muscle fibers (striated)

Many nuclei per cell (fiber)

Striations (cross-stripes)

A cell (fiber)

(B) Skeletal muscle fibers (striated)

FIGURE 7-24 Three main kinds of muscle.

leg, which attaches to the heelbone by the Achilles tendon. Other muscles attach by **fascia,** a tough, sheetlike membrane that covers and protects the tissue. Examples include the deep muscles of the trunk and back, which are surrounded by the lumbodorsal fascia. When a muscle attaches to a bone, the end that does not move is called the **origin.** The end that moves when the muscle contracts is called the **insertion.** For example, the origin of the shoulder muscle, called the *deltoid,* is by the clavicle and scapula. Its insertion is on the humerus. When the deltoid contracts, the area by the scapula remains stationary, but the area by the humerus moves and abducts the arm away from the body.

A variety of different actions or movements performed by muscles are shown in figure 7-25 and are described as follows:

♦ **Adduction:** moving a body part toward the midline

♦ **Abduction:** moving a body part away from the midline

♦ **Flexion:** decreasing the angle between two bones, or bending a body part

♦ **Extension:** increasing the angle between two bones, or straightening a body part

♦ **Rotation:** turning a body part around its own axis; for example, turning the head from side to side

♦ **Circumduction:** moving in a circle at a joint, or moving one end of a body part in a circle while the other end remains stationary, such as swinging an arm in a circle

The major superficial muscles of the body are shown in figure 7-26; the locations and actions of the major muscles are noted in table 7-2.

Muscles are partially contracted at all times, even when not in use. This state of partial contraction is called **muscle tone** and is sometimes described as a state of readiness to act. Loss of muscle tone can occur in severe illness such as paralysis. When muscles are not used for a long period, they can *atrophy* (shrink in size and lose strength). Lack of use can also result in a **contracture,** a severe tightening of a flexor muscle resulting in bending of a joint. Foot drop is a common contracture, but the fingers, wrists, knees, and other joints can also be affected.

DISEASES AND ABNORMAL CONDITIONS

Fibromyalgia

Fibromyalgia is chronic, widespread pain in specific muscle sites. Other symptoms include muscle stiffness, numbness or tingling in the arms or

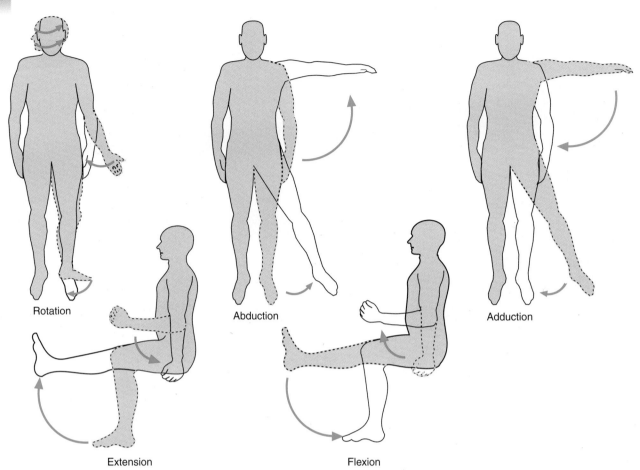

Rotation

Abduction

Adduction

Extension

Flexion

FIGURE 7-25 Types of muscle movement.

TABLE 7-2 Locations and Functions of Major Muscles of the Body

MUSCLE	LOCATION	FUNCTION
Sternocleidomastoid	Side of neck	Turns and flexes head
Trapezius	Upper back and neck	Extends head, moves shoulder
Deltoid	Shoulder	Abducts arm, injection site
Biceps brachii	Upper arm	Flexes lower arm and supinates hand
Triceps brachii	Upper arm	Extends and adducts lower arm
Pectoralis major	Upper chest	Adducts and flexes upper arm
Intercostals	Between ribs	Moves ribs for breathing
Rectus abdominus	Ribs to pubis (pelvis)	Compresses abdomen and flexes vertebral column
Latissimus dorsi	Spine around to chest	Extends and adducts upper arm
Gluteus maximus	Buttocks	Extends and rotates thigh, injection site
Sartorius	Front of thigh	Abducts thigh, flexes leg
Quadriceps femoris	Front of thigh	Extends leg, injection site
Tibialis anterior	Front of lower leg	Flexes and inverts foot
Gastrocnemius	Back of lower leg	Flexes and supinates sole of the foot

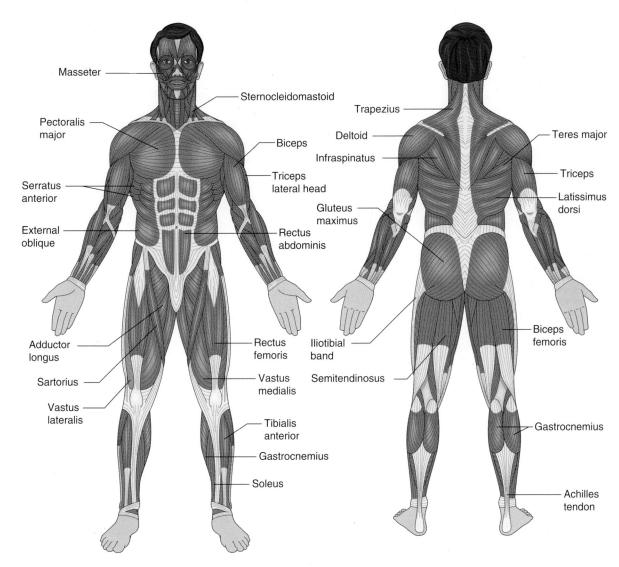

Masseter

Sternocleidomastoid

Pectoralis
major

Biceps

Triceps
lateral head

Serratus
anterior

External
oblique

Rectus
abdominis

Adductor
longus

Rectus
femoris

Sartorius

Vastus
medialis

Vastus
lateralis

Tibialis
anterior

Gastrocnemius

Soleus

Trapezius

Deltoid

Teres major

Infraspinatus

Triceps

Gluteus
maximus

Latissimus
dorsi

Iliotibial
band

Biceps
femoris

Semitendinosus

Gastrocnemius

Achilles
tendon

Anterior Surface Muscles

Posterior Surface Muscles

FIGURE 7-26 Main muscles of the body.

legs, fatigue, sleep disturbances, headaches, and depression. The cause is unknown, but stress, weather, and poor physical fitness affect the condition. Treatment is directed toward pain relief and includes physical therapy, massage, exercise, stress reduction, and medication to relax muscles and relieve pain.

Muscular Dystrophy

Muscular dystrophy is actually a group of inherited diseases that lead to chronic, progressive muscle atrophy. Muscular dystrophy usually appears in early childhood; most types result in total disability and early death. The most common type is Duchenne muscular dystrophy, which is caused by a genetic defect. At birth, the infant is healthy. As muscle cells die, the child

loses the ability to move. The onset usually occurs between 2 and 5 years of age. By age 9 to 12, the child is confined to a wheelchair. Eventually, the muscle weakness affects the heart and diaphragm, resulting in respiratory and/or cardiac failure that causes death. The life expectancy is usually from the late teens to the early twenties. Although there is no cure, physical therapy is used to slow the progress of the disease.

Myasthenia Gravis

Myasthenia gravis is a chronic condition where nerve impulses are not properly transmitted to the muscles. This leads to progressive muscular weakness and paralysis. If the condition affects the respiratory muscles, it can be fatal. Although the cause is unknown, myasthenia gravis is thought to be an autoimmune disease, with anti-bodies attacking the body's own tissues. There is no cure, and treatment is supportive.

Muscle Spasms

Muscle spasms, or cramps, are sudden, painful, involuntary muscle contractions. They usually occur in the legs or feet and may result from over-exertion, low electrolyte levels, or poor circula-tion. Gentle pressure and stretching of the muscle are used to relieve the spasm.

Strain

A strain is an overstretching of or injury to a mus-cle and/or tendon. Frequent sites include the back, arms, and legs. Prolonged or sudden muscle exer-tion is usually the cause. Symptoms include myal-gia (muscle pain), swelling, and limited movement. Treatment methods include rest, muscle relaxants or pain medications, elevating the extremity, and alternating hot and cold applications.

STUDENT: *Go to the workbook and complete the assignment sheet for 7:5, Muscular System.*

7:6 Nervous System

Objectives

After completing this section, you should be able to:

♦ Identify the four main parts of a neuron

♦ Name the two main divisions of the nervous system

♦ Describe the function of each of the five main parts of the brain

♦ Explain three functions of the spinal cord

♦ Name the three meninges

♦ Describe the circulation and function of cere-brospinal fluid

♦ Contrast the actions of the sympathetic and parasympathetic nervous systems

♦ Describe at least five diseases of the nervous system

♦ Define, pronounce, and spell all key terms

KEY TERMS

autonomic nervous system
brain
central nervous system (CNS)
cerebellum *(seh"-reh-bell'-um)*
cerebrospinal fluid *(seh-ree"-broh-spy'-nal fluid)*
cerebrum *(seh-ree'-brum)*
diencephalon

hypothalamus
medulla oblongata *(meh-due'-la ob-lawn-got'-ah)*
meninges (singular: meninx) *(meh-nin'-jeez)*
midbrain
nerves
nervous system
neuron *(nur'-on)*

parasympathetic *(par"-ah-sim"-pah-thet'-ik)*
peripheral nervous system (PNS) *(peh-rif'-eh-ral)*
pons *(ponz)*
somatic nervous system
spinal cord
sympathetic
thalamus
ventricles

RELATED HEALTH CAREERS

- ◆ Acupressurist
- ◆ Acupuncturist
- ◆ Anesthesiologist
- ◆ Chiropractor
- ◆ Diagnostic Imager
- ◆ Doctor of Osteopathic Medicine
- ◆ Electroencephalographic Technologist
- ◆ Electroneurodiagnostic Technologist
- ◆ Mental Health Technician
- ◆ Neurologist
- ◆ Neurosurgeon
- ◆ Physical Therapist
- ◆ Polysomnographic Technologist
- ◆ Psychiatrist
- ◆ Psychologist

7:6 INFORMATION

The **nervous system** is a complex, highly organized system that coordinates all the activities of the body. This system enables the body to respond and adapt to changes that occur both inside and outside the body.

The basic structural unit of the nervous system is the **neuron,** or nerve cell (figure 7-27). It consists of a cell body containing a nucleus; nerve fibers, called *dendrites* (which carry impulses toward the cell body); and a single nerve fiber, called an *axon* (which carries impulses away from the cell body). Many axons have a lipid (fat) covering called a *myelin sheath,* which increases the rate of impulse transmission and insulates and maintains the axon. The axon of one neuron lies close to the dendrites of many other neurons. The spaces between them are known as *synapses.*

Impulses coming from one axon "jump" the synapse to get to the dendrite of another neuron, which will carry the impulse in the right direction. Special chemicals, called *neurotransmitters,* located at the end of each axon, allow the nerve impulses to pass from one neuron to another. In this way, impulses can follow many different routes.

Nerves are a combination of many nerve fibers located outside the brain and spinal cord. *Afferent,* or sensory, nerves carry messages from all parts of the body to the brain and spinal cord. *Efferent,* or motor, nerves carry messages from the brain and spinal cord to the muscles and glands. *Associative,* or *internuncial,* nerves carry both sensory and motor messages.

There are two main divisions to the nervous system: the central nervous system and the peripheral nervous system (figure 7-28). The

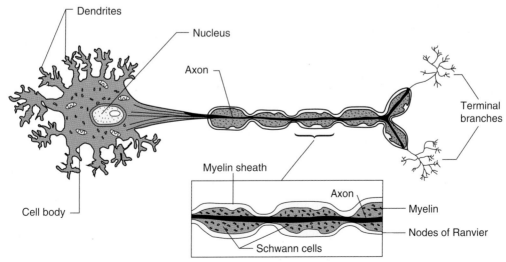

FIGURE 7-27 A neuron, the basic structural unit of the nervous system.

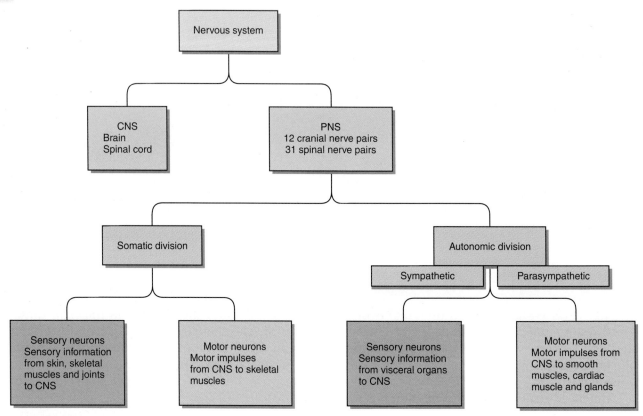

FIGURE 7-28 Divisions of the nervous system.

central nervous system (CNS) consists of the brain and spinal cord. The **peripheral nervous system (PNS)** consists of the nerves and has two divisions: the somatic nervous system and the autonomic nervous system. The **somatic nervous system** carries messages between the CNS and the body. The **autonomic nervous system** contains the sympathetic and parasympathetic nervous systems, which work together to control involuntary body functions.

CENTRAL NERVOUS SYSTEM

The **brain** is a mass of nerve tissue well protected by membranes and the cranium, or skull (figure 7-29). The main sections include:

♦ **Cerebrum:** the largest and highest section of the brain. The outer part is arranged in folds, called *convolutions,* and separated into lobes. The lobes include the frontal, parietal, temporal, and occipital, named from the skull bones that surround them (figure 7-30). The cere-

brum is responsible for reasoning, thought, memory, judgment, speech, sensation, sight, smell, hearing, and voluntary body movement.

♦ **Cerebellum:** the section below the back of the cerebrum. It is responsible for muscle coordination, balance, posture, and muscle tone.

♦ **Diencephalon:** the section located between the cerebrum and midbrain. It contains two structures: the thalamus and hypothalamus. The **thalamus** acts as a relay center and directs sensory impulses to the cerebrum. It also allows conscious recognition of pain and temperature. The **hypothalamus** regulates and controls the autonomic nervous system, temperature, appetite, water balance, sleep, and blood vessel constriction and dilation. The hypothalamus is also involved in emotions such as anger, fear, pleasure, pain, and affection.

♦ **Midbrain:** the section located below the cerebrum at the top of the brainstem. It is responsible for conducting impulses between

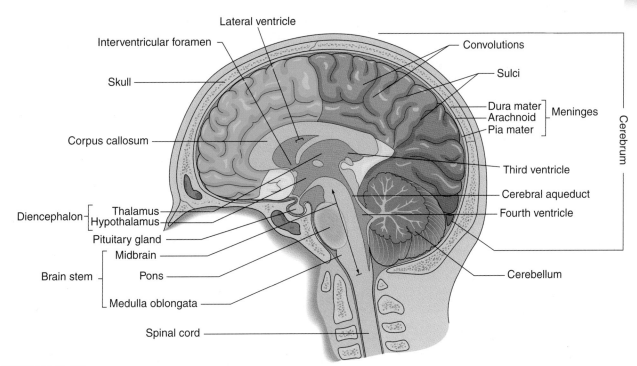

Lateral ventricle

Interventricular foramen

Skull

Corpus callosum

Diencephalon — Thalamus
Hypothalamus

Pituitary gland

Midbrain

Brain stem — Pons

Medulla oblongata

Spinal cord

Convolutions

Sulci

Dura mater ⎤
Arachnoid ⎬ Meninges
Pia mater ⎦

Third ventricle

Cerebral aqueduct

Fourth ventricle

Cerebellum

Cerebrum

FIGURE 7-29 The brain and spinal cord.

brain parts and for certain eye and auditory reflexes.

♦ **Pons:** the section located below the midbrain and in the brainstem. It is responsible for conducting messages to other parts of the brain; for certain reflex actions including chewing, tasting, and saliva production; and for assisting with respiration.

♦ **Medulla oblongata:** the lowest part of the brainstem. It connects with the spinal cord and is responsible for regulating heartbeat, respiration, swallowing, coughing, and blood pressure.

The **spinal cord** continues down from the medulla oblongata and ends at the first or second lumbar vertebrae (figure 7-31). It is surrounded and protected by the vertebrae. The spinal cord is responsible for many reflex actions and for carrying sensory (afferent) messages up to the brain and motor (efferent) messages from the brain to the nerves that go to the muscles and glands.

The **meninges** are three membranes that cover and protect the brain and spinal cord. The *dura mater* is the thick, tough, outer layer. The middle layer is delicate and weblike, and is called the *arachnoid membrane.* It is loosely attached to the other meninges to allow space for fluid to flow between the layers. The innermost layer, the *pia mater,* is closely attached to the brain and spinal cord, and contains blood vessels that nourish the nerve tissue.

The brain has four **ventricles,** hollow spaces that connect with each other and with the space under the arachnoid membrane (the subarachnoid space). The ventricles are filled with a clear, colorless fluid called **cerebrospinal fluid.** This fluid circulates continually between the ventricles and through the subarachnoid space. It serves as a shock absorber to protect the brain and spinal cord. It also carries nutrients to some parts of the brain and spinal cord and helps remove metabolic products and wastes. The fluid is produced in the ventricles of the brain by the special structures called *choroid plexuses.* After circulating, it is absorbed into the blood vessels of the dura mater and returned to the bloodstream through special structures called *arachnoid villi.*

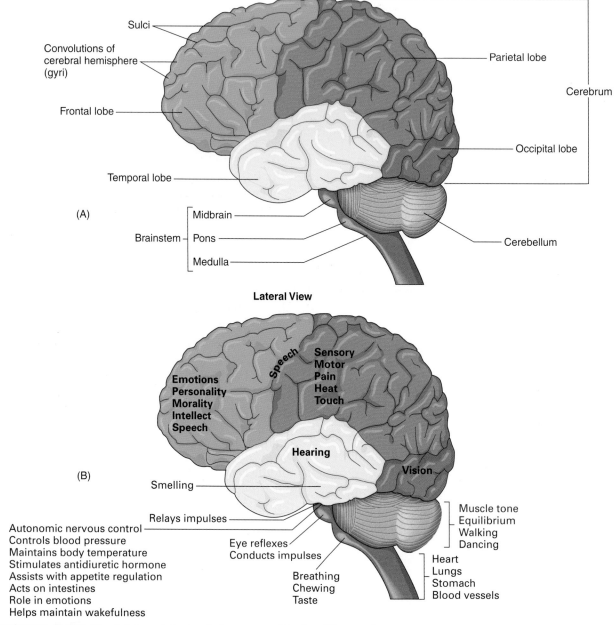

FIGURE 7-30 Each lobe of the brain is responsible for different functions.

PERIPHERAL NERVOUS SYSTEM

The peripheral nervous system consists of the somatic and the autonomic nervous systems.

Somatic Nervous System

The somatic nervous system consists of 12 pairs of cranial nerves and their branches, and 31 pairs of spinal nerves and their branches. Some of the cranial nerves are responsible for special senses such as sight, hearing, taste, and smell. Others receive general sensations such as touch, pressure, pain, and temperature, and send out impulses for involuntary and voluntary muscle control. The spinal nerves carry messages to and from the spinal cord and are mixed nerves, both sensory (afferent) and motor (efferent). There are 8 cervical, 12 thoracic, 5 lumbar, 5 sacral, and 1 pair of coccygeal spinal nerves. Each nerve goes

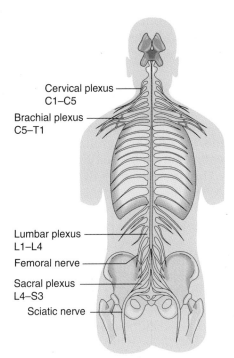

Cervical plexus
C1–C5

Brachial plexus
C5–T1

Lumbar plexus
L1–L4

Femoral nerve

Sacral plexus
L4–S3

Sciatic nerve

FIGURE 7-31 The spinal cord and nerves.

directly to a particular part of the body or networks with other spinal nerves to form a plexus that supplies sensation to a larger segment of the body.

Autonomic Nervous System

The autonomic nervous system is an important part of the peripheral nervous system. It helps maintain a balance in the involuntary functions of the body and allows the body to react in times of emergency. There are two divisions to the autonomic nervous system: the **sympathetic** and **parasympathetic** nervous systems. These two systems usually work together to maintain a balanced state, or *homeostasis,* in the body and to control involuntary body functions at proper rates. In times of emergency, the sympathetic nervous system prepares the body to act by increasing heart rate, respiration, and blood pressure, and slowing activity in the digestive tract. This is known as the *fight or flight response.* After the emergency, the parasympathetic nervous system counteracts the actions of the sympathetic system by slowing heart rate, decreasing respiration, lowering blood pressure, and increasing activity in the digestive tract.

DISEASES AND ABNORMAL CONDITIONSS

Amyotrophic Lateral Sclerosis

Amyotrophic lateral sclerosis (ALS), also known as Lou Gehrig's disease, is a chronic, degenerative neuromuscular disease. The cause is unknown, but genetic or viral-immune factors are suspected. Nerve cells in the CNS that control voluntary movement degenerate, resulting in a weakening and atrophy (wasting away) of the muscles they control. Initial symptoms include muscle weakness, abnormal reflexes, tripping and falling, impaired hand and arm movement, and difficulty in speaking or swallowing. As the disease progresses, more muscles are affected, resulting in total body paralysis. In the later stages, the patient loses all ability to communicate, breathe, eat, and move. Mental acuity is unaffected, so an active mind is trapped inside a paralyzed body. No treatment exists, but drugs such as Riluzole may slow the progress of the disease. ALS is usually fatal within 4 to 6 years of symptom onset, but some patients with slower rates of progression have survived 10–20 years after the onset of the disease.

Carpal Tunnel Syndrome

Carpal tunnel syndrome is a condition that occurs when the medial nerve and tendons that pass through a canal or "tunnel" on their way from the forearm to the hands and fingers are pinched. Repetitive movement of the wrist causes swelling around this tunnel, which puts pressure on the nerves and tendons. Symptoms include pain, muscle weakness in the hand, and impaired movement. A classic symptom is pain, numbness, and tingling in the thumb, ring finger, and middle finger. Initially, carpal tunnel is treated with anti-inflammatory medications, analgesics for pain, and splinting to immobilize the joint. Severe cases that do not respond to this treatment may require surgery to enlarge the "tunnel" and relieve the pressure on the nerves and tendons.

Cerebral Palsy

Cerebral palsy is a disturbance in voluntary muscle action and is caused by brain damage. Lack of oxygen to the brain, birth injuries, prenatal rubella (German measles), and infections can all cause cerebral palsy. Of the three forms—spastic, athetoid, and atactic—spastic is the most common. Symptoms include exaggerated reflexes, tense muscles, contracture development, seizures, speech impairment, spasms, tremors, and in some cases, mental retardation. Although there is no cure, physical, occupational, and speech therapy are important aspects of treatment. Muscle relaxants, anticonvulsive drugs, casts, braces, and/or orthopedic surgery (for severe contractures) are also used.

Cerebrovascular Accident

A cerebrovascular accident (CVA), also called a *brain attack, stroke,* or *apoplexy,* occurs when the blood flow to the brain is impaired, resulting in a lack of oxygen and a destruction of brain tissue. It can be caused by cerebral hemorrhage resulting from hypertension, an aneurysm, or a weak blood vessel; or by an occlusion, or blockage, caused by atherosclerosis or a thrombus (blood clot). Factors that increase the risk for a CVA include smoking, a high-fat diet, obesity, and a sedentary lifestyle. Symptoms vary depending on the area and amount of brain tissue damaged. Some common symptoms of an acute CVA include loss of consciousness, weakness or paralysis on one side of the body (hemiplegia), dizziness, dysphagia (difficult swallowing), visual disturbances, mental confusion, aphasia (speech and language impairment), and incontinence. When a CVA occurs, immediate care during the first 3 hours can help prevent brain damage. Treatment with thrombolytic or "clot-busting" drugs such as TPA (tissue plasminogen activator) or angioplasty of the cerebral arteries can dissolve a blood clot and restore blood flow to the brain. Computerized tomography (CT) scans (noninvasive computerized X-rays that show cross-sectional views of body tissue) are used to determine the cause of the CVA. Clot-busting drugs cannot be used if the CVA is caused by a hemorrhage. Neuroprotective agents, or drugs that help prevent injury to neurons, are also used initially to prevent permanent brain damage. Additional treatment depends on symptoms and is directed toward helping the person recover from or adapt to the symptoms that are present. Physical, occupational, and speech therapy are the main forms of treatment.

Encephalitis

Encephalitis is an inflammation of the brain and is caused by a virus, bacterium, chemical agent, or as a complication of measles, chicken pox, or mumps. The virus is frequently contracted from a mosquito bite because mosquitos can carry the encephalitis virus. Symptoms vary but may include fever, extreme weakness or lethargy, visual disturbances, headaches, vomiting, stiff neck and back, disorientation, seizures, and coma. Treatment methods are supportive and include antiviral drugs, maintenance of fluid and electrolyte balance, antiseizure medication, and monitoring of respiratory and kidney function.

Epilepsy

Epilepsy, or seizure syndrome, is a brain disorder associated with abnormal electrical impulses in the neurons of the brain. Although causes can include brain injury, birth trauma, tumors, toxins such as lead or carbon monoxide, and infections, many cases of epilepsy are idiopathic (spontaneous, or primary). Absence, or petit mal, seizures are milder and are characterized by a loss of consciousness lasting several seconds. They are common in children and frequently disappear by late adolescence. Generalized tonic-clonic, or grand mal, are the most severe seizures. They are characterized by a loss of consciousness lasting several minutes; convulsions accompanied by violent shaking and thrashing movements; hypersalivation, causing foaming at the mouth; and loss of body functions. Some individuals experience an *aura,* such as a particular smell, ringing in the ears, visual disturbances, or tingling in the fingers and/or toes just before a seizure occurs. Anticonvulsant drugs are effective in controlling epilepsy.

Hydrocephalus

Hydrocephalus is an excessive accumulation of cerebrospinal fluid in the ventricles and, in some cases, the subarachnoid space of the brain. It is usually caused by a congenital (at birth) defect, infection, or tumor that obstructs the flow of cerebrospinal fluid out of the brain. Symptoms include an abnormally enlarged head, prominent forehead, bulging eyes, irritability, distended scalp veins, and when pressure prevents proper development of the brain, retardation. The condition is treated by the surgical implantation of a shunt (tube) between the ventricles and the veins, heart, or abdominal peritoneal cavity to provide for drainage of the excess fluid.

Meningitis

Meningitis is an inflammation of the meninges of the brain and/or spinal cord and is caused by a bacterium, virus, fungus, or toxin such as lead or arsenic. Symptoms include high fever, headaches, back and neck pain and stiffness, nausea and vomiting, delirium, convulsions, and if untreated, coma and death. Treatment methods include antibiotics, antipyretics (for fever), anticonvulsants, and/or medications for pain and cerebral edema.

Multiple Sclerosis

Multiple sclerosis (MS) is a chronic, progressive, disabling condition resulting from a degeneration of the myelin sheath in the CNS. It usually occurs between the ages of 20 and 40 (figure 7-32). The cause is unknown but genetics or a viral infection of the immune system are suspected. The disease progresses at different rates and has periods of remission. Early symptoms include visual disturbances such as diplopia (double vision), weakness, fatigue, poor coordination, and tingling and

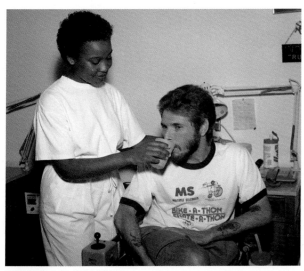

FIGURE 7-32 Multiple sclerosis usually occurs between the ages of 20 and 40.

numbness. As the disease progresses, tremors, muscle spasticity, paralysis, speech impairment, emotional swings, and incontinence occur. There is no cure. Treatment methods such as physical therapy, muscle relaxants, steroids, and psychological counseling are used to maintain functional ability as long as possible.

Neuralgia

Neuralgia is nerve pain. It is caused by inflammation, pressure, toxins, and other disease. Treatment is directed toward eliminating the cause of the pain.

Paralysis

Paralysis usually results from a brain or spinal cord injury that destroys neurons and results in a loss of function and sensation below the level of injury. *Hemiplegia* is paralysis on one side of the body and is caused by a tumor, injury, or CVA. *Paraplegia* is paralysis in the lower extremities or lower part of the body and is caused by a spinal cord injury. *Quadriplegia* is paralysis of the arms, legs, and body below the spinal cord injury. Currently, no cure exists, although much research is being directed toward repairing spinal cord damage. Treatment methods are supportive and include physical and occupational therapy.

Parkinson's Disease

Parkinson's disease is a chronic, progressive condition involving degeneration of brain cells, usually in persons over 50 years of age. Symptoms include tremors, stiffness, muscular rigidity, a forward leaning position, a shuffling gait, difficulty in stopping while walking, loss of facial expression, drooling, mood swings and frequent depression, and behavioral changes. Although no cure exists, a drug called levodopa is used to relieve the symptoms. In some cases, surgery can be performed to destroy selectively a small area of the brain and control involuntary movements. Physical therapy is also used to limit muscular rigidity.

Shingles

Shingles, or herpes zoster, is an acute inflammation of nerve cells and is caused by the herpes virus, which also causes chicken pox. It characteristically occurs in the thoracic area on one side of the body and follows the path of the affected nerves (figure 7-33). Fluid-filled vesicles appear on the skin, accompanied by severe pain, red-

ness, itching, fever, and abnormal skin sensations. Treatment is directed toward relieving pain and itching until the inflammation subsides, usually in 1–4 weeks.

STUDENT: *Go to the workbook and complete the assignment sheet for 7:6, Nervous System.*

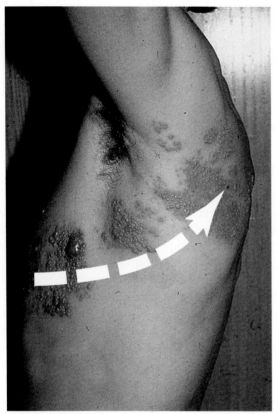

FIGURE 7-33 The vesicles of shingles follow the path of the affected nerves.

7:7 Special Senses

Objectives

After completing this section, you should be able to:

♦ Identify five special senses

♦ Label the major parts on a diagram of the eye

♦ Trace the pathway of light rays as they pass through the eye

♦ Label the major parts on a diagram of the ear

♦ Trace the pathway of sound waves as they pass through the ear

♦ Explain how the ear helps maintain balance and equilibrium

♦ State the locations of the four main taste receptors

♦ List at least four general senses located throughout the body

♦ Describe at least six diseases of the eye and ear

♦ Define, pronounce, and spell all key terms

KEY TERMS

aqueous humor
  (a'-kwee"-us hue-more)
auditory canal
auricle *(or'-eh-kul")*
choroid coat *(koh'-royd)*
cochlea *(co'-klee-ah)*
conjunctiva
  (kon-junk"-tye'-vah)
cornea
eustachian tube
  (you-stay'-she-en)

iris
lacrimal glands
  (lack'-rih"-mal)
lens
organ of Corti
ossicles *(os'-ick-uls)*
pinna *(pin'-nah)*
pupil
refracts

retina *(ret'-in-ah)*
sclera *(sklee'-rah)*
semicircular canals
tympanic membrane
  (tim-pan'-ik)
vestibule *(ves'-tih-bewl)*
vitreous humor
  (vit'-ree-us hue'-more)

RELATED HEALTH CAREERS

- ◆ Allergist
- ◆ Audiologist
- ◆ Eye, Ear, Nose, and Throat Specialist
- ◆ Ophthalmic Assistant
- ◆ Ophthalmic Laboratory Technician
- ◆ Ophthalmic Medical Technologist
- ◆ Ophthalmic Technician
- ◆ Ophthalmologist
- ◆ Optician
- ◆ Optometrist
- ◆ Otolaryngologist
- ◆ Otologist

7:7 INFORMATION

Special senses allow the human body to react to the environment by providing for sight, hearing, taste, smell, and balance maintenance. These senses are possible because the body has structures that receive sensations, nerves that carry sensory messages to the brain, and a brain that interprets and responds to sensory messages.

THE EYE

The eye is the organ that controls the special sense of sight. It receives light rays and transmits impulses from the rays to the optic nerve, which carries the impulses to the brain, where they are interpreted as vision, or sight.

The eye (figure 7-34A) is well protected. It is partially enclosed in a bony socket of the skull. Eyelids and eyelashes help keep out dirt and pathogens. **Lacrimal glands** in the eye produce tears, which constantly moisten and cleanse the eye. The tears flow across the eye and drain through the nasolacrimal duct into the nasal cavity. A mucous membrane, called the **conjunctiva,** lines the eyelids and covers the front of the eye to provide additional protection and lubrication.

There are three main layers to the eye (figure 7-34B). The outermost layer is the tough connective tissue called the **sclera.** It is frequently referred to as the "white" of the eye. The sclera maintains the shape of the eye. Extrinsic muscles, responsible for moving the eye within the socket, are attached to the outside of the sclera. The **cor-**

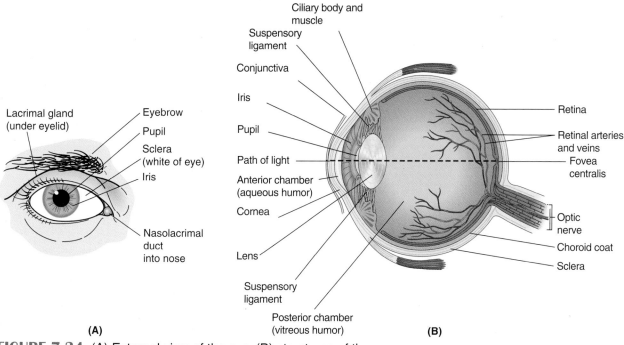

FIGURE 7-34 (A) External view of the eye; (B) structures of the eye.

nea is a circular, transparent part of the front of the sclera. It allows light rays to enter the eye. The middle layer of the eye, the **choroid coat,** is interlaced with many blood vessels that nourish the eyes. The innermost layer of the eye is the **retina.** It is made of many layers of nerve cells, which transmit the light impulses to the optic nerve. Two such special cells are *cones* and *rods.* Cones are sensitive to color and are used mainly for vision when it is light. Most of the cones are located in a depression located on the back surface of the retina called the *fovea centralis;* this is the area of sharpest vision. Rods are used for vision when it is dark or dim.

The **iris** is the colored portion of the eye. It is located behind the cornea on the front of the choroid coat. The opening in the center of the iris is called the **pupil.** The iris contains two muscles, which control the size of the pupil and regulate the amount of light entering the eye.

Other special structures are also located in the eye. The **lens** is a circular structure located behind the pupil and suspended in position by ligaments. It **refracts** (bends) light rays so the rays focus on the retina. The **aqueous humor** is a clear, watery fluid that fills the space between the cornea and iris. It helps maintain the forward curvature of the eyeball and refracts light rays. The **vitreous humor** is the jellylike substance that fills the area behind the lens. It helps maintain the shape of the eyeball and also refracts light rays. A series of muscles located in the eye provide for eye movement.

When light rays enter the eye, they pass through a series of parts that refract the rays so that the rays focus on the retina. These parts are the cornea, the aqueous humor, the pupil, the lens, and the vitreous humor. In the retina, the light rays (image) are picked up by the rods and cones, changed into nerve impulses, and transmitted by the optic nerve to the occipital lobe of the cerebrum, where sight is interpreted. If the rays are not refracted correctly by the various parts, vision can be distorted or blurred (figure 7-35).

Diseases and Abnormal Conditions

Amblyopia

Amblyopia, or lazy eye, commonly occurs in early childhood. It results in poor vision in one eye and is caused by the dominance of the other eye. Treatment methods include covering the good eye to stimulate development of the "lazy" eye, exercises to strengthen the weak eye, corrective lenses, and/or surgery. If the condition is not treated before 8 to 9 years of age, blindness of the affected eye may occur.

Astigmatism

Astigmatism is an abnormal shape or curvature of the cornea that causes blurred vision. Light rays focus on multiple areas of the retina (figure 7-35). Corrective lenses (glasses or contact lenses) correct the condition.

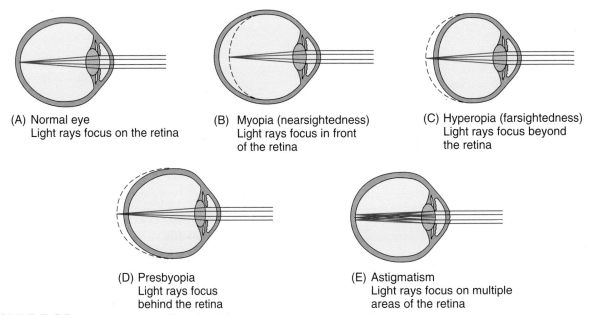

(A) Normal eye
Light rays focus on the retina

(B) Myopia (nearsightedness)
Light rays focus in front
of the retina

(C) Hyperopia (farsightedness)
Light rays focus beyond
the retina

(D) Presbyopia
Light rays focus
behind the retina

(E) Astigmatism
Light rays focus on multiple
areas of the retina

FIGURE 7-35 Improper refraction of light rays causes impaired vision.

Cataract

A cataract occurs when the normally clear lens becomes cloudy or opaque (figure 7-36). This occurs gradually, usually as a result of aging, but may be the result of trauma. Symptoms include blurred vision, halos around lights, gradual vision loss, and in later stages, a milky white pupil. Sight is restored by the surgical removal of the lens. An implanted intraocular lens or prescription glasses or contact lenses correct the vision and compensate for the removed lens.

Conjunctivitis

Conjunctivitis, or pink eye, is a contagious inflammation of the conjunctiva and is usually caused by a bacterium or virus. Symptoms include redness, swelling, pain, and, at times, pus formation in the eye. Antibiotics, frequently in the form of an eye ointment, are used to treat conjunctivitis.

Glaucoma

Glaucoma is a condition of increased intraocular (within the eye) pressure caused by an excess amount of aqueous humor. It is common after age 40 and is a leading cause of blindness. A tonometer (instrument that measures intraocular pressure) is usually used during regular eye examinations to check for this condition. Symptoms include loss of peripheral (side) vision, halos around lights, limited night vision, and mild aching. Glaucoma is usually controlled with medications that decrease the amount of fluid produced or improve the drainage. In some cases, surgery is performed to create an opening for the flow of the aqueous humor.

Hyperopia

Hyperopia is farsightedness. It occurs when the light rays are not refracted sharply enough and

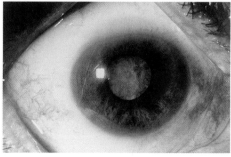

FIGURE 7-36 A cataract occurs when the lens of the eye becomes cloudy or opaque. *(Courtesy of National Eye Institute, NEH)*

the image focuses behind the retina (figure 7-35). Vision is corrected by the use of convex lenses.

Macular Degeneration

Macular degeneration, a major cause of vision loss and blindness, is a disease of the macula, the central and most sensitive section of the retina. It is an age-related disorder caused by damage to the blood vessels that nourish the retina. The most common type is dry macular degeneration that occurs as fatty deposits decrease the blood supply to the retina, resulting in a gradual thinning of the retina. It progresses slowly and results in blurred distorted vision with an absence of central vision. Peripheral (side) vision is usually not affected. No treatment currently exists, but optical aids such as special lighting or magnifiers may improve vision slightly. Wet macular degeneration is caused by an abnormal growth of blood vessels that leak blood and fluids that damage the retina. Laser treatment to coagulate or seal the leaking blood vessels can preserve sight. New research directed toward creation of an artificial retina or bionic eye may allow individuals with this disease to regain the ability to see light and large objects in the future.

Myopia

Myopia is nearsightedness. It occurs when the light rays are refracted too sharply and the image focuses in front of the retina (figure 7-35). Vision is corrected by the use of concave lenses. A newer method of treatment is a surgical procedure called *radial keratotomy* (RK). Small incisions are made in the cornea to flatten it so it can refract light rays correctly. In some cases, a laser is used to flatten the cornea without cutting. RK can correct myopia and eliminate the need for corrective lenses.

Presbyopia

Presbyopia is farsightedness caused by a loss of lens elasticity. Light rays focus behind the retina (figure 7-35). It results from the normal aging process and is treated by the use of corrective lenses or "reading" glasses.

Strabismus

Strabismus is a disorder in which the eyes do not move or focus together. The eyes may move inward (cross-eyed) or outward, or up or down. It is caused by muscle weakness in one or both eyes. Treatment methods include eye exercises, covering the good eye, corrective lenses, and/or surgery on the muscles that move the eye.

THE EAR

The ear is the organ that controls the special senses of hearing and balance. It transmits impulses from sound waves to the auditory nerve (vestibulocochlear), which carries the impulses to the brain for interpretation as hearing. The ear is divided into three main sections: the outer ear, the middle ear, and the inner ear (figure 7-37).

The outer ear contains the visible part of the ear, called the **pinna,** or **auricle.** The pinna is elastic cartilage covered by skin. It leads to a canal, or tube, called the *external auditory meatus,* or **auditory canal.** Special glands in this canal produce *cerumen,* a wax that protects the ear. Sound waves travel through the auditory canal until they reach the eardrum, or **tympanic membrane.** The tympanic membrane separates the outer ear from the middle ear. It vibrates when sound waves hit it and transmits the sound waves to the middle ear.

The middle ear is a small space, or cavity, in the temporal bone. It contains three small bones **(ossicles):** the malleus, the incus, and the stapes. The bones are connected and transmit sound waves from the tympanic membrane to the inner ear. The middle ear is connected to the pharynx, or throat, by a tube called the **eustachian tube.** This tube allows air to enter the middle ear and helps equalize air pressure on both sides of the tympanic membrane.

The inner ear is the most complex portion of the ear. It is separated from the middle ear by a membrane called the *oval window.* The first section is the **vestibule,** which acts as the entrance to the two other parts of the inner ear. The **cochlea,** shaped like a snail's shell, contains delicate, hairlike cells, which compose the **organ of Corti,** a receptor of sound waves. The organ of Corti transmits the impulses from sound waves to the auditory nerve. This nerve carries the impulses to the temporal lobe of the cerebrum, where they are interpreted as hearing. **Semicircular canals** are also located in the inner ear. These canals contain a liquid and delicate, hairlike cells that bend when the liquid moves with head and body movements. Impulses sent from the semicircular canals to the cerebellum of the brain help to maintain our sense of balance and equilibrium.

Diseases and Abnormal Conditions

Hearing Loss

Hearing loss is classified as either conductive or sensory. Conductive hearing loss or deafness occurs when sound waves are not conducted to the inner ear. Possible causes include a wax (cerumen) plug, a foreign body obstruction, otosclerosis, an infection, or a ruptured tympanic

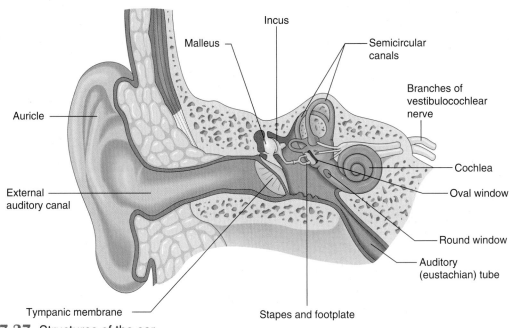

Incus

Malleus

Semicircular canals

Branches of vestibulocochlear nerve

Auricle

Cochlea

Oval window

External auditory canal

Round window

Auditory (eustachian) tube

Tympanic membrane

Stapes and footplate

FIGURE 7-37 Structures of the ear.

membrane. Treatment is directed toward eliminating the cause. Surgery and the use of hearing aids are common forms of treatment. Sensory hearing loss or deafness occurs when there is damage to the inner ear or auditory nerve. This type of hearing loss usually cannot be corrected, but cochlear implants can improve severe hearing loss.

Ménière's Disease

Ménière's disease results from a collection of fluid in the labyrinth of the inner ear and a degeneration of the hair cells in the cochlea and vestibule. Symptoms include severe vertigo (dizziness), tinnitus (ringing in the ears), nausea and vomiting, loss of balance, and a tendency to fall. Forms of treatment include drugs to reduce the fluid, draining the fluid, and antihistamines. In severe, chronic cases, surgery to destroy the cochlea may be performed; however, this causes permanent deafness.

Otitis Externa

Otitis externa is an inflammation of the external auditory canal. It is caused by a pathogenic organism such as a bacterium or virus. Swimmer's ear is one form. It is caused by swimming in contaminated water. Inserting bobby pins, fingernails, or cotton swabs into the ear can also cause this condition. Treatment methods include antibiotics; warm, moist compresses; and/or pain medications.

Otitis Media

Otitis media is an inflammation or infection of the middle ear that is caused by a bacterium or virus. It frequently follows a sore throat because organisms from the throat can enter the middle ear through the eustachian tube. Infants and young children are very susceptible to otitis media because the eustachian tube is angled differently than in adults. Secretions from the nose and throat accumulate in the middle ear, resulting in an inflammatory response that causes the eustachian tube to swell shut. Symptoms include severe pain, fever, vertigo (dizziness), nausea and vomiting, and fluid buildup in the middle ear. Treatment usually consists of administering antibiotics and pain medications. At times, a *myringotomy* (incision of the tympanic membrane) is performed, and tubes are inserted to relieve pressure and allow fluid to drain.

Otosclerosis

Otosclerosis occurs when the stapes becomes immobile, causing conductive hearing loss. Symptoms include gradual hearing loss, tinnitus, and at times, vertigo. Surgical removal of the stapes and insertion of an artificial stapes corrects the condition.

THE TONGUE AND SENSE OF TASTE

The tongue is a mass of muscle tissue with projections called *papillae* (figure 7-38). The papillae contain taste buds that are stimulated by the flavors of foods moistened by saliva. There are four main tastes: sweet tastes and salty tastes at the tip of the tongue; sour tastes at the sides of the tongue; and bitter tastes at the back of the tongue. Taste is influenced by the sense of smell.

THE NOSE AND SENSE OF SMELL

The nose is the organ of smell (figure 7-39). The sense of smell is made possible by olfactory receptors, which are located in the upper part of the nasal cavity. Impulses from these receptors are carried to the brain by the olfactory nerve. The human nose can detect more than 6,000 different smells. The sense of smell is more sensitive than taste, but is closely related to the sense of taste. This is clearly illustrated by the fact that food does not taste as good when you have a head cold and your sense of smell is impaired.

THE SKIN AND GENERAL SENSES

General sense receptors for pressure, heat, cold, touch, and pain are located throughout the body in the skin and connective tissue. Each receptor perceives only one type of sense. For example, the skin contains special receptors for heat and different receptors for cold. Messages from these receptors allow the human body to respond to its environment and help it react to conditions that can cause injury.

STUDENT: *Go to the workbook and complete the assignment sheet for 7:7, Special Senses.*

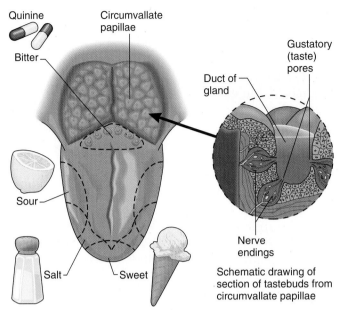

FIGURE 7-38 Locations of taste buds.

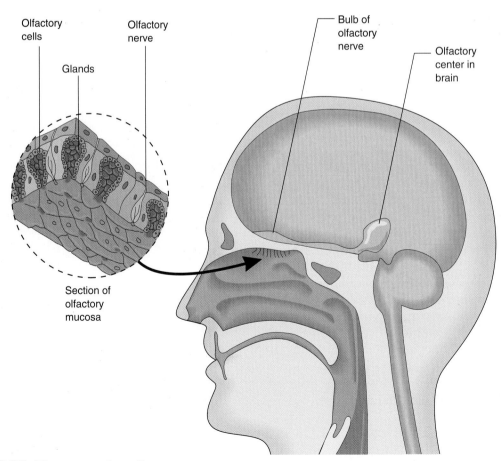

FIGURE 7-39 The sense of smell.

7:8 Circulatory System

Objectives

After completing this section, you should be able to:

♦ Label the layers, chambers, valves, and major blood vessels on a diagram of the heart

♦ Differentiate between systole and diastole by explaining what happens in the heart during each phase

♦ List the three major types of blood vessels and the action of each type

♦ Compare the three main types of blood cells by describing the function of each

♦ Describe at least five diseases of the circulatory system

♦ Define, pronounce, and spell all key terms

KEY TERMS

aortic valve *(ay-or'-tick)*
arrhythmias
arteries
blood
capillaries *(cap'-ih-lair-eez)*
circulatory system
diastole *(dy-az'-tah-lee")*
endocardium *(en-doe-car'-dee-um)*
erythrocytes *(eh-rith'-row-sitez)*

hemoglobin *(hee'-mow-glow"-bin)*
left atrium *(ay'-tree-um)*
left ventricle *(ven'tri"-kul)*
leukocytes *(lew'-coh-sitez")*
mitral valve *(my'-tral)*
myocardium
pericardium
plasma *(plaz'-ma)*

pulmonary valve
right atrium
right ventricle
septum
systole *(sis'-tah-lee")*
thrombocytes *(throm'-bow-sitez)*
tricuspid valve
veins

RELATED HEALTH CAREERS

♦ Cardiac Surgeon
♦ Cardiologist
♦ Cardiovascular Technologist
♦ Echocardiographer

♦ Electrocardiographic Technician
♦ Hematologist
♦ Internist
♦ Medical Laboratory Technologist/Technician

♦ Perfusionist
♦ Phlebotomist
♦ Radiology Technologist
♦ Thoracic Surgeon

7:8 INFORMATION

The **circulatory system,** also known as the cardiovascular system, is often referred to as the "transportation" system of the body. It consists of the heart, blood vessels, and blood. It transports oxygen and nutrients to the body cells, and carbon dioxide and metabolic materials away from the body cells.

THE HEART

The heart is a muscular, hollow organ often called the "pump" of the body (figure 7-40). Even though

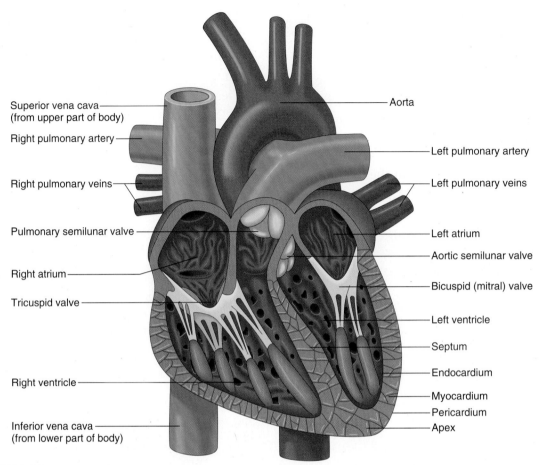

FIGURE 7-40 Basic structure of the heart.

it weighs less than one pound and is approximately the size of a closed fist, it contracts about 100,000 times each day to pump the equivalent of 2,000 gallons of blood through the body. The heart is located in the mediastinal cavity, between the lungs, behind the sternum, and above the diaphragm. Three layers of tissue form the heart. The **endocardium** is a smooth layer of cells that lines the inside of the heart and is continuous with the inside of blood vessels. It allows for the smooth flow of blood. The thickest layer is the **myocardium,** the muscular middle layer. The **pericardium** is a double-layered membrane, or sac, that covers the outside of the heart. A lubricating fluid, pericardial fluid, fills the space between the two layers to prevent friction and damage to the membranes as the heart beats or contracts.

The **septum** is a muscular wall that separates the heart into a right side and a left side. It prevents blood from moving between the right and left sides of the heart. The upper part of the sep-

tum is called the *interatrial septum,* and the lower part is called the *interventricular septum.*

The heart is divided into four parts, or chambers. The two upper chambers are called *atria,* and the two lower chambers are called *ventricles.* The **right atrium** receives blood as it returns from the body cells. The **right ventricle** receives blood from the right atrium and pumps the blood into the pulmonary artery, which carries the blood to the lungs for oxygen. The **left atrium** receives oxygenated blood from the lungs. The **left ventricle** receives blood from the left atrium and pumps the blood into the aorta for transport to the body cells.

One-way valves in the chambers of the heart keep the blood flowing in the right direction. The **tricuspid valve** is located between the right atrium and the right ventricle. It closes when the right ventricle contracts, allowing blood to flow to the lungs and preventing blood from flowing back into the right atrium. The **pulmonary valve** is located between the right ventricle and the pul-

At times it is necessary to use external or internal artificial pacemakers to regulate the heart's rhythm, (figure 7-43). The *pacemaker* is a small, battery-powered device with electrodes. The electrodes are threaded through a vein and positioned in the right atrium and in the apex of the right ventricle. The pacemaker monitors the heart's activity and delivers an electrical impulse through the electrodes to stimulate contraction. Fixed pacemakers deliver electrical impulses at a predetermined rate. Demand pacemakers, the most common type, deliver electrical impulses only when the heart's own conduction system is not responding correctly. Even though modern pacemakers are protected from electromagnetic forces, such as microwave ovens, most manufacturers still recommend that people with pacemakers avoid close contact with digital cellular telephones. For example, the cellular telephone should not be stored in a shirt pocket close to the pacemaker.

BLOOD VESSELS

When the blood leaves the heart, it is carried throughout the body in blood vessels. The heart and blood vessels form a closed system for the flow of blood. There are three main types of blood vessels: arteries, capillaries, and veins.

Arteries (figure 7-44) carry blood away from the heart. The aorta is the largest artery in the body; it receives the blood from the left ventricle of the heart. The aorta branches into all of the other arteries that supply blood to the body. The first branch of the aorta is the coronary artery, which divides into a right and left coronary artery to carry blood to the myocardium of the heart.

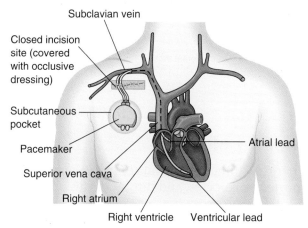

Subclavian vein

Closed incision site (covered with occlusive dressing)

Subcutaneous pocket

Pacemaker

Superior vena cava

Right atrium

Right ventricle

Atrial lead

Ventricular lead

FIGURE 7-43 Artificial pacemakers can help regulate the heart's rhythm.

Additional branches of the aorta carry blood to the head, neck, arms, chest, back, abdomen, and legs. The smallest branches of arteries are called *arterioles.* They join with capillaries. Arteries are more muscular and elastic than are the other blood vessels because they receive the blood as it is pumped from the heart.

Capillaries connect arterioles with *venules,* the smallest veins. Capillaries are located in close proximity to almost every cell in the body. They have thin walls that contain only one layer of cells. These thin walls allow oxygen and nutrients to pass through to the cells and allow carbon dioxide and metabolic products from the cells to enter the capillaries.

Veins (figure 7-45) are blood vessels that carry blood back to the heart. *Venules,* the smallest branches of veins, connect with the capillaries. The venules join together and, becoming larger, form veins. The veins continue to join together until they form the two largest veins: the superior vena cava and the inferior vena cava. The superior vena cava brings the blood from the upper part of the body, and the inferior vena cava brings the blood from the lower part of the body. Both vena cavae drain into the right atrium of the heart. Veins are thinner and have less muscle tissue than do arteries. Most veins contain valves, which keep the blood from flowing in a backward direction (figure 7-46).

BLOOD COMPOSITION

The **blood** that flows through the circulatory system is often called a *tissue* because it contains many kinds of cells. There are approximately 4–6 quarts of blood in the average adult. This blood circulates continuously throughout the body. It transports oxygen from the lungs to the body cells, carbon dioxide from the body cells to the lungs, nutrients from the digestive tract to the body cells, metabolic and waste products from the body cells to the organs of excretion, heat produced by various body parts, and hormones produced by endocrine glands to the body organs.

Plasma

Blood is made of the fluid called *plasma* and formed or solid elements called *blood cells* (figure 7-47). **Plasma** is approximately 90 percent water,

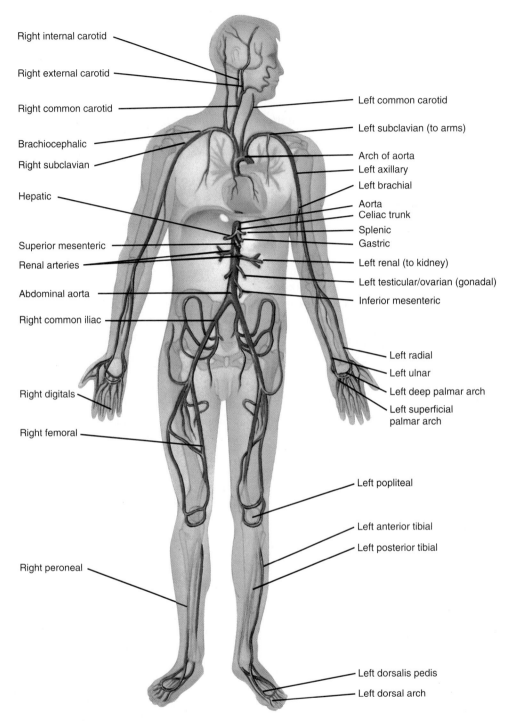

FIGURE 7-44 Major arteries of the body.

with many dissolved, or suspended, substances. Among these substances are blood proteins such as fibrinogen and prothrombin (both necessary for clotting); nutrients such as vitamins, carbohydrates, and proteins; mineral salts or electrolytes such as potassium, calcium, and sodium; gases such as carbon dioxide and oxygen; metabolic and waste products; hormones; and enzymes.

Blood Cells

There are three main kinds of blood cells: erythrocytes, leukocytes, and thrombocytes.

The **erythrocytes,** or red blood cells, are produced in the red bone marrow at a rate of about one million per minute. They live approximately 120 days before being broken down by the

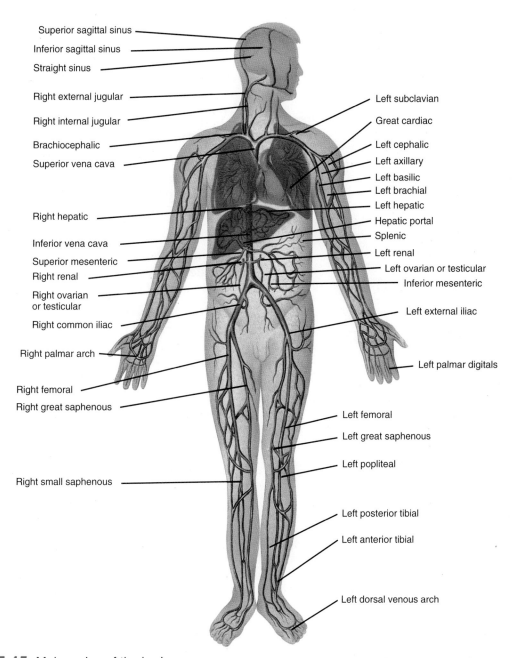

Superior sagittal sinus
Inferior sagittal sinus
Straight sinus
Right external jugular
Right internal jugular
Brachiocephalic
Superior vena cava
Right hepatic
Inferior vena cava
Superior mesenteric
Right renal
Right ovarian or testicular
Right common iliac
Right palmar arch
Right femoral
Right great saphenous
Right small saphenous

Left subclavian
Great cardiac
Left cephalic
Left axillary
Left basilic
Left brachial
Left hepatic
Hepatic portal
Splenic
Left renal
Left ovarian or testicular
Inferior mesenteric
Left external iliac
Left palmar digitals
Left femoral
Left great saphenous
Left popliteal
Left posterior tibial
Left anterior tibial
Left dorsal venous arch

FIGURE 7-45 Major veins of the body.

liver and spleen. There are 4.5–5.5 million erythrocytes per cubic millimeter (approximately one drop) of blood, or approximately 25 trillion in the body. The mature form circulating in the blood lacks a nucleus and is shaped like a disk with a thinner central area. The erythrocytes contain **hemoglobin,** a complex protein composed of the protein molecule called *globin* and the iron compound called *heme.* Hemoglobin carries both oxygen and carbon dioxide. When carrying oxygen, hemoglobin gives blood its characteristic red color. When blood contains a lot of oxygen, it is bright red; when blood contains less oxygen and more carbon dioxide, it is a much darker red with a bluish cast.

Leukocytes, or white blood cells, are not as numerous as are erythrocytes. They are formed in the bone marrow and lymph tissue and usually live about 3–9 days. A normal count is 5,000–9,000 leukocytes per cubic millimeter of blood. Leukocytes can pass through capillary walls and enter body tissue. Their main function is to fight infection. Some do this by engulfing, ingesting, and destroying pathogens, or germs, by a process

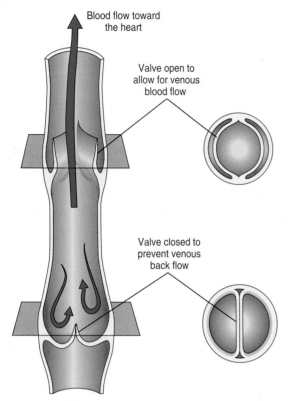

FIGURE 7-46 Most veins contain valves to prevent the backflow of blood.

called *phagocytosis.* The five types of leukocytes and their functions include:

♦ *Neutrophils*: phagocytize bacteria by secreting an enzyme called *lysozyme*

♦ *Eosinophils*: remove toxins and defend the body from allergic reactions by producing antihistamines

♦ *Basophils*: participate in the body's inflammatory response; produce histamine, a vasodilator, and heparin, an anticoagulant

♦ *Monocytes*: phagocytize bacteria and foreign materials

♦ *Lymphocytes*: provide immunity for the body by developing antibodies; protect against the formation of cancer cells

Thrombocytes, also called *platelets,* are usually described as fragments or pieces of cells because they lack nuclei and vary in shape and size. They are formed in the bone marrow and live for about 5–9 days. A normal thrombocyte count is 250,000–400,000 per cubic millimeter of blood. Thrombocytes are important for the clotting process, which stops bleeding. When a blood

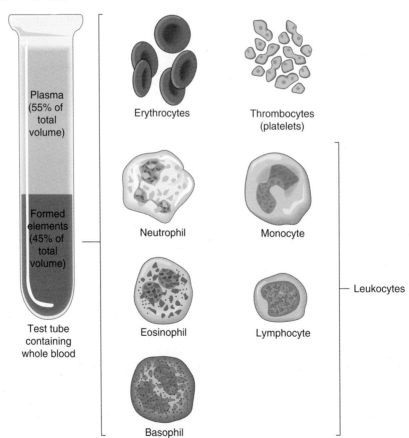

FIGURE 7-47 The major components of blood.

vessel is cut, the thrombocytes collect at the site to form a sticky plug. They secrete a chemical, serotonin, which causes the blood vessel to spasm and narrow, decreasing the flow of blood. At the same time, the thrombocytes release an enzyme, thromboplastin, which acts with calcium and other substances in the plasma to form thrombin. Thrombin acts on the blood protein fibrinogen to form fibrin, a gel-like net of fine fibers that traps erythrocytes, platelets, and plasma to form a clot. This is an effective method for controlling bleeding in smaller blood vessels. If a large blood vessel is cut, the rapid flow of blood can interfere with the formation of fibrin. In these instances, a doctor may have to insert sutures (stitches) to close the opening and control the bleeding.

DISEASES AND ABNORMAL CONDITIONS

Anemia

Anemia is an inadequate number of red blood cells, hemoglobin, or both. Symptoms include pallor (paleness), fatigue, dyspnea (difficult breathing), and rapid heart rate. Hemorrhage can cause rapid blood loss, resulting in acute-blood-loss anemia. Blood transfusions are used to correct this form of anemia. *Iron deficiency anemia* results when there is an inadequate amount of iron to form hemoglobin in erythrocytes. Iron supplements and increased iron intake in the diet from green leafy vegetables and other foods can correct this condition. *Aplastic anemia* is a result of injury to or destruction of the bone marrow, leading to poor or no formation of red blood cells. Common causes include chemotherapy, radiation, toxic chemicals, and viruses. Treatment includes eliminating the cause, blood transfusions, and in severe cases, a bone marrow transplant. Unless the damage can be reversed, it is frequently fatal. *Pernicious anemia* results in the formation of erythrocytes that are abnormally large in size, but inadequate in number. The cause is a lack of intrinsic factor (a substance normally present in the stomach), which results in inadequate absorption of vitamin B_{12}. Vitamin B_{12} and folic acid are required for the development of mature erythrocytes. Administering vitamin B_{12} injections can control and correct this condition. *Sickle cell anemia* is a chronic, inher-

ited anemia. It results in the production of abnormal, crescent-shaped erythrocytes that carry less oxygen, break easily, and block blood vessels (figure 7-48). Sickle cell anemia occurs almost exclusively among African Americans. Treatment methods include transfusions of packed cells and supportive therapy during crisis. Research directed toward bone marrow transplants, stem cell transplants from placental blood, and gene cell therapy may offer a cure for sickle cell anemia in the near future. Genetic counseling can lead to prevention of the disease if carriers make informed decisions not to have children.

Aneurysm

An aneurysm is a ballooning out of, or saclike formation on, an artery wall. Disease, congenital defects, and injuries leading to weakened arterial wall structure can cause this defect. Although some aneurysms cause pain and pressure, others generate no symptoms. Common sites are the cerebral, aortal, and abdominal arteries. If an aneurysm ruptures, hemorrhage, which can cause death, occurs. Treatment usually involves surgically removing the damaged area of blood vessel and replacing it with a plastic graft or another blood vessel.

Arteriosclerosis

Arteriosclerosis is a hardening or thickening of the arterial walls, resulting in a loss of elasticity and contractility. It commonly occurs as a result of aging. Arteriosclerosis causes high blood pressure, or hypertension, and can lead to an aneurysm or cerebral hemorrhage. The main focus of treatment is lowering blood pressure through the use of diet, medications, or both.

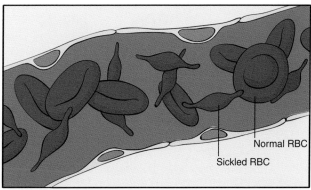

FIGURE 7-48 Sickle cell anemia is characterized by abnormal, crescent-shaped erythrocytes.

Atherosclerosis

Atherosclerosis occurs when fatty plaques (frequently cholesterol) are deposited on the walls of the arteries. This narrows the arterial opening, which reduces or eliminates blood flow. If plaques break loose, they can circulate through the bloodstream as *emboli*. A low-cholesterol diet, medications to lower cholesterol blood levels, abstaining from smoking, reduction of stress, and exercise are used to prevent atherosclerosis. Angioplasty (figure 7-49) may be used to remove or compress the deposits, or to insert a stent to allow blood flow. Bypass surgery is used when the arteries are completely blocked.

Congestive Heart Failure

Congestive heart failure (CHF) is a condition that occurs when the heart muscles do not beat adequately to supply the blood needs of the body. It may involve either the right side or the left side of the heart. Symptoms include edema (swelling); dypsnea; pallor or cyanosis; distention of the neck veins; a weak, rapid pulse; and a cough accompanied by pink, frothy sputum. Cardiotonic drugs (to slow and strengthen the heartbeat), diuretics (to remove retained body fluids), elastic support hose, oxygen therapy, bedrest, and/or a low-sodium diet are used as treatment methods.

Embolus

An embolus is a foreign substance circulating in the bloodstream. It can be air, a blood clot, bacterial clumps, a fat globule, or other similar substances. When an embolus enters an artery or capillary too small for passage, blockage of the blood vessel occurs.

(A) Conventional balloon angioplasty

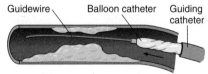

1. In conventional balloon angioplasty, a guiding catheter is positioned in the opening of the coronary artery. The physician then pushes a thin, flexible guidewire down the vessel and through the narrowing. The balloon catheter is then advanced over this guidewire.

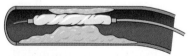

2. The balloon catheter is positioned next to the atherosclerotic plaque.

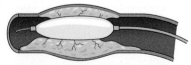

3. The balloon is inflated stretching and cracking the plaque.

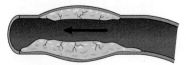

4. When the balloon is withdrawn, blood flow is re-established through the widened vessel.

(B) Coronary atherectomy

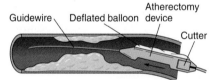

1. In coronary atherectomy procedures, a special cutting device with a deflated balloon on one side and an opening on the other is pushed over a wire down the coronary artery.

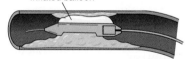

2. When the device is within a coronary artery narrowing, the balloon is inflated, so that part of the atherosclerotic plaque is "squeezed" into the opening of the device.

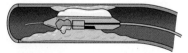

3. When the physician starts rotating the cutting blade, pieces of plaque are shaved off into the device.

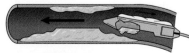

4. The catheter is withdrawn, leaving a larger opening for blood flow.

(C) Coronary stent

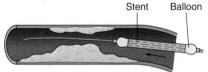

1. To place a coronary stent within a vessel narrowing, physicians use a special catheter with a deflated balloon and the stent at the tip.

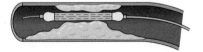

2. The catheter is positioned so that the stent is within the narrowed region of the coronary artery.

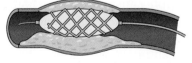

3. The balloon is then inflated, causing the stent to expand and stretch the coronary artery.

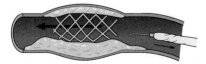

4. The balloon catheter is then withdrawn, leaving the stent behind to keep the vessel open.

FIGURE 7-49 Ways to open clogged arteries: (A) balloon angioplasty, (B) coronary atherectomy, and (C) coronary stent.

Hemophilia

Hemophilia is an inherited disease that occurs almost exclusively in male individuals but can be carried by female individuals. Because of the lack of a plasma protein required for the clotting process, the blood is unable to clot. A minor cut can lead to prolonged bleeding, and a minor bump can cause internal bleeding. Treatment involves transfusing whole blood, or plasma, and administering the missing protein factor.

Hypertension

Hypertension is high blood pressure. A systolic pressure above 140 and a diastolic pressure above 90 millimeters of mercury (mmHg) is usually regarded as hypertension. Risk factors that increase the incidence of hypertension include family history, race (higher in African Americans), obesity, stress, smoking, aging (higher in postmenopausal women), and a diet high in saturated fat. Although there is no cure, hypertension can usually be controlled with antihypertensive drugs, diuretics (to remove retained body fluids), limited stress, avoidance of tobacco, and/or a low-sodium or low-fat diet. If hypertension is not treated, it can cause permanent damage to the heart, blood vessels, and kidneys.

Leukemia

Leukemia is a malignant disease of the bone marrow or lymph tissue. It results in a high number of immature white blood cells. There are different types of leukemia, some acute and some chronic. Symptoms include fever, pallor, swelling of lymphoid tissues, fatigue, anemia, bleeding gums, excessive bruising, and joint pain. Treatment methods vary with the type of leukemia but can include chemotherapy, radiation, and/or bone marrow transplant.

Myocardial Infarction

A myocardial infarction, or heart attack, occurs when a blockage in the coronary arteries cuts off the supply of blood to the heart. The affected heart tissue dies and is known as an *infarct.* Death can occur immediately. Symptoms include severe crushing pain (angina pectoris) that radiates to the arm, neck, and jaw; pressure in the chest; perspiration and cold, clammy skin; dypsnea; and a change in blood pressure. If the heart stops, cardiopulmonary resuscitation should be started immediately. Immediate treatment with a thrombolytic or "clot-busting" drug such as streptokinase or TPA, tissue plasminogen activator, may open the blood vessel and restore blood flow to the heart. However, the clot-busting drug must be used within the first several hours, and its use is prohibited if bleeding is present. Additional treatment methods include complete bed rest, pain medications, vasodilators, cardiotonic drugs (to slow and strengthen the heartbeat), oxygen therapy, anticoagulants (to prevent additional clots), and control of arrhythmias (abnormal heart rhythms). Long-term care includes control of blood pressure, a diet low in cholesterol and saturated fat, avoidance of tobacco and stress, regular exercise, and weight control.

Phlebitis

Phlebitis is an inflammation of a vein, frequently in the leg. If a thrombus, or clot, forms, the condition is termed *thrombophlebitis.* Symptoms include pain, edema, redness, and discoloration at the site. Treatment methods include anticoagulants; pain medication; elevation of the affected area; antiembolism or support hose; and if necessary, surgery to remove the clot.

Varicose Veins

Varicose veins are dilated, swollen veins that have lost elasticity and cause stasis, or decreased blood flow. They frequently occur in the legs and result from pregnancy, prolonged sitting or standing, and hereditary factors. Treatment methods include exercise, antiembolism or support hose, and avoidance of prolonged sitting or standing and tight-fitting or restrictive clothing. In severe cases, surgery can be performed to remove the vein.

STUDENT: *Go to the workbook and complete the assignment sheet for 7:8, Circulatory System.*

7:9 Lymphatic System

Objectives

After completing this section, you should be able to:

♦ Explain the function of lymphatic vessels

♦ List at least two functions of lymph nodes

♦ Identify the two lymphatic ducts and the areas of the body that each drains

♦ List at least three functions of the spleen

♦ Describe the function of the thymus

♦ Describe at least three diseases of the lymphatic system

♦ Define, pronounce, and spell all key terms

KEY TERMS

cisterna chyli *(sis-tern'-uh-kye'-lee)*

lacteals

lymph *(limf')*

lymph nodes

lymphatic capillaries *(lim-fat'-ik)*

lymphatic system

lymphatic vessels

right lymphatic duct

spleen

thoracic duct *(tho-rass'-ik)*

thymus

tonsils

RELATED HEALTH CAREERS

♦ Immunologist

♦ Internist

7:9 INFORMATION

The **lymphatic system** consists of lymph, lymph vessels, lymph nodes, and lymphatic tissue. This system works in conjunction with the circulatory system to remove wastes and excess fluids from the tissues (figure 7-50).

Lymph is a thin, watery fluid composed of *intercellular,* or *interstitial,* fluid, which forms when plasma diffuses into tissue spaces. It is composed of water, digested nutrients, salts, hormones, oxygen, carbon dioxide, lymphocytes, and metabolic wastes such as urea. When this fluid enters the lymphatic system, it is known as lymph.

Lymphatic vessels are located throughout the body in almost all of the tissues that have blood vessels. Small, open-ended lymph vessels act like drainpipes and are called **lymphatic capillaries.** The lymphatic capillaries pick up lymph at tissues throughout the body. The capillaries then join together to form larger lymphatic vessels, which pass through the lymph nodes. Contrac-

tions of skeletal muscles against the lymph vessels cause the lymph to flow through the vessels. Lymphatic vessels also have valves that keep the lymph flowing in only one direction. In the area of the small intestine, specialized lymphatic capillaries, called **lacteals,** pick up digested fats or lipids. When lymph is mixed with the lipids it is called *chyle.* The lacteals transport the chyle to the bloodstream through the thoracic duct.

Lymph nodes, popularly called "glands," are located all over the body, usually in groups or clusters. They are small, round, or oval masses ranging in size from that of a pinhead to that of an almond. Lymph vessels bring lymph to the nodes. The nodes filter the lymph and remove impurities such as carbon, cancer cells, pathogens (disease-producing organisms), and dead blood cells. In addition, the lymphatic tissue in the nodes produces lymphocytes (a type of leukocyte, or white blood cell) and antibodies (substances used to combat infection). The purified lymph, with lymphocytes and antibodies added, leaves the lymph node by a single lymphatic vessel.

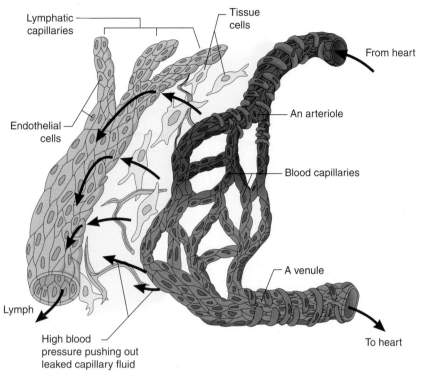

FIGURE 7-50 The lymphatic system works with the circulatory system to remove metabolic waste and excess fluid from the tissues.

As lymphatic vessels leave the lymph nodes, they continue to join together to form larger lymph vessels (figure 7-51). Eventually, these vessels drain into one of two lymphatic ducts: the right lymphatic duct or the thoracic duct. The **right lymphatic duct** is the short tube that receives all of the purified lymph from the right side of the head and neck, the right chest, and the right arm. It empties into the right subclavian vein, returning the purified lymph to the blood. The **thoracic duct,** a much larger tube, drains the lymph from the rest of the body. It empties into the left subclavian vein. At the start of the thoracic duct, an enlarged pouchlike structure called the **cisterna chyli** serves as a storage area for purified lymph before this lymph returns to the bloodstream. The cisterna chyli also receives chyle from the intestinal lacteals.

In addition to being found in the lymph nodes, lymphatic tissue is located throughout the body. The tonsils, spleen, and thymus are examples of lymphatic tissue.

The **tonsils** are masses of lymphatic tissue that filter interstitial fluid. There are three pairs of tonsils:

♦ *Palatine tonsils*: located on each side of the soft palate

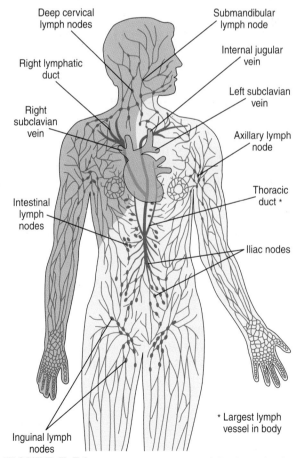

FIGURE 7-51 Main components of the lymphatic system.

♦ *Pharyngeal tonsils*: (also called *adenoids*) located in the nasopharynx (the upper part of the throat)

♦ *Lingual tonsils*: located on the back of the tongue

The **spleen** is an organ located beneath the left side of the diaphragm and in back of the upper part of the stomach. It produces leukocytes and antibodies, destroys old erythrocytes (red blood cells), stores erythrocytes to release into the bloodstream if excessive bleeding occurs, destroys thrombocytes (platelets), and filters metabolites and wastes from body tissues.

The **thymus** is a mass of lymph tissue located in the center of the upper chest. It atrophies (wastes away) after puberty and is replaced by fat and connective tissue. During early life, it produces antibodies and manufactures lymphocytes to fight infection. Its function is taken over by the lymph nodes.

DISEASES AND ABNORMAL CONDITIONS

Adenitis

Adenitis is an inflammation or infection of the lymph nodes. It occurs when large quantities of harmful substances, such as pathogens or cancer cells, enter the lymph nodes and infect the tissue. Symptoms include fever and swollen, painful nodes. If the infection is not treated, an abscess may form in the node. Usually treatment methods are antibiotics and warm, moist compresses. If an abscess forms, it is sometimes necessary to incise and drain the node.

Hodgkin's Disease

Hodgkin's disease is a chronic, malignant disease of the lymph nodes. It is the most common form of lymphoma (tumor of lymph tissue). Symptoms include painless swelling of the lymph nodes, fever, night sweats, weight loss, fatigue, and pru-ritus (itching). Chemotherapy and radiation are usually effective forms of treatment.

Lymphangitis

Lymphangitis is an inflammation of lymphatic vessels, usually resulting from an infection in an extremity. Symptoms include a characteristic red streak extending up an arm or leg from the source of infection, fever, chills, and tenderness or pain. Treatment methods include antibiotics, rest, elevation of the affected part, and/or warm, moist compresses.

Splenomegaly

Splenomegaly is an enlargement of the spleen. It can result from an abnormal accumulation of red blood cells, mononucleosis, and cirrhosis of the liver. The main symptoms are swelling and abdominal pain. An increased destruction of blood cells can lead to anemia (low red blood cell count), leukopenia (low white blood cell count), and thrombocytopenia (low thrombocyte count). If the spleen ruptures, intraperitoneal hemorrhage and shock can lead to death. In severe cases, where the underlying cause cannot be treated, a splenectomy (surgical removal of the spleen) is performed.

Tonsillitis

Tonsillitis is an inflammation or infection of the tonsils. It usually involves the pharyngeal (adenoid) and palatine tonsils. Symptoms include throat pain, dysphagia (difficulty swallowing), fever, white or yellow spots of exudate on the tonsils, and swollen lymph nodes near the mandible. Antibiotics, warm throat irrigations, rest, and analgesics for pain are the main forms of treatment. Chronic, frequent infections or hypertrophy (enlargement) that causes obstruction are indications for a tonsillectomy, or surgical removal of the tonsils.

STUDENT: *Go to the workbook and complete the assignment sheet for 7:9, Lymphatic System.*

7:10 Respiratory System

Objectives

After completing this section, you should be able to:

♦ Label a diagram of the respiratory system

♦ List five functions of the nasal cavity

♦ Identify the three sections of the pharynx

♦ Explain how the larynx helps create sound and speech

♦ Describe the function of the epiglottis

♦ Compare the processes of inspiration and expiration, including the muscle action that occurs during each process

♦ Differentiate between external and internal respiration

♦ Describe at least five diseases of the respiratory system

♦ Define, pronounce, and spell all key terms

KEY TERMS

alveoli *(ahl-vee'-oh''-lie)*
bronchi *(bron'-kie)*
bronchioles *(bron'-key''-ohlz)*
cellular respiration
cilia *(sil'-lee-ah)*
epiglottis *(ep-ih-glot'-tiss)*
expiration
external respiration

inspiration
internal respiration
larynx *(lar'-inks)*
lungs
nasal cavities
nasal septum
nose
pharynx *(far'-inks)*

pleura
respiration
respiratory system *(res'-peh-reh-tor'-ee)*
sinuses
trachea *(tray'-key''-ah)*
ventilation

RELATED HEALTH CAREERS

♦ Internist

♦ Otolaryngologist

♦ Perfusionist

♦ Pulmonologist

♦ Respiratory Therapist

♦ Respiratory Therapy Technician

♦ Thoracic Surgeon

7:10 INFORMATION

The **respiratory system** consists of the lungs and air passages. This system is responsible for taking in oxygen, a gas needed by all body cells, and removing carbon dioxide, a gas that is a metabolic waste product produced by the cells when the cells convert food into energy. Because the body has only a 4–6-minute supply of oxygen, the respiratory system must work continuously to prevent death.

The parts of the respiratory system are the nose, pharynx, larynx, trachea, bronchi, alveoli, and lungs (figure 7-52).

RESPIRATORY ORGANS AND STRUCTURES

The **nose** has two openings, called *nostrils* or *nares*, through which air enters. A wall of cartilage, called the **nasal septum,** divides the nose into two hollow spaces, called **nasal cavities.** The nasal cavities are lined with a mucous membrane and have a rich blood supply. As air enters the cavities, it is warmed, filtered, and moistened. Mucus, produced by the mucous membranes, moistens the air and helps trap pathogens and dirt. Tiny, hairlike structures, called **cilia,** filter

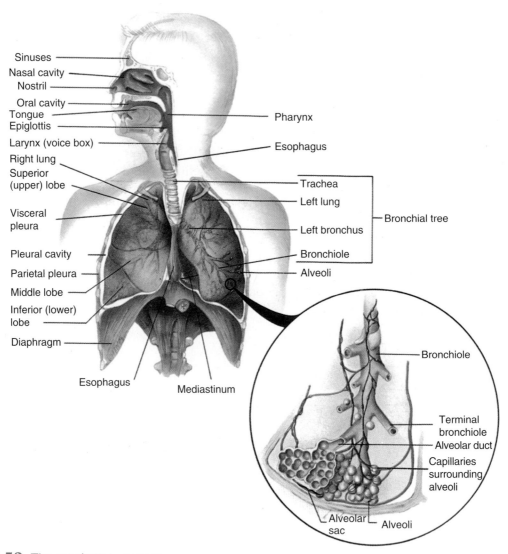

FIGURE 7-52 The respiratory system.

inhaled air to trap dust and other particles. The cilia then help move the mucous layer that lines the airways to push trapped particles toward the esophagus, where they can be swallowed. The *olfactory receptors* for the sense of smell are also located in the nose. The *nasolacrimal ducts* drain tears from the eye into the nose to provide additional moisture for the air.

Sinuses are cavities in the skull that surround the nasal area. They are connected to the nasal cavity by short ducts. The sinuses are lined with a mucous membrane that warms and moistens air. The sinuses also provide resonance for the voice.

The **pharynx,** or throat, lies directly behind the nasal cavities. As air leaves the nose, it enters the pharynx. The pharynx is divided into three sections. The *nasopharynx* is the upper portion, located behind the nasal cavities. The pharyngeal tonsils, or adenoids (lymphatic tissue), and the eustachian tube (tube to middle ear) openings are located in this section. The *oropharynx* is the middle section, located behind the oral cavity (mouth). This section receives both air from the nasopharynx and food and air from the mouth. The *laryngopharynx* is the bottom section of the pharynx. The esophagus, which carries food to the stomach, and the trachea, which carries air to and from the lungs, branch off the laryngopharynx.

The **larynx,** or voice box, lies between the pharynx and trachea. It has nine layers of cartilage. The largest, the thyroid cartilage, is commonly called the *Adam's apple.* The larynx contains two folds, called *vocal cords*. The opening between the vocal cords is called the *glottis*. As air leaves the lungs, the vocal cords vibrate and produce sound. The tongue and lips act on the sound to produce speech. The **epiglottis,** a special leaflike piece of cartilage, closes the opening into the larynx during swallowing. This prevents food and liquids from entering the respiratory tract.

The **trachea** (windpipe) is a tube extending from the larynx to the center of the chest. It carries air between the pharynx and the bronchi. A series of C-shaped cartilages (which are open on the dorsal, or back, surfaces) help keep the trachea open.

The trachea divides into two **bronchi** near the center of the chest, a right bronchus and a left bronchus. The right bronchus is shorter, wider, and extends more vertically than the left bronchus. Each bronchus enters a lung and carries air from the trachea to the lung. In the lungs, the bronchi continue to divide into smaller and smaller bronchi until, finally, they divide into the smallest branches, called **bronchioles.** The smallest bronchioles, called *terminal bronchioles,* end in air sacs, called *alveoli.*

The **alveoli** resemble a bunch of grapes. An adult lung contains approximately 500 million alveoli. They are made of one layer of squamous epithelial tissue and contain a rich network of blood capillaries. The capillaries allow oxygen and carbon dioxide to be exchanged between the blood and the lungs. The inner surfaces of the alveoli are covered with a lipid (fatty) substance, called *surfactant,* to help prevent them from collapsing.

The divisions of the bronchi and the alveoli are found in organs called **lungs.** The right lung has three sections, or lobes: the superior, the middle, and the inferior. The left lung has only two lobes: the superior and the inferior. The left lung is smaller because the heart is located toward the left side of the chest. Each lung is enclosed in a membrane, or sac, called the **pleura.** The pleura consists of two layers of serous membrane: a visceral pleura attached to the surface of the lung, and a parietal pleura attached to the chest wall. A pleural space, located between the two layers, is filled with a thin layer of pleural fluid that lubricates the membranes and prevents friction as the lungs expand during breathing. Both of the lungs, along with the heart and major blood vessels, are located in the thoracic cavity.

PROCESS OF BREATHING

Ventilation is the process of breathing. It involves two phases: inspiration and expiration. **Inspiration** (inhalation) is the process of breathing in air. The diaphragm (dome-shaped muscle between the thoracic and abdominal cavities) and the intercostal muscles (between the ribs) contract and enlarge the thoracic cavity to create a vacuum. Air rushes in through the airways to the alveoli, where the exchange of gases takes place. When the diaphragm and intercostal muscles relax, the process of **expiration** (exhalation) occurs. Air is forced out of the lungs and air passages. This process of inspiration and expiration is known as **respiration.** The process of respiration is controlled by the respiratory center in the medulla oblongata of the brain. An increased amount of carbon dioxide in the blood, or a decreased amount of oxygen as seen in certain diseases (asthma, congestive heart failure, or emphysema), causes the center to increase the rate of respiration. Although this process is usually involuntary, a person can control the rate of breathing by breathing faster or slower.

STAGES OF RESPIRATION

There are two main stages of respiration: external respiration and internal respiration (figure 7-53). **External respiration** is the exchange of oxygen and carbon dioxide between the lungs and bloodstream. Oxygen, breathed in through the respiratory system, enters the alveoli. Because the oxygen concentration in the alveoli is higher than the oxygen concentration in the blood capillaries, oxygen leaves the alveoli and enters the capillaries and the bloodstream. Carbon dioxide, a metabolic waste product, is carried in the bloodstream. Because the carbon dioxide concentration in the capillaries is higher than the carbon dioxide concentration in the alveoli, carbon dioxide leaves the capillaries and enters the alveoli, where it is expelled from the body during exhalation. **Internal respiration** is the exchange of carbon dioxide and oxygen between the tissue cells and the bloodstream. Oxygen is carried to the tissue cells by the blood. Because the oxygen

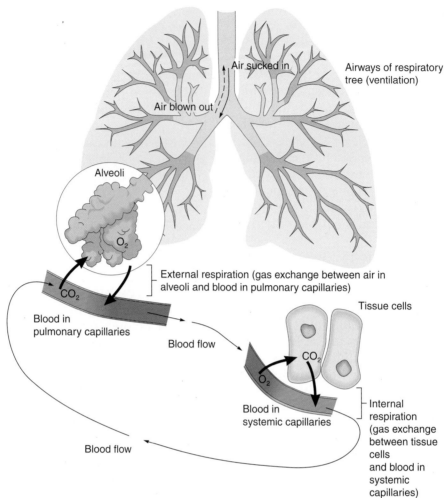

FIGURE 7-53 External and internal respiration.

concentration is higher in the blood than in the tissue cells, oxygen leaves the blood capillaries and enters the tissue cells. The cells then use the oxygen and nutrients to produce energy, water, and carbon dioxide. This process is called **cellular respiration.** Because the carbon dioxide concentration is higher in tissue cells than in the bloodstream, carbon dioxide leaves the cells and enters the bloodstream to be transported back to the lungs, where external respiration takes place.

DISEASES AND ABNORMAL CONDITIONS

Asthma

Asthma is a respiratory disorder usually caused by a sensitivity to an allergen such as dust, pollen, an animal, medications, or a food. Stress, overex-

ertion, and infection can also cause an asthma attack, during which bronchospasms narrow the openings of the bronchioles, mucus production increases, and edema develops in the mucosal lining. Symptoms of an asthma attack include dyspnea (difficult breathing), wheezing, coughing accompanied by expectoration of sputum, and tightness in the chest. Treatment methods include bronchodilators (to enlarge the bronchioles), anti-inflammatory medications, epinephrine, and oxygen therapy. Identification and elimination of or disensitization to allergens are important in preventing asthma attacks.

Bronchitis

Bronchitis is an inflammation of the bronchi and bronchial tubes. *Acute bronchitis* is usually caused by infection and is characterized by a productive cough, dyspnea, rales (bubbly or noisy breath sounds), chest pain, and fever. It is treated with antibiotics, expectorants (to remove excessive mucus), rest, and drinking large amounts of water. *Chronic bronchitis* results from frequent attacks of acute bronchitis and long-term exposure to pollutants or smoking. It is characterized by chronic inflammation, damaged cilia, and enlarged mucous glands. Symptoms include excessive mucus resulting in a productive cough, wheezing, dyspnea, chest pain, and prolonged air expiration. Although there is no cure, antibiotics, bronchodilators, and/or respiratory therapy are used in treatment.

Chronic Obstructive Pulmonary Disease

Chronic obstructive pulmonary disease (COPD) is a term used to describe any chronic lung disease that results in obstruction of the airways. Disorders such as chronic asthma, chronic bronchitis, emphysema, and tuberculosis lead to COPD. Smoking is the primary cause, but allergies and chronic respiratory infections are also factors. Treatment methods include bronchodilators, mucolytics (loosen mucus secretions), and cough medications. The prognosis is poor because damage to the lungs causes a deterioration of pulmonary function, leading to respiratory failure and death.

Emphysema

Emphysema is a noninfectious, chronic respiratory condition that occurs when the walls of the alveoli deteriorate and lose their elasticity (figure 7-54). Carbon dioxide remains trapped in the alveoli, and there is poor exchange of gases. The most common causes are heavy smoking and prolonged exposure to air pollutants. Symptoms include dyspnea, a feeling of suffocation, pain, barrel chest, chronic cough, cyanosis, rapid respirations accompanied by prolonged expirations, and eventual respiratory failure and death. Although there is no cure, treatment methods include bronchodilators, breathing exercises, prompt treatment of respiratory infections, oxygen therapy, respiratory therapy, and avoidance of smoking.

Epistaxis

Epistaxis, or a nosebleed, occurs when capillaries in the nose become congested and bleed. It can be caused by an injury or blow to the nose, hyper-

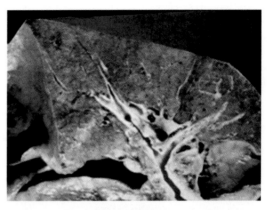
Normal lung

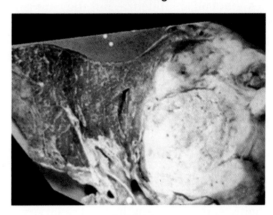
Cancer

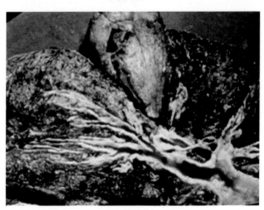
Emphysema

FIGURE 7-54 Two common lung diseases are emphysema and cancer. *(Reprinted by the permission of the American Cancer Society, Inc. All rights reserved.)*

tension, chronic infection, anticoagulant drugs, and blood diseases such as hemophilia and leukemia. Compressing the nostrils toward the septum; elevating the head and tilting it slightly forward; and applying cold compresses will usually control epistaxis, although it is sometimes necessary to insert nasal packs or cauterize (burn and destroy) the bleeding vessels. Treatment of any underlying cause, such as hypertension, is important in preventing epistaxis.

Influenza

Influenza, or flu, is a highly contagious viral infection of the upper respiratory system. Onset is sudden, and symptoms include chills, fever, a cough, sore throat, runny nose, muscle pain, and fatigue. Treatment methods include bed rest, fluids, analgesics (for pain), and antipyretics (for fever). Antibiotics are not effective against the viruses that cause influenza, but they are sometimes given to prevent secondary infections such as pneumonia. Immunization with a flu vaccine is recommended for the elderly, individuals with chronic diseases, pregnant women, and health care workers. Because many different viruses cause influenza, vaccines are developed each year to immunize against the most common viruses identified.

Laryngitis

Laryngitis is an inflammation of the larynx and vocal cords. It frequently occurs in conjunction with other respiratory infections. Symptoms include hoarseness or loss of voice, sore throat, and dysphagia (difficult swallowing). Treatment methods include rest, limited voice use, fluids, and medication, if an infection is present.

Lung Cancer

Lung cancer is the leading cause of cancer death in both men and women (figure 7-54). It is a preventable disease because the main cause is exposure to carcinogens in tobacco, either through smoking or through exposure to "second-hand" smoke. Three common types of lung cancer include small cell, squamous cell, and adenocarcinoma. In the early stages, there are no symptoms. In later stages, symptoms include a chronic cough, hemoptysis (coughing up blood-tinged sputum), dyspnea, fatigue, weight loss, and chest pain. The prognosis (outcome) for lung cancer patients is poor because the disease is usually advanced before it is diagnosed. Treatment includes surgical removal of the cancerous sections of the lung, radiation, and/or chemotherapy.

Pleurisy

Pleurisy is an inflammation of the pleura, or membranes, of the lungs. It usually occurs in conjunction with pneumonia or other lung infections. Symptoms include sharp, stabbing pain while breathing; crepitation (grating sounds in the lungs); dyspnea; and fever. Treatment methods include rest and medications to relieve pain and inflammation. If fluid collects in the pleural space, a *thoracentesis* (withdrawal of fluid through a needle) is performed to remove the fluid and prevent compression of the lungs.

Pneumonia

Pneumonia is an inflammation or infection of the lungs characterized by exudate (a buildup of fluid) in the alveoli. It is usually caused by bacteria, viruses, protozoa, or chemicals. Symptoms include chills, fever, chest pain, productive cough, dyspnea, and fatigue. Treatment methods include bed rest, oxygen therapy, fluids, antibiotics (if indicated), respiratory therapy, and/or pain medication.

Rhinitis

Rhinitis is an inflammation of the nasal mucous membrane, resulting in a runny nose, watery eyes, sneezing, soreness, and congestion. Common causes are infections and allergens. Treatment consists of administering fluids and medications to relieve congestion. Rhinitis is usually self-limiting.

Sinusitis

Sinusitis is an inflammation of the mucous membrane lining the sinuses. One or more sinuses may be affected. Sinusitis is usually caused by a bacterium or virus. Symptoms include headache or pressure, dizziness, thick nasal discharge, congestion, and loss of voice resonance. Treatment methods include analgesics (for pain), antibiotics (if indicated), decongestants (medications to loosen secretions), and moist inhalations. Surgery is used in cases of chronic sinusitis to open the cavities and encourage drainage.

Sleep Apnea

Sleep apnea is a condition in which an individual stops breathing while asleep, causing a measurable decrease in blood oxygen levels. There are two main kinds of sleep apnea: obstructive and central. *Obstructive sleep apnea* is caused by a blockage in the air passage that occurs when the muscles that keep the airway open relax and allow the tongue and palate to block the airway. *Central sleep apnea* is caused by a disorder in the respiratory control center of the brain. The condition is more common in men. Factors such as obesity, hypertension, smoking, alcohol ingestion, and/or the use of sedatives may increase the severity. Sleep apnea is diagnosed when more than 5 periods of apnea lasting at least 10 seconds each occur during 1 hour of sleep. The periods of apnea reduce the blood oxygen level. This causes the brain to awaken the individual, who then gasps for air and snores loudly. This interruption of the sleep cycle leads to excessive tiredness and drowsiness during the day. Treatment involves losing weight, abstaining from smoking and the use of alcohol or sedatives, and sleeping on the side or stomach. In more severe cases of obstructive sleep apnea, a continuous positive airway pressure, or CPAP (pronounced see-pap), is used to deliver pressure to the airway to keep the airway open while the individual sleeps (figure 7-55). The CPAP consists of a mask that is fit securely against the face. Tubing connects the mask with a blower device that can be adjusted to deliver air at different levels of pressure. Treatment of central sleep apnea usually involves the use of medications to stimulate breathing.

Tuberculosis

Tuberculosis (TB) is an infectious lung disease caused by the bacterium *Mycobacterium tuberculosis*. At times, white blood cells surround the invading TB organisms and wall them off, creating nodules, called *tubercles,* in the lungs. The TB organisms remain dormant in the tubercles but can cause an active case of TB later, if body resistance is lowered. Symptoms of an active case of TB include fatigue, fever, night sweats, weight loss, hemoptysis (coughing up blood-tinged sputum), and chest pain. Treatment includes administering drugs for one or more years to destroy the bacteria. Good nutrition and rest are also important. In recent years, a new strain of the TB bacteria resistant to drug therapy has created concern that TB will become a widespread infectious disease.

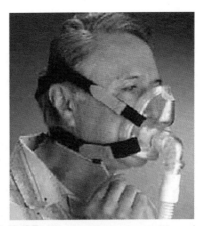

FIGURE 7-55 The continuous positive airway pressure (CPAP) mask attaches to a blower device that uses air pressure to keep the airway open and prevent sleep apnea.

Upper Respiratory Infection

An upper respiratory infection (URI), or common cold, is an inflammation of the mucous membrane lining the upper respiratory tract. Caused by viruses, URIs are highly contagious. Symptoms include fever, runny nose, watery eyes, congestion, sore throat, and hacking cough. There is no cure, and symptoms usually last approximately one week. Analgesics (for pain), antipyretics (for fever), rest, increased fluid intake, and antihistamines (to relieve congestion) are used to treat the symptoms.

STUDENT: *Go to the workbook and complete the assignment sheet for 7:10, Respiratory System.*

7:11 Digestive System

Objectives

After completing this section, you should be able to:

♦ Label the major organs on a diagram of the digestive system

♦ Identify at least three organs that are located in the mouth and aid in the initial breakdown of food

♦ Cite two functions of the salivary glands

♦ Describe how the gastric juices act on food in the stomach

♦ Explain how food is absorbed into the body by the villi in the small intestine

♦ List at least three functions of the large intestine

♦ List at least four functions of the liver

♦ Explain how the pancreas helps digest foods

♦ Describe at least five diseases of the digestive system

♦ Define, pronounce, and spell all key terms

KEY TERMS

alimentary canal *(ahl-ih-men'-tar"-ee)*
anus
colon *(coh'-lun)*
digestive system
duodenum *(dew-oh-deh'-num)*
esophagus *(ee"-sof'-eh-gus)*
gallbladder

hard palate
ileum *(ill'-ee"-um)*
jejunum *(jeh-jew'-num)*
large intestine
liver
mouth
pancreas *(pan'-cree"-as)*
peristalsis *(pair"-ih-stall"-sis)*
pharynx *(far'-inks)*

rectum
salivary glands
small intestine
soft palate
stomach
teeth
tongue
vermiform appendix
villi *(vil'-lie)*

RELATED HEALTH CAREERS

♦ Dental Assistant

♦ Dental Hygienist

♦ Dentist

♦ Dietetic Assistant

♦ Dietitian

♦ Enterostomal RN or Technician

♦ Gastroenterologist

♦ Hepatologist

♦ Internist

♦ Proctologist

7:11 INFORMATION

The **digestive system,** also known as the *gastrointestinal system,* is responsible for the physical and chemical breakdown of food so that it can be taken into the bloodstream and used by body cells and tissues. The system consists of the alimentary canal and accessory organs (figure 7-56). The **alimentary canal** is a long, muscular tube that begins at the mouth and includes the mouth (oral cavity), pharynx, esophagus, stomach, small intestine, large intestine, and anus. The accessory organs are the salivary glands, tongue, teeth, liver, gallbladder, and pancreas.

PARTS OF THE ALIMENTARY CANAL

The **mouth,** also called the *buccal cavity* (figure 7-57) receives food as it enters the body. While food is in the mouth, it is tasted, broken down physically by the teeth, lubricated and partially digested by saliva, and swallowed. The **teeth** are special structures in the mouth that physically break down food by chewing and grinding. This process is called *mastication.* The **tongue** is a muscular organ that contains special receptors called *taste buds.* The taste buds allow a person to taste sweet, salty, sour, and bitter sensations. The

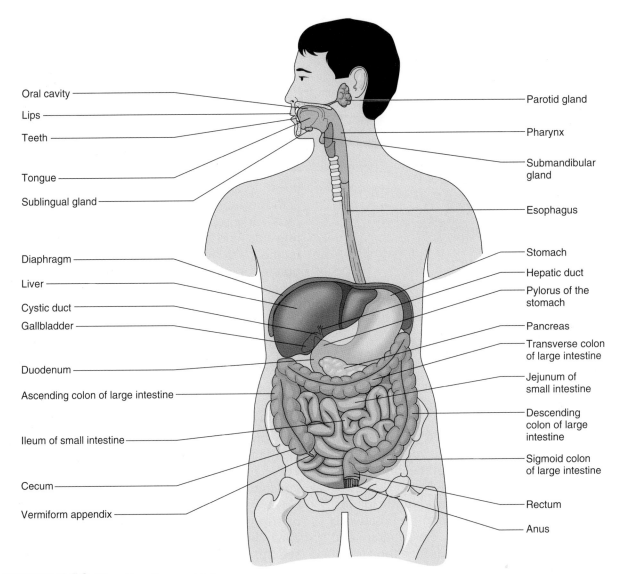

Oral cavity

Lips

Teeth

Tongue

Sublingual gland

Diaphragm

Liver

Cystic duct

Gallbladder

Duodenum

Ascending colon of large intestine

Ileum of small intestine

Cecum

Vermiform appendix

Parotid gland

Pharynx

Submandibular gland

Esophagus

Stomach

Hepatic duct

Pylorus of the stomach

Pancreas

Transverse colon of large intestine

Jejunum of small intestine

Descending colon of large intestine

Sigmoid colon of large intestine

Rectum

Anus

FIGURE 7-56 The digestive system.

tongue also aids in chewing and swallowing food. The **hard palate** is the bony structure that forms the roof of the mouth and separates the mouth from the nasal cavities. Behind the hard palate is the **soft palate,** which separates the mouth from the nasopharynx. The *uvula,* a cone-shaped muscular structure, hangs from the middle of the soft palate. It prevents food from entering the nasopharynx during swallowing. Three pairs of **salivary glands,** the parotid, sublingual, and submandibular, produce a liquid called *saliva.* Saliva lubricates the mouth during speech and chewing and moistens food so that it can be swallowed easily. Saliva also contains an enzyme (a substance that speeds up a chemical reaction) called *salivary amylase,* formerly known as *ptyalin.* Salivary amylase begins the chemical break-

down of carbohydrates, or starches, into sugars that can be taken into the body.

After the food is chewed and mixed with saliva, it is called a *bolus.* When the bolus is swallowed, it enters the **pharynx** (throat). The pharynx is a tube that carries both air and food. It carries the air to the trachea, or windpipe, and food to the esophagus. When a bolus is being swallowed, muscle action causes the epiglottis to close over the larynx, preventing the bolus from entering the respiratory tract and causing it to enter the esophagus.

The **esophagus** is the muscular tube dorsal to (behind) the trachea. This tube receives the bolus from the pharynx and carries the bolus to the stomach. The esophagus, like the remaining part of the alimentary canal, relies on a rhythmic,

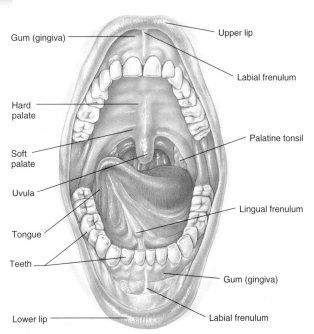

Gum (gingiva)

Upper lip

Labial frenulum

Hard palate

Palatine tonsil

Soft palate

Uvula

Lingual frenulum

Tongue

Teeth

Gum (gingiva)

Lower lip

Labial frenulum

FIGURE 7-57 Parts of the oral cavity, or mouth.

wavelike, involuntary movement of its muscles called **peristalsis** to move the food in a forward direction.

The **stomach** is an enlarged part of the alimentary canal. It receives the food from the esophagus. The mucous membrane lining of the stomach contains folds, called *rugae.* These disappear as the stomach fills with food and expands. The cardiac sphincter, a circular muscle between the esophagus and stomach, closes after food enters the stomach and prevents food from going back up into the esophagus. The pyloric sphincter, a circular muscle between the stomach and small intestine, keeps food in the stomach until the food is ready to enter the small intestine. Food usually remains in the stomach for approximately 2–4 hours. During this time, food is converted into a semifluid material, called *chyme,* by gastric juices produced by glands in the stomach. The gastric juices contain hydrochloric acid and enzymes. Hydrochloric acid kills bacteria, facilitates iron absorption, and activates the enzyme pepsin. The enzymes in gastric juices include lipase, which starts the chemical breakdown of fats, and pepsin, which starts protein digestion. In infants, the enzyme rennin is also secreted to aid in the digestion of milk. Rennin is not present in adults.

When the food, in the form of chyme, leaves the stomach, it enters the small intestine. The **small intestine** is a coiled section of the ali-

mentary canal. It is approximately 20 feet in length and 1 inch in diameter, and is divided into three sections: the duodenum, the jejunum, and the ileum. The **duodenum** is the first 9–10 inches of the small intestine. Bile (from the gallbladder and liver) and pancreatic juice (from the pancreas) enter this section through ducts, or tubes. The **jejunum** is approximately 8 feet in length and forms the middle section of the small intestine. The **ileum** is the final 12 feet of the small intestine, and it connects with the large intestine at the cecum. The circular muscle called the *ileocecal valve* separates the ileum and cecum and prevents food from returning to the ileum. While food is in the small intestine, the process of digestion is completed, and the products of digestion are absorbed into the bloodstream for use by the body cells. Intestinal juices, produced by the small intestine, contain the enzymes maltase, sucrase, and lactase, which break down sugars into simpler forms. The intestinal juices also contain enzymes known as *peptidases,* which complete the digestion of proteins, and *steapsin (lipase),* which aids in the digestion of fat. Bile from the liver and gallbladder emulsifies (physically breaks down) fats. Enzymes from the pancreatic juice complete the process of digestion. These enzymes include pancreatic *amylase* or *amylopsin* (which acts on sugars), *trypsin* and *chymotrypsin* (which act on proteins), and *lipase* or *steapsin* (which acts on fats). After food has been digested, it is absorbed into the bloodstream. The walls of the small intestine are lined with fingerlike projections called **villi** (figure 7-58). The villi contain blood capillaries and lacteals. The blood capillaries absorb the digested nutrients and carry them to the liver, where they are either stored or released into general circulation for use by the body cells. The lacteals absorb most of the digested fats and carry them to the thoracic duct in the lymphatic system, which releases them into the circulatory system. When food has completed its passage through the small intestine, only wastes, indigestible materials, and excess water remain.

The **large intestine** is the final section of the alimentary canal. It is approximately 5 feet in length and 2 inches in diameter. Functions include absorption of water and any remaining nutrients; storage of indigestible materials before they are eliminated from the body; synthesis (formation) and absorption of some B-complex vitamins and vitamin K by bacteria present in the

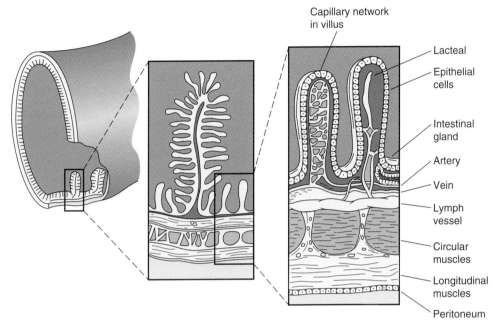

Capillary network
in villus

Lacteal

Epithelial
cells

Intestinal
gland

Artery

Vein

Lymph
vessel

Circular
muscles

Longitudinal
muscles

Peritoneum

FIGURE 7-58 Lymphatic and blood capillaries in the villi of the small intestine provide for the absorption of the products of digestion.

intestine; and transportation of waste products out of the alimentary canal. The large intestine is divided into a series of connected sections. The *cecum* is the first section and is connected to the ileum of the small intestine. It contains a small projection, called the **vermiform appendix.** The next section, the **colon,** has several divisions. The *ascending colon* continues up on the right side of the body from the cecum to the lower part of the liver. The *transverse colon* extends across the abdomen, below the liver and stomach and above the small intestine. The *descending colon* extends down the left side of the body. It connects with the *sigmoid colon,* an S-shaped section that joins with the rectum. The **rectum** is the final 6–8 inches of the large intestine and is a storage area for indigestibles and wastes. It has a narrow canal, called the *anal canal,* which opens at a hole, called the **anus.** Fecal material, or stool, the final waste product of the digestive process, is expelled through this opening.

ACCESSORY ORGANS

The **liver** (figure 7-59), is the largest gland in the body and is an accessory organ to the digestive system. It is located under the diaphragm and in the upper right quadrant of the abdomen. The liver secretes bile, which is used to emulsify fats in the digestive tract. Bile also makes fats water

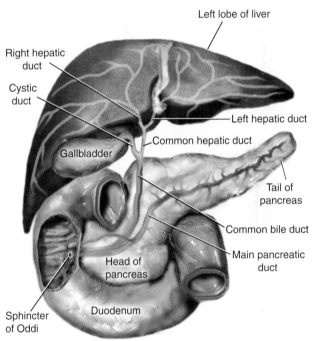

Left lobe of liver

Right hepatic
duct

Cystic
duct

Left hepatic duct

Common hepatic duct

Gallbladder

Tail of
pancreas

Common bile duct

Main pancreatic
duct

Head of
pancreas

Sphincter
of Oddi

Duodenum

FIGURE 7-59 The liver, gallbladder, and pancreas.

soluble, which is necessary for absorption. The liver stores sugar in the form of glycogen. The glycogen is converted to glucose and released into the bloodstream when additional blood sugar is needed. The liver also stores iron and certain vitamins. It produces heparin, which prevents clotting of the blood; blood proteins such as fibrinogen and prothrombin, which aid in clotting of the blood; and cholesterol. Finally, the liver detoxifies (renders less harmful) substances such as alcohol and pesticides, and destroys bacteria that have been taken into the blood from the intestine.

The **gallbladder** is a small, muscular sac located under the liver and attached to it by connective tissue. It stores and concentrates bile, which it receives from the liver. When the bile is needed to emulsify fats in the digestive tract, the gallbladder contracts and pushes the bile through the cystic duct into the common bile duct, which drains into the duodenum.

The **pancreas** is a glandular organ located behind the stomach. It produces pancreatic juices, which contain enzymes to digest food. These juices enter the duodenum through the pancreatic duct. The enzymes in the juices include pancreatic amylase or amylopsin (to break down sugars), trypsin and chymotrypsin (to break down proteins), and lipase or steapsin (to act on fats). The pancreas also produces insulin, which is secreted into the bloodstream. Insulin regulates the metabolism, or burning, of carbohydrates to convert glucose (blood sugar) to energy.

DISEASES AND ABNORMAL CONDITIONS

Appendicitis

Appendicitis is an acute inflammation of the appendix, usually resulting from an obstruction and infection. Symptoms include generalized abdominal pain that later localizes at the lower right quadrant, nausea and vomiting, mild fever, and elevated white blood cell count. If the appendix ruptures, the infectious material will spill into the peritoneal cavity and cause peritonitis, a serious condition. Appendicitis is treated by an appendectomy (surgical removal of the appendix).

Cholecystitis

Cholecystitis is an inflammation of the gallbladder. When gallstones form from crystallized cholesterol, bile salts, and bile pigments, the condition is known as *cholelithiasis.* Symptoms frequently occur after eating fatty foods and include indigestion, nausea and vomiting, and

pain that starts under the rib cage and radiates to the right shoulder. If a gallstone blocks the bile ducts, the gallbladder can rupture and cause peritonitis. Treatment methods include a low-fat diet, lithotripsy (shock waves that are used to shatter the gallstones), and/or a cholecystectomy (surgical removal of the gallbladder).

Cirrhosis

Cirrhosis is a chronic destruction of liver cells accompanied by the formation of fibrous connective and scar tissue. Causes include hepatitis, bile duct disease, chemical toxins, and malnutrition associated with alcoholism. Symptoms vary and become more severe as the disease progresses. Some common symptoms are liver enlargement, anemia, indigestion, nausea, edema in the legs and feet, hematemesis (vomiting blood), nosebleeds, jaundice (yellow discoloration), and ascites (an accumulation of fluid in the abdominal peritoneal cavity). When the liver fails, disorientation, hallucinations, hepatic coma, and death occur. Treatment is directed toward preventing further damage to the liver. Alcohol avoidance, proper nutrition, vitamin supplements, diuretics (to reduce ascites and edema), rest, infection prevention, and appropriate exercise are encouraged. A liver transplant may be performed if too much of the liver is destroyed.

Constipation

Constipation is when fecal material remains in the colon too long, causing excessive reabsorption of water. The feces or stool becomes hard, dry, and difficult to eliminate. Causes include poor bowel habits, chronic laxative use leading to a "lazy" bowel, a diet low in fiber, and certain digestive diseases. The condition is usually corrected by a high-fiber diet, adequate fluids, and exercise. Although laxatives are sometimes used to stimulate defecation, frequent laxative use may be habit forming and lead to chronic constipation.

Diarrhea

Diarrhea is a condition characterized by frequent watery stools. Causes include infection, stress, diet, an irritated colon, and toxic substances. Diarrhea can be extremely dangerous in infants and small children because of the excessive fluid loss. Treatment is directed toward eliminating the cause, providing adequate fluid intake, and modifying the diet.

Diverticulitis

Diverticulitis is an inflammation of the diverticula, pouches (or sacs) that form in the intestine as the mucosal lining pushes through the surrounding muscle. When fecal material and bacteria become trapped in the diverticula, inflammation occurs. This can result in an abscess or rupture, leading to peritonitis. Symptoms vary depending on the amount of inflammation but may include abdominal pain, irregular bowel movements, flatus (gas), constipation or diarrhea, abdominal distention (swelling), low-grade fever, and nausea and vomiting. Treatment methods include antibiotics, stool-softening medications, pain medications, high-fiber diet, and in severe cases, surgery to remove the affected section of colon.

Gastroenteritis

Gastroenteritis is an inflammation of the mucous membrane that lines the stomach and intestinal tract. Causes include food poisoning, infection, and toxins. Symptoms include abdominal cramping, nausea, vomiting, fever, and diarrhea. Usual treatment methods are rest and increased fluid intake. In severe cases, antibiotics, intravenous fluids, and medications to slow peristalsis may be used.

Hemorrhoids

Hemorrhoids are painful dilated or varicose veins of the rectum and/or anus. They may be caused by straining to defecate, constipation, pressure during pregnancy, insufficient fluid intake, laxative abuse, and prolonged sitting or standing. Symptoms include pain, itching, and bleeding. Treatment methods include a high-fiber diet; increased fluid intake; stool softeners; sitz baths or warm, moist compresses; and in some cases, a hemorrhoidectomy (surgical removal of the hemorrhoids).

Hepatitis

Hepatitis is a viral inflammation of the liver. *Type A, HAV* or infectious hepatitis, is highly contagious and is transmitted in food or water con-taminated by the feces of an infected person. It is the most benign form of hepatitis and is usually self-limiting. A vaccine is available to prevent hepatitis A. *Type B, HBV,* or serum hepatitis, is transmitted by body fluids including blood, serum, saliva, urine, semen, vaginal secretions, and breast milk. It is more serious than type A and can lead to chronic hepatitis or to cirrhosis of the liver. A vaccine developed to prevent hepatitis B is recommended for all health care workers. *Type C,* or *HCV,* is also spread through contact with blood or body fluids. The main methods of transmission include sharing needles while injecting drugs, getting stuck with a contaminated needle or sharps while on the job, or passing the virus from an infected mother to the infant during birth. Hepatitis C is much more likely to progress to chronic hepatitis, cirrhosis, or both. There is no vaccine for type C. Other strains of the hepatitis virus that have been identified include types D and E. Symptoms include fever, anorexia (lack of appetite), nausea, vomiting, fatigue, dark-colored urine, clay-colored stool, myalgia (muscle pain), enlarged liver, and jaundice. Treatment methods include rest and a diet high in protein and calories and low in fat. A liver transplant may be necessary if the liver is severely damaged.

Hernia

A hernia, or rupture, occurs when an internal organ pushes through a weakened area or natural opening in a body wall. A hiatal hernia is when the stomach protrudes through the diaphragm and into the chest cavity through the opening for the esophagus (figure 7-60). Symptoms include heartburn, stomach distention, chest pain, and difficult swallowing. Treatment methods include a bland diet, small frequent meals, staying upright after eating, and surgical repair. An inguinal hernia is when a section of the small intestine protrudes through the inguinal rings of the lower abdominal wall. If the hernia cannot be reduced (pushed back in place), a herniorrhaphy (surgical repair) is performed.

Pancreatitis

Pancreatitis is an inflammation of the pancreas. The pancreatic enzymes begin to digest the pancreas itself, and the pancreas becomes necrotic, inflamed, and edematous. If the damage extends

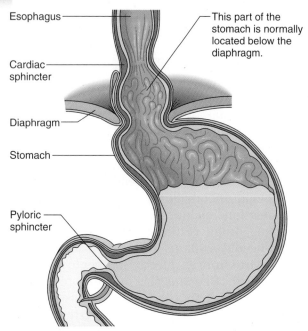

Esophagus

This part of the stomach is normally located below the diaphragm.

Cardiac sphincter

Diaphragm

Stomach

Pyloric sphincter

FIGURE 7-60 A hiatal hernia occurs when the stomach protrudes through the diaphragm.

to blood vessels in the pancreas, hemorrhage and shock occur. Pancreatitis may be caused by excessive alcohol consumption or blockage of pancreatic ducts by gallstones. Many cases are *idiopathic*, or of unknown cause. Symptoms include severe abdominal pain that radiates to the back, nausea, vomiting, diaphoresis (excessive perspiration), and jaundice if swelling blocks the common bile duct. Treatment depends on the cause. A cholecystectomy, removal of the gall bladder, is performed if gallstones are the cause. Analgesics for pain and nutritional support are used if the cause of pancreatitis is alcoholism or idiopathic. This type of pancreatitis has a poor prognosis and often results in death.

Peritonitis

Peritonitis, an inflammation of the abdominal peritoneal cavity, usually occurs when a rupture in the intestine allows the intestine contents to enter the peritoneal cavity. A ruptured appendix or gallbladder can cause this condition. Symptoms include abdominal pain and distention, fever, nausea, and vomiting. Treatment methods include antibiotics and, if necessary, surgical repair of the damaged intestine.

Ulcer

An ulcer is an open sore on the lining of the digestive tract. Peptic ulcers include gastric (stomach) ulcers and duodenal ulcers. The major cause is a bacterium, *Helicobacter pylori (H. pylori)*, that burrows into the stomach membranes, allowing stomach acids and digestive juices to create an ulcer. Symptoms include burning pain, indigestion, hematemesis (bloody vomitus), and melena (dark, tarry stool). Usual treatment methods are antacids, a bland diet, decreased stress, and avoidance of irritants such as alcohol, fried foods, tobacco, and caffeine. If the *H. pylori* bacteria are present, treatment with antibiotics and a bismuth preparation, such as Pepto-Bismol, usually cures the condition. In severe cases, surgery is performed to remove the affected area.

Ulcerative Colitis

Ulcerative colitis is a severe inflammation of the colon accompanied by the formation of ulcers and abscesses. It is thought to be caused by stress, food allergy, or an autoimmune reaction. The main symptom is diarrhea containing blood, pus, and mucus. Other symptoms include weight loss, weakness, abdominal pain, anemia, and anorexia. Periods of remission and exacerbation are common. Treatment is directed toward controlling inflammation, reducing stress with mild sedation, maintaining proper nutrition, and avoiding substances that aggravate the condition. In some cases, surgical removal of the affected colon and creation of a colostomy (an artificial opening in the colon that allows fecal material to be excreted through the abdominal wall) is necessary.

STUDENT: *Go to the workbook and complete the assignment sheet for 7:11, Digestive System.*

7:12 Urinary System

Objectives

After completing this section, you should be able to:

♦ Label a diagram of the urinary system

♦ Explain the action of the following parts of a nephron: glomerulus, Bowman's capsule, convoluted tubule, and collecting tubule

- State the functions of the ureter, bladder, and urethra
- Explain why the urethra is different in male and female individuals
- Interpret at least five terms used to describe conditions that affect urination
- Describe at least three diseases of the urinary system
- Define, pronounce, and spell all key terms

KEY TERMS

bladder
Bowman's capsule
cortex *(core'-tex)*
excretory system *(ex'-kreh-tor"-ee)*
glomerulus *(glow"-mare'-you-luss)*

hilum
homeostasis
kidneys
medulla *(meh-due'-la)*
nephrons *(nef'-ronz)*
renal pelvis
ureters *(you'-reh"-turz)*

urethra *(you"-wreath'-rah)*
urinary meatus *(you'-rih-nah-ree" me-ate'-as)*
urinary system
urine
void

RELATED HEALTH CAREERS

- Dialysis Technician
- Medical Laboratory Technologist/Technician
- Nephrologist
- Urologist

7:12 INFORMATION

The **urinary system,** also known as the **excretory system,** is responsible for removing certain wastes and excess water from the body and for maintaining the body's acid–base balance. It is one of the major body systems that maintains **homeostasis,** a state of equilibrium or constant state of natural balance in the internal environment of the body. The parts of the urinary system are two kidneys, two ureters, one bladder, and one urethra (figure 7-61).

The **kidneys** (figure 7-62) are two bean-shaped organs located on either side of the vertebral column, behind the upper part of the abdominal cavity, and separated from this cavity by the peritoneum. Their location is often described as retroperitoneal. The kidneys are protected by the ribs and a heavy cushion of fat.

Connective tissue helps hold the kidneys in position. Each kidney is enclosed in a mass of fatty tissue, called an *adipose capsule,* and covered externally by a tough, fibrous tissue, called the *renal fascia,* or *fibrous capsule.*

Each kidney is divided into two main sections: the cortex and the medulla. The **cortex** is the outer section of the kidney. It contains most of the nephrons, which aid in the production of urine. The **medulla** is the inner section of the kidney. It contains most of the collecting tubules, which carry the urine from the nephrons through the kidney. Each kidney has a **hilum,** a notched or indented area through which the ureter, nerves, blood vessels, and lymph vessels enter and leave the kidney.

Nephrons (figure 7-63) are microscopic filtering units located in the kidneys. There are more than one million nephrons per kidney. Each

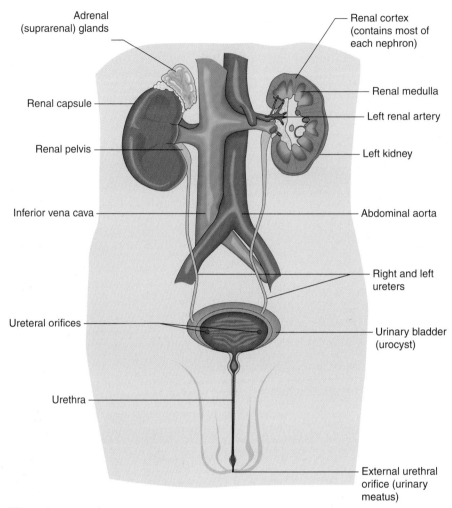

Adrenal
(suprarenal) glands

Renal cortex
(contains most of
each nephron)

Renal capsule

Renal medulla

Left renal artery

Renal pelvis

Left kidney

Inferior vena cava

Abdominal aorta

Right and left
ureters

Ureteral orifices

Urinary bladder
(urocyst)

Urethra

External urethral
orifice (urinary
meatus)

FIGURE 7-61 The urinary system.

nephron consists of a glomerulus, a Bowman's capsule, a proximal convoluted tubule, a distal convoluted tubule, and a collecting duct (tubule). The renal artery carries blood to the kidney. Branches of the renal artery pass through the medulla to the cortex, where the blood enters the first part of the nephron, the **glomerulus,** which is a cluster of capillaries. As blood passes through the glomerulus, water, mineral salts, glucose (sugar), metabolic products, and other substances are filtered out of the blood. Red blood cells and proteins are not filtered out. The filtered blood leaves the glomerulus and eventually makes its way to the renal vein, which carries it away from the kidney. The substances filtered out in the glomerulus enter the next section of the nephron, the **Bowman's capsule.** The Bowman's capsule is a C-shaped structure that surrounds the glomerulus and is the start of the convoluted tubule. It picks up the materials filtered from the blood in the glomerulus and passes

them into the convoluted tubule. As these materials pass through the various sections of the tubule, substances needed by the body are reabsorbed and returned to the blood capillaries. By the time the filtered materials pass through the tubule, most of the water, glucose, vitamins, and mineral salts have been reabsorbed. Excess glucose and mineral salts, some water, and wastes (including urea, uric acid, and creatinine) remain in the tubule and become known as the concentrated liquid called *urine.* The urine then enters collecting ducts, or tubules, located in the medulla. These collecting ducts empty into the **renal pelvis** (renal basin), a funnel-shaped structure that is the first section of the ureter.

The **ureters** are two muscular tubes approximately 10–12 inches in length. One extends from the renal pelvis of each kidney to the bladder. Peristalsis (a rhythmic, wavelike motion of muscle) moves the urine through the ureter from the kidney to the bladder.

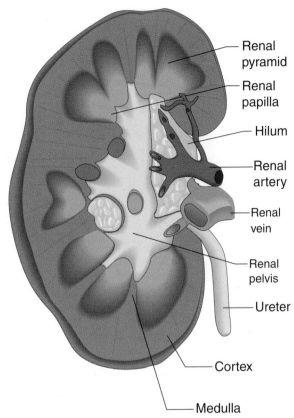

Renal pyramid

Renal papilla

Hilum

Renal artery

Renal vein

Renal pelvis

Ureter

Cortex

Medulla

FIGURE 7-62 A cross section of the kidney.

The **bladder** is a hollow, muscular sac that lies behind the symphysis pubis and at the midline of the pelvic cavity. It has a mucous membrane lining arranged in a series of folds, called *rugae.* The rugae disappear as the bladder expands to fill with urine. Three layers of visceral (smooth) muscle form the walls of the bladder, which receives the urine from the ureters and stores the urine until it is eliminated from the body. Although the urge to **void** (urinate, or micturate) occurs when the bladder contains approximately 250 milliliters (mL) (1 cup) of urine, the bladder can hold much more. A circular sphincter muscle controls the opening to the bladder to prevent emptying. When the bladder is full, receptors in the bladder wall send out a reflex action, which opens the muscle. Infants cannot control this reflex action. As children age, however, they learn to control the reflex.

The **urethra** is the tube that carries the urine from the bladder to the outside. The external opening is called the **urinary meatus.** The urethra is different in female individuals and male individual. In females, it is a tube approximately 3.75 cm (1.5 inches) in length that opens in front of the vagina and carries only urine to the outside. In males, the urethra is approximately 20 cm (8 inches) in length and passes through the prostate gland and out through the penis. It carries both urine (from the urinary system) and semen (from the reproductive system), although not at the same time.

Urine is the liquid waste product produced by the urinary system. It is approximately 95 percent water. Waste products dissolved in this liquid are urea, uric acid, creatinine, mineral salts, and various pigments. Excess useful products, such as sugar, can also be found in the urine, but their presence usually indicates disease. Approximately 1,500–2,000 milliliters (mL) (1.5–2 quarts) of urine are produced daily from the approximately 150 quarts of liquid that is filtered through the kidneys.

Terms used to describe conditions that affect urination include:

♦ *Polyuria:* excessive urination

♦ *Oliguria:* below normal amounts of urination

♦ *Anuria:* absence of urination

♦ *Hematuria:* blood in the urine

♦ *Pyuria:* pus in the urine

♦ *Nocturia:* urination at night

♦ *Dysuria:* painful urination

♦ *Retention:* inability to empty the bladder

♦ *Incontinence:* involuntary urination

♦ *Proteinuria:* protein in the urine

♦ *Albuminuria:* albumin (a blood protein) in the urine

DISEASES AND ABNORMAL CONDITIONS

Cystitis

Cystitis is an inflammation of the bladder, usually caused by pathogens entering the urinary meatus. It is more common in female individuals because of the shortness of the urethra. Symptoms include frequent urination, dysuria, a burning sensation during urination, hematuria, lower back pain, bladder spasm, and fever. Treatment methods are antibiotics and increased fluid intake.

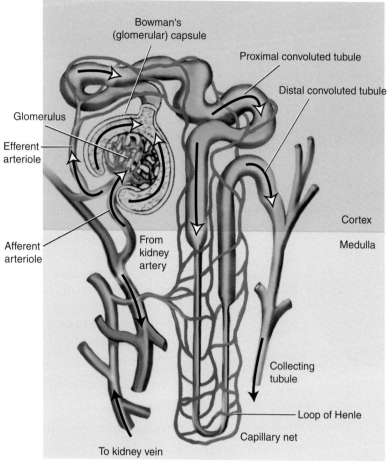

FIGURE 7-63 A nephron unit.

Glomerulonephritis

Glomerulonephritis, or nephritis, is an inflammation of the glomerulus of the kidney. *Acute glomerulonephritis* usually follows a streptococcal infection such as strep throat, scarlet fever, or rheumatic fever. Symptoms include chills, fever, fatigue, edema, oliguria, hematuria, and albuminuria (protein in the urine). Treatment methods include rest, restriction of salt, maintenance of fluid and electrolyte balance, antipyretics (for fever), diuretics (for edema), and at times, antibiotics. With treatment, kidney function is usually restored, and the prognosis is good. Repeated attacks can cause a chronic condition. *Chronic glomerulonephritis* is a progressive disease that causes scarring and sclerosing of the glomeruli. Early symptoms include hematuria, albuminuria, and hypertension. As the disease progresses and additional glomeruli are destroyed, edema, fatigue, anemia, hypertension, anorexia (loss of appetite), weight loss, congestive heart failure, pyuria, and finally, renal failure and death occur. Treatment is directed at treating the symptoms, and treatment methods include a low-sodium diet, antihypertensive drugs, maintenance of fluids and electrolytes, and hemodialysis (removal of the waste products from the blood by a hemodialysis machine) (figure 7-64). When both kidneys are severely damaged, a kidney transplant can be performed.

Pyelonephritis

Pyelonephritis is an inflammation of the kidney tissue and renal pelvis (upper end of the ureter), usually caused by pyogenic (pus-forming) bacteria. Symptoms include chills, fever, back pain, fatigue, dysuria, hematuria, and pyuria (pus in the urine). Treatment methods are antibiotics and increased fluid intake.

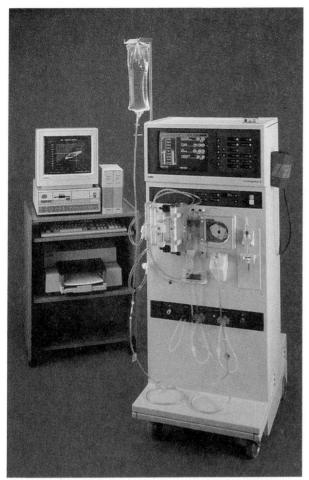

FIGURE 7-64 A hemodialysis machine helps remove waste products from the blood when the kidneys are not functioning correctly.

Renal Calculus

A renal calculus, or urinary calculus, is a kidney stone. A calculus is formed when salts in the urine precipitate (settle out of solution). Some small calculi may be eliminated in the urine, but larger stones often become lodged in the renal pelvis or ureter. Symptoms include sudden, intense pain (renal colic); hematuria; nausea and vomiting; a frequent urge to void; and in some cases, urinary retention. Initial treatment consists of increasing fluids, providing pain medication, and straining all urine through gauze or filter paper to determine whether stones are being eliminated. Extracorporeal shock-wave lithotripsy is a procedure where high-energy pressure waves are used to crush the stones so that they can be eliminated through the urine. In some cases, surgery is required to remove the calculi.

Renal Failure

Renal failure is when the kidneys stop functioning. *Acute renal failure (ARF)* can be caused by hemorrhage, shock, injury, poisoning, nephritis, or dehydration. Symptoms include oliguria or anuria, headache, an ammonia odor to the breath, edema, cardiac arrhythmia, and uremia. Prompt treatment involving dialysis, restricted fluid intake, and correction of the condition causing renal failure results in a good prognosis. *Chronic renal failure (CRF)* results from the progressive loss of kidney function. It can be caused by chronic glomerulonephritis, hypertension, toxins, and endocrine disease such as diabetes mellitus. Long-term substance abuse and alcoholism can also lead to renal failure. Waste products accumulate in the blood and affect many body systems. Symptoms include nausea, vomiting, diarrhea, weight loss, decreased mental ability, convulsions, muscle irritability, an ammonia odor to the breath, uremic frost (deposits of white crystals on the skin), and in later stages, coma prior to death. Treatment methods are dialysis, diet modifications and restrictions, careful skin and mouth care, and control of fluid intake. A kidney transplant is the only cure.

Uremia

Uremia, also called *azotemia,* is a toxic condition that occurs when the kidneys fail and urinary waste products are present in the bloodstream. It can result from any condition that affects the proper functioning of the kidneys, such as renal failure, chronic glomerulonephritis, and hypotension. Symptoms include headache, dizziness, nausea, vomiting, an ammonia odor to the breath, oliguria or anuria, mental confusion, convulsions, coma, and eventually, death. Treatment consists of a restricted diet, cardiac medications to increase blood pressure and cardiac output, and dialysis until a kidney transplant can be performed.

Urethritis

Urethritis is an inflammation of the urethra, usually caused by bacteria (such as gonococcus), viruses, or chemicals (such as bubble bath solutions). It is more common in male than female individuals. Symptoms include frequent and painful urination, redness and itching at the urinary meatus, and a purulent (pus) discharge. Treatment methods include sitz baths or warm, moist compresses; antibiotics; and/or increased fluid intake.

STUDENT: *Go to the workbook and complete the assignment sheet for 7:12, Urinary System.*

7:13 Endocrine System

Objectives

After completing this section, you should be able to:

◆ Label a diagram of the main endocrine glands

◆ Describe how hormones influence various body functions

◆ Describe at least five diseases of the endocrine glands

◆ Define, pronounce, and spell all key terms

KEY TERMS

adrenal glands *(ah"-dree'-nal)*
endocrine system *(en'-doh"-krin)*
hormones
ovaries

pancreas *(pan-kree-as)*
parathyroid glands
pineal body *(pin'-knee"-ahl)*
pituitary gland *(pih"-too'-ih-tar-ee)*

placenta
testes *(tess'-tees)*
thymus
thyroid gland

RELATED HEALTH CAREERS

◆ Endocrinologist

◆ Nuclear Medicine Technologist

7:13 INFORMATION

The **endocrine system** consists of a group of ductless (without tubes) glands that secrete substances directly into the bloodstream. These substances are called *hormones.* The endocrine system consists of the pituitary gland, thyroid gland, parathyroid gland, adrenal glands, pancreas, ovaries, testes, thymus, pineal body, and placenta (figure 7-65).

Hormones, chemical substances produced and secreted by the endocrine glands, are frequently called "chemical messengers." They are transported throughout the body by the bloodstream and perform many functions including:

◆ Stimulate exocrine glands (glands with ducts, or tubes) to produce secretions

◆ Stimulate other endocrine glands

◆ Regulate growth and development

◆ Regulate metabolism

◆ Maintain fluid and chemical balance

◆ Control various sex processes

Table 7-3 lists the main hormones produced by each endocrine gland and the actions they perform.

PITUITARY GLAND

The **pituitary gland** is often called the "master gland" of the body because it produces many hormones that affect other glands. It is located at

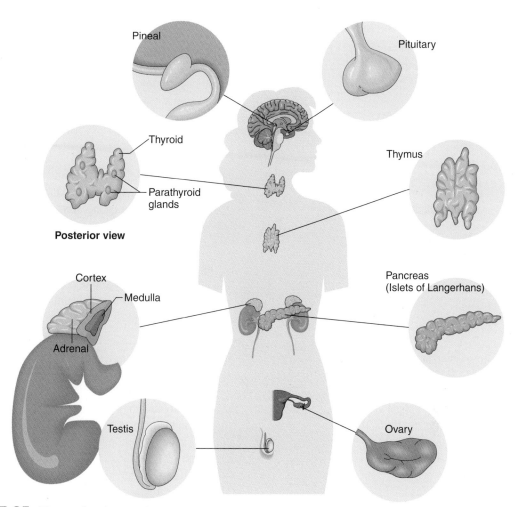

FIGURE 7-65 The endocrine system.

TABLE 7-3 Hormones Produced by the Endocrine Glands and Their Actions

GLAND	HORMONE	ACTION
Pituitary		
Anterior lobe	ACTH—adrenocorticotropic	Stimulates growth and secretion of the cortex of the adrenal gland
	TSH—thyrotropin	Stimulates growth and secretion of the thyroid gland
	GH—somatotropin	Growth hormone, stimulates normal body growth
	FSH—follicle stimulating	Stimulates growth and hormone production in the ovarian follicles of female individuals, production of sperm in male individuals
	LH—luteinizing (female) *or*	Causes ovulation and secretion of progesterone in female individuals
	ICSH—interstitial cell stimulating (male)	Stimulates testes to secrete testosterone
	LTH—lactogenic or prolactin	Stimulates secretion of milk from mammary glands after delivery of an infant
	MSH—melanocyte stimulating	Stimulates production and dispersion of melanin pigment in the skin

(continues)

TABLE 7-3 Hormones Produced by the Endocrine Glands and Their Actions *(Continued)*

GLAND	HORMONE	ACTION
Posterior lobe	ADH—vasopressin	Antidiuretic hormone, promotes reabsorption of water in kidneys, constricts blood vessels
	Oxytocin (pitocin)	Causes contraction of uterus during childbirth, stimulates milk flow from the breasts
Thyroid		
	Thyroxine and tri-iodothyronine	Increase metabolic rate; stimulate physical and mental growth; regulate metabolism of carbohydrates, fats, and proteins
	Thyrocalcitonin (calcitonin)	Accelerates absorption of calcium by the bones and lowers blood calcium level
Parathyroid		
	Parathormone (PTH)	Regulates amount of calcium and phosphate in the blood, increases reabsorption of calcium and phosphates from bones, stimulates kidneys to conserve blood calcium, stimulates absorption of calcium in the intestine
Adrenal		
Cortex	Mineralocorticoids Aldosterone	Regulate the reabsorption of sodium in the kidney and the elimination of potassium, increase the reabsorption of water by the kidneys
	Glucocorticoids Cortisol-hydrocortisone Cortisone	Aid in metabolism of proteins, fats, and carbohydrates; increase amount of glucose in blood; provide resistance to stress; and depress immune responses (anti-inflammatory)
	Gonadocorticoids	Act as sex hormones
	Estrogens	Stimulate female sexual characteristics
	Androgens	Stimulate male sexual characteristics
Medulla	Epinephrine (adrenaline)	Activates sympathetic nervous system, acts in times of stress to increase cardiac output and increase blood pressure
	Norepinephrine	Activates body in stress situations
Pancreas		
	Insulin	Used in metabolism of glucose (sugar) by promoting entry of glucose into cells to decrease blood glucose levels, promotes transport of fatty acids and amino acids (proteins) into the cells
	Glucagon	Maintains blood level of glucose by stimulating the liver to release stored glycogen in the form of glucose
Ovaries		
	Estrogen	Promotes growth and development of sex organs in female individuals
	Progesterone	Maintains lining of uterus
Testes		
	Testosterone	Stimulates growth and development of sex organs in male individuals, stimulates maturation of sperm
Thymus		
	Thymosin (thymopoietin)	Stimulates production of lymphocytes and antibodies in early life

(continues)

TABLE 7-3 Hormones Produced by the Endocrine Glands and Their Actions *(Continued)*

GLAND	HORMONE	ACTION
Pineal		
	Melatonin	May delay puberty by inhibiting gonadotropic (sex) hormones, may regulate sleep/wake cycles
	Adrenoglomerulotropin	May stimulate adrenal cortex to secrete aldosterone
	Serotonin	May prevent vasoconstriction of blood vessels in the brain, inhibits gastric secretions
Placenta		
	Estrogen	Stimulates growth of reproductive organs
	Chorionic gonadotropin	Causes corpus luteum of ovary to continue secretions
	Progesterone	Maintains lining of uterus to provide fetal nutrition

the base of the brain in the sella turcica, a small, bony depression of the sphenoid bone. It is divided into two sections, or lobes: the anterior lobe and the posterior lobe. Each lobe secretes certain hormones, as shown in table 7-3.

Diseases and Abnormal Conditions

Acromegaly

Acromegaly results from an oversecretion of somatotropin (growth hormone) in an adult and is usually caused by a benign (noncancerous) tumor of the pituitary called an *adenoma*. Bones of the hands, feet, and face enlarge and create a grotesque appearance. The skin and tongue thicken, and slurred speech develops. Surgical removal and/or radiation of the tumor is the usual treatment, but the tumor frequently recurs. Acromegaly eventually causes cardiovascular and respiratory diseases that shorten life expectancy.

Giantism

Giantism results from an oversecretion of somatotropin before puberty (figure 7-66). It causes excessive growth of long bones, extreme tallness, decreased sexual development, and at times, retarded mental development. If a tumor of the pituitary is the cause, surgical removal or radiation is the treatment.

Diabetes Insipidus

Diabetes insipidus is caused by decreased secretion of vasopressin, or antidiuretic hormone (ADH). A low level of ADH prevents water from being reabsorbed in the kidneys. Symptoms

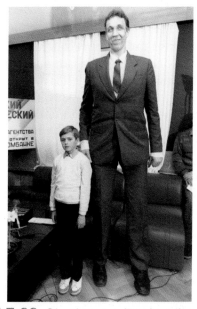

FIGURE 7-66 Giantism results when the pituitary gland secretes excessive amounts of somatotropin (growth hormone) before puberty.

include polyuria (excessive urination), polydipsia (excessive thirst), dehydration, weakness, constipation, and dry skin. The condition is corrected by administering ADH.

Dwarfism

Dwarfism results from an undersecretion of somatotropin and can be caused by a tumor, infection, genetic factors, or injury (figure 7-67). It is characterized by small body size, short extremities, and lack of sexual development. Mental development is usually normal. If the condition is diagnosed early, it can be treated with injections of somatotropic hormone for 5 or more years until long bone growth is complete.

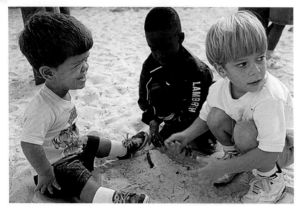

FIGURE 7-67 Dwarfism results from an undersecretion of somatotropin (growth hormone).

THYROID GLAND

The **thyroid gland** synthesizes hormones that regulate the body's metabolism and control the level of calcium in the blood. It is located in front of the upper part of the trachea (windpipe) in the neck. It has two lobes, one on either side of the larynx (voice box), connected by the isthmus, a small piece of tissue. To produce its hormones, the thyroid gland requires iodine, which is obtained from certain foods and iodized salt. The hormones secreted by the thyroid gland are shown in table 7-3.

Diseases and Abnormal Conditions

Goiter
A goiter is an enlargement of the thyroid gland. Causes can include a hyperactive thyroid, an iodine deficiency, an oversecretion of thyroid-stimulating hormone on the part of the pituitary gland, or a tumor. Symptoms include thyroid enlargement, dysphagia (difficult swallowing), a cough, and a choking sensation. Treatment is directed toward eliminating the cause. For example, iodine is given if a deficiency exists. Surgery may be performed to remove very large goiters.

Hyperthyroidism
Hyperthyroidism is an overactivity of the thyroid gland, which causes increased production of thyroid hormones and increased basal metabolic rate (BMR). Symptoms include extreme nervousness, tremors, irritability, rapid pulse, diarrhea, diaphoresis (excessive perspiration), heat intolerance, polydipsia (excessive thirst), goiter formation, and hypertension. An excessive appetite with extreme weight loss is a classic symptom. Treatment consists of either radiation to destroy part of the thyroid or a thyroidectomy (surgical removal of the thyroid). If the thyroid is removed, thyroid hormones are given for the lifetime of the individual.

Graves' Disease
Graves' disease is a severe form of hyperthyroidism more common in women than men. Symptoms include a strained and tense facial expression, exophthalmia (protruding eyeballs), goiter, nervous irritability, emotional instability, tachycardia, a tremendous appetite accompanied by weight loss, and diarrhea. Treatment methods include medication to inhibit the synthesis of thyroxine, radioactive iodine to destroy thyroid tissue, and/or a thyroidectomy.

Hypothyroidism
Hypothyroidism is an underactivity of the thyroid gland and a deficiency of thyroid hormones. Two main forms exist: *cretinism* and *myxedema.* Cretinism develops in infancy or early childhood and results in a lack of mental and physical growth, leading to mental retardation and an abnormal, dwarfed stature. If diagnosed early, oral thyroid hormone can be given to minimize mental and physical damage. Myxedema occurs in later childhood or adulthood. Symptoms include coarse, dry skin; slow mental function; fatigue; weakness; intolerance of cold; weight gain; edema; puffy eyes; and a slow pulse. Treatment consists of administering oral thyroid hormone to restore normal metabolism. In some countries where iodized salt is not available, myxedema may be caused by an iodine deficiency. Adding iodine to the diet corrects this type of myxedema.

PARATHYROID GLANDS

The **parathyroid glands** are four small glands located behind and attached to the thyroid gland. Their hormone, parathormone, regulates the amount of calcium in the blood (see table 7-3). It stimulates bone cells to break down bone tissue and release calcium and phosphates into the blood, causes the kidneys to conserve and reabsorb calcium, and activates intestinal cells to absorb calcium from digested foods. Although most of the body's calcium is in the bones, the calcium circulating in the blood is important for blood clotting, the tone of heart muscle, and muscle contraction. Because there is a constant exchange of calcium and phosphate between the bones and blood, the parathyroid hormone plays an important function in maintaining the proper level of circulating calcium.

Diseases and Abnormal Conditions

Hyperparathyroidism

Hyperparathyroidism is an overactivity of the parathyroid gland resulting in an overproduction of parathormone. This results in hypercalcemia (increased calcium in the blood), which leads to renal calculi (kidney stones) formation, lethargy, gastrointestinal disturbances, and calcium deposits on the walls of blood vessels and organs. Because the calcium is drawn from the bones, they become weak, deformed, and likely to fracture. This condition is often caused by an adenoma (glandular tumor), and removal of the tumor usually results in normal parathyroid function. Other treatments include surgical removal of the parathyroids followed by administration of parathormone, diuretics to increase the excretion of water and calcium, and a low-calcium diet.

Hypoparathyroidism

Hypoparathyroidism is an underactivity of the parathyroid gland, which causes a low level of calcium in the blood. Causes include the surgical removal of or injury to the parathyroid and/or thyroid glands. Symptoms include tetany (a sustained muscular contraction), hyperirritability of the nervous system, and convulsive twitching. Death can occur if the larynx and respiratory muscles are involved. The condition is easily treated with calcium, vitamin D (which increases the absorption of calcium from the digestive tract), and parathormone.

ADRENAL GLANDS

The **adrenal glands** are frequently called the *suprarenal* glands because one is located above each kidney. Each gland has two parts: the outer portion, or cortex, and the inner portion, or medulla. The adrenal cortex secretes many steroid hormones, which are classified into three groups: mineralocorticoids, glucocorticoids, and gonadocorticoids. The groups and the main hormones in each group are listed in table 7-3. The adrenal medulla secretes two main hormones: epinephrine and norepinephrine. These hormones are sympathomimetic; that is, they mimic the sympathetic nervous system and cause the fight or flight response.

Diseases and Abnormal Conditions

Addison's Disease

Addison's disease is caused by decreased secretion of aldosterone on the part of the adrenal cortex. This interferes with the reabsorption of sodium and water and causes an increased level of potassium in the blood. Symptoms include dehydration, diarrhea, fatigue, hypotension (low blood pressure), mental lethargy, weight loss, muscle weakness, excessive pigmentation leading to a "bronzing" (yellow-brown color) of the skin, hypoglycemia (low blood sugar), and edema. Treatment methods include administering corticosteroid hormones, controlled intake of sodium, and fluid regulation to combat dehydration.

Cushing's Syndrome

Cushing's syndrome results from an oversecretion of glucocorticoids on the part of the adrenal cortex. It can be caused by either a tumor of the adrenal cortex or excess production of ACTH on the part of the pituitary gland. Symptoms include hyperglycemia (high blood sugar), hypertension, muscle weakness, fatigue, hirsutism (excessive growth and/or an abnormal distribution of hair), poor wound healing, a tendency to bruise easily, a "moon" face, and obesity (figure 7-68). If a tumor is causing the disease, treatment is removal of the tumor. If the glands are removed, hormonal therapy is required to replace the missing hormones. Cushing's syndrome can also occur in patients receiving long-term steroid therapy such as prednisone. These patients must be monitored closely, and steroid therapy must be reduced gradually if symptoms of Cushing's syndrome develop.

PANCREAS

The **pancreas** is a fish-shaped organ located behind the stomach. It is both an exocrine gland and an endocrine gland. As an exocrine gland, it

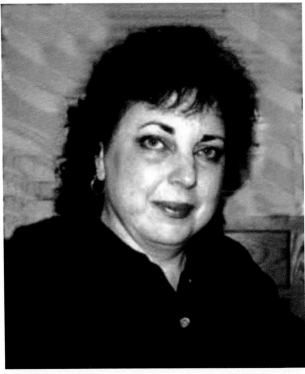 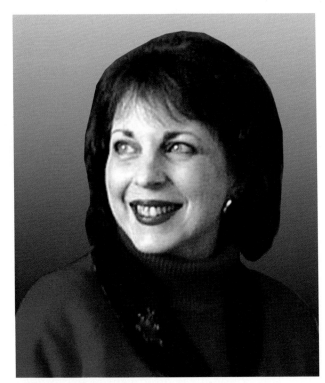

FIGURE 7-68 Cushing's syndrome. (A) The classic "moon face" of Cushing's syndrome. (B) The same individual after treatment. *(Courtesy of Ruth Jones)*

secretes pancreatic juices, which are carried to the small intestine by the pancreatic duct to aid in the digestion of food. Special B, or beta, cells located throughout the pancreas in patches of tissue called *islets of Langerhans* produce the hormone insulin, which is needed for the cells to absorb sugar from the blood. Insulin also promotes the transport of fatty acids and amino acids (proteins) into the cells. Alpha, or A, cells produce the hormone glucagon, which increases the glucose level in blood (see table 7-3).

Disease

Diabetes Mellitus

Diabetes mellitus is a chronic disease caused by decreased secretion of insulin. The metabolism of carbohydrates, proteins, and fats is affected. There are two main types of diabetes mellitus, named according to the age of onset and need for insulin. Insulin-dependent diabetes mellitus (IDDM), or Type 1, usually occurs early in life, is more severe, and requires insulin. Noninsulin-dependent diabetes mellitus (NIDDM), or Type 2, is the mature-onset form of diabetes mellitus. It frequently occurs in obese adults and is usually controlled with diet and/or oral hypoglycemic (lower-blood-sugar) medications. The main symptoms include hyperglycemia (high blood sugar), polyuria (excessive urination), polydipsia (excessive thirst), polyphagia (excessive hunger), glycosuria (sugar in the urine), weight loss, fatigue, slow healing of skin infections, and vision changes. If the condition is not treated, diabetic coma and death may occur. Treatment methods are a carefully regulated diet to control the blood sugar level, regulated exercise, and oral hypoglycemic drugs or insulin injections. Newer medications that increase insulin production, increase the sensitivity to insulin, or slow the absorption of glucose into cells are also available. External and implantable insulin pumps that monitor blood glucose levels and deliver the required amount of insulin can be used to replace insulin injections. A new form of therapy is an inhaled form of insulin. However, this is expensive and has not been approved for use in children.

Estimates indicate that more than 16 million Americans have diabetes, and as many as 40–50 percent might not know they have the disease. Researchers have proved that weight control (avoiding obesity) and moderate exercise can reduce the risk for development of diabetes by as much as 55–70 percent. Preventing diabetes is important because diabetes can cause atherosclerosis, myocardial infarctions (heart attacks), cerebrovascular accidents (strokes), peripheral vascular disease leading to poor wound healing and gangrene in the legs and feet, diabetic retinopathy causing blindness, and kidney disease or failure.

OTHER ENDOCRINE GLANDS

The **ovaries** are the gonads, or sex glands, of the female. They are located in the pelvic cavity, one on each side of the uterus. They secrete hormones that regulate menstruation and secondary sexual characteristics (see table 7-3).

The **testes** are the gonads of the male. They are located in the scrotal sac and are suspended outside the body. They produce hormones that regulate sexual characteristics of the male (see table 7-3).

7:14 Reproductive System

Objectives

After completing this section, you should be able to:

♦ Label a diagram of the male reproductive system

♦ Trace the pathway of sperm from where they are produced to where they are expelled from the body

The **thymus** is a mass of tissue located in the upper part of the chest and under the sternum. It contains lymphoid tissue. The thymus is active in early life, activating cells in the immune system, but atrophies (wastes away) during puberty, when it becomes a small mass of connective tissue and fat. It produces one hormone, thymosin (see table 7-3).

The **pineal body** is a small structure attached to the roof of the third ventricle in the brain. Knowledge regarding the physiology of this gland is limited. Three main hormones secreted by this gland are listed in table 7-3.

The **placenta** is a temporary endocrine gland produced during pregnancy. It acts as a link between the mother and infant, provides nutrition for the developing infant, and promotes lactation (the production of milk in the breasts). It is expelled after the birth of the child (when it is called *afterbirth*). Three hormones secreted by this gland are listed in table 7-3.

STUDENT: *Go to the workbook and complete the assignment sheet for 7:13, Endocrine System.*

♦ Identify at least three organs of the male reproductive system that secrete fluids added to semen

♦ Label a diagram of the female reproductive system

♦ Describe how an ovum is released from an ovary

♦ Explain the action of the endometrium

♦ Describe at least six diseases of the reproductive systems

♦ Define, pronounce, and spell all key terms

KEY TERMS

Bartholin's glands *(Bar'-tha-lens)*
breasts
Cowper's (bulbourethral) glands *(Cow'-purrs)*
ejaculatory ducts *(ee-jack'-you-lah-tore"-ee)*
endometrium *(en"-doe-me'-tree-um)*

epididymis *(eh"-pih-did'-ih-muss)*
fallopian tubes *(fah-low'-pea"-an)*
fertilization *(fur"-til-ih-zay'-shun)*
labia majora *(lay'-bee"-ah mah"-jore'-ah)*

labia minora *(lay'-bee"-ah ma-nore'-ah)*
ovaries
penis
perineum *(pear"-ih-knee'-um)*
prostate gland
reproductive system
scrotum *(skrow'-tum)*

KEY TERMS

seminal vesicles *(sem'-ih-null ves'-ik-ullz)*
testes *(tes'-tees)*
urethra

uterus
vagina *(vah-jie'-nah)*
vas (ductus) deferens *(vass deaf'-eh-rens)*

vestibule
vulva *(vull'-vah)*

RELATED HEALTH CAREERS

- ◆ Embryologist
- ◆ Genetic Counselor
- ◆ Geneticist

- ◆ Gynecologist
- ◆ Midwife
- ◆ Obstetrician

- ◆ Ultrasound Technologist (Sonographer)

7:14 INFORMATION

The function of the **reproductive system** is to produce new life. Although the anatomic parts differ in male and female individuals, the reproductive systems of both have the same types of organs: gonads (sex glands); ducts (tubes) to carry the sex cells and secretions; and accessory organs.

MALE REPRODUCTIVE SYSTEM

The male reproductive system consists of the testes, epididymis, vas deferens, seminal vesicles, ejaculatory ducts, urethra, prostate gland, Cowper's glands, and penis (figure 7-69).

The male gonads are the **testes.** The two testes are located in the **scrotum,** a sac suspended between the thighs. The testes produce the male sex cells called *sperm,* or *spermatozoa,* in seminiferous tubules located within each testis. Because the scrotum is located outside the body, the temperature in the scrotum is lower than that inside the body. This lower temperature is essential for the production of sperm. The testes also produce male hormones. The main hormone is testosterone, which aids in the maturation of the sperm and also is responsible for the secondary male sex characteristics such as body hair, facial hair, large muscles, and a deep voice.

After the sperm develop in the seminiferous tubules in the testes, they enter the **epididymis.** The epididymis is a tightly coiled tube approximately 20 feet in length and located in the scrotum and above the testes. It stores the sperm while they mature and become motile (able to move by themselves). It also produces a fluid that becomes part of the semen (fluid released during ejaculation). The epididymis connects with the next tube, the vas deferens.

The **vas (ductus) deferens** receives the sperm and fluid from the epididymis. On each side, a vas deferens joins with the epididymis and extends up into the abdominal cavity, where it curves behind the urinary bladder and joins with a seminal vesicle. Each vas deferens acts as both a passageway and a temporary storage area for sperm. The vas deferens are also the tubes that are cut during a *vasectomy* (procedure to produce sterility in the male).

The **seminal vesicles** are two small pouch-like tubes located behind the bladder and near the junction of the vas deferens and the ejaculatory ducts. They contain a glandular lining. This lining produces a thick, yellow fluid that is rich in sugar and other substances and provides nourishment for the sperm. This fluid composes a large part of the semen.

The **ejaculatory ducts** are two short tubes formed by the union of the vas deferens and the seminal vesicles. They carry the sperm and fluids known collectively as *semen* through the prostate gland and into the urethra.

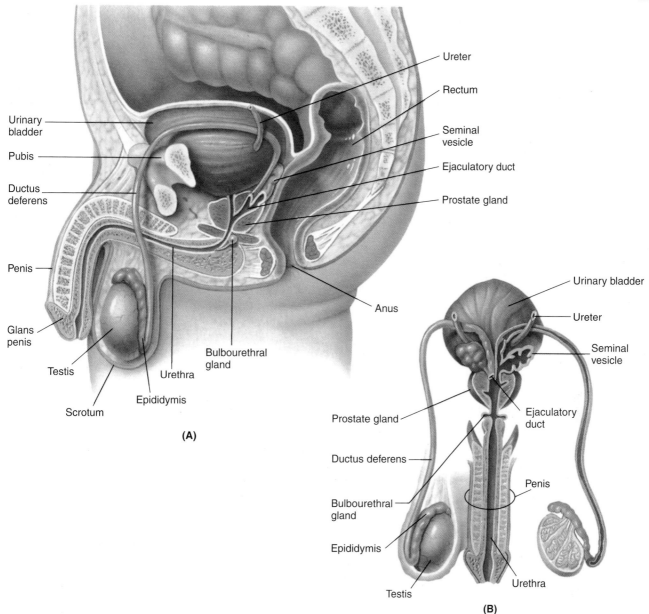

Urinary bladder

Pubis

Ductus deferens

Penis

Glans penis

Testis

Scrotum

Epididymis

Urethra

Bulbourethral gland

Ureter

Rectum

Seminal vesicle

Ejaculatory duct

Prostate gland

Anus

(A)

Urinary bladder

Ureter

Seminal vesicle

Ejaculatory duct

Prostate gland

Ductus deferens

Bulbourethral gland

Epididymis

Testis

Penis

Urethra

(B)

FIGURE 7-69 The male reproductive system. (A) Lateral view. (B) Anterior view.

The **prostate gland** is a doughnut-shaped gland located below the urinary bladder and on either side of the urethra. It produces an alkaline secretion that both increases sperm motility and neutralizes the acidity in the vagina, providing a more favorable environment for the sperm. The muscular tissue in the prostate contracts during ejaculation (expulsion of the semen from the body) to aid in the expulsion of the semen into the urethra. When the prostate contracts, it also closes off the urethra, preventing urine passage through the urethra.

Cowper's (bulbourethral) glands are two small glands located below the prostate and con-

nected by small tubes to the urethra. They secrete mucus, which serves as a lubricant for intercourse, and an alkaline fluid, which decreases the acidity of the urine residue in the urethra, providing a more favorable environment for the sperm.

The **urethra** is the tube that extends from the urinary bladder, through the penis, and to the outside of the body. It carries urine from the urinary bladder and semen from the reproductive tubes.

The **penis** is the external male reproductive organ and is located in front of the scrotum. At the distal end is an enlarged structure, called the *glans penis.* The glans penis is covered with a prepuce (foreskin), which is sometimes removed surgically in a procedure called *circumcision.* The penis is made of spongy, erectile tissue. During sexual arousal, the spaces in this tissue fill with blood, causing the penis to become erect. The penis functions as the male organ of copulation, or intercourse; deposits the semen in the vagina; and provides for the elimination of urine from the bladder through the urethra.

Diseases and Abnormal Conditions

Epididymitis

Epididymitis is an inflammation of the epididymis, usually caused by a pathogenic organism such as gonococcus, streptococcus, or staphylococcus. It frequently occurs with a urinary tract or prostate infection, mumps, or sexually transmitted diseases (STDs). If epididymitis is not treated promptly, it can cause scarring and sterility. Symptoms include intense pain in the testes, swelling, and fever. Treatment methods include antibiotics, cold applications, scrotal support, and pain medication.

Orchitis

Orchitis is an inflammation of the testes, usually caused by mumps, pathogens, or injury. It can lead to atrophy of the testes and cause sterility. Symptoms include swelling of the scrotum, pain, and fever. Treatment methods include antibiotics (if indicated), antipyretics (for fever), scrotal support, and pain medication. Prevention methods include mumps vaccinations and observing measures to prevent sexually transmitted diseases (STDs).

Prostatic Hypertrophy and Cancer

Prostatic hypertrophy, or hyperplasia, is an enlargement of the prostate gland. Common in men over age 50, prostatic hypertrophy can be a benign condition, caused by inflammation, a tumor, or a change in hormonal activity, or a malignant (cancerous) condition. Symptoms of prostatic hypertrophy include difficulty in starting to urinate, frequent urination, nocturia (voiding at night), dribbling, urinary infections, and when the urethra is blocked, urinary retention. Initial treatment methods include fluid restriction, antibiotics (for infections), and prostatic massage. When hypertrophy causes urinary retention, a prostatectomy (surgical removal of all or part of the prostate) is necessary. A transurethral resection (TUR), or removal of part of the prostate, is performed by inserting a scope into the urethra and resecting, or removing, the enlarged area. A prostatectomy can also be done by a perineal, or suprapubic (above the pubis bone), incision. Prostatic carcinoma (cancer) can have the same symptoms as prostatic hypertrophy or it may not have any symptoms. A screening blood test, called a *prostatic-specific antigen (PSA) test,* can detect a substance released by cancer cells and aid in an early diagnosis. A digital rectal examination may show a hard, abnormal mass in the prostate gland. A tissue biopsy of the prostate is usually performed to diagnose cancer.

If the condition is malignant, prostatectomy, radiation, and estrogen therapy (to decrease the effects of testosterone) are the main treatments. In some cases, an orchiectomy, surgical removal of the testes, is performed to stop the production of testosterone. Radioactive seeds can also be implanted in the prostate to destroy the cancerous cells without affecting the organs and tissue surrounding the prostate. If prostate cancer is detected early, the prognosis (expected outcome) is good. All men older than 50 years are encouraged to have annual prostate examinations.

Testicular Cancer

Testicular cancer, or cancer of the testes, occurs most frequently in men from ages 20 to 35. It is a highly malignant form of cancer and can metastasize, or spread, rapidly. Symptoms include a painless swelling of the testes, a heavy feeling, and an accumulation of fluid. Treatment includes an *orchiectomy,* or surgical removal of the testis, chemotherapy, and/or radiation. It has been recommended that male individuals begin monthly testicular self-examinations at the age of 15. To perform the examination, the male individuals should examine the testicles after a warm shower when scrotal skin is relaxed. Each testicle should be examined separately with both hands by placing the index and middle fingers under the testicle and the thumbs on top. The testicle should be rolled gently between the fingers to feel for lumps, nodules, or extreme tenderness. In addition, the male should examine the testes for any signs of swelling or changes in appearance. If any abnormalities are noted, the male should be examined by a physician as soon as possible.

FEMALE REPRODUCTIVE SYSTEM

The female reproductive system consists of the ovaries, fallopian tubes, uterus, vagina, Bartholin's glands, vulva, and breasts (figure 7-70).

The **ovaries** are the female gonads (figure 7-71). They are small, almond-shaped glands located in the pelvic cavity and attached to the uterus by ligaments. The ovaries contain thousands of small sacs called *follicles.* Each follicle contains an immature ovum, or female sex cell. When an ovum matures, the follicle enlarges and then ruptures to release the mature ovum. This process, called *ovulation,* usually occurs once every 28 days. The ovaries also produce hormones that aid in the development of the reproductive organs and produce secondary sexual characteristics.

The **fallopian tubes** are two tubes, each approximately 5 inches in length and attached to the upper part of the uterus. The lateral ends of these tubes are located above the ovaries but are not directly connected to the ovaries. These ends have fingerlike projections, called *fimbriae.* The fimbriae help move the ovum, which is released by the ovary, into the fallopian tube. Each fallopian tube serves as a passageway for the ovum as the ovum moves from the ovary to the uterus. The muscle layers of the tube move the ovum by peristalsis. Cilia, hairlike structures on the lining of the tubes, also keep the ovum moving toward the uterus. **Fertilization,** the union of the ovum and a sperm to create a new life, usually takes place in the fallopian tubes.

The **uterus** is a hollow, muscular, pear-shaped organ located behind the urinary bladder and in front of the rectum. It is divided into three parts: the *fundus* (the top section, where the fallopian tubes attach); the body, or *corpus* (the middle section); and the *cervix* (the narrow, bottom section, which attaches to the vagina). The uterus is the organ of menstruation, allows for the development and growth of the fetus, and contracts to aid in expulsion of the fetus during birth. The uterus has three layers. The inner layer is called the **endometrium.** This layer of specialized epithelium provides for implantation of a fertilized ovum and aids in the development of

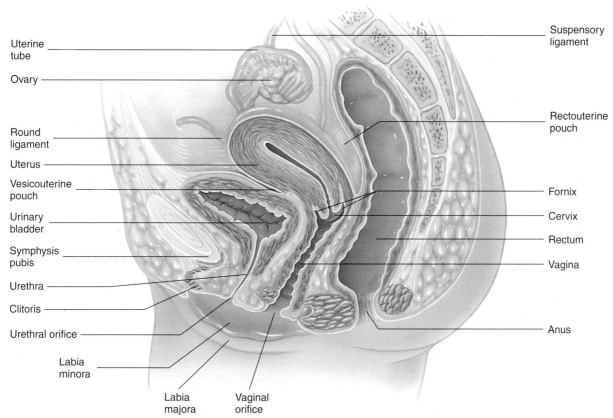

FIGURE 7-70 The female reproductive system.

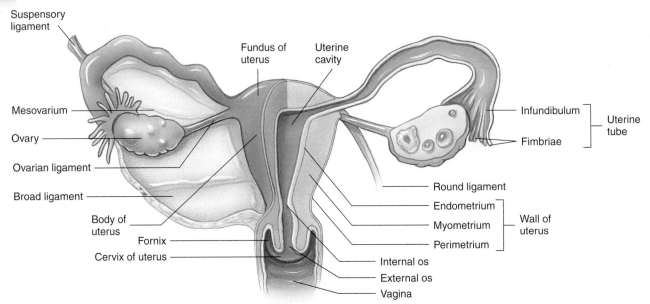

FIGURE 7-71 Anterior view of the female reproductive system.

the fetus. If fertilization does not occur, the endometrium deteriorates and causes the bleeding known as *menstruation.* The middle layer of the uterus, the *myometrium,* is a muscle layer. It allows for the expansion of the uterus during pregnancy and contracts to expel the fetus during birth. The outer layer, the *perimetrium,* is a serous membrane.

The **vagina** is a muscular tube that connects the cervix of the uterus to the outside of the body. It serves as a passageway for the menstrual flow, receives the sperm and semen from the male, is the female organ of copulation, and acts as the birth canal during delivery of the infant. The vagina is lined with a mucous membrane arranged in folds called *rugae.* The rugae allow the vagina to enlarge during childbirth and intercourse.

Bartholin's glands, also called *vestibular glands,* are two small glands located one on each side of the vaginal opening. They secrete mucus for lubrication during intercourse.

The **vulva** is the collective name for the structures that form the external female genital area (figure 7-72). The *mons veneris,* or mons pubis, is the triangular pad of fat that is covered with hair and lies over the pubic area. The **labia majora** are the two large folds of fatty tissue that are covered with hair on their outer surfaces; they enclose and protect the vagina. The **labia minora** are the two smaller hairless folds of tissue that are located within the labia majora. The area of the vulva located inside the labia minora is called the **vestibule.** It contains the openings

to the urethra and the vagina. An area of erectile tissue, called the *clitoris,* is located at the junction of the labia minora. It produces sexual arousal when stimulated directly or indirectly during intercourse. The **perineum** is defined as the area between the vagina and anus in the female body, although it can be used to describe the entire pelvic floor in both the male and female individual.

The **breasts,** or mammary glands, contain lobes separated into sections by connective and fatty tissue. Milk ducts located in the tissue exit on the surface at the nipples. The main function of the glands is to secrete milk (lactate) after childbirth.

Diseases and Abnormal Conditions

Breast Tumors

Breast tumors can be benign or malignant. Symptoms include a lump or mass in the breast tissue, a change in breast size or shape (flattening or bulging of tissue), and a discharge from the nipple. Breast self-examination (BSE) can often detect tumors early (figure 7-73). The American Cancer Society recommends that an adult woman should do a BSE every month at the end of menstruation, or on a scheduled day of the month after menopause. The breasts should be examined in front of a mirror to observe for changes in appearance, in a warm shower after soaping the

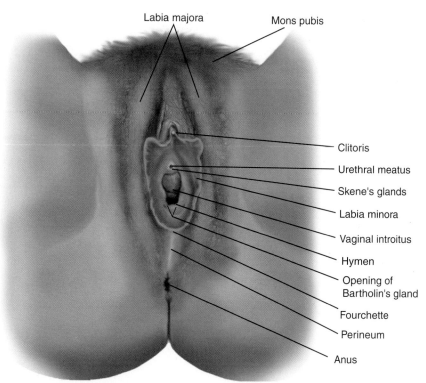

Labia majora

Mons pubis

Clitoris

Urethral meatus

Skene's glands

Labia minora

Vaginal introitus

Hymen

Opening of
Bartholin's gland

Fourchette

Perineum

Anus

FIGURE 7-72 The external female genital area.

breasts, and while lying flat in a supine position. A physician should be contacted immediately if any abnormalities are found. In addition, the American Cancer Society recommends that women between the ages of 35 and 40 years should have a baseline mammogram. Between ages 40 and 49, women should have a mammogram every 1–2 years, and after age 50, women should have a mammogram every year. Mammograms and ultrasonography can often detect tumors or masses up to 2 years before the tumor or mass could be felt. Treatment methods for breast tumors include a lumpectomy (removal of the tumor), a simple mastectomy (surgical removal of the breast), or a radical mastectomy (surgical removal of the tissue, underlying muscles, and axillary lymph nodes). If the tumor is malignant, chemotherapy and/or radiation are usually used in addition to surgery.

Cervical or Uterine Cancer

Cancer of the cervix and/or uterus is common in women. Cervical cancer can be detected early by a Pap smear. Symptoms of cervical cancer include abnormal vaginal discharge and bleeding. Symptoms of uterine cancer include an enlarged uterus, a watery discharge, and abnormal bleeding. Treatment methods include a hysterectomy (surgical removal of the uterus and cervix) or

panhysterectomy (surgical removal of the uterus, ovaries, and fallopian tubes); chemotherapy; and/or radiation.

Endometriosis

Endometriosis is the abnormal growth of endometrial tissue outside the uterus. The tissue can be transferred from the uterus by the fallopian tubes, blood, or lymph, or during surgery. It usually becomes embedded in a structure in the pelvic area, such as the ovaries or the peritoneal tissues, and constantly grows and sheds. Endometriosis can cause sterility if the fallopian tubes become blocked with scar tissue. Symptoms include pelvic pain, abnormal bleeding, and dysmenorrhea (painful menstruation). Treatment methods vary with the age of the patient and the degree of abnormal growth but can include hormonal therapy, pain medications, and/or surgical removal of affected organs.

Ovarian Cancer

Ovarian cancer is one of the most common causes of cancer deaths in women. It frequently occurs between ages 40 and 65. Initial symptoms are vague and include abdominal discomfort and mild gastrointestinal disturbances such as constipation and/or diarrhea. As the disease progresses, pain, abdominal distention, and urinary

HOW TO DO BSE

1. Lie down and put a pillow under your right shoulder. Place your right arm behind your head.
2. Use the finger pads of the three middle fingers on your left hand to feel for lumps or thickening. Your finger pads are the top third of each finger.

4. Move around the breast in a set way. You can choose either the circle (A), the up and down (B), or the wedge (C). Do it the same way every time. It will help you to make sure that you've gone over the entire breast area and to remember how your breast feels each month.

5. Now, examine your left breast using right hand finger pads.
   You might want to check your breasts while standing in front of a mirror right after you do your BSE each month. You might also want to do an extra BSE while you're in the shower. Your soapy hands will glide over the wet skin making it easy to check how your breasts feel.

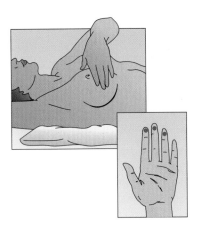

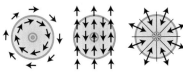

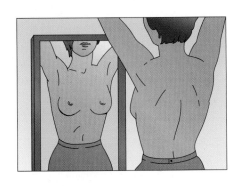

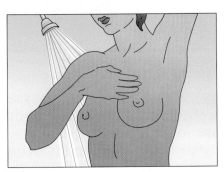

3. Press hard enough to know how your breast feels. If you are not sure how hard to press, ask your health care provider. Or try to copy the way your health care provider uses the finger pads during a breast exam. Learn what your breast feels like most of the time. A firm ridge in the lower curve of each breast is normal.

FIGURE 7-73 Breast self-examination (BSE) can often detect tumors early. *(Reprinted by the permission of the American Cancer Society, Inc. All rights reserved.)*

frequency occur. Treatment includes surgical removal of all of the reproductive organs and affected lymph nodes, chemotherapy, and radiation in some cases.

Pelvic Inflammatory Disease

Pelvic inflammatory disease (PID) is an inflammation of the cervix (cervicitis) the endometrium of the uterus (endometritis), fallopian tubes (salpingitis), and at times, the ovaries (oophoritis). It is usually caused by pathogenic organisms such as bacteria, viruses, and fungi. Symptoms include pain in the lower abdomen, fever, and a purulent (pus) vaginal discharge. Treatment methods include antibiotics, increased fluid intake, rest, and/or pain medication.

Premenstrual Syndrome

Premenstrual syndrome (PMS) is actually a group of symptoms that appear 3–14 days before menstruation. A large percentage of women experi-

ence some degree of PMS. The cause is unknown but may be related to a hormonal or biochemical imbalance, poor nutrition, or stress. Symptoms vary and may include nervousness, irritability, depression, headache, edema, backache, constipation, abdominal bloating, temporary weight gain, and breast tenderness and enlargement. Treatment is geared mainly toward relieving symptoms, and methods include diet modification, exercise, stress reduction, diuretics to remove excess fluids, analgesics for pain, and/or medications to relieve the emotional symptoms.

SEXUALLY TRANSMITTED DISEASES

Sexually transmitted diseases (STDs), or *sexually transmitted infections (STIs)*, affect both men and women. The incidence of these diseases has increased greatly in recent years, especially among young people. If not treated, STDs can cause serious chronic conditions and, in some cases, sterility or death.

Acquired Immune Deficiency Syndrome

Acquired immune deficiency syndrome (AIDS) is caused by a virus called the *human immunodeficiency virus (HIV)*. This virus attacks the body's immune system, rendering the immune system unable to fight off certain infections and diseases, and eventually causing death. The virus is spread through sexual secretions or blood, and from an infected mother to her infant during pregnancy or childbirth.

The HIV virus does not live long outside the body and is not transmitted by casual, nonsexual contact. Individuals infected with HIV can remain free of any symptoms for years after infection. During this asymptomatic period, infected individuals can transmit the virus to any other individual with whom they exchange sexual secretions, blood, or blood products. After this initial asymptomatic period, many individuals develop HIV symptomatic infection, formerly called AIDS-related complex (ARC). Symptoms include a positive blood test for antibodies to the HIV virus, lack of infection resistance, appetite loss, weight loss, recurrent fever, night sweats, skin rashes, diarrhea, fatigue, and swollen lymph nodes. When the HIV virus causes a critical low level (below 200 cells per cubic millimeter of blood) of special leukocytes (white blood cells) called CD4 or T cells, and/or opportunistic diseases appear, AIDS is diagnosed. Three of the most common opportunistic diseases include the rare type of pneumonia called *Pneumocystis carinii,* a yeast infection called *Candidiasis,* and the slow-growing cancer called *Kaposi's sarcoma* (figure 7-74).

Currently, there is no cure for AIDS, although much research is being directed toward developing a vaccine to prevent and drugs to cure AIDS. Treatment with a combination of drugs, commonly called a *drug cocktail,* is used to slow the progression of the disease. These drugs, however, do not cure the disease. Although several experimental drugs are currently being tested, many patients cannot tolerate the side effects and bone marrow toxicity of these drugs. Prevention is the best method in dealing with AIDS. Standard pre-

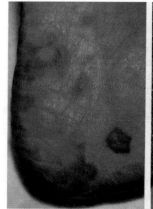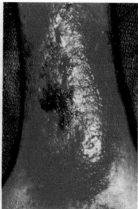

FIGURE 7-74 A common opportunistic disease that occurs in AIDS patients is Kaposi's sarcoma. *(Courtesy of the Centers for Disease Control and Prevention, Atlanta, GA)*

cautions should be followed while handling blood, body secretions, and sexual secretions. High-risk sexual activities, such as having multiple partners, should be avoided. A condom and an effective spermicide should be used to form a protective barrier during intercourse. The use of drugs and sharing of intravenous (IV) needles should be avoided. Females infected with HIV should avoid pregnancy. *Everyone* must concern themselves with eliminating the transmission of AIDS.

Chlamydia

Chlamydia (klah-mid-e-ah) is one of the most frequently occurring STDs and is caused by several strains of the chlamydia organism, a specialized bacterium that lives as an intracellular parasite. Symptoms are similar to those of gonorrhea. Male individuals experience burning when urinating and a mucoid discharge. Female individuals are frequently asymptomatic, although some may have a vaginal discharge. The disease frequently causes pelvic inflammatory disease and sterility in women, if not treated. Chlamydia can be treated with tetracycline or erythromycin antibiotics.

Gonorrhea

Gonorrhea (gon-oh-re-ah) is caused by the gonococcus bacterium *neisseria gonorrhoeae.* Symptoms in male individuals include a greenish-yellow discharge, burning when urinating, sore throat, and swollen glands. Female individuals are frequently asymptomatic but may experience

TODAY'S RESEARCH: TOMORROW'S HEALTH CARE

Body organs that are grown in the laboratory?

Organ transplants have become a common type of surgery. Hearts, lungs, livers, kidneys, and many other organs are transplanted daily to save lives. The big problem is the major shortage of organs to transplant. Today, almost 100,000 Americans are on the national waiting list for an organ. Statistics show that almost 20 percent, or 1 in every 5 patients, will die before they can receive an organ.

Researchers are trying to grow human organs by using a patient's own cells. Already, researchers in Boston have created a urinary bladder that functions in dogs. They molded a biodegradable material (substance that will dissolve inside the body) in the shape of a bladder. They then coated the outside of the structure with layers of muscle cells and the inside with layers of urothelial cells obtained from a dog's bladder. After the cells grew and multiplied, the dog's own bladder was removed, and the new artificial organ was transplanted. Within a month, the organ performed like a normal urinary bladder, storing urine until it was expelled to the outside. The chance of the dog rejecting the new organ was also slim because the cells that produced it were the dog's own cells.

Israeli scientists are using stem cells to grow human kidneys. Stem cells are obtained from a developing fetus. These cells are capable of transforming themselves into any of the body's specialized cells. The scientists transplanted the stem cells into mice and grew human kidneys in the mice. The kidneys filtered the blood and produced urine. Scientists hope that the chance of rejection is decreased because the stem cells are immature and less likely to carry characteristics of a specific individual. Many more trials are needed before these laboratory produced "organs" will be used in humans. However, the future for individuals needing transplants will be much better when scientists can "grow" the organs the individuals need.

dysuria, pain in the lower abdomen, and greenish-yellow vaginal discharge. An infected woman can transmit the gonococcus organism to her infant's eyes during childbirth, causing blindness. To prevent this, a drop of silver nitrate or antibiotic is routinely placed in the eyes of newborn babies. Gonorrhea is treated with large doses of antibiotics.

Herpes

Herpes is a viral disease caused by the herpes simplex virus type II. Symptoms include a burning sensation, fluid-filled vesicles (blister-like sores) that rupture and form painful ulcers, and painful urination. After the sores heal, the virus becomes dormant. Many people have repeated attacks, but the attacks are milder. There is no cure, and treatment is directed toward promoting healing and easing discomfort. Antiviral medications are used to decrease the number and severity of recurrences.

Pubic Lice

Pubic lice are parasites that are usually transmitted sexually, although they can be spread by contact with clothing, bed linen, or other items containing the lice. Symptoms include an intense itching and redness of the perineal area. Medications that kill the lice are used as treatment. To prevent a recurrence, it is essential to wash all clothing and bed linen to destroy any lice or nits (eggs).

Syphilis

Syphilis is caused by a spirochete bacterium. The symptoms occur in stages. During the primary stage, a painless chancre (shang-ker), or sore, appears, usually on the penis of the male and in the vulva or on the cervix of the female. This chancre heals within several weeks. During the second stage, which occurs if the chancre is not treated, the organism enters the bloodstream and causes a rash that does not itch, a sore throat, a fever, and swollen glands. These symptoms also disappear within several weeks. The third stage occurs years later after the spirochete has damaged vital organs. Damage to the heart and blood vessels causes cardiovascular disease; damage to the spinal cord causes a characteristic gait and paralysis; and brain damage causes mental disorders, deafness, and blindness. At this stage, damage is irreversible, and death occurs. Early diagnosis and treatment with antibiotics can cure syphilis during the first two stages.

Trichomoniasis

Trichomoniasis is caused by a parasitic protozoan, *Trichomonas vaginalis.* The main symptom is a large amount of a frothy, yellow-green, foul-smelling discharge. Men are frequently asymptomatic but may experience urethral itching. The antiparasitic oral medication Flagyl is used to treat this disease. Both sexual partners must be treated to prevent reinfection.

STUDENT: *Go to the workbook and complete the assignment sheet for 7:14, Reproductive System.*

CHAPTER 7 SUMMARY

A health care worker must understand normal functioning of the human body to understand disease processes. A study of anatomy, the form and structure of an organism, and physiology, the processes of living organisms, adds to this understanding.

The basic structural unit of the human body is the cell. Cells join together to form tissues. Tissues join together to form organs, which work together to form body systems.

Systems work together to provide for proper functioning of the human body. The integumentary system, or skin, provides a protective covering for the body. The skeletal and muscular systems provide structure and movement. The circulatory system transports oxygen and nutrients to all body cells and carries carbon dioxide and metabolic materials away from the cells. The lymphatic system assists the circulatory system in removing wastes and excess fluid from the cells and tissues. The nervous system coordinates the many activities that occur in the body and allows the body to respond and adapt to changes. Special senses provided by organs such as the eyes and ears also allow the body to react to the environment. The respiratory system takes in oxygen for use by the body and eliminates carbon dioxide, a waste product produced by body cells. The digestive system is responsible for the physical and chemical breakdown of food so it can be used by body cells. The urinary system removes certain wastes and excess water from the body. The endocrine system, composed of a group of glands, controls many body functions. The reproductive system allows the human body to create new life.

All of the systems are interrelated, working as a unit to maintain a constant balance (homeostasis) within the human body. When disease occurs, this balance frequently is disturbed. Some of the major diseases and disorders of each system were also discussed in this chapter.

INTERNET SEARCHES

Use the suggested search engines in Chapter 17:4 of this textbook to search the Internet for additional information on the following topics:

1. *Anatomy and physiology*: search the name of a body system, organ, and/or tissue to obtain additional information on the structure and function of the system, organ, or tissue

2. *Pathophysiology*: search the name of specific diseases discussed in each subunit to obtain additional information on occurrence, prognosis, signs and symptoms, and current methods of treatment

3. *American Cancer Society*: search this information base to obtain information on cancer in various parts of the body, breast self-examination, testicular self-examination, and statistics on cancer

4. *Tutorials*: search publishers, software providers, and bookstore sites to find a variety of materials that can be used to learn the anatomy and physiology of the human body

REVIEW QUESTIONS

1. Differentiate between anatomy, physiology, and pathophysiology.

2. Name the four (4) main groups of tissues. By each tissue, list three (3) body systems that contain the tissue.

3. List at least ten (10) body systems and state the main function(s) of each system.

4. Identify the main bones or groups of bones in both the axial and the appendicular skeleton.

5. Describe the five (5) main actions or movements of muscles and provide a specific example for each type of movement.

6. Create a diagram showing the divisions of the nervous system and list the main parts in each division of the system.

7. List four (4) special senses and the organ that is required for each of the senses.

8. Trace a drop of blood as it enters the heart, goes through pulmonary circulation, returns to the heart, and goes to body cells. Name each chamber and valve in the heart, each blood vessel or type of vessel, and any organs blood passes through. Make sure all parts are in correct order.

9. Name all parts of the alimentary canal in correct order. Begin at the mouth and end at the anus.

10. Differentiate between endocrine and exocrine glands. Give five (5) examples of each type of gland and list the main function for each gland.

11. Evaulate three (3) sexually transmitted diseases (STDs) and describe how symptoms are the same or different in male versus female individuals.

12. Body systems are interrelated and work together to perform specific functions. For example, the circulatory and respiratory systems perform a joint function of obtaining oxygen for the body and eliminating carbon dioxide. Describe five (5) other examples of interrelationships between body systems.

CHAPTER 8

Human Growth and Development

Chapter Objectives

After completing this chapter,
you should be able to:

♦ Identify at least two physical, mental, emotional, and social developments that occur during each of the seven main life stages

♦ Explain the causes and treatments for eating disorders and chemical abuse

♦ Identify methods used to prevent suicide and list common warning signs

♦ Recognize ways that life stages affect an individual's needs

♦ Describe the five stages of grieving that occur in the dying patient and the role of the health care worker during each stage

♦ List two purposes of hospice care and provide justifications for the "right to die"

♦ Create examples for each of Maslow's Hierarchy of Needs

♦ Name the two main methods people use to meet or satisfy needs

♦ Describe a situation that shows the use of each of the following defense mechanisms: rationalization, projection, displacement, compensation, daydreaming, repression, suppression, denial, and withdrawal

♦ Define, pronounce, and spell all key terms

 Observe Standard Precautions

 Instructor's Check—Call Instructor at This Point

 Safety—Proceed with Caution

 OBRA Requirement—Based on Federal Law

 Math Skill

 Legal Responsibility

 Science Skill

 Career Information

 Communications Skill

 Technology

KEY TERMS

acceptance
adolescence
affection
Alzheimer's disease *(Altz'-high-merz)*
anger
anorexia nervosa *(an-oh-rex'-see-ah ner-voh'-sah)*
arteriosclerosis *(ar-tear''-ee-oh-skleh-row'-sis)*
bargaining
bulimarexia *(byou-lee''-mah-rex'-ee-ah)*
bulimia *(byou-lee'-me-ah)*
chemical abuse
cognitive
compensation *(cahm''-pen-say'-shun)*
daydreaming
defense mechanisms

denial
depression
development
displacement
early adulthood
early childhood
emotional
esteem
growth
hospice *(hoss'-pis)*
infancy
late adulthood
late childhood
life stages
mental
middle adulthood
motivated
needs
physical

physiological needs *(fizz''-ee-oh-lodg'-ih-kal)*
projection
puberty *(pew'-burr''-tee)*
rationalization *(rash''-en-nal-ih-zay'-shun)*
repression
right to die
safety
satisfaction
self-actualization
sexuality
social
suicide
suppression
tension
terminal illness
withdrawal

INTRODUCTION

Human growth and development is a process that begins at birth and does not end until death. **Growth** refers to the measurable physical changes that occur throughout a person's life. Examples include height, weight, body shape, head circumference, physical characteristics, development of sexual organs, and dentition (dental structure). **Development** refers to the changes in intellectual, mental, emotional, social, and functional skills that occur over time. Development is more difficult to measure, but usually proceeds from simple to complex tasks as maturation, or the process of becoming fully grown and developed, occurs. During all stages of growth and development, individuals have certain tasks that must be accomplished and needs that must be met. A health care worker must be aware of the various life stages and of individual needs to provide quality health care (figure 8-1).

8:1 INFORMATION

Life Stages

Even though individuals differ greatly, each person passes through certain stages of growth and development from birth to death. These stages are frequently called **life stages.** A common method of classifying life stages is as follows:

- ◆ **Infancy:** birth to 1 year
- ◆ **Early childhood:** 1–6 years
- ◆ **Late childhood:** 6–12 years
- ◆ **Adolescence:** 12–18 years
- ◆ **Early adulthood:** 19–40 years
- ◆ **Middle adulthood:** 40–65 years
- ◆ **Late adulthood:** 65 years and older

As individuals pass through these life stages, four main types of growth and development

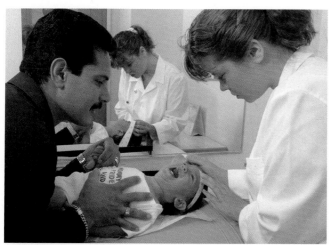 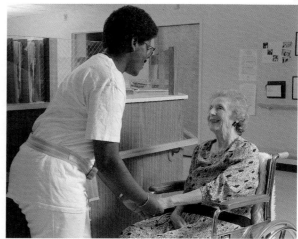

FIGURE 8-1 An understanding of life stages is important for the health care worker, who may provide care to individuals of all ages; from the very young (left) to the elderly (right).

occur: physical, mental or cognitive, emotional, and social. **Physical** refers to body growth and includes height and weight changes, muscle and nerve development, and changes in body organs. **Mental** or **cognitive** refers to intellectual development and includes learning how to solve problems, make judgments, and deal with situations. **Emotional** refers to feelings and includes dealing with love, hate, joy, fear, excitement, and other similar feelings. **Social** refers to interactions and relationships with other people.

Each stage of growth and development has its own characteristics and has specific developmental tasks that an individual must master. These tasks progress from the simple to the more complex. For example, an individual first learns to sit, then crawl, then stand, then walk, and then, finally, run. Each stage establishes the foundation for the next stage. In this way, growth and development proceeds in an orderly pattern. It is important to remember, however, that the rate of progress varies among individuals. Some children master speech early, others master it later. Similarly, an individual may experience a sudden growth spurt and then maintain the same height for a period of time.

Erik Erikson, a psychoanalyst, has identified eight stages of psychosocial development. His eight stages of development, the basic conflict or need that must be resolved at each stage, and ways to resolve the conflict are shown in table 8-1. Erikson believes that if an individual is not able to resolve a conflict at the appropriate stage, the individual will struggle with the same conflict later in life. For example, if a toddler is not allowed

to learn and become independent by mastering basic tasks, the toddler may develop a sense of doubt in his or her abilities. This sense of doubt will interfere with later attempts at mastering independence.

Health care providers must understand that each life stage creates certain needs in individuals. Likewise, other factors can affect life stages and needs. An individual's sex, race, heredity (factors inherited from parents, such as hair color and body structure) culture, life experiences, and health status can influence needs. Injury or illness usually has a negative effect and can change needs or impair development.

INFANCY

Physical Development

The most dramatic and rapid changes in growth and development occur during the first year of life. A newborn baby usually weighs approximately 6–8 pounds (2.7–3.6 kg) and measures 18–22 inches (46–55 cm) (figure 8-2). By the end of the first year of life, weight has usually tripled, to 21–24 pounds (9.5–11 kg), and height has increased to approximately 29–30 inches (74–76 cm).

Muscular system and nervous system developments are also dramatic. The muscular and nervous systems are very immature at birth. Certain reflex actions present at birth allow the infant to respond to the environment. These include the Moro, or startle, reflex to a loud noise or sudden

TABLE 8-1 Erikson's Eight Stages of Psychosocial Development

STAGE OF DEVELOPMENT	BASIC CONFLICT	MAJOR LIFE EVENT	WAYS TO RESOLVE CONFLICT
Infancy Birth to 1 Year Oral–Sensory	Trust versus Mistrust	Feeding	Infant develops trust in self, others, and the environment when caregiver is responsive to basic needs and provides comfort; if needs are not met, infant becomes uncooperative and aggressive, and shows a decreased interest in the environment
Toddler 1–3 Years Muscular–Anal	Autonomy versus Shame/Doubt	Toilet Training	Toddler learns control while mastering skills such as feeding, toileting, and dressing when caregivers provide reassurance but avoid overprotection; if needs are not met, toddler feels ashamed and doubts own abilities, which leads to lack of self-confidence in later stages
Preschool 3–6 Years Locomotor	Initiative versus Guilt	Independence	Child begins to initiate activities in place of just imitating activities; uses imagination to play; learns what is allowed and what is not allowed to develop a conscience; caregivers must allow child to be responsible while providing reassurance; if needs are not met, child feels guilty and thinks everything he or she does is wrong, which leads to a hesitancy to try new tasks in later stages
School-Age 6–12 Years Latency	Industry versus Inferiority	School	Child becomes productive by mastering learning and obtaining success; child learns to deal with academics, group activities, and friends when others show acceptance of actions and praise success; if needs are not met, child develops a sense of inferiority and incompetence, which hinders future relationships and the ability to deal with life events
Adolescence 12–18 Years	Identity versus Role Confusion	Peer	Adolescent searches for self-identity by making choices about occupation, sexual orientation, lifestyle, and adult role; relies on peer group for support and reassurance to create a self-image separate from parents; if needs are not met, adolescent experiences role confusion and loss of self-belief
Young Adulthood 19–40 Years	Intimacy versus Isolation	Love Relationships	Young adult learns to make a personal commitment to others and share life events with others; if self-identity is lacking, adult may fear relationships and isolate self from others
Middle Adulthood 40–65 Years	Generativity versus Stagnation	Parenting	Adult seeks satisfaction and obtains success in life by using career, family, and civic interests to provide for others and the next generation; if adult does not deal with life issues, feels lack of purpose to life and sense of failure
Older Adulthood 65 Years to Death	Ego Integrity versus Despair	Reflection on and Acceptance of Life	Adult reflects on life in a positive manner, feels fulfillment with his or her own life and accomplishments, deals with losses, and prepares for death; if fulfillment is not felt, adult feels despair about life and fear of death

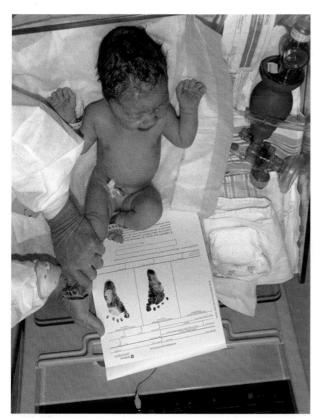

FIGURE 8-2 A newborn baby usually weighs approximately 6–8 pounds and measures 18–22 inches in length.

movement; the rooting reflex, in which a slight touch on the cheek causes the mouth to open and the head to turn; the sucking reflex, caused by a slight touch on the lips; and the grasp reflex, in which infants can grasp an object placed in the hand. Muscle coordination develops in stages. At first, infants are able to lift the head slightly. By 2–4 months, they can usually roll from side to back, support themselves on their forearms when prone, and grasp or try to reach objects. By 4–6 months, they can turn the body completely around, accept objects handed to them, grasp stationary objects such as a bottle, and with support, hold the head up while sitting. By 6–8 months, infants can sit unsupported, grasp moving objects, transfer objects from one hand to the other, and crawl on the stomach. By 8–10 months, they can crawl using their knees and hands, pull themselves to a sitting or standing position, and use good hand–mouth coordination to put things in their mouths. By 12 months, infants frequently can walk without assistance, grasp objects with the thumb and fingers, and throw small objects.

Other physical developments are also dramatic. Most infants are born without teeth, but usually have 10–12 teeth by the end of the first year of life. At birth, vision is poor and may be limited to black and white, and eye movements are not coordinated. By 1 year of age, however, close vision is good, in color, and can readily focus on small objects. Sensory abilities such as those of smell, taste, sensitivity to hot and cold, and hearing, while good at birth, become more refined and exact.

Mental Development

Mental development is also rapid during the first year. Newborns respond to discomforts such as pain, cold, or hunger by crying. As their needs are met, they gradually become more aware of their surroundings and begin to recognize individuals associated with their care. As infants respond to stimuli in the environment, learning activities grow. At birth, they are unable to speak. By 2–4 months, they coo or babble when spoken to, laugh out loud, and squeal with pleasure. By 6 months of age, infants understand some words and can make basic sounds, such as "mama" and "dada." By 12 months, infants understand many words and use single words in their vocabularies.

Emotional Development

Emotional development is observed early in life. Newborns show excitement. By 4–6 months of age, distress, delight, anger, disgust, and fear can often be seen. By 12 months of age, elation and affection for adults is evident. Events that occur in the first year of life when these emotions are first exhibited can have a strong influence on an individual's emotional behavior during adulthood.

Social Development

Social development progresses gradually from the self-centeredness concept of the newborn to the recognition of others in the environment. By 4 months of age, infants recognize their caregivers, smile readily, and stare intently at others (figure 8-3). By 6 months of age, infants watch the activities of others, show signs of possessiveness, and may become shy or withdraw when in the presence of strangers. By 12 months of age, infants may still be shy with strangers, but they socialize freely with familiar people, and mimic and imitate gestures, facial expressions, and vocal sounds.

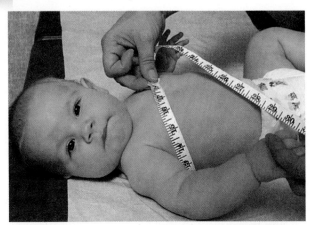

FIGURE 8-3 By 4 months of age, infants recognize their caregivers and stare intently at others.

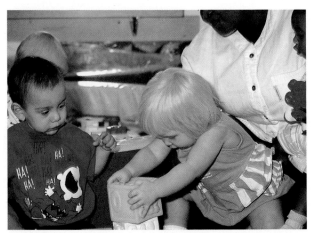

FIGURE 8-4 One to two-year-olds are interested in many different activities, but they have short attention spans.

Needs

Infants are dependent on others for all needs. Food, cleanliness, and rest are essential for physical growth. Love and security are essential for emotional and social growth. Stimulation is essential for mental growth.

EARLY CHILDHOOD

Physical Development

During early childhood, from 1–6 years of age, physical growth is slower than during infancy. By age 6, the average weight is 45 pounds (20.4 kg), and the average height is 46 inches (116 cm). Skeletal and muscle development helps the child assume a more adult appearance. The legs and lower body tend to grow more rapidly than do the head, arms, and chest. Muscle coordination allows the child to run, climb, and move freely. As muscles of the fingers develop, the child learns to write, draw, and use a fork and knife. By age 2 or 3, most teeth have erupted, and the digestive system is mature enough to handle most adult foods. Between 2 and 4 years of age, most children learn bladder and bowel control.

Mental Development

Mental development advances rapidly during early childhood. Verbal growth progresses from the use of several words at age 1 to a vocabulary of 1,500–2,500 words at age 6. Two-year-olds have short attention spans but are interested in many different activities (figure 8-4). They can remem-

ber details and begin to understand concepts. Four-year-olds ask frequent questions and usually recognize letters and some words. They begin to make decisions based on logic rather than on trial and error. By age 6, children are very verbal and want to learn how to read and write. Memory has developed to the point where the child can make decisions based on both past and present experiences.

Emotional Development

Emotional development also advances rapidly. At ages 1–2, children begin to develop self-awareness and to recognize the effect they have on other people and things. Limits are usually established for safety, leading the 1- or 2-year-old to either accept or defy such limits. By age 2, most children begin to gain self-confidence and are enthusiastic about learning new things (figure 8-5). However, children can feel impatient and frustrated as they try to do things beyond their abilities. Anger, often in the form of "temper tantrums," occurs when they cannot perform as desired. Children at this age also like routine and become stubborn, angry, or frustrated when changes occur. From ages 4–6, children begin to gain more control over their emotions. They understand the concept of right and wrong, and because they have achieved more independence, they are not frustrated as much by their lack of ability. By age 6, most children also show less anxiety when faced with new experiences, because they have learned they can deal with new situations.

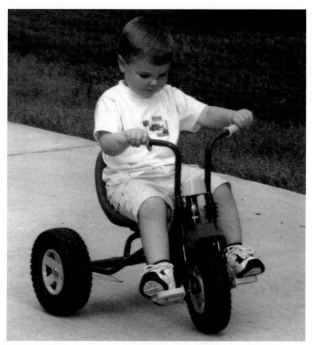

FIGURE 8-5 By age two, most children begin to gain some self-confidence and are enthusiastic about learning new things.

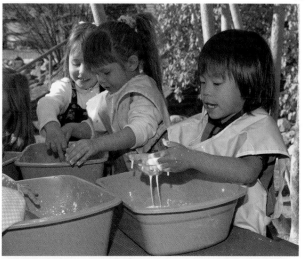

FIGURE 8-6 Playing alongside and with other children allows preschoolers to learn how to interact with others.

Social Development

Social development expands from a self-centered 1-year-old to a sociable 6-year-old. In the early years, children are usually strongly attached to their parents (or to the individuals who provide their care), and they fear any separation. They begin to enjoy the company of others, but are still very possessive. Playing alongside other children is more common than playing with other children (figure 8-6). Gradually, children learn to put "self" aside and begin to take more of an interest in others. They learn to trust other people and make more of an effort to please others by becoming more agreeable and social. Friends of their own age are usually important to 6-year-olds.

Needs

The needs of early childhood still include food, rest, shelter, protection, love, and security. In addition, children need routine, order, and consistency in their daily lives. They must be taught to be responsible and must learn how to conform to rules. This can be accomplished by making reasonable demands based on the child's ability to comply.

LATE CHILDHOOD

Physical Development

The late childhood life stage, which covers ages 6–12, is also called *preadolescence*. Physical development is slow but steady. Weight gain averages 4–7 pounds (2.3–3.2 kg) per year, and height usually increases approximately 2–3 inches (5–7.5 cm) per year. Muscle coordination is well developed, and children can engage in physical activities that require complex motor-sensory coordination. During this age, most of the primary teeth are lost, and permanent teeth erupt. The eyes are well developed, and visual acuity is at its best. During ages 10–12, secondary sexual characteristics may begin to develop in some children.

Mental Development

Mental development increases rapidly because much of the child's life centers around school. Speech skills develop more completely, and reading and writing skills are learned. Children learn to use information to solve problems, and the memory becomes more complex. They begin to understand more abstract concepts such as loyalty, honesty, values, and morals. Children use more active thinking and become more adept at making judgments (figure 8-7).

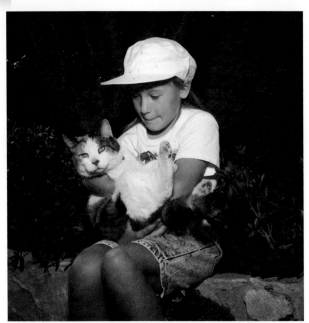

FIGURE 8-7 In late childhood (ages 6–12), children become more adept at making judgments.

Emotional Development

Emotional development continues to help the child achieve a greater independence and a more distinct personality. At age 6, children are often frightened and uncertain as they begin school. Reassuring parents and success in school help children gain self-confidence. Gradually, fears are replaced by the ability to cope. Emotions are slowly brought under control and dealt with in a more effective manner. By ages 10–12, sexual maturation and changes in body functions can lead to periods of depression followed by periods of joy. These emotional changes can cause children to be restless, anxious, and difficult to understand.

Social Development

Social changes are evident during these years. Seven-year-olds tend to like activities they can do by themselves and do not usually like group activities. However, they want the approval of others, especially their parents and friends. Children from ages 8–10 tend to be more group oriented, and they typically form groups with members of their own sex. They are more ready to accept the opinions of others and learn to conform to rules and standards of behavior followed by the group. Toward the end of this period, children tend to make friends more easily, and they begin to develop an increasing awareness of the opposite sex. As children spend more time with others their own age, their dependency on their parent(s) lessens, as does the time they spend with their parents.

Needs

Needs of children in this age group include the same basic needs of infancy and early childhood, together with the need for reassurance, parental approval, and peer acceptance.

ADOLESCENCE

Physical Development

Adolescence, ages 12 to 18, is often a traumatic life stage. Physical changes occur most dramatically in the early period. A sudden "growth spurt" can cause rapid increases in weight and height. A weight gain of up to 25 pounds (11 kg) and a height increase of several inches can occur in a period of months. Muscle coordination does not advance as quickly. This can lead to awkwardness or clumsiness in motor coordination. This growth spurt usually occurs anywhere from ages 11 to 13 in girls and ages 13 to 15 in boys.

The most obvious physical changes in adolescents relate to the development of the sexual organs and secondary sexual characteristics, frequently called **puberty.** Secretion of sex hormones leads to the onset of menstruation in girls and the production of sperm and semen in boys. Secondary sexual characteristics in females include growth of pubic hair, development of breasts and wider hips, and distribution of body fat leading to the female shape. The male develops a deeper voice; attains more muscle mass and broader shoulders; and grows pubic, facial, and body hair.

Mental Development

Since most of the foundations have already been established, mental development primarily involves an increase in knowledge and a sharpening of skills. Adolescents learn to make decisions and to accept responsibility for their actions. At times, this causes conflict because they are treated as both children and adults, or are told to "grow up" while being reminded that they are "still children."

Emotional Development

Emotional development is often stormy and in conflict. As adolescents try to establish their identities and independence, they are often uncertain and feel inadequate and insecure. They worry about their appearance, their abilities, and their relationships with others. They frequently respond more and more to peer group influences. At times, this leads to changes in attitude and behavior and conflict with values previously established. Toward the end of adolescence, self-identity has been established. At this point, teenagers feel more comfortable with who they are and turn attention toward what they may become. They gain more control of their feelings and become more mature emotionally.

Social Development

Social development usually involves spending less time with family and more time with peer groups. As adolescents attempt to develop self-identity and independence, they seek security in groups of people their own age who have similar problems and conflicts (figure 8-8). If these peer relationships help develop self-confidence through the approval of others, adolescents become more secure and satisfied. Toward the end of this life stage, adolescents develop a more mature attitude and begin to develop patterns of

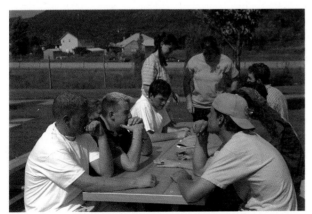

FIGURE 8-8 Adolescents use the peer group as a safety net as they try to establish their identities and independence.

behavior that they associate with adult behavior or status.

Needs

In addition to basic needs, adolescents need reassurance, support, and understanding. Many problems that develop during this life stage can be traced to the conflict and feelings of inadequacy and insecurity that adolescents experience. Examples include eating disorders, drug and alcohol abuse, and suicide. Even though these types of problems also occur in earlier and later life stages, they are frequently associated with adolescence.

Eating disorders often develop from an excessive concern with appearance. Two common eating disorders are anorexia nervosa and bulimia. **Anorexia nervosa,** commonly called *anorexia,* is a psychological disorder in which a person drastically reduces food intake or refuses to eat at all. This results in metabolic disturbances, excessive weight loss, weakness, and if not treated, death. **Bulimia** is a psychological disorder in which a person alternately binges (eats excessively) and then fasts, or refuses to eat at all. When a person induces vomiting or uses laxatives to get rid of food that has been eaten, the condition is called **bulimarexia.** All three conditions are more common in female than male individuals. Psychological or psychiatric help is usually needed to treat these conditions.

Chemical abuse is the use of substances such as alcohol or drugs and the development of a physical and/or mental dependence on these chemicals. Chemical abuse can occur in any life stage, but it frequently begins in adolescence. Reasons for using chemicals include anxiety or stress relief, peer pressure, escape from emotional or psychological problems, experimentation with feelings the chemicals produce, desire for "instant gratification," hereditary traits, and cultural influences. Chemical abuse can lead to physical and mental disorders and disease. Treatment is directed toward total rehabilitation that allows the chemical abuser to return to a productive and meaningful life.

Suicide, found in many life stages, is one of the leading causes of death in adolescents. Suicide is always a permanent solution to a temporary problem. Reasons for suicide include depression, grief over a loss or love affair, failure in school, inability to meet expectations, influence of suicidal friends, or lack of self-esteem. The risk for suicide increases with a family history of suicide, a major loss or disappointment, previous suicide attempts, and/or the recent suicide of friends, family, or role models (heroes or idols). The impulsive nature of adolescents also increases the possibility of suicide. Most individuals who are thinking of suicide give warning signs such as verbal statements like "I'd rather be dead" or "You'd be better off without me." Other warning signs include:

♦ sudden changes in appetite and sleep habits

♦ withdrawal, depression, and moodiness

♦ excessive fatigue or agitation

♦ neglect of personal hygiene

♦ alcohol or drug abuse

♦ losing interest in hobbies and other aspects of life

♦ preoccupation with death

♦ injuring one's body

♦ giving away possessions

♦ social withdrawal from family and friends

These individuals are calling out for attention and help, and usually respond to efforts of assistance. Their direct and indirect pleas should never be ignored. Support, understanding, and psychological or psychiatric counseling are used to prevent suicide.

EARLY ADULTHOOD

Physical Development

Early adulthood, ages 19–40, is frequently the most productive life stage. Physical development is basically complete, muscles are developed and strong, and motor coordination is at its peak. This is also the prime childbearing time and usually produces the healthiest babies (figure 8-9). Both male and female sexual development is at its peak.

Mental Development

Mental development usually continues throughout this stage. Many young adults pursue additional education to establish and progress in their chosen careers. Frequently, formal education

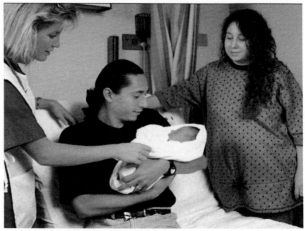

FIGURE 8-9 Early adulthood is the prime child-bearing time and usually produces the healthiest babies.

continues for many years. The young adult often also deals with independence, makes career choices, establishes a lifestyle, selects a marital partner, starts a family, and establishes values, all of which involve making many decisions and forming many judgments.

Emotional Development

Emotional development usually involves preserving the stability established during previous stages. Young adults are subjected to many emotional stresses related to career, marriage, family, and other similar situations. If emotional structure is strong, most young adults can cope with these worries. They find satisfaction in their achievements, take responsibility for their actions, and learn to accept criticism and to profit from mistakes.

Social Development

Social development frequently involves moving away from the peer group. Instead, young adults tend to associate with others who have similar ambitions and interests, regardless of age. The young adult often becomes involved with a mate and forms a family. Young adults do not necessarily accept traditional sex roles and frequently adopt nontraditional roles. For example, male individuals fill positions as nurses and secretaries, and female individuals enter administrative or construction positions. Such choices have caused and will continue to cause changes in the traditional patterns of society.

MIDDLE ADULTHOOD

Physical Development

Middle adulthood, ages 40–65, is frequently called *middle age.* Physical changes begin to occur during these years. The hair tends to gray and thin, the skin begins to wrinkle, muscle tone tends to decrease, hearing loss starts, visual acuity declines, and weight gain occurs. Women experience *menopause,* or the end of menstruation, along with decreased hormone production that causes physical and emotional changes. Men also experience a slowing of hormone production. This can lead to physical and psychological changes, a period frequently referred to as the *male climacteric.* However, except in cases of injury, disease, or surgery, men never lose the ability to produce sperm or to reproduce.

Mental Development

Mental ability can continue to increase during middle age, a fact that has been proved by the many individuals in this life stage who seek formal education. Middle adulthood is a period when individuals have acquired an understanding of life and have learned to cope with many different stresses. This allows them to be more confident in making decisions and to excel at analyzing situations.

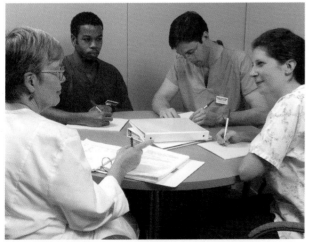

FIGURE 8-10 Job stability and enjoyment during middle adulthood contribute to emotional satisfaction.

Emotional Development

Emotionally, middle age can be a period of contentment and satisfaction, or it can be a time of crisis. The emotional foundation of previous life stages and the situations that occur during middle age determine emotional status during this period. Job stability, financial success, the end of child rearing, and good health can all contribute to emotional satisfaction (figure 8-10). Stress, created by loss of job, fear of aging, loss of youth and vitality, illness, marital problems, or problems with children or aging parents, can contribute to emotional feelings of depression, insecurity, anxiety, and even anger. Therefore, emotional status varies in this age group and is largely determined by events that occur during this period.

Social Development

Social relationships also depend on many factors. Family relationships often see a decline as children begin lives of their own and parents die. Work relationships frequently replace family. Relationships between husband and wife can become stronger as they have more time together and opportunities to enjoy success. However, divorce rates are also high in this age group, as couples who have remained together "for the children's sake" now separate. Friendships are usually with people who have the same interests and lifestyles.

LATE ADULTHOOD

Physical Development

Late adulthood, age 65 and older, has many different terms associated with it. These include "elderly," "senior citizen," "golden ager," and "retired citizen." Much attention has been directed toward this life stage in recent years because people are living longer, and the number of people in this age group is increasing daily.

Physical development is on the decline. All body systems are usually affected. The skin becomes dry, wrinkled, and thinner. Brown or yellow spots (frequently called "age spots") appear. The hair becomes thin and frequently loses its luster or shine. Bones become brittle and porous, and are more likely to fracture or break. Cartilage between the vertebrae thins and can lead to a stooping posture. Muscles lose tone and strength, which can lead to fatigue and poor coordination. A decline in the function of the nervous system leads to hearing loss, decreased visual acuity, and decreased tolerance for temperatures that are too hot or too cold. Memory loss can occur, and reasoning ability can diminish. The heart is less efficient, and circulation decreases. The kidney and bladder are less efficient. Breathing capacity decreases and causes shortness of breath. However, it is important to note that these changes usually occur slowly over a long period. Many individuals, because of better health and living conditions, do not show physical changes of aging until their seventies and even eighties.

Mental Development

Mental abilities vary among individuals. Elderly people who remain mentally active and are willing to learn new things tend to show fewer signs of decreased mental ability (figure 8-11). Although some 90-year-olds remain alert and well oriented, other elderly individuals show decreased mental capacities at much earlier ages. Short-term memory is usually first to decline. Many elderly individuals can clearly remember events that occurred 20 years ago, but do not remember yesterday's events. Diseases such as **Alzheimer's disease** can lead to irreversible loss of memory, deterioration of intellectual functions, speech and gait disturbances, and disorientation. **Arteriosclerosis,** a thickening and hardening of the walls of the arteries, can also decrease the blood supply to the brain and cause a decrease in mental

abilities. These diseases are discussed in greater detail in Chapter 10:4.

Emotional Development

Emotional stability also varies among individuals in this age group. Some elderly people cope well with the stresses presented by aging and remain happy and able to enjoy life. Others become lonely, frustrated, withdrawn, and depressed. Emotional adjustment is necessary throughout this cycle. Retirement, death of a spouse and friends, physical disabilities, financial problems, loss of independence, and knowledge that life must end all can cause emotional distress. The adjustments that the individual makes during this life stage are similar to those made throughout life.

Social Development

Social adjustment also occurs during late adulthood. Retirement can lead to a loss of self-esteem, especially if work is strongly associated with self-identity: "I am a teacher," instead of "I am Sandra Jones." Less contact with coworkers and a more limited circle of friends usually occur. Many elderly adults engage in other activities and continue to make new social contacts (figure 8-12). Others limit their social relationships. Death of a spouse and friends, and moving to a new environment can also cause changes in social rela-

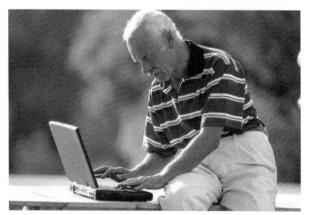

FIGURE 8-11 Elderly adults who are willing to learn new things show fewer signs of decreased mental ability.

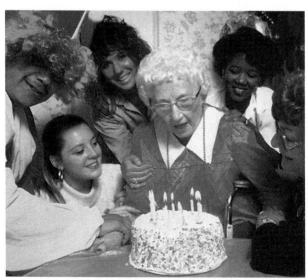

FIGURE 8-12 Social contacts and activities are important during late adulthood.

tionships. Development of new social contacts is important at this time. Senior centers, golden age groups, churches, and many other organizations help provide the elderly with the opportunity to find new social roles.

Needs

Needs of this life stage are the same as those of all other life stages. In addition to basic needs, the elderly need a sense of belonging, self-esteem, financial security, social acceptance, and love.

STUDENT: *Go to the workbook and complete the assignment sheet for 8:1, Life Stages.*

8:2 INFORMATION

Death and Dying

Death is often referred to as "the final stage of growth." It is experienced by everyone and cannot be avoided. In our society, the young tend to ignore its existence. It is usually the elderly, having lost spouses and/or friends, who begin to think of their own deaths.

When a patient is told that he or she has a **terminal illness,** a disease that cannot be cured and will result in death, the patient may react in different ways. Some patients react with fear and anxiety. They fear pain, abandonment, and loneliness. They fear the unknown. They become anxious about their loved ones and about unfinished work or dreams. Anxiety diminishes in patients who feel they have had full lives and who have strong religious beliefs regarding life after death. Some patients view death as a final peace. They know it will bring an end to loneliness, pain, and suffering.

STAGES OF DYING AND DEATH

Dr. Elizabeth Kübler-Ross has done extensive research on the process of death and dying, and is known as a leading expert on this topic. Because of her research, most medical personnel now believe patients should be told of their approaching deaths. However, patients should be left with "some hope" and the knowledge that they will "not be left alone." It is important that all staff members who provide care to the dying patient know both the extent of information given to the patient and how the patient reacted.

Dr. Kübler-Ross has identified five stages of grieving that dying patients and their families/ friends may experience in preparation for death. The stages may not occur in order, and they may overlap or be repeated several times. Some patients may not progress through all of the stages before death occurs. Other patients may be in several stages at the same time. The stages are denial, anger, bargaining, depression, and acceptance.

Denial is the "No, not me!" stage, which usually occurs when a person is first told of a terminal illness. It occurs when the person cannot accept the reality of death or when the person feels loved ones cannot accept the truth. The person may make statements such as "The doctor does not know what he is talking about" or "The tests have to be wrong." Some patients seek second medical opinions or request additional tests. Others refuse to discuss their situations and avoid any references to their illnesses. It is important for patients to discuss these feelings. The health care worker should listen to a patient and try to provide support without confirming or denying. Statements such as "It must be hard for you" or "You feel additional tests will help?" will allow the patient to express feelings and move on to the next stage.

Anger occurs when the patient is no longer able to deny death. Statements such as "Why me?" or "It's your fault" are common. Patients may strike out at anyone who comes in contact with them and become hostile and bitter. They may blame themselves, their loved ones, or health care personnel for their illnesses. It is important for the health care worker to understand that this anger is not a personal attack; the anger is caused by the situation the patient is experiencing. Providing understanding and support, listening, and making every attempt to respond to the patient's demands quickly and with kindness is essential during this stage. This stage continues until the anger is exhausted or the patient must attend to other concerns.

Bargaining occurs when patients accept death but want more time to live. Frequently, this is a period when patients turn to religion and spiritual beliefs. At this point, the will to live is strong, and patients fight hard to achieve goals set. They want to see their children graduate or get married, they want time to arrange care for their families, they want to hold new grandchildren, or other similar desires. Patients make promises to God to obtain more time. Health care workers must again be supportive and be good listeners. Whenever possible, they should help patients meet their goals.

Depression occurs when patients realize that death will come soon and they will no longer be with their families or be able to complete their goals. They may express these regrets, or they may withdraw and become quiet (figure 8-13). They experience great sadness and, at times, overwhelming despair. It is important for health care workers to let patients know that it is "OK" to be depressed. Providing quiet understanding, support, and/or a simple touch, and allowing patients to cry or express grief are important during this stage.

Acceptance is the final stage. Patients understand and accept the fact that they are going to die. Patients may complete unfinished business and try to help those around them deal with the oncoming death. Gradually, patients separate themselves from the world and other people. At the end, they are at peace and can die with dignity. During this final stage, patients still need emotional support and the presence of others, even if it is just the touch of a hand (figure 8-14).

HOSPICE CARE

Providing care to dying patients can be very difficult, but very rewarding. Providing supportive care when families and patients require it most

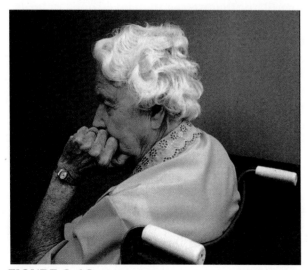

FIGURE 8-13 Depression can be a normal stage of grieving in a dying patient.

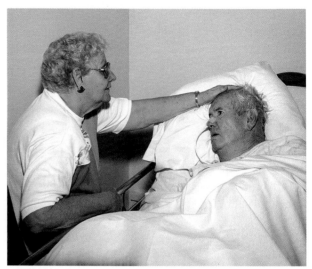

FIGURE 8-14 The support and presence of others is important to the dying person.

can be one of the greatest satisfactions a health care worker can experience. To be able to provide this care, however, health care workers must first understand their own personal feelings about death and come to terms with these feelings. Feelings of fear, frustration, and uncertainty about death can cause workers to avoid dying patients or provide superficial, mechanical care. With experience, health care workers can find ways to deal with their feelings and learn to provide the supportive care needed by the dying.

Hospice care can play an important role in meeting the needs of the dying patient. Hospice care offers *palliative care,* or care that provides support and comfort. It can be offered in hospitals, medical centers, and special facilities, but most frequently it is offered in the patient's home. Hospice care is not limited to a specific time period in a patient's life. Usually it is not started until a physician declares that the patient has 6 months or less to live, but it can be started sooner. Most often patients and their families are reluctant to begin hospice care because they feel that this action recognizes the end of life. They seem to feel that if they do not use hospice care until later, death will not be as near as it actually is. The philosophy behind hospice care is to allow the patient to die with dignity and comfort. Using palliative measures of care and the philosophy of death with dignity provides patients and families with many comforts and provides an opportunity to find closure. Some of the comforts provided by hospice may include providing hospital equipment such as beds, wheelchairs, and bedside commodes; offering psychological, spiritual, social, and financial counseling; and providing free or less expensive pain medication. Pain is controlled so that the patient can remain active as long as possible. In medical facilities, personal care of the patient is provided by the staff; in the home situation, this care is provided by home health aides and other health care professionals. Specially trained volunteers are an important part of many hospice programs. They make regular visits to the patient and family, stay with the patient while the family leaves the home for brief periods of time, and help provide the support and understanding that the patient and family need. When the time for death arrives, the patient is allowed to die with dignity and in peace. After the death of the patient, hospice personnel often maintain contact with the family during the initial period of mourning.

RIGHT TO DIE

The **right to die** is another issue that health care workers must understand. Because health care workers are ethically concerned with promoting life, allowing patients to die can cause conflict. However, a large number of surveys have shown that most people feel that an individual who has a terminal illness, with no hope of being cured, should be allowed to refuse measures that would prolong life. This is called the *right to die*. Most states have passed, or are now creating, laws that allow adults who have terminal illnesses to instruct their doctors, in writing, to withhold treatments that might prolong life. Most of the laws involve the use of advance directives, discussed in Chapter 5:4. Under these laws, specific actions to end life cannot be taken. However, the use of respirators, pacemakers, and other medical devices can be withheld, and the person can be allowed to die with dignity.

Hospices throughout the nation are encouraging individuals to make their end-of-life wishes known through the *LIVE* promise. This promise encourages individuals to:

♦ **L**earn about end-of-life services and care

♦ **I**mplement plans or advanced directives to ensure wishes are honored

♦ **V**oice decisions

♦ **E**ngage others in conversations about end-of-life care options

Health care workers must be aware that a dying person has rights that must be honored. A Dying Person's Bill of Rights was created at a workshop sponsored by the South Western Michigan Inservice Education Council. This bill of rights states:

♦ I have the right to be treated as a living human being until I die.

♦ I have the right to maintain a sense of hopefulness, however changing its focus may be.

♦ I have the right to be cared for by those who can maintain a sense of hopefulness, however challenging this might be.

♦ I have the right to express my feelings and emotions about my approaching death in my own way.

♦ I have the right to participate in decisions concerning my care.

♦ I have the right to expect continuing medical and nursing attention even though "cure" goals must be changed to "comfort" goals.

♦ I have the right not to die alone.

♦ I have the right to be free from pain.

♦ I have the right to have my questions answered honestly.

♦ I have the right not to be deceived.

♦ I have the right to have help from and for my family in accepting my death.

♦ I have the right to die in peace and with dignity.

♦ I have the right to maintain my individuality and not be judged for my decisions, which may be contrary to the beliefs of others.

♦ I have the right to expect that the sanctity of the human body will be respected after death.

♦ I have the right to be cared for by caring, sensitive, knowledgeable people who will attempt to understand my needs and will be able to gain some satisfaction in helping me face my death.

♦ I have the right to discuss and enlarge my religious and/or spiritual experiences, whatever these may mean to others.

Health care workers deal with death and with dying patients because death is a part of life. By understanding the process of death and by thinking about the needs of dying patients, the health care worker will be able to provide the special care needed by these individuals.

STUDENT: *Go to the workbook and complete the assignment sheet for 8:2, Death and Dying.*

8:3 INFORMATION
Human Needs

Needs are frequently defined as "a lack of something that is required or desired." From the moment of birth to the moment of death, every human being has needs. Needs motivate the individual to behave or act so that these needs will be met, if at all possible.

Certain needs have priority over other needs. For example, at times a need for food may take priority over a need for social approval, or the approval of others. If individuals have been without food for a period of time, they will direct most of their actions toward obtaining food. Even though they want social approval and the respect of others, they may steal for food, knowing that stealing may cause a loss of social approval or respect.

MASLOW'S HIERARCHY OF NEEDS

Abraham Maslow, a noted psychologist, developed a hierarchy of needs (figure 8-15). According to Maslow, the lower needs should be met before an individual can strive to meet higher needs. Only when satisfaction has been obtained at one level is an individual motivated toward meeting needs at a higher level. The levels of needs include physiological needs, safety, affection, esteem, and self-actualization.

Physiological Needs

Physiological needs are often called "physical," "biological," or "basic" needs. These needs are required by every human being to sustain life. They include food, water, oxygen, elimination of waste materials, sleep, and protection from extreme temperatures. These needs must be met for life to continue. If any of these needs goes unmet, death will occur. Even among these needs, a priority exists. For example, because lack of oxygen will cause death in a matter of minutes, the need for oxygen has priority over the need for

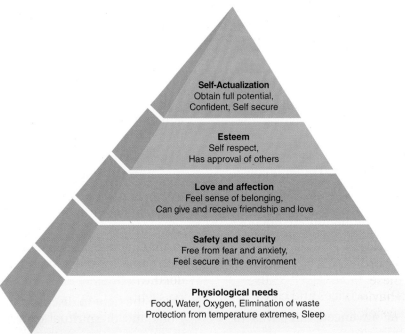

FIGURE 8-15 Maslow's Hierarchy of Needs: the lower needs should be met before the individual can try to meet higher needs.

food. A patient with severe lung disease who is gasping for every breath will not be concerned with food intake. This individual's main concern will be to obtain enough oxygen to live through the next minute.

Other physiological needs include sensory and motor needs. If these needs are not met, individuals may not die, but their body functions will be affected. Sensory needs include hearing, seeing, feeling, smelling, tasting, and mental stimulation. When these needs are met, they allow the individual to respond to the environment. If these needs are not met, the person may lose contact with the environment or with reality. An example is motor needs, which include the ability to move and respond to the individual's environment. If muscles are not stimulated, they will atrophy (waste away), and function will be lost.

Many of the physiological needs are automatically controlled by the body. The process of breathing is usually not part of the conscious thought process of the individual until something occurs to interfere with breathing. Another example is the functioning of the urinary bladder. The bladder fills automatically, and the individual only becomes aware of the bladder when it is full. If the individual does not respond and go to the restroom to empty the bladder, eventually control will be lost and the bladder will empty itself.

Health care workers must be aware of how an illness interferes with meeting physiological needs. A patient scheduled for surgery or laboratory tests may not be allowed to eat or drink before the procedure. Anxiety about an illness may interfere with a patient's sleep or elimination patterns. Medications may affect a patient's appetite. Elderly individuals are even more likely to have difficulty meeting physiological needs. A loss of vision or hearing due to aging may make it difficult for an elderly person to communicate with others. A decreased sense of smell and taste can affect appetite. Deterioration of muscles and joints can lead to poor coordination and difficulty in walking. Any of these factors can cause a change in a person's behavior. If health care workers are aware that physiological needs are not being met, they can provide understanding and support to the patient and make every effort to help the patient satisfy the needs.

Safety

Safety becomes important when physiological needs have been met. Safety needs include the need to be free from anxiety and fear, and the need to feel secure in the environment. The need for order and routine is another example of an individual's effort to remain safe and secure. Individuals often prefer the familiar over the unknown. New environments, a change in routine, marital problems, job loss, injury, disease, and other similar events can threaten an individual's safety.

Illness is a major threat to an individual's security and well-being. Health care workers are familiar with laboratory tests, surgeries, medications, and therapeutic treatments. Patients are usually frightened when they are exposed to them and their sense of security is threatened. If health care workers explain the reason for the tests or treatments and the expected outcomes to the patient, this can frequently alleviate the patient's anxieties. Patients admitted to a health care facility or long-term care facility must adapt to a strange and new environment. They frequently experience anxiety or depression. Patients may also experience depression over the loss of health or loss of a body function. Health care workers must be aware of the threats to safety and security that patients are experiencing, and make every effort to explain procedures, provide support and understanding, and help patients adapt to the situation.

Love and Affection

The need for love and **affection,** a warm and tender feeling for another person, occupies the third level of Maslow's Hierarchy of Needs. When an individual feels safe and secure, and after all physiological needs have been met, the individual next strives for social acceptance, friendship, and to be loved. The need to belong, to relate to others, and to win approval of others motivates an individual's actions at this point. The individual may now attend a social function that was avoided when safety was more of a priority. Individuals who feel safe and secure are more willing to accept and adapt to change and are more willing to face unknown situations. The need for love and affection is satisfied when friends are made, social contacts are established, acceptance by others is received, and the individual is able to both give and receive affection and love (figure 8-16).

Maslow states that sexuality is both a part of the need for love and affection, as well as a physiological need. **Sexuality** in this context is defined by people's feelings concerning their masculine/feminine natures, their abilities to give and receive love and affection, and finally, their roles in reproduction of the species. It is important to note that in all three of these areas, sexuality involves a person's feelings and attitudes, not just the person's sexual relationships.

It is equally important to note that a person's sexuality extends throughout the life cycle. At conception, a person's sexual organs are determined. Following birth, a person is given a name, at least generally associated with the person's sex. Studies have shown that children receive treatment according to gender from early childhood and frequently are rewarded for behavior that is deemed "gender appropriate." With the onset of puberty, adolescents become more aware of their emerging sexuality and of the standards that society places on them. During both childhood and adolescence, much of what is learned about sexuality comes from observing adult role models. As the adolescent grows into young adulthood, society encourages a reexamination of sexuality and the role it plays in helping to fulfill the need for love and affection. In adulthood, sexuality develops new meanings according to the roles that the adult takes on. Sexuality needs do not

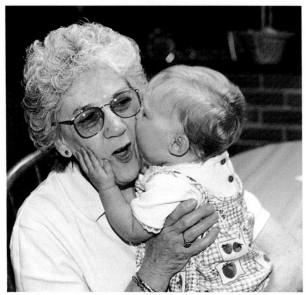

FIGURE 8-16 Individuals of all ages need love and affection. *(Courtesy of Sandy Clark)*

cease in late adulthood. Long-term care facilities are recognizing this fact by allowing married couples to share a room, instead of separating people according to sex. Even after the death of a spouse, an individual may develop new relationships. Determining what role sexuality will play in a person's life is a dynamic process that allows people to meet their need for love and affection throughout their life.

Sexuality, in addition to being related to the satisfaction of needs, is also directly related to an individual's moral values. Issues such as the appropriateness of sex before marriage, the use of birth control, how to deal with pregnancy, and how to deal with sexually transmitted diseases all require individuals to evaluate their moral beliefs. These beliefs then serve as guidelines to help people reach decisions on their behaviors.

Some individuals use sexual relationships as substitutes for love and affection. Individuals who seek to meet their needs only in this fashion cannot successfully complete Maslow's third level.

Esteem

Maslow's fourth level includes the need for **esteem.** Esteem includes feeling important and worthwhile. When others show respect, approval, and appreciation, an individual begins to feel esteem and gains self-respect. The self-concept, or beliefs, values, and feelings people have about themselves, becomes positive. Individuals will engage in activities that bring achievement, success, and recognition in an effort to maintain their need for esteem. Failure in an activity can cause a loss of confidence and lack of esteem. When esteem needs are met, individuals gain confidence in themselves and begin to direct their actions toward becoming what they want to be.

Illness can have a major effect on esteem. When self-reliant individuals, competent at making decisions, find themselves in a health care facility and dependent on others for basic care such as bathing, eating, and elimination, they can experience a severe loss of esteem. They may also worry about a lack of income, possible job loss, the well-being of their family, and/or the possibility of permanent disability or death. Patients may become angry and frustrated or quiet and withdrawn. Health care workers must recognize this loss of esteem and make every attempt to listen to the patient, encourage as much independence as possible, provide supportive care, and allow the person to express anger or fear.

Self-Actualization

Self-actualization, frequently called *self-realization,* is the final need in Maslow's hierarchy. All other needs must be met, at least in part, before self-actualization can occur. **Self-actualization** means that people have obtained their full potentials, or that they are what they want to be. People at this level are confident and willing to express their beliefs and stick to them. They feel so strongly about themselves that they are willing to reach out to others to provide assistance and support.

MEETING NEEDS

When needs are felt, individuals are **motivated** (stimulated) to act. If the action is successful and the need is met, **satisfaction,** or a feeling of pleasure or fulfillment, occurs. If the need is not met, **tension,** or frustration, an uncomfortable inner sensation or feeling, occurs. Several needs can be felt at the same time, so individuals must decide which needs are stronger. For example, if individuals need both food and sleep, they must decide which need is most important, because an individual cannot eat and sleep at the same time.

Individuals feel needs at different levels of intensity. The more intense a need, the greater the desire to meet or reduce the need. Also, when an individual first experiences a need, the individual may deal with it by trying different actions in a trial-and-error manner, a type of behavior frequently seen in very young children. As they grow older, children learn more effective means of meeting the need and are able to satisfy the need easily.

METHODS OF SATISFYING HUMAN NEEDS

Needs can be satisfied by direct or indirect methods. Direct methods work at meeting the need and obtaining satisfaction. Indirect methods work at reducing the need or relieving the tension and frustration created by the unmet need.

Direct Methods

Direct methods include:

♦ hard work

♦ realistic goals

♦ situation evaluation

♦ cooperation with others

All these methods are directed toward meeting the need. Students who constantly fail tests but who want to pass a course have a need for success. They can work harder by listening more in class, asking questions on points they do not understand, and studying longer for the tests. They can set realistic goals that will allow them to find success. By working on one aspect of the course at a time, by concentrating on new material for the next test, by planning to study a little each night rather than studying only the night before a test, and by working on other things that will enable them to pass, they can establish goals they can achieve. They can evaluate the situation to determine why they are failing and to try to find other ways to pass the course. They may determine that they are always tired in class and that by getting more sleep, they will be able to learn the material. They can cooperate with others. By asking the teacher to provide extra assistance, by having parents or friends question them on the material, by asking a counselor to help them learn better study habits, or by having a tutor provide extra help, they may learn the material, pass the tests, and achieve satisfaction by meeting their need.

Indirect Methods

Indirect methods of dealing with needs usually reduce the need and help relieve the tension created by the unmet need. The need is still present, but its intensity decreases. **Defense mechanisms,** unconscious acts that help a person deal with an unpleasant situation or socially unacceptable behavior, are the main indirect methods used. Everyone uses defense mechanisms to some degree. Defense mechanisms provide methods for maintaining self-esteem and relieving discomfort. Some use of defense mechanisms is helpful because it allows individuals to cope with certain situations. However, defense mechanisms can be unhealthy if they are used all the time and individuals substitute them for more effective ways of dealing with situations. Being aware of the use of defense mechanisms and the reason for using them is a healthy use. This allows the individual to relieve tension while modifying habits, learning to accept reality, and striving to find more efficient ways to meet needs.

Examples of defense mechanisms include:

♦ **Rationalization:** This involves using a reasonable excuse or acceptable explanation for behavior to avoid the real reason or true motivation. For example, a patient who fears having laboratory tests performed may tell the health worker, "I can't take time off from my job," rather than admit fear.

♦ **Projection:** This involves placing the blame for one's own actions or inadequacies on someone else or on circumstances rather than accepting responsibility for the actions. Examples include, "The teacher failed me because she doesn't like me," rather than "I failed because I didn't do the work"; and "I'm late because the alarm clock didn't go off," rather than "I forgot to set the alarm clock, and I overslept." When people use projection to blame others, they avoid having to admit that they have made mistakes.

♦ **Displacement:** This involves transferring feelings about one person to someone else. Displacement usually occurs because individuals cannot direct the feelings toward the person who is responsible. Many people fear directing hostile or negative feelings toward their bosses or supervisors because they fear job loss. They then direct this anger toward coworkers and/or family members. The classic example is the man who is mad at his boss. When the man gets home, he yells at his wife or children. In such a case, a constructive talk with the boss may solve the problem. If not, or if this is not possible, physical activity can help work off hostile or negative feelings.

♦ **Compensation:** This involves the substitution of one goal for another goal to achieve success. If a substitute goal meets needs, this can be a healthy defense mechanism. For example, Joan wanted to be a doctor, but she did not have enough money for a medical education. So she changed her educational plans and became a physician's assistant. Compensation was an efficient defense mechanism because she enjoyed her work and found satisfaction.

♦ **Daydreaming:** This is a dreamlike thought process that occurs when a person is awake. Daydreaming provides a means of escape when a person is not satisfied with reality. If it allows a person to establish goals for the future and leads to a course of action to accomplish those goals, it is a good defense mechanism. However, if daydreaming is a substitute for reality, and the dreams become more satisfying than actual life experiences, it can contribute to a poor adjustment to life. For example, if a person dreams about becoming a dental hygienist and takes courses and works toward this goal, daydreaming is effective. If the person dreams about the goal but is satisfied by the thoughts and takes no action, the person will not achieve the goal and is simply escaping from reality.

♦ **Repression:** This involves the transfer of unacceptable or painful ideas, feelings, and thoughts into the unconscious mind. An individual is not aware that this is occurring. When feelings or emotions become too painful or frightening for the mind to deal with, repression allows the individual to continue functioning and to "forget" the fear or feeling. Repressed feelings do not vanish, however. They can resurface in dreams or affect behavior. For example, a person is terrified of heights but does not know why. It is possible that a frightening experience regarding heights happened in early childhood and that the experience was repressed.

♦ **Suppression:** This is similar to repression, but the individual is aware of the unacceptable feelings or thoughts and refuses to deal with them. The individual may substitute work, a hobby, or a project to avoid the situation. For example, a woman ignores a lump in her breast and refuses to go to a doctor. She avoids thinking about the lump by working overtime and joining a health club to exercise during her spare time. This type of behavior creates excessive stress, and eventually the individual will be forced to deal with the situation.

♦ **Denial:** This involves disbelief of an event or idea that is too frightening or shocking for a

TODAY'S RESEARCH: TOMORROW'S HEALTH CARE

An artificial bone that grows?

   Bone cancer is rare, but when it occurs, it usually happens in children and young adults. Common sites are the knee or leg bones. Amputation of the leg was once the only hope for a cure. Then surgeons began to cut out the tumors and use metal rods to replace the damaged bones. The only problem with this treatment was that the bones did not grow with the child. Every few years, additional surgery was required to replace the metal rods with longer rods.

   Now researchers in France have invented Repiphysis, a "growable" metal rod. Repiphysis contains a spring that is held together by a polymer sleeve hooked to an antenna. Harmless electromagnetic rays are beamed at the leg. These rays cause the antenna to create heat. The heat softens the polymer sleeve and the spring loosens. This allows the ends of the metal rod to extend slowly. When the rod has "grown" to the correct length, and the leg matches the growth of the child's other leg, the electromagnetic beam is turned off. In seconds, the polymer sleeve hardens and the metal rod is frozen at its new length. The best feature of the procedure is that it is painless and can be done in a physician's office.

person to cope with. Often, an individual is not aware that denial is occurring. Denial frequently occurs when a terminal illness is diagnosed. The individual will say that the doctor is wrong and seek another opinion. When the individual is ready to deal with the event or idea, denial becomes acceptance.

♦ **Withdrawal:** There are two main ways withdrawal can occur: individuals can either cease to communicate or remove themselves physically from a situation (figure 8-17). Withdrawal is sometimes a satisfactory means of avoiding conflict or an unhappy situation. For example, if you are forced to work with an individual you dislike and who is constantly criticizing your work, you can withdraw by avoiding any and all communication with this individual, quitting your job, or asking for a transfer to another area. At times, interpersonal conflict cannot be avoided, however. In these cases, an open and honest communication with the individual may lead to improved understanding in the relationship.

   It is important for health care workers to be aware of both their own and patients' needs. By recognizing needs and understanding the actions individuals take to meet needs, more efficient and higher quality care can be provided. Health

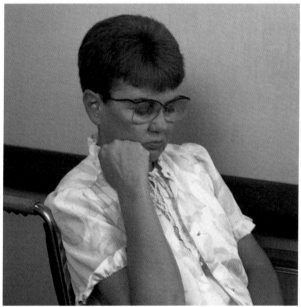

FIGURE 8-17 Refusing to communicate is a sign of withdrawal.

care workers will be better able to understand their own behavior and the behavior of others.

STUDENT: *Go to the workbook and complete the assignment sheet for 8:3, Human Needs.*

CHAPTER 8 SUMMARY

Human growth and development is a process that begins at birth and does not end until death. Each individual passes through certain stages of growth and development, frequently called *life stages.* Each stage has its own characteristics and has specific developmental tasks that an individual must master. Each stage also establishes the foundation for the next stage.

Death is often called "the final stage of growth." Dr. Elizabeth Kübler-Ross has identified five stages that dying patients and their families may experience before death. These stages are denial, anger, bargaining, depression, and acceptance. The health care worker must be aware of these stages to provide supportive care to the dying patient. In addition, the health care worker must understand the concepts represented by hospice care and the right to die.

Each life stage creates needs that must be met by the individual. Abraham Maslow, a noted psychologist, developed a hierarchy of needs that is frequently used to classify and define the needs experienced by human beings. The needs are classified into five levels, and according to Maslow, the lower needs must be met before an individual can strive to meet the higher needs. The needs, beginning at the lowest level and progressing to the highest, are physiological, or physical, needs; safety and security; love and affection; esteem; and self-actualization.

Needs are met or satisfied by direct and indirect methods. Direct methods meet and eliminate a need. Indirect methods, usually the use of defense mechanisms, reduce the need and help relieve the tension created by the unmet need.

Mastering these concepts will allow health care workers to develop good interpersonal relationships and provide more effective health care.

INTERNET SEARCHES

Use the suggested search engines in Chapter 17:4 of this textbook to search the Internet for additional information on the following topics:

1. *Erikson's stages of psychosocial development*: search for more details and examples of the stages of development

2. *Stages of human growth and development*: search words such as infancy, childhood, adolescence, puberty, and adulthood to obtain information on each stage

3. *Eating disorders*: search for statistics; signs and symptoms; and treatment of anorexia nervosa, bulimia, and bulimarexia

4. *Chemical or drug abuse*: search for statistics, signs/symptoms, and treatment of chemical and drug abuse (*Hint*: use words such as alcoholism and cocaine.)

5. *Suicide*: search for statistics, signs/symptoms, and ways to prevent suicide

6. *Death and dying*: search for information on Dr. Kübler-Ross, hospice care, palliative treatment, advance directives, and the right to die

7. *Maslow's hierarchy of needs*: search for additional information on each of the five levels of needs

8. *Defense mechanisms*: search for specific information on rationalization, projection, displacement, compensation, daydreaming, repression, suppression, denial, and withdrawal

REVIEW QUESTIONS

1. Differentiate between growth and development.

2. List the seven (7) life stages and at least two (2) physical, mental, emotional, and social developments that occur in each stage.

3. Create an example for what a patient and/or family member might say or do during each of the five (5) stages of death and dying.

4. Explain what is meant by the "right to die." Do you believe in this right? Why or why not?

5. Identify each level of Maslow's Hierarchy of Needs and give examples of specific needs at each level.

6. Create a specific example for each of the following defense mechanisms: rationalization, projection, displacement, compensation, daydreaming, repression, suppression, denial, and withdrawal.

CHAPTER 9

Nutrition and Diets

Observe Standard Precautions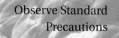

Instructor's Check—Call Instructor at This Point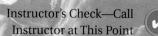

Safety—Proceed with Caution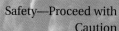

OBRA Requirement—Based on Federal Law

Math Skill

Legal Responsibility

Science Skill

Career Information

Communications Skill

Technology

Chapter Objectives

After completing this chapter, you should be able to:

◆ Define the term *nutrition* and list the effects of good and bad nutrition

◆ Name the six groups of essential nutrients and their functions and sources

◆ Differentiate between the processes of digestion, absorption, and metabolism

◆ Create a sample daily menu using the five major food groups and recommendations on *My Pyramid*

◆ Use the body mass index (BMI) graph to determine an individual's BMI

◆ Calculate an individual's daily required caloric intake to maintain current weight

◆ Name, describe, and explain the purposes of at least eight therapeutic diets

◆ Define, pronounce, and spell all key terms

KEY TERMS

absorption	essential nutrients	nutritional status
anorexia *(an-oh-rex'-ee"-ah)*	fat-restricted diets	obesity
antioxidants	fats	osteoporosis *(os-tee"-oh-*
atherosclerosis *(ath-eh-row"-*	hypertension *(high"-purr-*	*pour-oh'-sis)*
skleh-row'-sis)	*ten'-shun)*	overweight
basal metabolic rate (BMR)	kilocalorie (kcal) *(kill'-oh-*	peristalsis *(per-eh-stall"-sis)*
(base'-al met"-ah-ball'-ik)	*kall"-oh-ree)*	protein diets
bland diet	lipids	proteins
body mass index (BMI)	liquid diets	regular diet
calorie	low-cholesterol diet	sodium-restricted diets
calorie-controlled diets	low-residue diet	soft diet
carbohydrates	malnutrition	therapeutic diets *(ther"-ah-*
cellulose	metabolism *(meh-tab'-oh-*	*pew'-tick)*
cholesterol *(co"-less'-ter-all)*	*liz"-em)*	underweight
diabetic diet	minerals	vitamins
digestion	nutrition	wellness

9:1 Information

Fundamentals of Nutrition

People enjoy food and like to discuss it. Most people know that there is an important relationship between food and good health. However, many people do not know which nutrients are needed or why they are necessary. They are not able to select proper foods in their daily diets in order to promote optimum health. Therefore, it is important for every health care worker to have a solid understanding of basic nutrition. With this understanding, the health care worker can both practice and promote good nutrition.

Nutrition includes all body processes relating to food. These include digestion, absorption, metabolism, circulation, and elimination. These processes allow the body to use food for energy, maintenance of health, and growth. **Nutritional status** refers to the state or condition of one's nutrition. The goal is, of course, to be in a state of good nutrition and to maintain **wellness,** a state of good health with optimal body function. To do this, one must choose foods that are needed by the body, and not just foods that taste good.

Nutrition plays a large role in determining height, weight, strength, skeletal and muscular development, physical agility, resistance to dis-

ease, appetite, posture, complexion, mental ability, and emotional and psychological health. The immediate effects of good nutrition include a healthy appearance, a well-developed body, a good attitude, proper sleep and bowel habits, a high energy level, enthusiasm, and freedom from anxiety. In addition, the effects of good nutrition accumulate throughout life and may prevent or delay diseases or conditions such as the following:

♦ **Hypertension:** high blood pressure; may be caused by an excess amount of fat or salt in the diet; can lead to diseases of the heart, blood vessels, and kidneys

♦ **Atherosclerosis:** condition in which arteries are narrowed by the accumulation of fatty substances on their inner surfaces; thought to be caused by a diet high in saturated fats and cholesterol; can lead to heart attack or stroke

♦ **Osteoporosis:** condition in which bones become porous (full of tiny openings) and break easily; one cause is long-term deficiencies of calcium, magnesium, and vitamin D

♦ **Malnutrition:** the state of poor nutrition; may be caused by poor diet or illness. Symptoms include fatigue, depression, poor posture, being overweight or underweight, poor

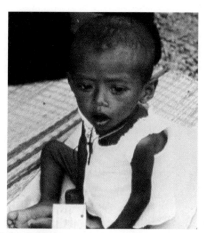

FIGURE 9-1 This child shows many of the signs of severe malnutrition. *(Courtesy of the Centers for Disease Control and Prevention, Public Health Image Library)*

TABLE 9-1 The Six Essential Nutrient Groups

NUTRIENT GROUPS	FUNCTIONS
Carbohydrates	Provide heat and energy Supply fiber for good digestion and elimination
Lipids (Fats)	Provide fatty acids needed for growth and development Provide heat and energy Carry fat-soluble vitamins (A, D, E, and K) to body cells
Proteins	Build and repair body tissue Provide heat and energy Help produce antibodies
Vitamins	Regulate body functions Build and repair body tissue
Minerals	Regulate body functions Build and repair body tissue
Water	Carries nutrients and wastes to and from body cells Regulates body functions

complexion, lifeless hair, and irritability (figure 9-1). It can cause deficiency diseases, poor muscular and skeletal development, reduced mental abilities, and even death. Malnutrition is most likely to affect individuals living in extreme poverty, patients undergoing drug therapy such as treatment for cancer, infants, young children, adolescents, and the elderly. Obesity is also a form of malnutrition, caused by excess food consumption.

9:2 INFORMATION

Essential Nutrients

Essential nutrients are composed of chemical elements found in food. They are used by the body to perform many different body functions. As the body uses the elements, they are replaced by elements in the food one eats. The essential nutrients are divided into six groups. The six groups and the specific functions of each group are shown in table 9-1.

CARBOHYDRATES

Carbohydrates are the major source of readily usable human energy. They are commonly called *starches* or *sugars*. Carbohydrates are a cheaper source of energy than are proteins and fats because they are mainly produced by plants. They are easily digested, grow well in most climates, and keep well without refrigeration. They are made of carbon, hydrogen, and oxygen.

The main sources of carbohydrates are breads, cereals, noodles or pastas, crackers, potatoes, corn, peas, beans, grains, fruits, sugar, and syrups.

Cellulose is the fibrous, indigestible form of plant carbohydrate. It is important because it provides bulk in the digestive tract and causes regular bowel movements. The best sources of cellulose are bran, whole-grain cereals, and fibrous fruits and vegetables.

LIPIDS (FATS)

Lipids, commonly called **fats** and oils, are organic compounds. Three of the most common lipids found in both food and the human body are *triglycerides* (fats and fatty acids), *phospholipids* (lecithin), and *sterols* (cholesterol). Lipids are also made of carbon, hydrogen, and oxygen, but they contain more oxygen than carbohydrates. Fats provide the most concentrated form of energy but are a more expensive source of energy than carbohydrates. Fats also maintain body temperature by providing insulation, cushion organs and bones, aid in the absorption of fat-soluble vitamins, and provide flavor to meals. The main sources of fats include butter, margarine, oils, cream, fatty meats, cheeses, and egg yolk.

Fats are also classified as saturated or polyunsaturated. *Saturated fats* are usually solid at room temperature. Examples include the fats in meats, eggs, whole milk, cream, butter, and cheeses. *Polyunsaturated fats* are usually soft or oily at room temperature. Examples include vegetable oils, margarines and other products made from vegetable oils, fish, and peanuts.

Cholesterol is a sterol lipid found in body cells and animal products. It is used in the production of steroid hormones, vitamin D, and bile acids. Cholesterol is also a component of cell membranes. Common sources are egg yolk, fatty meats, shellfish, butter, cream, cheeses, whole milk, and organ meats (liver, kidney, and brains). In addition, cholesterol is synthesized (manufactured) by the liver. Cholesterol is transported in the bloodstream mainly by two carrier molecules called *lipoproteins*. They are known as HDL and LDL, or high-density and low-density lipoprotein. HDL, commonly called "good" cholesterol, tends to transport cholesterol back to the liver and prevents plaque from accumulating on the walls of arteries. LDL, commonly called "bad" cholesterol, tends to contribute to plaque buildup and an excess amount leads to atherosclerosis. Consequently, it is advisable to limit the intake of foods that contain fats from animal sources.

PROTEINS

Proteins are the basic components of all body cells. They are essential for building and repairing tissue, regulating body functions, and providing energy and heat. They are made of carbon, hydrogen, oxygen, and nitrogen, and some also contain sulfur, phosphorus, iron, and iodine.

Proteins are made up of 22 "building blocks" called *amino acids*. Nine of these amino acids are essential to life. The proteins that contain these nine are called *complete proteins*. The best sources of complete proteins are animal foods such as meats, fish, milk, cheeses, and eggs. Proteins that contain any of the remaining 13 amino acids and some of the 9 essential amino acids are called *incomplete proteins*. Sources of incomplete proteins are usually vegetable foods such as cereals, soybeans, dry beans, peas, corn, and nuts. Choosing plant foods carefully can provide a mixture of amino acids from incomplete proteins that contain all the essential amino acids. It is important for a vegetarian to select foods that meet these dietary needs.

VITAMINS

Vitamins are organic compounds that are essential to life. They are important for metabolism, tissue building, and regulation of body processes. They allow the body to use the energy provided by carbohydrates, fats, and proteins. Only small amounts of vitamins are required, and a well-balanced diet usually provides the required vitamins. An excess amount of vitamins or a deficiency of vitamins can cause poor health.

Some vitamins are **antioxidants,** organic molecules that help protect the body from harmful chemicals called *free radicals*. In the body, oxygen used during metabolism causes free radicals to form. Free radicals can damage tissues, cells, and even genes in the same way that oxygen causes metals to rust or apples to become brown. Research is indicating that free radicals can lead to the development of chronic diseases such as cancer, heart disease, and arthritis. Antioxidants, found mainly in fruits and vegetables, deactivate the free radicals and prevent them from damaging body cells. The main antioxidant vitamins are vitamins A, C, and E.

Vitamins are usually classified as water soluble or fat soluble. *Water-soluble* vitamins dissolve in water, are not normally stored in the body, and are easily destroyed by cooking, air, and light. *Fat-soluble* vitamins dissolve in fat, can be stored in the body, and are not easily destroyed by cooking, air, and light. Some of the vitamins along with their sources and functions are listed in table 9-2.

MINERALS

Minerals are inorganic (nonliving) elements found in all body tissues. They regulate body fluids, assist in various body functions, contribute to growth, and aid in building tissues. Some minerals, such as selenium, zinc, copper, and manganese, are antioxidants. Table 9-3 lists some of the minerals essential to life, their sources, and their main functions.

TABLE 9-2 Vitamins

Vitamins	Best Sources	Functions
Fat-Soluble Vitamins		
Vitamin A (Retinol)	Liver, fatty fish Butter, margarine Whole milk, cream, cheese Egg yolk Leafy green and yellow vegetables	Growth and development Health of eyes Structure and functioning of the cells of the skin and mucous membranes Antioxidant to protect cells from free radicals
Vitamin D (Calciferol)	Sunshine (stimulates production in skin) Fatty fish, liver Egg yolk Butter, cream, fortified milk	Growth Regulates calcium and phosphorous absorption and metabolism Builds and maintains bones and teeth
Vitamin E (Tocopherol)	Vegetable oils, butter, margarine Peanuts Egg yolk Dark green leafy vegetables Soybeans and wheat germ	Necessary for protection of cell structure, especially red blood cells and epithelial cells Antioxidant to inhibit breakdown of vitamin A and some unsaturated fatty acids
Vitamin K	Spinach, kale, cabbage, broccoli Liver Soybean oil Cereals	Normal clotting of blood Formation of prothrombin
Water-Soluble Vitamins		
Thiamine (B_1)	Enriched bread and cereals Liver, heart, kidney, lean pork Potatoes, legumes	Carbohydrate metabolism Promotes normal appetite and digestion Normal function of nervous system
Riboflavin (B_2)	Milk, cheese, yogurt, eggs Enriched breads and cereals Dark green leafy vegetables Liver, kidney, heart, fish	Carbohydrate, fat, and protein metabolism Health of mouth tissue Healthy eyes
Niacin (Nicotinic Acid)	Meats (especially organ meats) Poultry and fish Enriched breads and cereals Peanuts and legumes	Carbohydrate, fat, and protein metabolism Healthy skin, nerves, and digestive tract
Pyridoxine (B_6)	Liver, kidney, pork Poultry and fish Enriched breads and cereals	Protein synthesis and metabolism Production of antibodies
Vitamin B_{12} (Cobalamin)	Liver, kidney, muscle meats, seafood Milk, cheese Eggs	Metabolism of proteins Production of healthy red blood cells Maintains nerve tissue
Vitamin C (Ascorbic Acid)	Citrus fruits, pineapple Melons, berries, tomatoes Cabbage, broccoli, green peppers	Healthy gums Aids in wound healing Aids in absorption of iron Formation of collagen
Folic Acid (Folacin)	Green leafy vegetables Citrus fruits Organ meats, liver Whole-grain cereals, yeast	Protein metabolism Maturation of red blood cells Formation of hemoglobin Synthesis of DNA Reduces risk for neural tube defect (spina bifida) in fetus—important for pregnant women to consume recommended daily amount

TABLE 9-3 Minerals

Minerals	Best Sources	Functions
Calcium (Ca)	Milk and milk products Cheese Salmon and sardines Some dark green leafy vegetables	Develops/maintains bones and teeth Clotting of the blood Normal heart and muscle action Nerve function
Phosphorus (P)	Milk and cheese Meat, poultry, fish Nuts, legumes Whole-grain cereals	Develops/maintains bones and teeth Maintains blood acid–base balance Metabolism of carbohydrates, fats, and proteins Constituent of body cells
Magnesium (Mg)	Meat, seafood Nuts and legumes Milk and milk products Cereal grains Fresh green vegetables	Constituent of bones, muscles, and red blood cells Healthy muscles and nerves Metabolism of carbohydrates and fats
Sodium (Na)	Salt Meat and fish Poultry and eggs Milk, cheese	Fluid balance, acid–base balance Regulates muscles and nerves Glucose (sugar) absorption
Potassium (K)	Meat Milk and milk products Vegetables Oranges, bananas, prunes, raisins Cereals	Fluid balance Regular heart rhythm Cell metabolism Proper nerve function Regulates contraction of muscles
Chlorine (Cl) (Chloride)	Salt Meat, fish, poultry Milk, eggs	Fluid balance Acid–base balance Formation of hydrochloric acid
Sulfur (S)	Meat, poultry, fish Eggs	Healthy skin, hair, and nails Activates energy-producing enzymes
Iron (Fe)	Liver, muscle meats Dried fruits Egg yolk Enriched breads and cereals Dark green leafy vegetables	Formation of hemoglobin in red blood cells Part of cell enzymes Aids in production of energy
Iodine (I)	Saltwater fish Iodized salt	Formation of hormones in thyroid gland Regulates basal metabolic rate
Copper (Cu)	Liver, organ meats, seafood Nuts, legumes Whole-grain cereals	Utilization of iron Component of enzymes Formation of hemoglobin in red blood cells
Fluorine (Fl) (Fluoride)	Fluoridated water Fish, meat, seafood	Healthy teeth and bones
Zinc (Zn)	Seafood, especially oysters Eggs Milk and milk products	Component of enzymes and insulin Essential for growth and wound healing
Selenium (Se)	Organ meats Seafood	Metabolism of fat Acts as antioxidant

WATER

Water is found in all body tissues. It is essential for the digestion (breakdown) of food, makes up most of the blood plasma and cytoplasm of cells, helps body tissues absorb nutrients, and helps move waste material through the body. Although water is found in almost all foods, the average person should still drink six to eight glasses of water each day to provide the body with the water it needs.

9:3 INFORMATION

Utilization of Nutrients

Before the body is able to use nutrients, it must break down the foods that are eaten to obtain the nutrients and then absorb them into the circulatory system. These processes are called *digestion* and *absorption* (figure 9-2). The actual use of the nutrients by the body is called *metabolism*. These processes are discussed in greater detail in Chapter 7:11 of this textbook.

DIGESTION

Digestion is the process by which the body breaks down food into smaller parts, changes the food chemically, and moves the food through the digestive system. There are two types of digestive action: mechanical and chemical. During mechanical digestion, food is broken down by the teeth and moved through the digestive tract by a process called **peristalsis,** a rhythmic, wavelike motion of the muscles. During chemical digestion, food is mixed with digestive juices secreted by the mouth, stomach, small intestine, and pancreas. The digestive juices contain enzymes, which break down the food chemically so the nutrients can be absorbed into the blood.

ABSORPTION

After the food is digested, absorption occurs. **Absorption** is the process in which blood or lymph capillaries pick up the digested nutrients. The nutrients are then carried by the circulatory system to every cell in the body. Most absorption occurs in the small intestine, but water, salts, and some vitamins are absorbed in the large intestine.

METABOLISM

After nutrients have been absorbed and carried to the body cells, **metabolism** occurs. This is the process in which nutrients are used by the cells

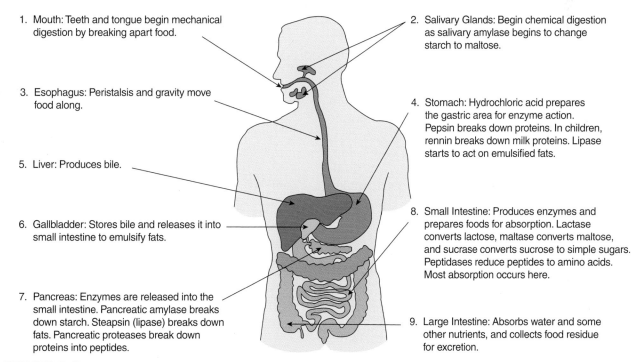

1. Mouth: Teeth and tongue begin mechanical digestion by breaking apart food.

2. Salivary Glands: Begin chemical digestion as salivary amylase begins to change starch to maltose.

3. Esophagus: Peristalsis and gravity move food along.

4. Stomach: Hydrochloric acid prepares the gastric area for enzyme action. Pepsin breaks down proteins. In children, rennin breaks down milk proteins. Lipase starts to act on emulsified fats.

5. Liver: Produces bile.

6. Gallbladder: Stores bile and releases it into small intestine to emulsify fats.

7. Pancreas: Enzymes are released into the small intestine. Pancreatic amylase breaks down starch. Steapsin (lipase) breaks down fats. Pancreatic proteases break down proteins into peptides.

8. Small Intestine: Produces enzymes and prepares foods for absorption. Lactase converts lactose, maltase converts maltose, and sucrase converts sucrose to simple sugars. Peptidases reduce peptides to amino acids. Most absorption occurs here.

9. Large Intestine: Absorbs water and some other nutrients, and collects food residue for excretion.

FIGURE 9-2 The processes of digestion and absorption.

for building tissue, providing energy, and regulating various body functions. During this process, nutrients are combined with oxygen, and energy and heat are released. Energy is required for voluntary work, such as swimming or housecleaning, and for involuntary work, such as breathing and digestion. The rate at which the body uses energy just for maintaining its own tissue, without doing any voluntary work, is called the **basal metabolic rate,** or **BMR.** The body needs energy continuously, so it stores some nutrients for future use. These stored nutrients are used to provide energy when food intake is not adequate for energy needs.

9:4 INFORMATION

Maintenance of Good Nutrition

Good health is everyone's goal, and good nutrition is the best way of achieving and maintaining it. Normally, this is accomplished by eating a balanced diet in which all of the required nutrients are included in correct amounts. The simplest guide for planning healthy meals is the *U.S. Department of Agriculture (USDA) Food Guide*, which classifies foods into five major food groups. Foods are arranged in groups containing similar nutrients. This is known as *My Pyramid* (figure 9-3). The pyramid has rainbow-hued bands running vertically. Each color represents a different food group. The width of the bands represents the relative proportionate amount of each group that an individual should consume every day. The importance of exercise is emphasized by the person climbing the side of the pyramid. *My Pyramid* stresses that one size does not fit everyone. Individuals are encouraged to utilize the *My Pyramid* Web site (*www.mypyramid.gov*) to develop a customized food plan based on age, sex, and physical activity. This helps an individual to make smart choices from every food group, determine the required balance between food and physical activity, and gain optimal nutrition from calories consumed.

An example of a food plan for an individual requiring 2,000 calories per day is shown in table 9-4. It lists the five major food groups, recommended daily amount, average serving size, and nutrient contents of the foods. A sample menu using these recommendations is shown in table 9-5.

Although the major food groups are a key to healthy meal plans, variety, taste, color, aroma, texture, and general food likes and dislikes must also be considered. If food is not appealing, people will usually not eat it even though it is healthy.

Sound and sensible nutritional principles can be found in the booklet published by the U.S. Department of Agriculture (USDA) and entitled *Finding Your Way to a Healthier You: Dietary Guidelines for Americans*. Some guidelines discussed in greater detail in the booklet include:

♦ *Make smart choices from every food group.* Eat a variety of foods. Choose different foods from each of the five major food groups each day. Adjust the number and size of portions based on body weight and nutritional needs. This helps provide the wide variety of nutrients required for good health.

♦ *Find your balance between food and physical activity.* Be physically active for at least 30 minutes most days of the week. Children, teenagers, and adults trying to lose weight should be physically active for 60 minutes each day. Maintain healthy weight. Determine your proper body weight and try to maintain this weight by proper eating habits and exercise.

♦ *Limit fats.* Choose a diet low in fat, saturated fat, and cholesterol. Eat lean meat, poultry without skin, fish, and low-fat dairy products. Use fats and oils sparingly and limit fried foods.

♦ *Get the most nutrition out of your calories.* Determine the correct number of calories you should eat daily. Then choose nutritionally rich foods that are high in nutrients but lower in calories. Choose a diet with plenty of vegetables, fruits, and grain products.

♦ *Don't sugarcoat it.* Use sugars only in moderation. Limit cookies, candy, cakes, and soft drinks. Brush and floss your teeth after eating sweet foods.

♦ *Reduce sodium (salt) and increase potassium.* Use salt and sodium only in moderation. Flavor foods with herbs and spices. Reduce the amount of salty foods. Eat foods high in potassium to counteract some of the effect of sodium on blood pressure.

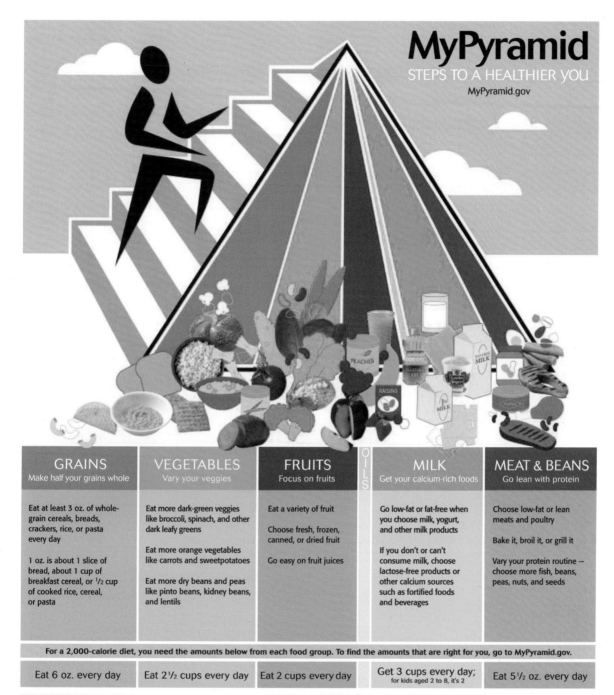

FIGURE 9-3 *My Pyramid* provides the guidelines for a healthier you. *(Courtesy of the U.S. Department of Agriculture, www.mypyramid.gov)*

TABLE 9-4 *My Pyramid* for a 2,000 Calorie Diet

FOOD GROUP	RECOMMENDED DAILY AMOUNT	AVERAGE RECOMMENDED PORTION SIZE	NUTRIENT CONTENT
Grains (Breads, Cereals, Rice, & Pasta)	6 ounces	1 slice bread 1/2 bagel or English muffin 1/2 cup cooked cereal 1/2 cup cooked pasta or rice 1 cup dry cereal	Carbohydrates; phosphorus; magnesium; potassium; iron; vitamins B, K, and folic acid
Vegetables	2 1/2 cups	1 cup raw leafy vegetables 1/2 cup cooked vegetables 3/4 cup vegetable juice	Carbohydrates; iron; calcium; potassium; magnesium; vitamins A, B, C, E, K, and folic acid
Fruits	2 cups	1 medium size fruit 1/2 cup canned/cooked fruit 1/4 cup dried fruit 1 cup fruit juice 1 cup fresh fruit	Carbohydrates; potassium; vitamin C and folic acid
Milk, Milk Products, Yogurt, & Cheese	3 cups	1 cup milk, yogurt, pudding 1 1/2 ounces cheese 1 cup cottage cheese 1 cup ice cream	Protein; carbohydrate; fat; calcium; potassium; sodium; magnesium; phosphorus; vitamins A, B_{12}, D, and riboflavin
Meats, Fish, Poultry, Dry Beans, Eggs, & Nuts	5 1/2 ounces	1 ounce meat, fish, or poultry 1/4 cup dry beans 1/2 cup cooked beans 1 egg 1 tablespoon peanut butter 1/2 ounce nuts	Proteins; fats; iron; sulfur; copper; iodine; sodium; magnesium; zinc; potassium; phosphorus; chlorine; fluorine; vitamins A, B, and D

TABLE 9-5 Sample Menu Using *My Pyramid* Guidelines

BREAKFAST	LUNCH	DINNER

1 cup orange juice
1 cup dry cereal
1 slice whole-grain toast
1 teaspoon margarine
1 cup fat-free milk
1 small banana
	Tuna fish sandwich:
	  2 slices wheat bread
	  3 ounces tuna
	  2 slices tomato
	  1 lettuce leaf
	8 small raw carrots
	1 oatmeal cookie
	1 unsweetened beverage
		3 ounces roasted chicken
		1/2 cup rice
		1/2 cup broccoli
		1 cup green salad
		1 tablespoon vinegar/oil dressing
		1 small dinner roll
		1/2 teaspoon margarine
		1 cup fat-free milk
		1 cup low-fat fruit yogurt

Suggested snacks: 1/4 cup dried fruit, 1/2 ounce nuts, 2 tablespoons raisins, 1 cup popcorn, 1 medium fruit

♦ *Read food labels to know the facts about the foods you eat.* Most foods have a Nutrition Facts label (figure 9-4). Check the label to determine the serving size and number of servings in the container. Evaluate the number of calories per serving to determine whether the food is a low- or high-calorie food. Calculate the amount of fat and try to keep total fat intake between 20 and 35 percent of total caloric intake. Look at the daily value percentage for each nutrient listed to determine whether the food is nutritious and worth eating. Avoid empty calories or high-caloric foods with no vitamins, minerals, carbohydrates, and/or proteins.

Nutrition Facts

Serving Size 1/2 cup (114g)
Servings Per Container 4

Amount Per Serving

Calories 90   Calories from Fat 30

	% Daily Value
Total Fat 3g	**5%**
Saturated Fat 0g	**0%**
Cholesterol 0mg	**0%**
Sodium 300mg	**13%**
Total Carbohydrate 13g	**4%**
Dietary Fiber 3g	**12%**
Sugars 3g	
Protein 3g	

Vitamin A	80%	•	Vitamin C	60%
Calcium	4%	•	Iron	4%

• Percent Daily Values are based on a 2,000 calorie diet. Your daily values may be higher or lower depending on your calorie needs:

		Calories	2,000	2,500
Total Fat	Less than		65g	80g
Sat Fat	Less than		20g	25g
Cholesterol	Less than		300mg	300mg
Sodium	Less than		2,400mg	2,400mg
Total Carbohydrate			300g	375g
Fiber			25g	30g

Calories per gram:
Fat 9   •   Carbohydrate 4   •   Protein 4

FIGURE 9-4 It is important to check food labels to determine the caloric and nutrient content of the food. *(Courtesy of the Food and Drug Administration)*

♦ *Be aware that alcohol can be harmful to your health.* If alcohol is consumed, it should be in moderation. Alcohol should be avoided by pregnant women, individuals using medications, children and adolescents, and individuals who are driving or engaging in an activity that requires attention or skill.

Following the preceding guidelines will result in a diet that will maintain and may even improve health.

Food habits also affect nutrition. At times, habits are based on cultural or religious beliefs. Different cultures and races have certain food preferences. Some religions require certain dietary restrictions that must be observed (see table 9-6). Unusual habits are not necessarily bad. They should be evaluated using the five major food groups as a guide. When habits do require changing in order to improve nutrition, the person making suggestions must use tact, patience, and imagination. Many food habits are formed during youth, and changing them is a difficult and slow process.

9:5 INFORMATION

Weight Management

Good nutrition and adequate exercise allow an individual to maintain a *normal* weight, or body weight that is in proportion to body height. Many charts are available to provide suggested ranges of weight based on an individual's height. In addition, a general formula can be used to calculate an approximate desired weight for adults. Basic principles include:

♦ *Male individuals*: For the first 60 inches (5 feet) of height, a male individual should weigh 106 pounds. For each inch over 60 inches, 6 pounds should be added. For example, a man measuring 74 inches (6 feet 2 inches) should weigh approximately 190 pounds: 106 pounds plus 84 pounds (6 pounds × 14 inches = 84) equals 190 pounds.

♦ *Female individuals*: For the first 60 inches of height, a female individual should weigh 100 pounds. For each inch over 60 inches, 5 pounds should be added. For example, a woman measuring 68 inches (5 feet 8 inches) should weigh approximately 140 pounds: 100 pounds plus 40 pounds (5 pounds × 8 inches) equals 140 pounds.

♦ *Large-boned individuals*: Increase the weight by 10 percent for individuals of either sex who have a large bone structure.

♦ *Small-boned individuals*: Decrease the weight by 10 percent for individuals of either sex who have a small bone structure.

Even though the above formulas provide a basic desired weight, most research has shown that a better indication of an individual's health status is body mass index. **Body mass index**

TABLE 9-6 Religious Dietary Restrictions

RELIGION	COFFEE & TEA	ALCOHOL	DAIRY PRODUCTS	PORK & PORK PRODUCTS	MEAT	SPECIAL RESTRICTIONS
Baptist (Strict)	Restricted	Prohibited				Some groups drink coffee and tea Many are ovolactovegetarians (use eggs and milk, but no meat)
Buddhist	Some sects prohibit	Some sects prohibit		Some sects abstain	Some sects abstain	Many sects are vegetarians Some sects eat beef and pork Some may refuse strong spices
Christian Scientist	Most avoid	Most avoid				
Greek Orthodox (Eastern Orthodox)			Wednesdays and Fridays during Lent and other Holy Days		Wednesdays and Fridays during Lent and other Holy Days	Avoid food and beverages before communion
Hindu		Most avoid		Prohibited	Beef prohibited because cow is sacred	Most are vegetarians Many do not use eggs as they represent life
Islamic, Muslim		Prohibited		Prohibited		Do not eat or drink during daylight hours in month of Ramadan Shellfish forbidden Meat must be slaughtered according to specific rules
Jewish (Orthodox)			Must not be prepared or eaten with meat	Prohibited	Must not be prepared or eaten with dairy products	Forbids cooking on Sabbath Shellfish forbidden Food must be prepared according to Kosher rules May fast on certain holy days
Mormon (Latter Day Saints)	Prohibited	Prohibited			Encouraged to eat sparingly	Cola and other caffeine drinks prohibited Some fast on the first Sunday of each month
Roman Catholic					Refrain from meat on Ash Wednesday and Fridays during Lent	Many avoid food and beverages 1 hour prior to communion
Seventh Day Adventist	Prohibited	Prohibited		Prohibited		Vegetarian diet is encouraged Avoid shellfish Prohibit foods containing caffeine

(BMI) is a calculation that measures weight in relation to height and correlates this with body fat. It is determined by dividing a person's weight in kilograms by height in meters squared. A graphic chart showing BMI ranges is the easiest way to determine BMI (figure 9-5). The ideal range is 18.5–24.9. A BMI less than 18.5 indicates the individual is underweight. A BMI greater than 25 is indicative of excess weight and more health risks.

UNDERWEIGHT AND OVERWEIGHT

Weight management is used to achieve and maintain the desired body weight. The major conditions that occur due to poor nutrition and improper exercise are underweight, overweight, and obesity.

Underweight is a body weight that is 10 to 15 percent less than the desired weight. Underweight individuals are much more likely to have nutritional deficiencies. Causes can include inadequate intake of food, excessive exercise, severe infections, eating disorders, diseases that cause anorexia (lack of appetite), and/or starvation. Treatment involves gradually increasing the amount of food consumed, eating higher calorie foods, counseling and medical treatment for eating disorders or diseases, and decreasing exercise if excessive exercise is a cause.

Overweight is a body weight that is 10–20 percent greater than the average recommended weight for a person's height. **Obesity** is excessive body weight 20 percent or more above the average recommended weight. Obesity has become a major health concern in the United States. Research by the National Center for Health Statistics shows that more than 30 percent of adults are obese. This means that more than 60 million adults in the United States are obese. Statistics also show that more than 15 percent of young people aged 6 to 17 are overweight. The main causes of obesity are excessive calorie consumption and inadequate physical activity. Genetic, psychological, biochemical (metabolic), socioeconomic, cultural, and environmental factors can contribute to these conditions. Treatment involves modifying eating habits and increasing physical activity. In more severe cases, medical intervention with medications, counseling, and even surgery may be necessary. If obesity is not controlled, an individual is at high risk for development of hypertension, diabetes mellitus, coronary heart disease, high cholesterol, cerebrovascular accident (stroke), osteoarthritis, gallbladder disease, breathing problems such as sleep apnea, and many other similar conditions. Research has also shown that obesity decreases life span and causes many early deaths.

Following the principles shown on *My Pyramid* and in the USDA dietary guidelines is the easiest way to manage weight. Every person should become familiar with these principles and make every attempt to follow them on a daily basis. Even though poor food habits are hard to break, it can be done if an individual is motivated to change his or her behavior.

MEASURING FOOD ENERGY

Foods vary in the amount of energy they contain. For example, a candy bar provides more energy than does an apple. When the body metabolizes nutrients to produce energy, heat is also released. The amount of heat produced during metabolism is the way the energy content of food is measured. This heat is measured by a unit called a **kilocalorie (kcal),** or just **calorie.** The number of kilocalories, or calories, in a certain food is known as that food's *caloric value.* Carbohydrates and proteins provide four calories per gram. Fat provides nine calories per gram. Vitamins, minerals, and water do not provide any calories.

An individual's caloric requirement is the number of kilocalories, or calories, needed by the body during a 24-hour period. Caloric requirements vary from person to person, depending on activity, age, size, sex, physical condition, and climate. The amount of physical activity or exercise is usually the main factor determining caloric requirement, because energy used must be replaced. An individual who wants to gain weight can decrease activity and increase caloric intake. An individual who wants to lose weight can increase activity and decrease caloric intake.

MANAGING WEIGHT

Most people know that maintaining desired body weight can lead to a longer and healthier life. For this reason, many individuals try many different

ARE YOU A HEALTHY WEIGHT?

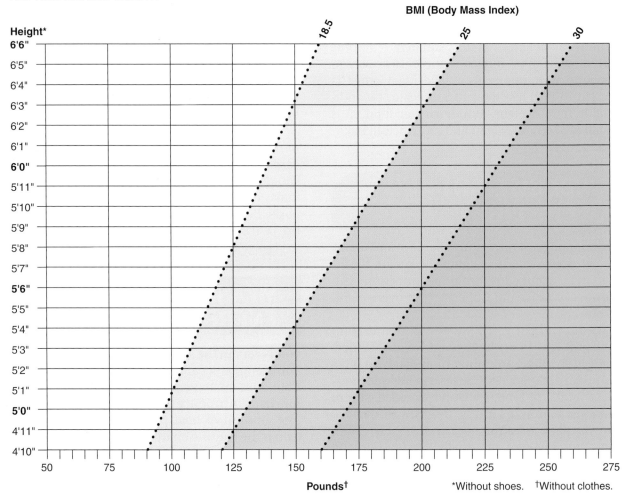

BMI measures weight in relation to height. The BMI ranges shown above are for adults. They are not exact ranges of healthy and unhealthy weights. However, they show that health risk increases at higher levels of overweight and obesity. Even within the healthy BMI range, weight gains can carry health risks for adults.

Directions: Find your weight on the bottom of the graph. Go straight up from that point until you come to the line that matches your height. Then look to find your weight group.

☐ **Healthy Weight** BMI from 18.5 up to 25 refers to healthy weight.

☐ **Overweight** BMI from 25 up to 30 refers to overweight.

☐ **Obese** BMI 30 or higher refers to obesity. Obese persons are also overweight.

Source: *Report of the Dietary Guidelines Advisory Committee on the Dietary Guidelines for Americans, 2000.*

FIGURE 9-5 Body mass index (BMI) helps individuals determine healthy weight ranges. *(From Report of the Dietary Guidelines Advisory Committee on the Dietary Guidelines for Americans, 2000)*

types of diets to lose weight. Research has shown that even though these diets might lead to weight loss, they usually do not allow an individual to maintain weight when the diet is no longer used. Most fad diets require eating specific foods, limiting certain food groups, eating large amounts of one type of food, or using liquid supplements in place of food. When individuals resume their normal eating habits, the weight that was lost is quickly regained.

The best method for weight control is to make desired changes slowly. Research has shown that gradual weight loss with a change in habits is much healthier and more likely to be sustained. For example, a person never exercises but knows that it is important. Initially, the person may walk at a slow pace for 15 minutes every day. Gradually, the time and rate can be increased until the person is walking at a brisk pace for 30 minutes 5 days a week. At the same time that exercise increases, the number of calories consumed must change.

Before starting any weight management plan, a physician should be consulted. The physician may perform a physical examination, order blood or other laboratory tests to check for diseases that could affect weight, run an electrocardiogram, and/or order a stress test to determine cardiovascular fitness. The physician can then recommend a nutrition plan and exercise program that is customized to the individual's needs.

⊕ A general guideline for weight loss or gain is that 1 pound of body fat equals approximately 3,500 calories. To lose 1 pound, a decrease of 3,500 calories is required, either by consuming 3,500 fewer calories or by using 3,500 calories through increased exercise. To gain 1 pound, an increase of 3,500 calories is required. A general guideline to maintain weight is that a person consume 15 calories per pound per day. For example, if a person weighs 120 pounds, maintaining this weight would require a daily intake of 15×120, or 1,800, calories daily. By decreasing caloric intake by 500 calories per day, a person would lose 1 pound per week (500 calories per day times 7 days equals 3,500 calories, or 1 pound of fat). By increasing caloric intake by 500 calories per day, a person would gain 1 pound per week. It is important to note that increasing or decreasing exercise along with controlling calorie intake is essential. Also, a slow, steady gain or loss of 1–2 pounds per week is an efficient and safe form of weight control.

The USDA *Dietary Guidelines* recommendations for managing weight include:

♦ Balance calories from foods and beverages with calories expended

♦ Prevent gradual weight gain by making small decreases in daily calories and small increases in physical activity

♦ Engage in at least 30 minutes or more of moderate-intensity physical activity most days of the week

♦ Consume less than 10 percent of calories from saturated fatty acids and less than 300 milligrams of cholesterol daily

♦ Keep daily total fat intake to between 20 and 35 percent of calories consumed

♦ Select lean, low-fat, or fat-free foods whenever possible

♦ Eat more fiber-rich fruits, vegetables, and whole grains

♦ Limit foods high in sugar and salt

Following these recommendations can help an individual obtain and maintain a healthy weight. This will help reduce the risk factor for heart disease, hypertension, diabetes mellitus, high cholesterol, osteoarthritis, and many other diseases. It will also allow the individual to enjoy a longer and healthier life span.

9:6 Information

Therapeutic Diets

Therapeutic diets are modifications of the normal diet and are used to improve specific health conditions. They are normally prescribed by a doctor and planned by a dietitian. These diets may change the nutrients, caloric content, and/or texture of the normal diet. They may seem strange and even unpleasant to patients. In addition, a patient's appetite may be affected by **anorexia** (loss of appetite), weakness, illness, loneliness, self-pity, and other factors. Therefore, it is essential that the health care worker use patience and tact to convince the patient to eat the foods on the diet. An understanding of the purposes of the various diets will also help the health care worker provide simple explanations to patients.

REGULAR DIET

A **regular diet** is a balanced diet usually used for the patient with no dietary restrictions. At times, it has a slightly reduced calorie content. Foods such as rich desserts, cream sauces, salad dressings, and fried foods may be decreased or omitted.

LIQUID DIETS

Liquid diets include both clear liquids and full liquids. Both are nutritionally inadequate and should be used only for short periods of time. All foods served must be liquid at body temperature. Foods included on the clear-liquid diet are mainly carbohydrates and water, including apple or grape juice, fat-free broths, plain gelatin, fruit ice, ginger ale, and tea or black coffee with sugar (figure 9-6). The full-liquid diet includes the liquids allowed on the clear-liquid diet plus strained soups and cereals, fruit and vegetable juices, yogurt, hot cocoa, custard, ice cream, pudding, sherbet, and eggnog. These diets may be used after surgery, for patients with acute infections or digestive problems, to replace fluids lost by vomiting or diarrhea, and before some X-rays of the digestive tract.

SOFT DIET

A **soft diet** is similar to the regular diet, but foods must require little chewing and be easy to digest (figure 9-7). Foods to avoid include meat and shellfish with tough connective tissue, coarse cereals, spicy foods, rich desserts, fried foods, raw fruits and vegetables, nuts, and coconut. This diet may be used following surgery or for patients with infections, digestive disorders, or chewing problems.

DIABETIC DIET

A **diabetic diet** is used for patients with diabetes mellitus. In this condition, the body does not produce enough of the hormone insulin to metabolize carbohydrates. Patients frequently take insulin by injection. The diet contains exchange lists that group foods according to type, nutrients, and caloric content. Patients are allowed a certain number of items from each exchange list according to their individual needs. Sugar-heavy foods such as candy, soft drinks, desserts, cookies, syrup, honey, condensed milk, chewing gum, and jams and jellies are usually avoided.

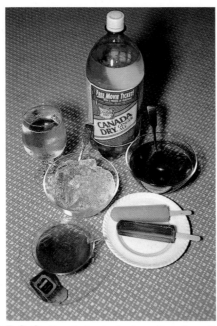

FIGURE 9-6 Foods included on the clear-liquid diet are mainly carbohydrates and water.

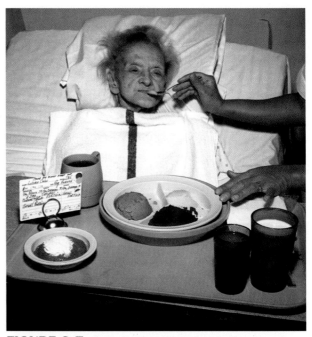

FIGURE 9-7 Soft diets include foods that require little chewing and are easy to digest.

CALORIE-CONTROLLED DIETS

Calorie-controlled diets include both low-calorie and high-calorie diets. Low-calorie diets are frequently used for patients who are overweight. High-calorie foods are either avoided or very limited. Examples of such foods include butter, cream, whole milk, cream soups or gravies, sweet soft drinks, alcoholic beverages, salad dressings, fatty meats, candy, and rich desserts. High-calorie diets are used for patients who are underweight or have anorexia nervosa, hyperthyroidism (overactivity of thyroid gland), or cancer. Extra proteins and carbohydrates are included. High-bulk foods such as green salads, watermelon, and fibrous fruits are avoided because they fill up the patient too soon. High-fat foods such as fried foods, rich pastries, and cheese cake are avoided because they digest slowly and spoil the appetite.

LOW-CHOLESTEROL DIET

A **low-cholesterol diet** restricts foods that contain cholesterol. It is used for patients with atherosclerosis and heart disease. Foods high in saturated fat, such as beef, liver, pork, lamb, egg yolk, cream cheese, natural cheeses, shellfish (crab, shrimp, lobster), and whole milk, are limited, as are coconut and palm oil products.

FAT-RESTRICTED DIETS

Fat-restricted diets are also called *low-fat diets*. Examples of foods to avoid include cream, whole milk, cheeses, fats, fatty meats, rich desserts, chocolate, nuts, coconut, fried foods, and salad dressings. Fat-restricted diets may be used for obese patients or patients with gallbladder and liver disease or atherosclerosis.

SODIUM-RESTRICTED DIETS

Sodium-restricted diets are also called *low-sodium* or *low-salt diets*. Frequently, patients use low-sodium-diet lists similar to the carbohydrate-exchange lists used by diabetic patients. Patients should avoid or limit adding salt to food, smoked meats or fish, processed foods, pickles, olives, sauerkraut, and some processed cheeses. This diet reduces salt intake for patients with cardiovascular diseases (such as hypertension or congestive heart failure), kidney disease, and edema (retention of fluids).

PROTEIN DIETS

Protein diets include both low-protein and high-protein diets. Protein-rich foods include meats, fish, milk, cheeses, and eggs. These foods would be limited or decreased in low-protein diets and increased in high-protein diets. Low-protein diets are ordered for patients with certain kidney or renal diseases and certain allergic conditions. High-protein diets may be ordered for children and adolescents, if growth is delayed; for pregnant or lactating (milk-producing) women; before and/or after surgery; and for patients suffering from burns, fevers, or infections.

BLAND DIET

A **bland diet** consists of easily digested foods that do not irritate the digestive tract. Foods to be avoided include coarse foods, fried foods, highly seasoned foods, pastries, candies, raw fruits and vegetables, alcoholic and carbonated beverages, smoked and salted meats or fish, nuts, olives, avocados, coconut, whole-grain breads and cereals, and usually, coffee and tea. It is used for patients with ulcers, colitis, and other diseases of the digestive system.

LOW-RESIDUE DIET

A **low-residue diet** eliminates or limits foods that are high in bulk and fiber. Examples of such foods include raw fruits and vegetables, whole-grain breads and cereals, nuts, seeds, beans, peas, coconut, and fried foods. It is used for patients with digestive and rectal diseases, such as colitis or diarrhea.

OTHER DIETS

Other therapeutic diets that restrict or increase certain nutrients may also be ordered. The health care worker should always check the prescribed

TODAY'S RESEARCH: TOMORROW'S HEALTH CARE

A daily pill that prevents heart attacks and strokes?

Heart disease is the main cause of death in the United States. The American Heart Association estimates that in the United States alone, 70.1 million people have some form of cardiovascular (heart and blood vessel) disease. Each year more than 1 million people have a heart attack. More than 800,000 people die of heart disease. Stroke is the third largest cause of death in the United States. Each year about 700,000 people have a stroke; of these, almost 275,000 die.

In Europe, researchers are evaluating a pill that will reduce heart attacks and strokes by almost 80 percent. It has been called a "super vitamin" because it is a once-daily pill. The pill contains six different types of medicines: aspirin, a cholesterol-lowering drug, three blood pressure–lowering drugs, and folic acid. Aspirin is used to regulate the level of platelets (blood cells that aid in the clotting of blood). Cholesterol is a type of fat found in animal products. Its presence in high amounts can cause fatty deposits on the walls of blood vessels. The three blood pressure–lowering drugs are used in small amounts, but each has a different way to reduce blood pressure. Folic acid, a vitamin, is used to reduce the amount of a protein that may contribute to blocked arteries.

The current problem is to ensure that all of the combined ingredients do not cause other chemical reactions. The drug must be stable over a period of time, and care must be taken so that the products do not break down or deteriorate. Researchers are also experimenting with the "ideal" amount of each ingredient. It may even be necessary to create "super pills" with different amounts of the six ingredients to account for individual differences. However, if these problems can be solved, people could stay much healthier by taking one "super vitamin" each day. Thousands of lives could be saved each year through the prevention of heart attacks and strokes.

---

diet and ask questions if foods seem incorrect. Every effort should be made to include foods the patient likes if they are allowed on a particular diet. If a patient will not eat the foods on a prescribed therapeutic diet, the diet will not contribute to good nutrition.

STUDENT: *Go to the workbook and complete the assignment sheet for Chapter 9, Nutrition and Diets.*

CHAPTER 9 SUMMARY

An understanding of basic nutrition is essential for health care workers. Good nutrition helps maintain wellness, a state of good health with optimal body function.

Essential nutrients are used by the body to perform many different functions. There are six groups of essential nutrients: carbohydrates, fats, proteins, vitamins, minerals, and water.

Daily food intake should provide an individual with proper amounts of the essential nutrients.

Before the body can obtain the essential nutrients from food, the body must digest the food. After digestion, the nutrients are absorbed and carried by the circulatory system to every cell in the body. Metabolism then occurs, and the nutrients are used by cells for body functions.

The simplest guide for planning healthy meals that provide the required essential nutrients is to eat a variety of foods from the five major food groups. Portion sizes should vary according to the individual's caloric requirements. Maintaining healthy weight, choosing foods low in fat, using sugar and salt in moderation, and limiting alcoholic beverages are also important aspects of proper nutrition.

Weight management is used to achieve and maintain the desired body weight. The major conditions that occur because of poor nutrition and improper exercise are underweight, overweight, and obesity. Careful control of caloric intake and regular physical exercise are the key methods for obtaining and maintaining normal weight, or body weight that is in proportion to body height. Good weight management reduces the risk factor for many diseases and allows an individual to enjoy a longer and healthier life span.

Therapeutic diets are modifications of the normal diet. They are used to improve specific health conditions. Examples of therapeutic diets include liquid, diabetic, calorie-controlled, low-cholesterol, fat- or sodium-restricted, high- or low-protein, and bland diets. An understanding of these diets will allow the health care worker to encourage patients to follow prescribed diets.

INTERNET SEARCHES

Use the suggested search engines in Chapter 17:4 of this textbook to search the Internet for additional information on the following topics:

1. *Nutritional status*: search words such as nutrition, diet, and nutritional status

2. *Diseases*: search for more detailed information on nutritional diseases such as hypertension, atherosclerosis, osteoporosis, and malnutrition

3. *Essential nutrients*: search for information on daily nutritional requirements for nutrients such as carbohydrates, proteins, lipids or fats, vitamins, and minerals

4. *Utilization of nutrients*: search for information on the processes of digestion, absorption, and metabolism

5. *Food energy*: use words such as weight loss, weight gain, and diet to learn more about weight control by proper nutrition

6. *Organizations*: obtain additional information on nutrition from organizations such as the U.S. Department of Agriculture and the American Dietetic Association

7. *Therapeutic diets*: determine foods allowed or foods that must be avoided in diabetic, calorie-controlled, low-cholesterol, fat-restricted, sodium-restricted, low-residue, bland, and high- or low-protein diets

REVIEW QUESTIONS

1. List the six (6) essential nutrients and the main function of each nutrient.

2. Differentiate between digestion, absorption, and metabolism.

3. What is BMR?

4. List all of the foods you have eaten today. Be sure to include all snacks. Compare your list with the recommended daily intake of various foods from *My Pyramid*. Is your diet adequate or deficient? Explain why.

5. Differentiate between overweight and obesity. List six (6) conditions that can develop as a result of obesity.

6. What is BMI? Calculate your BMI.

7. Calculate the number of calories you require per day to maintain your present weight. How many calories should you ingest per day to gain one pound per week? How many calories should you ingest per day to lose one pound per week?

8. Identify the type of therapeutic diet that may be ordered for patients with the following conditions:
   a. gallbladder or liver disease
   b. diabetes mellitus
   c. hypertension or heart disease
   d. ulcers, colitis, or diseases of the digestive tract
   e. pregnant or lactating women
   f. severe nausea, vomiting, and/or diarrhea

PART 3

Special Considerations in Health Care

CHAPTER 10 Cultural Diversity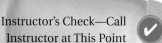

Chapter Objectives

After completing this chapter,
you should be able to:

- ♦ List the four basic characteristics of culture

- ♦ Differentiate between culture, ethnicity, and race

- ♦ Identify some of the major ethnic groups in the United States

- ♦ Provide an example of acculturation in the United States

- ♦ Create an example of how a bias, prejudice, or stereotype can cause a barrier to effective relationships with others

- ♦ Describe at least five ways to avoid bias, prejudice, and stereotyping

- ♦ Differentiate between a nuclear family and an extended family

- ♦ Identify ways in which language, personal space, touching, eye contact, and gestures are affected by cultural diversity

- ♦ Compare and contrast the diverse health beliefs of different ethnic/cultural groups

- ♦ List five ways health care providers can show respect for an individual's religious beliefs

- ♦ Identify methods that can be used to show respect for cultural diversity

- ♦ Define, pronounce, and spell all key terms

Observe Standard Precautions

Instructor's Check—Call Instructor at This Point

Safety—Proceed with Caution

OBRA Requirement—Based on Federal Law

Math Skill

Legal Responsibility

Science Skill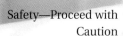

Career Information

Communications Skill

Technology

KEY TERMS

acculturation	ethnocentric	personal space
agnostic	extended family	prejudice
atheist	holistic care	race
bias	matriarchal *(may'-tree-ar"-kel)*	religion
cultural assimilation		sensitivity
cultural diversity	nuclear family	spirituality
culture	patriarchal *(pay'-tree-ar"-kel)*	stereotyping
ethnicity		

10:1 INFORMATION

Culture, Ethnicity, and Race

Health care providers must work with and provide care to many different people. At the same time, they must respect the individuality of each person. Therefore, every health care provider must be aware of the factors that cause each individual to be unique. Uniqueness is influenced by many things including physical characteristics (sex, body size, and hair, nail, and skin color), family life, socioeconomic status, religious beliefs, geographical location, education, occupation, and life experiences. A major influence on any individual's uniqueness is the person's cultural/ethnic heritage.

Culture is defined as the values, beliefs, attitudes, languages, symbols, rituals, behaviors, and customs unique to a particular group of people and passed from one generation to the next. It is often defined as a set of rules, because culture provides an individual with a blueprint or general design for living. Family relations, child rearing, education, occupational choice, social interactions, spirituality, religious beliefs, food preferences, health beliefs, and health care are all influenced by culture. Culture is not uniform among all members within a cultural group, but it does provide a foundation for behavior. Even though differences exist between cultural groups and in individuals within a cultural group, all cultures have four basic characteristics:

♦ *Culture is learned*: Culture does not just happen. It is taught to others. For example, children learn patterns of behavior by imitating

adults and developing attitudes accepted by others.

♦ *Culture is shared*: Common practices and beliefs are shared with others in a cultural group.

♦ *Culture is social in nature*: Individuals in the cultural group understand appropriate behavior based on traditions that have been passed from generation to generation.

♦ *Culture is dynamic and constantly changing*: New ideas may generate different standards for behavior. This allows a cultural group to meet the needs of the group by adapting to environmental changes.

Ethnicity is a classification of people based on national origin and/or culture. Members of an ethnic group may share a common heritage, geographic location, social customs, language, and beliefs. Even though every individual in an ethnic group may not practice all of the beliefs of the group, the individual is still influenced by other members of the group. There are many different ethnic groups in the United States (figure 10-1). Some of the common ethnic groups and their countries of origin include:

♦ *African American*: Central and South African countries, Dominican Republic, Haiti, and Jamaica

♦ *Asian/Pacific American*: Cambodia, China, Guam, Hawaii, India, Indonesia and Pacific Island countries, Japan, Korea, Laos, Philippines, Samoa, and Vietnam

♦ *European American*: England, France, Germany, the Netherlands, Ireland, Italy, Norway,

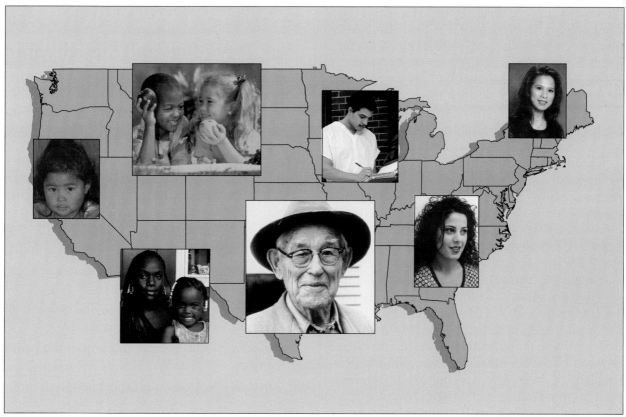

FIGURE 10-1 The many faces of the United States.

Poland, Russia, Scandinavia, Scotland, and Switzerland

♦ *Hispanic American*: Cuba, Mexico, Puerto Rico, Spain, and Spanish-speaking countries in Central and South America

♦ *Middle Eastern/Arabic Americans*: Egypt, Iran, Iraq, Jordan, Kuwait, Lebanon, Palestine, Saudi Arabia, Yemen, and other North African and Middle Eastern countries

♦ *Native American*: more than 500 tribes of American Indians and Eskimos

It is important to recognize that within each of the ethnic groups, there are numerous subgroups, each with its own lifestyle and beliefs. For example, the European American group includes Italians and Germans, two groups with different languages and lifestyles.

Race is a classification of people based on physical or biological characteristics such as the color of skin, hair, and eyes; facial features; blood type; and bone structure. Race is frequently used to label a group of people and explain patterns of behavior. In reality, race cuts across multiple ethnic/cultural groups, and it is the values, beliefs, and behaviors learned from the ethnic/cultural group that generally account for the behaviors attributed to race. For example, blacks from Africa and blacks from the Caribbean both share many of the same physical characteristics, but they have different cultural beliefs and values. In addition, there are different races present in most ethnic groups. For example, there are white and black Hispanics, white Africans and Caribbeans, and white and black Asians.

Culture, ethnicity, and race do influence an individual's behavior, self-perception, judgment of others, and interpersonal relationships. These differences based on cultural, ethnic, and racial factors are called **cultural diversity.** It is important to remember that differences exist within ethnic/cultural groups and in individuals within a group. In previous times, the United States has often been called a "melting pot" to represent the absorption of many cultures into the dominant culture through a process called **cultural assimilation.** Cultural assimilation requires that the newly arrived cultural group alter unique beliefs and behaviors and adopt the ways of the dominant culture. In reality, the United States is striving to be more like a "salad bowl" where cultural differences are appreciated and respected. The simultaneous existence of various ethnic/cultural groups gives rise to a "multicultural" society that must recognize and respect many different beliefs. **Acculturation,** or the process of learning the beliefs and behaviors of a dominant culture and assuming some of the characteristics, does occur. However, acculturation occurs slowly over a long period, usually many years. Recent immigrants to the United States are more likely to use the language and follow the patterns of behavior of the country from which they emigrated. Second- and third-generation Americans are more likely to use English as their main language and follow the patterns of behavior prevalent in the United States (figure 10-2).

Because they provide care to culturally diverse patients in a variety of settings, health care providers must be aware of these factors and remember that no individual is 100 percent anything! Every individual has and will continue to create new and changing blends of values and beliefs. **Sensitivity,** the ability to recognize and appreciate the personal characteristics of others, is essential in health care. For example, in some cultures such as Native Americans or Asians, calling an adult by a first name is not acceptable except for close friends or relatives. Sensitive health care workers will address patients by their last names unless they are asked to use a patient's first name.

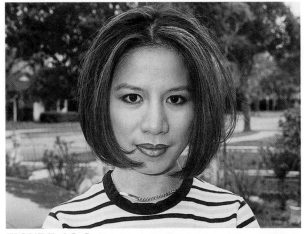

FIGURE 10-2 Second- or third-generation individuals in the same ethnic/cultural group will adopt many patterns of behavior dominant in the United States.

10:2 INFORMATION

Bias, Prejudice, and Stereotyping

Bias, prejudice, and stereotyping can interfere with acceptance of cultural diversity. A **bias** is a preference that inhibits impartial judgment. For example, individuals who believe in the supremacy of their own ethnic group are called **ethnocentric.** These individuals believe that their cultural values are better than the cultural values of others, and may antagonize and alienate people from other cultures. Individuals may also be biased with regard to other factors. Examples of common biases include:

◆ *Age:* Young people are physically and mentally superior to older people.

◆ *Education:* College-educated individuals are superior to uneducated individuals.

◆ *Economic:* Rich people are superior to poor people.

◆ *Physical size:* Obese and short people are inferior.

◆ *Occupation:* Nurses are inferior to doctors.

◆ *Sexual preference:* Homosexuals are inferior to heterosexuals.

◆ *Gender:* Women are inferior to men.

Prejudice means to prejudge. A prejudice is a strong feeling or belief about a person or subject that is formed without reviewing facts or information. Prejudiced individuals regard their ideas or behavior as right and other ideas or behavior as wrong. They are frequently afraid of things that are different. Prejudice causes fear and distrust and interferes with interpersonal relationships. Every individual is prejudiced to some degree. We all want to feel that our beliefs are correct. In health care, however, it is important to be aware of our prejudices and to make every effort to obtain as much information about a situation as possible. This allows us to learn about other individuals, understand their beliefs, and communicate successfully.

Stereotyping occurs when an assumption is made that everyone in a particular group is the same. A stereotype ignores individual characteristics and "labels" an individual. A classic example is, "All blondes are dumb." This stereotype has been perpetuated by "blonde jokes" detrimental to individuals who have light colored hair. Similar stereotypes exist with regard to race, sex, body size (thin, obese, short, or tall), occupation, and ethnic/cultural group. It is essential to remember that everyone is a unique individual. Each person will have different life experiences and exposure to other cultures and ideas. This allows a person to develop a unique personality and lifestyle.

Bias, prejudice, and stereotyping are barriers to effective relationships with others. Health care providers must be alert to these barriers and make every effort to avoid them. Some ways to avoid bias, prejudice, and stereotyping include:

♦ Know and be consciously aware of your own personal and professional values and beliefs.

♦ Obtain as much information as possible about different ethnic/cultural groups.

♦ Be sensitive to behaviors and practices different from your own.

♦ Remember that you are not being pressured to adopt other beliefs, but that you must respect them.

♦ Develop friendships with a wide variety of people from different ethnic/cultural groups.

♦ Ask questions and encourage questions from others to share ideas and beliefs.

♦ Evaluate all information before you form an opinion.

♦ Be open to differences.

♦ Avoid jokes that may offend.

♦ Remember that mistakes happen. Apologize if you hurt another person, and forgive if another person hurts you.

10:3 INFORMATION

Understanding Cultural Diversity

The cultural and ethnic beliefs of an individual will affect the behavior of the individual. Health care providers must be aware of these beliefs in order to provide **holistic care;** that is, care that provides for the well-being of the whole person and meets not only physical needs, but also social, emotional, and mental needs. Some areas of cultural diversity include family organization, language, personal space, touching, eye contact, gestures, health care beliefs, spirituality, and religion.

FAMILY ORGANIZATION

Family organization refers to the structure of a family and the dominant or decision-making person in a family. Families vary in their composition and in the roles assumed by family members. A **nuclear family** usually consists of a mother, father, and children (figure 10-3). It may also consist of a single parent and child(ren). An **extended family** includes the nuclear family plus grandparents, aunts, uncles, and cousins (figure 10-4). The nuclear family is usually the basic unit in European American families, but the extended family is important. The basic unit for Asian, Hispanic, and Native Americans is generally the extended family, and frequently, several different generations live in the same household. This affects care of children, the sick, and the elderly. In extended family cultures, families tend

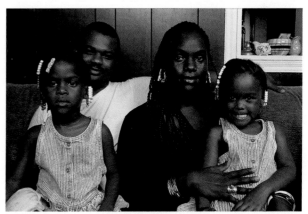

FIGURE 10-3 A nuclear family usually consists of a mother, father, and children.

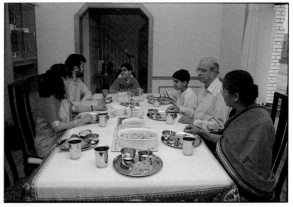

FIGURE 10-4 An extended family includes grandparents, aunts, uncles, and cousins in addition to the nuclear family.

to take care of their children and sick or elderly relatives in their home. For example, most Asian families have great respect for their elders and consider it a privilege to care for them. In some nuclear family cultures, people outside the family frequently care for children and sick or elderly relatives. Never assume anything about a family's organization. It is important to ask questions and observe the family.

Some families are **patriarchal** and the father or oldest male is the authority figure. In a **matriarchal** family, the mother or oldest female is the authority figure. This also affects health care. In a patriarchal family, the dominant male will make most health care decisions for all family members. For example, in some Asian and Middle Eastern families, men have the power and authority, and women are expected to be obedient. Husbands frequently accompany their wives to medical appointments and expect to make all the medical care decisions. In a matriarchal family, the dominant female may assume this responsibility. For example, if the mother or other female is the dominant figure in a family, she will make the health decisions for all members of the family. In many families, both the mother and father share the decisions. Regardless of who the decision maker is, respect for the individual and the family must be the primary concern for the health care worker. Health care providers must respect patients who state, "I have to check with my husband (wife) before I decide if I should have the surgery."

Recognition and acceptance of family organization is essential for health care providers. Patients who have extended families as basic units may have many visitors in a hospital or long-term care center. Everyone will be concerned with the care provided, and all family members may help make decisions regarding care. At times, family members may even insist on providing basic personal care to the patient, such as bathing or hair care. Health care providers must adapt to these situations and allow the family to assist as much as possible.

To determine a patient's family structure and learn about a patient's preferences, the health care provider should talk with the patient or ask questions. Examples of questions that can be asked include:

♦ Who are the members of your family?

♦ Do you have any children? Who will care for them while you are sick?

♦ Do you have extended family? For example, aunts, uncles, cousins, nephews, nieces?

♦ Who will be caring for you while you are sick?

♦ Who is the head of the household?

♦ Where do you and your family live?

♦ Was your entire family born in the United States?

♦ What do you and your family do together for recreation?

♦ Do you have family members who will be visiting you? (If patient is admitted to a health care facility)

LANGUAGE

In the United States, the dominant language is English, but many other languages are also spoken. Statistics from the U.S. Census Bureau verified that more than 20 percent of the population younger than age 65 speaks a language other than English at home. There are even variations within a language caused by different dialects. For example, the German taught in school may differ from the language spoken by Germans from different areas of Germany. Health care providers frequently encounter patients who do not use English as a dominant language. The health care provider must determine the patient's ability to communicate by talking with the patient or a relative and asking questions such as:

♦ Do you speak English as your primary language?

♦ What language is spoken at home?

♦ Do you read English? Do you read another language?

♦ Do you have a family member or friend who can interpret information for you?

Whenever possible, try to find an interpreter who speaks the language of the patient (figure 10-5). Frequently, another health care worker, a consultant, or a family member may be able to assist in the communication process. Most health care facilities have a roster of employees who speak other languages.

When providing care to people who have limited English-speaking abilities, speak slowly, use simple words, use gestures or pictures to clarify the meaning of words, and use nonver-

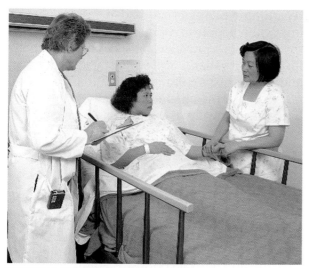

FIGURE 10-5 Whenever possible, try to find an interpreter to assist in communicating with a non-English-speaking patient.

bal communication in the form of a smile or gentle touch if it is culturally appropriate. Avoid the tendency to speak louder because this does not improve comprehension. Whenever possible, try to obtain feedback from the patient to determine whether the patient understands the information that has been provided.

Most patients appreciate it when a health care worker can speak even a few words in the patient's language. Make every attempt to try to learn some words or phrases in the patient's language. Even a few words allow you to show the patient that you are trying to communicate. If you work with many patients who speak a common language, such as Spanish, try to master the basics of that language by taking an introductory course or by using an audiotape.

Other resources are also available to help a health care provider meet the needs of a non-English-speaking patient. Many health care facilities have health care information or questions printed in several languages. Cards can be purchased that explain basic health care procedures or treatments in many other languages.

Most states require that any medical permit requiring a written signature be printed in the patient's language to ensure that the patient understands what he or she is signing. Health care providers must be aware of legal requirements for non-English-speaking patients and make sure that these requirements are met.

PERSONAL SPACE AND TOUCH

Personal space, often called *territorial space,* describes the distance people require to feel comfortable while interacting with others. This varies greatly among different ethnic/cultural groups. Some cultures are called "close contact" and others are called "distant contact." Individuals from close-contact cultures are comfortable standing very close to and even touching the person with whom they are interacting. For example, Arabs are a very close-contact group; they touch, feel, and smell people with whom they interact. French and Latin Americans tend to stand very close together while talking. Hispanic Americans are also comfortable with close contact and use hugs and handshakes to greet others. Even within a cultural group, there are variations. For example, women tend to stand closer together than men do, and children stand closer together than adults do. European and African Americans prefer some space (approximately 2–6 feet) during interactions, but do not hesitate to shake hands as a greeting. Asian Americans will stand closer, but usually do not touch during a conversation. Kissing or hugging is reserved for intimate relationships and is never done in public view. In Cambodia, members of the opposite sex may never touch each other in public, not even brothers and sisters. In addition, only a parent can touch the head of a child. The Vietnamese allow only the elderly to touch the head of a child because the head is considered sacred. In some Middle Eastern countries, men may not touch female individuals who are not immediate family members, and only men may shake hands with other men. This may cause a female from one of these countries to refuse personal health care provided by a male health care provider. For Native Americans, personal space is important, but they will lightly touch another person's hand during greetings. It is important to understand that these situations are examples. You must never assume anything about an individual's personal space and touch preferences. You need to question the individual. Sample questions can be found at the end of this section.

Health care providers have to use touch and invade personal space to give many types of care. For example, taking blood pressure involves palpation of arteries, wrapping a cuff around a person's arm, and placing a stethoscope on the skin. If a health care provider uses a slow, relaxed approach, explains the procedure, and encourages the patient to relax, this may help alleviate fear and eliminate the discomfort and panic that can occur when personal space is invaded. Always be alert to the patient's verbal and nonverbal communication, as well as inconsistencies between them. For example, a patient may give verbal permission for a procedure, but may seem anxious when personal space is invaded and demonstrate nonverbal behavior such as tensing muscles, turning or pulling away, or shaking when touched. An alert health care provider can try to move away from the patient periodically to give the patient "breathing room" and encourage the patient to relax.

When personal care must be provided to a patient, the health care provider should determine the patient's preferences by talking with the patient or asking questions. Examples of questions may include:

♦ Do you prefer to do as much of your own personal care as possible, or would you like assistance?

♦ Would you like a family member to assist with your personal care?

♦ Are there any special routines you would like followed while receiving personal care?

♦ Do you prefer to bathe in the morning or evening?

♦ Is there anything I can do to make you more comfortable?

EYE CONTACT

Eye contact is also affected by different cultural beliefs. Most European Americans regard eye contact during a conversation as indicative of interest and trustworthiness. They feel that individuals who look away are either not trustworthy or not paying attention. Some Asian Americans consider direct eye contact to be rude. Native Americans may use peripheral (side) vision and avoid direct eye contact. They may regard direct stares as hostile and threatening. Hispanic and African Americans may use brief eye contact, but then look away to indicate respect and attentiveness. Muslim women may avoid eye contact as a sign of modesty. In India, people of different socioeconomic classes may avoid eye contact with each other. The many different beliefs

regarding eye contact can lead to misunderstandings when people of different cultures interact.

Health care providers must be alert to the comfort levels of patients while using direct eye contact and recognize the cultural diversity that exists. Lack of eye contact is often interpreted as "not listening," when in reality, it can indicate respect.

GESTURES

Gestures are used to communicate many things. A common gesture in the United States is nodding the head up and down for "yes," and side to side for "no." In India, the head motions for "yes" and "no" are the exact opposite. Pointing at someone is also a common gesture in the United States and is frequently used to stress a specific idea. To Asian and Native Americans, this can represent a strong threat. Even the hand gesture for "OK" can be found insulting to some Asians.

Again, health care providers must be aware of how patients respond to hand gestures. If a patient seems uncomfortable with hand gestures, they should be avoided.

HEALTH CARE BELIEFS

The most common health care system in the United States is the biomedical health care system or the "Western" system. This system of health care bases the cause of disease on such things as microorganisms, diseased cells, and the process of aging. When the cause of disease is determined, heath care is directed toward eliminating the microorganisms, conquering the disease process, and/or preventing the effects of aging. Health care providers in the United States receive biomedical training and are licensed to practice as professionals. Some beliefs of this system of care include encouraging patients to learn as much as possible about their illnesses, informing patients about terminal diseases, teaching self-care, using medications and technology to cure or decrease the effects of a disease or illness, and teaching preventive care.

Health care beliefs vary greatly. These beliefs can affect an individual's response to health care. Most cultures have common conceptions regarding the cause of illness, ways to maintain health, appropriate response to pain, and effective methods of treatment. Some of the common beliefs are shown in table 10-1. It is important to remem-

TABLE 10-1 Health Care Beliefs

CULTURE	HEALTH CONCEPTS	CAUSE OF ILLNESS	TRADITIONAL HEALERS	METHODS OF TREATMENT	RESPONSE TO PAIN
South African	Maintain harmony of body, mind, and spirit Harmony with nature Illness can be prevented by diet, rest, and cleanliness	Supernatural cause Spirits and demons Punishment from God Conflict or disharmony in life	Root doctor Folk practitioners (community "mother" healer, spiritualist)	Restore harmony Prayer or meditation Herbs, roots, poultices, and oils Religious rituals Charms, talismans, and amulets	Tolerating pain is a sign of strength Some may express pain
Asian	Health is a state of physical and spiritual harmony with nature Balance of two energy forces: yin (cold) and yang (hot)	Imbalance between yin and yang Supernatural forces such as God, evil spirits, or ancestral spirits Unhealthy environment	Herbalist Physician Shaman healer (physician–priest)	Cold remedies if yang is overpowering and hot remedies if yin is overpowering Herbal remedies Acupuncture and acupressure Energy to restore balance between yin and yang	Pain must be accepted and endured silently Displaying pain in public brings disgrace May refuse pain medication
European	Health can be maintained by diet, rest, and exercise Immunizations and preventive practices help maintain health Good health is a personal responsibility	Outside sources such as germs, pollutants, or contaminants Punishment for sins Lack of cleanliness Self-abuse (drugs, alcohol, tobacco)	Physician Nurse	Medications and surgery Diet and exercise Home remedies and self-care for minor illnesses Prayer and religious rituals	Some express pain loudly and emotionally Others value self-control in response to pain Pain can be helped by medications
Hispanic	Health is a reward from God Health is good luck Balance between "hot" and "cold" forces	Punishment from God for sins Susto (fright), mal ojo (evil eye), or envidia (envy) Imbalance between hot and cold	Native healers (Curandero, Espiritualista, Yerbero or herbalist, Brujo)	Hot and cold remedies to restore balance Prayers, medals, candles, and religious rituals Herbal remedies, especially teas Massage Anointing with oil Wearing an Azabache (black stone) to ward off the evil eye	Many will express pain verbally and accept treatment Others feel pain is a part of life and must be endured

(continues)

TABLE 10-1 Health Care Beliefs (continued)

CULTURE	HEALTH CONCEPTS	CAUSE OF ILLNESS	TRADITIONAL HEALERS	METHODS OF TREATMENT	RESPONSE TO PAIN
Middle Eastern	Health is caused by spiritual causes Cleanliness essential for health Male individuals dominate and make decisions on health care	Spiritual causes Punishment for sins Evil spirits or evil "eye"	Traditional healers Physician	Meditation Charms and amulets Medications and surgery Male health professionals prohibited from touching or examining female patients	Tolerating pain is a sign of strength Self-inflicted pain is used as a sign of grief
Native American	Health is harmony between man and nature Balance among body, mind, and spirit Spiritual powers control body's harmony	Supernatural forces and evil spirits Violation of a taboo Imbalance between man and nature	Shaman Medicine Man	Rituals, charms, and masks Prayer and meditation to restore harmony with nature Plants and herbs Medicine bag or bundle filled with herbs and blessed by medicine man	Pain is a normal part of life and tolerance of pain signifies strength and power

ber that not all individuals in a specific ethnic/cultural group will believe and follow all of the customs. The customs, however, might still influence an individual's response to a different type of care.

Health care providers must understand that every culture has a system for health care based on values and beliefs that have existed for generations. Individuals may use herbal remedies, religious rites, and other forms of ethnic/cultural health care even while receiving biomedical health care. A major change in the practice of health care in the United States is the increase in the use of alternative health care methods. Many individuals are using alternative health care in addition to, or as a replacement for, biomedical care. Alternative health care providers include chiropractors, homeopaths, naturopaths, and hypnotists. Some types of treatments discussed in more detail in table 1-8 of Chapter 1:2, include:

♦ *Nutritional methods*: organic foods, herbs, vitamins, and antioxidants

♦ *Mind and body control methods*: relaxation, meditation, biofeedback, hypnotherapy, and imagery

♦ *Energetic touch therapy*: massage, acupuncture, acupressure, and therapeutic touch

♦ *Body-movement methods*: chiropractic, yoga, and tai chi

♦ *Spiritual methods*: faith healing, prayer, and spiritual counseling

It is important to remember that every individual has the right to choose the type of health care system and method of treatment he or she feels is best. Health care providers must respect this right.

To determine a patient's health care preferences the health care provider should talk with the patient and ask questions. Examples of questions may include:

♦ What do you do to stay healthy?

♦ Except for this current illness, do you feel that you are reasonably healthy?

♦ What do you feel is a healthy diet? Do you try to follow this diet?

♦ What do you do for exercise?

♦ Is there anything else that you do to stay healthy?

- Why do you think people become ill?
- What health care treatment method do you use when you are ill?
- Why do you think you have become ill?
- Were you born in the United States? Were your parents born in the United States?
- Do you or your parents still follow the traditions of your native land (or culture)? (If a patient and/or parents were not born in the United States)

SPIRITUALITY AND RELIGION

Spirituality and religion are an inherent part of every ethnic or cultural group. **Spirituality** is defined as the beliefs individuals have about themselves, their connections with others, and their relationship with a higher power. It is also described as an individual's need to find meaning and purpose in life (figure 10-6). When a person's

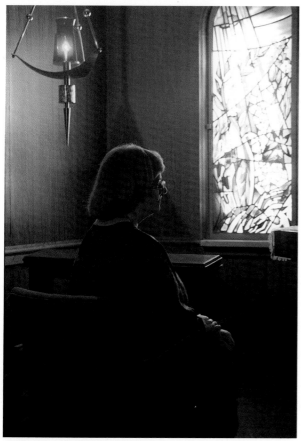

FIGURE 10-6 Spirituality is an individual's need to find meaning and purpose in life.

spiritual beliefs are firmly established, the individual has a basis for understanding life, finding sources of support when they are needed, and drawing on inner and/or external resources and strength to deal with situations that arise. Spirituality is often expressed through religious practices, but spirituality and religion are *not* the same. Spirituality is an individualized and personal set of beliefs and practices that evolves and changes throughout an individual's life.

Religion is an organized system of belief in a superhuman power or higher power. Religious beliefs and practices are associated with a particular form or place of worship. Beliefs about birth, life, illness, and death usually have a religious origin. Some of the more common religious beliefs are shown in table 10-2. Religious beliefs that affect dietary practices are discussed in Chapter 9 in table 9-6.

Even though a religion may establish certain beliefs and rituals, it is important to remember that not everyone follows all of the beliefs or rituals of their own religion. In addition, some individuals are non-believers. For example, an **atheist** is a person who does not believe in any deity. An **agnostic** is an individual who believes that the existence of God cannot be proved or disproved. Health care providers must determine what an individual personally believes to be important and respect that individual's beliefs.

To determine an individual's spiritual and religious needs, the health care provider should talk with the patient and ask questions. Examples of questions that may be asked include:

- Do you have a religious affiliation?
- Are there any spiritual practices that help you feel better (prayer, meditation, reading scriptures)?
- Do you normally pray at certain times of the day?
- Would you like a visit from a representative of your religion?
- Do you consult a religious healer?
- Do you observe any special religious days?
- Do you wear clothing or jewelry with a religious significance?
- Do you have any religious objects that require special care?
- Do your beliefs restrict any specific food or drink?

TABLE 10-2 Major Religious Beliefs

RELIGION	BELIEFS ABOUT BIRTH	BELIEFS ABOUT DEATH	HEALTH CARE BELIEFS	SPECIAL SYMBOLS, BOOKS, RELIGIOUS PRACTICES
Baptist (Christian)*	No infant baptism Baptism after person reaches age of understanding	Clergy provides prayer and counseling to patient and family Autopsy, organ donation, and cremation are an individual's choice No last rites	Oppose abortion Some believe in the healing power of "laying on of hands" May respond passively to medical treatment, believing that illness is "God's will" Physician is instrument for God's intervention	Bible is holy book Rite of Communion important Baptism by full immersion in water after a person reaches an age of understanding and accepts Jesus Christ Some use cross as symbol
Buddhism	No infant baptism but have infant presentation to dedicate child to Buddha	Believe in reincarnation Desire calm environment and limited touching during the process of death Buddhist priest must be present at death Last rites chanted at bedside immediately after death Autopsy and organ donation are controversial but usually regarded as an individual's choice Cremation is common	Suffering is an inevitable part of life Illness is the result of negative Karma (a person's acts and their ethical consequences) Cleanliness is important to maintain health	Belief in Buddha, the "enlightened one" Tipitaka, three collections of writings, are Buddhist canon Nirvana, the state of greater inner freedom, is the goal of existence Emphasize practice and personal enlightenment rather than doctrine or study of scripture May use pictures or statues of Buddha as religious symbols Some wear mala beads around the left wrist that may be removed only if absolutely necessary
Christian Scientist (Christian)*	No infant baptism	No last rites Autopsy only when required by law Organ donation discouraged but can be an individual's decision	Illness can be eliminated through prayer and spiritual understanding May not use medicine or surgical procedures May refuse blood transfusions Will accept legally mandated immunizations	Bible is holy book Rite of Communion important *Science and Health* by Mary Baker Eddy is basic textbook of Christian Science Prayer and faith will maintain health and prevent disease
Episcopal (Christian)*	Infant baptism (may be performed by anyone in an emergency)	Some observe last rites by priest Autopsy and organ donation encouraged Cremation is an individual's choice	May use Holy Unction or anointing of the sick with oil as a healing sacrament	Bible is holy book Rite of Communion important Book of Common Prayer Use cross as symbol

*Any religion that is designated as "Christian" has the following beliefs:
  God is one in three parts: Father, Son, and Holy Spirit
  Jesus Christ is the Son of God
  By accepting Jesus Christ, a person may be saved and inherit eternal life

(continues)

TABLE 10-2 Major Religious Beliefs (continued)

RELIGION	BELIEFS ABOUT BIRTH	BELIEFS ABOUT DEATH	HEALTH CARE BELIEFS	SPECIAL SYMBOLS, BOOKS, RELIGIOUS PRACTICES
Hinduism	No ritual at birth Naming ceremony is performed 10–11 days after birth to obtain blessings from gods and goddesses	Believe in reincarnation as humans, animals, or even plants Ultimate goal is freedom from the cycle of rebirth and death Priest ties thread around the neck or wrist of the deceased and may pour water in the mouth Only family and friends may touch and wash the body Autopsy and organ donation discouraged but regarded as individual's decision Cremation preferred	Some believe illness is punishment for sins Some believe in faith healing Will accept most medical interventions Abortion and birth control are discouraged	Vedas, four books, are the sacred scripture Brahma is principal source of universe and center of all things All forms of nature and life are sacred Person's Karma is determined by accumulated merits and demerits that result from all the actions the soul has committed in its past life or lives Cows are sacred and feeding a cow is an act of worship May use symbols such as statues of various gods, flat stones, incense, or sandalwood
Islam (Muslim)	Believe that first words an infant should hear at birth are "There is no God but Allah, and Mohammed is His prophet." Circumcision performed when 7 days old	Family must be with dying person Dying person must confess sins and ask forgiveness Only family touches or washes body after death Body is turned toward Mecca after death Autopsy only when required by law Organ donation is permitted if donor consents in writing Cremation not permitted	Illness is an atonement for sins May face city of Mecca (southeast direction if in United States) five times a day to pray to Allah Ritual washing before and after prayer Must take medications with right hand since left hand considered dirty	Allah is supreme deity Mohammed, founder of Islam, is chief prophet Holy Day of Worship is sunset Thursday to sunset Friday Koran is holy book of Islam (do not touch or place anything on top) Prayer rug is sacred Fast during daylight hours in month of Ramadan and during other religious holidays May wear item with words from Koran on arm, neck, or waist; do not remove or allow item to get wet An Imam is a Muslim preacher and teacher

(continues)

TABLE 10-2 Major Religious Beliefs (continued)

RELIGION	BELIEFS ABOUT BIRTH	BELIEFS ABOUT DEATH	HEALTH CARE BELIEFS	SPECIAL SYMBOLS, BOOKS, RELIGIOUS PRACTICES
Jehovah's Witness (Christian)*	No infant baptism Baptism by immersion done when child accepts beliefs	No last rites Autopsy only when required by law and body parts may not be removed Organ donation discouraged but decision is an individual's choice All organs and tissues must be drained of blood before transplantation Cremation permitted	Prohibited from receiving blood or blood products Elders of church will pray and read scriptures to promote healing Medications accepted if not derived from blood products	Name for God is Jehovah Bible is holy book: New World Bible Rite of Communion important Church elders provide guidance Each witness is a minister who must spread the group's teachings Acknowledge allegiance only to kingdom of Jesus Christ and refuse allegiance to any government
Judaism (Orthodox)	No infant baptism Male circumcision performed on 8th day after birth by Mohel (circumcisor), child's father, or Jewish physician	Person should never die alone Body is ritually cleaned after death May bury dead before sundown on day of death and usually within 24 hours Autopsy only when required by law Organ donation only after consultation with rabbi Cremation forbidden	May refuse surgical procedure or diagnostic tests on Sabbath or holy days Family may want surgically removed body parts for burial Ritual handwashing upon awakening and prior to eating	Lord God Jehovah is one Sabbath is sunset Friday to sunset Saturday Sabbath is devoted to prayer, study, and rest Torah is basis of religion (five books of Moses) Rabbi is spiritual leader Cantor often leads prayer services, performs marriages, and conducts funerals Star of David is symbol of Judaism Fast (no food or drink) during some holy days Men may wear kippah or yarmulke (small cap) and a tallith (prayer shawl)
Lutheran (Christian)*	Infant baptism by sprinkling (may be performed by any baptized Christian in an emergency)	No last rites Autopsy and organ donation allowed Cremation permitted	Communion often administered by clergy to sick or prior to surgery	Bible is holy book Rite of Communion important Use cross as symbol
Methodist (United) (Christian)*	Infant baptism	No last rites Organ donations encouraged Cremation permitted	May request communion before surgery or while ill	Bible is holy book Rite of Communion important Religion is a matter of personal belief and provides a guide for living Use cross as symbol

(continues)

TABLE 10-2 Major Religious Beliefs (continued)

RELIGION	BELIEFS ABOUT BIRTH	BELIEFS ABOUT DEATH	HEALTH CARE BELIEFS	SPECIAL SYMBOLS, BOOKS, RELIGIOUS PRACTICES
Mormon (Latter Day Saints)	Infant blessed by clergy in church as soon as possible after birth Baptism at 8 years of age	May want church elders present at death No last rites Autopsy and organ donation is individual's decision Cremation discouraged	May believe in divine healing with "laying on of hands" by church elders Anointing with oil can promote healing	Mormon refers to the four holy books: The Bible, *The Book of Mormon, The Doctrine and Covenants,* and *Pearl of Great Price* Special undergarment may be worn to symbolize dedication to God and should not be removed unless necessary Fast on first Sunday of each month Avoid medications containing alcohol or caffeine
Presbyterian (Christian)*	Infant baptism	No last rites Autopsy and organ donation permitted Cremation permitted	Prayer and counseling an important part of healing May request communion while ill or before surgery	Bible is holy book Rite of Communion important Salvation is a gift from God Use cross as symbol
Roman Catholic (Christian)*	Infant baptism mandatory Baptism necessary for salvation (any baptized Christian may perform an emergency baptism)	Sacrament of the Sick (last rites) performed by priest Autopsy and organ donation permitted Cremation permitted	Sacrament of the Sick and anointing with oil Life is sacred: abortion and contraceptive use prohibited Believe embryos are human beings and should not be destroyed or used for research	Bible is holy book Rite of Holy Eucharist (Communion) important May use prayer books, crucifix, rosary beads, religious medals, pictures and statues of saints Confession used as a rite for forgiveness of sins Use cross as symbol
Russian Orthodox (Christian)*	Infant baptism by priest	Last rites by ordained priest mandatory Arms of deceased are crossed Autopsy only if required by law Organ donations not encouraged Cremation prohibited	Holy Unction and anointing body with oil used for healing Will accept most medical treatments but believe in divine healing	Bible is holy book Rite of Communion important May wear a cross necklace that should not be removed unless absolutely necessary Use cross as symbol
Seventh Day Adventist (Christian)*	No infant baptism (baptize individuals when they reach the age of accountability)	No last rites Autopsy only when required by law Organ donation is an individual's decision	May avoid over-the-counter medications and caffeine May anoint body with oil Use prayer for healing Some believe only in divine healing Will accept required immunizations	Literal acceptance of Holy Bible Rite of Communion important Sabbath worship is sunset on Friday to sunset on Saturday

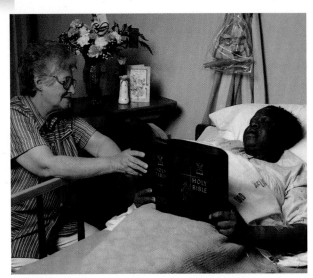

FIGURE 10-7 Always respect the patient's religious symbols and books.

♦ Do you fast or abstain from eating certain foods?

♦ Should food be prepared in a certain way?

♦ Do you prefer certain types of foods (vegetarian diet, diet free from pork)?

As long as it will not cause harm, every effort must be made to allow an individual to express his or her beliefs, practice any rituals, and/or follow a special diet. To show respect for an individual's beliefs and practices, the health care worker should:

♦ Be a willing listener.

♦ Provide support for spiritual and religious practices.

♦ Respect religious symbols and books (figure 10-7).

♦ Allow privacy for the patient during clergy visits or while the patient is observing religious customs such as communion, prayer, and meditation.

♦ Refrain from imposing your own beliefs on the patient.

10:4 INFORMATION

Respecting Cultural Diversity

The key to respecting cultural diversity is to regard each person as a unique individual. Every individual adopts beliefs and forms a pattern of behavior based on culture, ethnicity, race, life experiences, spirituality, and religion. Even though this pattern of behavior and beliefs may change based on new exposures and experiences, they are still an inherent part of the individual.

Health care workers must be aware of the needs of each individual to provide total care. They must learn to appreciate and respect the personal characteristics of others. Some ways to achieve this goal include:

♦ Listen to patients as they express their beliefs.

♦ Appreciate differences in people.

♦ Learn more about the cultural and ethnic groups that you see frequently.

♦ Recognize and avoid bias, prejudice, and stereotyping.

♦ Ask questions to determine a person's beliefs.

♦ Evaluate all information before forming an opinion.

♦ Allow patients to practice and express their beliefs as much as possible.

♦ Remember that you are not expected to adopt another's beliefs, just accept and respect them.

♦ Recognize and promote the patient's interactions with family.

♦ Be sensitive to how patients respond to eye contact, touch, and invasion of personal space.

♦ Respect spirituality, religious beliefs, symbols, and rituals.

STUDENT: *Go to the workbook and complete the assignment sheet for Chapter 10, Cultural Diversity.*

CHAPTER 10 SUMMARY

Because health care providers work with and care for many different people, they must be aware of the factors that cause each individual to be unique. These factors include culture, ethnicity, and race. Culture is defined as the values, beliefs, attitudes, languages, symbols, rituals, behaviors, and customs unique to a group of people and passed from one generation to the next.

TODAY'S RESEARCH: TOMORROW'S HEALTH CARE

A computer microchip that allows a physician to know what medication a person needs?

A major problem in health care today is determining what drug and what dosage should be used for a patient. Individuals react to medications in different ways. Some individuals need large amounts of pain medication; others need smaller quantities. A blood pressure medication works well for one individual, but is not effective for another patient. An antibiotic cures an infection in one person but causes an allergic reaction that kills another person. *Pharmacogenetics,* or prescribing medicine based on a person's unique genetic makeup, is the start of a revolution in personalizing treatment for a particular individual.

Researchers are using genetic information about individuals to try to determine their reactions to different medications. Scientists have proved that there is a gene in a person's body that controls how a drug is absorbed, used, and eliminated. This gene may be different from person to person. By learning an individual's genetic makeup, a physician could prescribe the exact medication and dosage that would be most beneficial to a patient.

Imagine a future where people will have a computer chip that contains all of their genetic information. Before any medication is given to a patient, the genetic information will be scanned to make sure it is compatible with the chemical properties of the medication. A computer will analyze the information and determine the exact dosage needed by the patient. Even though this process raises concerns about patient confidentiality, privacy, and legal regulations, it has the potential to save lives. If a medicine given to a patient is based on that person's specific needs, diseases will be cured because they will be treated correctly.

Ethnicity is a classification of people based on national origin and/or culture. Race is a classification of people based on physical or biological characteristics. The differences among people resulting from cultural, ethnic, and racial factors are called *cultural diversity.* Health care providers must show sensitivity, or recognize and appreciate the personal characteristics of others, because America is a multicultural society.

Bias, prejudice, and stereotyping can interfere with acceptance of cultural diversity. A bias is a preference that inhibits impartial judgment. A prejudice is a strong feeling or belief about a person or subject that is formed without reviewing facts or information. Stereotyping occurs when an assumption is made that everyone in a particular group is the same. Bias, prejudice, and stereotyping are barriers to effective relationships with others. Health care providers must be alert to these barriers and make every effort to avoid them.

An understanding of cultural diversity allows health care providers to give holistic care; that is, care that provides for the well-being of the whole person and meets not only physical, but also social, emotional, and mental needs.

Some areas of cultural diversity include family organization, language, personal space, touching, eye contact, gestures, health care beliefs, spirituality, and religion.

The key to respecting cultural diversity is to regard each person as a unique individual. Health care providers must learn to appreciate and respect the personal characteristics of others.

INTERNET SEARCHES

Use the suggested search engines in Chapter 17:4 of this textbook to search the Internet for additional information on the following topics:

1. *Cultural diversity*: search words such as culture, ethnicity, and race to obtain additional information on characteristics and examples for each

2. *Ethnic groups*: search countries of origin for information on different ethic groups or on your own ethnic group; for example, if you are German–Irish, search for information on both Germany and Ireland

3. *Cultural assimilation and acculturation*: search for additional information on these two topics

4. *Bias, prejudice, and stereotyping*: use these key words to search for more detailed information

5. *Family structure*: search words such as extended or nuclear family, patriarchal, and/or matriarchal

6. *Health care beliefs*: search by country of origin for health care beliefs, or search words such as yin and yang or shaman

7. *Alternative health care*: search for additional information on chiropractor, homeopath, naturopath, hypnotist, hypnotherapy, meditation, biofeedback, acupuncture, acupressure, therapeutic touch, yoga, tai chi, and/or faith healing

8. *Spirituality and religion*: search for additional information on spirituality; use the name of a religion to obtain more information about the beliefs and practices of the religion

REVIEW QUESTIONS

1. Differentiate between culture, ethnicity, and race.

2. Name five (5) common ethnic groups and at least two (2) countries of origin for each group.

3. Create examples of how a bias, prejudice, and stereotype may interfere with providing quality health care.

4. Describe your family structure. Is it a nuclear or extended family? Is it patriarchal or matriarchal or neither? Why?

5. Do you feel acculturation occurs in the United States? Why or why not?

6. Describe at least three (3) different health care practices that you have seen or heard about. Do you feel they are beneficial or harmful? Why?

7. Differentiate between spirituality and religion.

8. List six (6) specific ways to respect cultural diversity.

NOTE: The cultural assessment questions presented in this unit were adapted from Joan Luckmann's *Transcultural Communication in Health Care,* which adapted them from Fong's CONFHER model and Rosenbaum.

CHAPTER 11 Geriatric Care

Chapter Objectives

After completing this chapter,
you should be able to:

Observe Standard
Precautions

Instructor's Check—Call
Instructor at This Point

Safety—Proceed with
Caution

OBRA Requirement—Based
on Federal Law

Math Skill

Legal Responsibility

Science Skill

Career Information

Communications Skill

Technology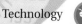

◆ Differentiate between the myths and facts of six aspects of aging

◆ Identify at least two physical changes of aging in each body system

◆ Demonstrate at least ten methods of providing care to the elderly individual who is experiencing physical changes of aging

◆ List five factors that cause psychosocial changes of aging

◆ Describe at least six methods to assist an elderly individual in adjusting to psychosocial changes

◆ Recognize the causes and effects of confusion and disorientation in the elderly

◆ Create a reality orientation program

◆ Justify the importance of respecting cultural and religious differences

◆ Explain the role of an ombudsman

◆ Define, pronounce, and spell all key terms

KEY TERMS

Alzheimer's disease (AD)
  (*Altz'-high-merz"*)
arteriosclerosis
  (*r-tear-ee-o-skleh-row'-sis*)
arthritis
atherosclerosis (*ath-eh-row"-skleh-row'-sis*)
bronchitis
cataracts
cerebrovascular accident
culture
delirium

dementia (*d-men'-she-a*)
disability
disease
dysphagia (*dis-fay'-gee-ah*)
emphysema
geriatric care
gerontology
  (*jer-un-tahl'-oh-gee*)
glaucoma (*glaw-ko'-mah*)
incontinence
myths
nocturia (*nok-tur'-ee-ah*)

ombudsman
osteoporosis
  (*os-tee'-oh-pour-oh'-sis*)
reality orientation (RO)
religion
senile lentigines
  (*seen'-ile len-ti'-jeans*)
thrombus
transient ischemic attacks
  (TIAs)
  (*tran'-z-ent is-ke'mik*)

INTRODUCTION

Just as they experienced the "baby boom," the United States and most other countries are now experiencing an "aging boom." In 1900, most individuals died before age 60, and there were only 3.1 million people older than 65 in the United States. In 2000, there were 34.7 million people older than 65 and 4.2 million people older than 85 years in the United States. U.S. government statistics prepared by the National Council on Aging project that by 2010, 40.2 million Americans will be older than 65 and 5.7 million will be older than 85. By 2020, 54.6 million Americans will be older than 65 and 7.3 million will be older than 85. By 2030, projections estimate that there will be 70.3 million people older than 65, including 8 million older than 85, in the United States. In addition, by 2030, the National Council on Aging predicts that almost 20 percent of the total population in the United States will be older than 65. These statistics truly indicate an "aging boom."

Today, most individuals can expect to live into their 70s, and many individuals enjoy healthy and happy lives as 80- and 90-year-olds. This age group uses health care services frequently, so it is essential for a health care worker to understand the special needs of the elderly population.

11:1 INFORMATION

Myths on Aging

Aging is a process that begins at birth and ends at death. It is a normal process and leads to normal changes in body structure and function. Even though few people want to grow old, it is a natural event in everyone's life. **Gerontology** is the scientific study of aging and the problems of the old. **Geriatric care** is care provided to elderly individuals. Through the study of the aging process and the elderly, many facts on aging have been established. However, many **myths,** or false beliefs, still exist regarding aging and elderly individuals. It is essential for the health care worker to be able to distinguish fact from myth when providing geriatric care.

♦ *Myth*: Most elderly individuals are cared for in institutions or long-term care facilities.

♦ *Fact*: Only approximately 5 percent of the elderly population lives in long-term care facilities. Most elderly individuals live in their own homes or apartments, or with other family members (figure 11-1). Others may choose to live in retirement communities or in independent-living or assisted-living facilities. These facilities provide assistance with meals,

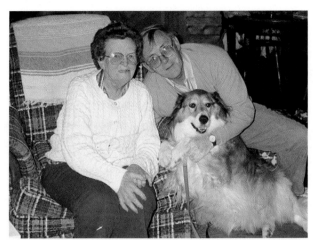

FIGURE 11-1 Most elderly individuals live in their own homes or apartments.

transportation, housekeeping, social activities, and medical care. By purchasing or renting a home or apartment in one of these facilities, the individual can obtain the degree of assistance needed while still living independently.

♦ *Myth*: Anyone over a certain set age, such as 65, is "old."

♦ *Fact*: Old is determined less by the number of years lived and more by how an individual thinks, feels, and behaves. For example, to a 10-year-old, a 35-year-old is old. It is important to remember that many individuals are active, productive, and self-sufficient into their 80s and even 90s. Too often the term *old* becomes synonymous with *worthless* or *worn-out*. A better term would be *experienced* or *mature*.

♦ *Myth*: Elderly people are incompetent and incapable of making decisions or handling their own affairs.

♦ *Fact*: Even though some experience confusion and disorientation, the majority of elderly individuals remain mentally competent until they die. In fact, older individuals may make better decisions and judgments because they frequently base their decisions on many years of experience and knowledge. In addition, studies have proved that older people are able to concentrate, learn new skills, and evaluate new information. Colleges and adult education programs recognize this fact and often provide tuition-free access that allows elderly individuals to participate in a wide variety of educational programs.

♦ *Myth*: All elderly people live in poverty.

♦ *Fact*: Recent statistics provided by the U.S. government show that less than 10 percent of adults older than 65 live at the poverty level. Even though many older individuals have limited incomes, most also have comparatively low expenses. Many own their own homes, and their children are raised and out on their own. With social security, savings, retirement pensions, and other sources of income, some elderly individuals are financially secure and enjoy comfortable lifestyles. Although it is true that some elderly individuals live in poverty, this is true of some individuals in all age groups. The financial status of the elderly varies just as the financial status of young or middle-aged people varies.

♦ *Myth*: Older people are unhappy and lonely.

♦ *Fact*: Studies have shown that most elderly individuals live with someone and/or associate frequently with friends or family members. Many elderly individuals are active in civic groups, charities, social activities, and volunteer programs. Others provide care for grandchildren and remain active as heads of extended families (figure 11-2). Although it is true that some elderly individuals are lonely and unhappy, the percentage is small, and many social agencies exist to assist these individuals.

♦ *Myth*: Elderly individuals do not want to work—that is, the goal of the elderly is to retire and, prior to retirement, they lose interest in work.

♦ *Fact*: Many individuals remain employed and productive into their 70s and even 80s (figure 11-3). Studies have shown that the older worker has good attendance, performs efficiently, readily learns new skills, and shows job satisfaction. Employers, desiring good work ethics and experience, frequently recruit and hire older workers. In addition, if projections from the National Council on Aging prove accurate, by 2030, one of every five people in the United States will be older than 65. Employers will have to rely on older workers to fill job vacancies. Many retired individuals do not want a full-time job, but they return to part-time positions or serve as consultants or volunteer workers.

♦ *Myth*: Retired people are bored and have nothing to do with their lives.

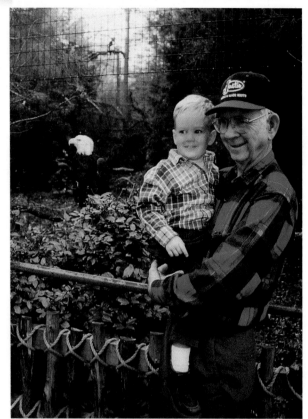

FIGURE 11-2 Caring for grandchildren is a very satisfying social relationship for many elderly individuals.

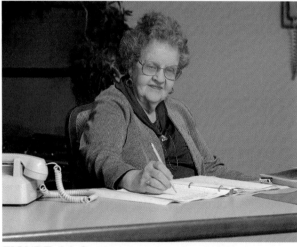

FIGURE 11-3 Many individuals remain employed and productive into their 70s and even 80s.

♦ *Fact*: Many retired people enjoy full and active lives. They engage in travel, hobbies, sports, social activities, family events, and church or community activities. In fact, many retired individuals say, "I don't know how I found time to work."

Many other myths also exist. It is important for the health care worker both to recognize problems that do exist for the elderly and to understand that the needs of the elderly vary according to many circumstances. Even the fact that only 5 percent of the elderly are in long-term care facilities means that more than 3 million people will be in these facilities by the year 2020. Many health care workers at all levels will provide needed services for these individuals. Geriatric care is and will continue to be a major aspect of health care.

STUDENT: *Go to the workbook and complete the assignment sheet for 11:1, Myths on Aging.*

11:2 INFORMATION

Physical Changes of Aging

As aging occurs, certain physical changes also occur in all individuals (figure 11-4). These changes are a normal part of the aging process. It is important to note that most of the changes are gradual and take place over a long period. In addition, the rate and degree of change varies among individuals. Factors such as disease can increase the speed and degree of the changes. Lifestyle, nutrition, economic status, social environment, and limited access to medical care can also have effects.

Most physical changes of aging involve a decrease in the function of body systems. Body processes slow down. There is a corresponding decrease in energy level. If an individual can recognize these changes as a normal part of aging,

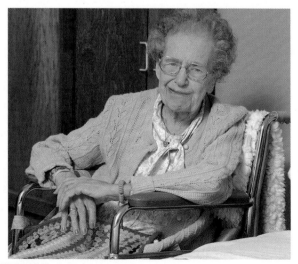

FIGURE 11-4 Note the physical signs of aging.

the individual can usually learn to adapt to and cope with the changes.

INTEGUMENTARY SYSTEM

Some of the most obvious effects of aging are seen in the integumentary system (figure 11-5). Production of new skin cells decreases with age. The sebaceous (oil) and sudoriferous (sweat) glands become less active. Circulation to the skin decreases and causes coldness, dryness, and poor healing of injured tissue. The hair loses color, and hair loss occurs.

The decreases in body function lead to the physical changes. The skin becomes less elastic and dry. Itching is common. Dark yellow or brown colored spots, called **senile lentigines,** appear. Although these are frequently called "liver spots," they are not related to the liver. When the fatty tissue layer of the skin diminishes, lines and wrinkles develop. The nails become thick, tough, and brittle. An increased sensitivity to temperature develops, and the elderly adult frequently feels cold. Hypothermia, a below normal body temperature, can be a serious problem for the elderly.

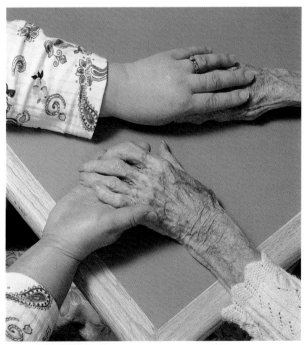

FIGURE 11-5 Some of the most obvious effects of aging are seen on the skin.

Good skin, nail, and hair care are essential. Mild soaps should be used because many soaps cause dryness. Frequently, bath oils or moisturizing lotions are recommended to combat dryness and itching. Daily baths can also contribute to dry, itchy skin; baths or showers two or three times a week with partial baths on other days are recommended. Brushing of the hair helps stimulate circulation and production of oil. Shampooing is usually done less frequently, but should be done as often as needed for cleanliness and comfort. Any sores or injuries to the skin should be cared for immediately. It is important to keep injured areas clean and free from infection. When elderly people notice sores or injuries that do not heal, they should get medical help. Frequently, the elderly person requires a room temperature that is higher than normal and free from drafts. Socks, sweaters, lap blankets, and layers of clothing can all help alleviate the feeling of coldness. The use of hot water bottles or heating pads is not recommended because the decreased sensitivity to temperature can result in burns.

Proper diet, exercise, good hygiene, decreased sun exposure, and careful skin care can help slow and even decrease the normal physical changes in the integumentary system.

MUSCULOSKELETAL SYSTEM

As aging occurs, muscles lose tone, volume, and strength. **Osteoporosis,** a condition in which calcium and other minerals are lost from the bones, causes the bones to become brittle and more likely to fracture or break. **Arthritis,** an inflammation of the joints, causes the joints to become stiff, less flexible, and painful. The rib cage becomes more rigid, and the bones in the vertebral column press closer together (compress).

These changes cause the elderly individual to experience a gradual loss in height, decreased mobility, and weakness. Movement is slower, and the sense of balance is less sure. Falls occur easily and often result in fractures of the hips, arms, and/or legs. Fine finger movements, such as those required when buttoning clothes or tying shoes, are often difficult for the elderly individual.

Elderly individuals should be encouraged to exercise as much as their physical conditions permit (figure 11-6). This helps keep muscles active and joints as flexible as possible. Even slow, daily walks help maintain muscle tone. Range-of-motion exercises can also maintain muscle strength. A diet rich in protein, calcium, and vitamins can slow the loss of minerals from the bones and maintain muscle structure. Extra attention must be paid to the environment so it is safer for the elderly person. Grab bars in the bathroom, hand rails in halls and on stairs, and other similar devices aid in ambulation. When the sense of balance is poor, an elderly person may need assistance and support during ambulation. The use of walkers and quad canes is frequently recommended. In addition, well-fitting shoes with non-slip soles and flat heels can help prevent falls. Self-stick strips and bands can replace buttons and shoestrings to make dressing easier. A consultation with a physician, physical therapist, and/or occupational therapist can provide an elderly individual with information on the latest and most effective adaptive devices to maintain independence.

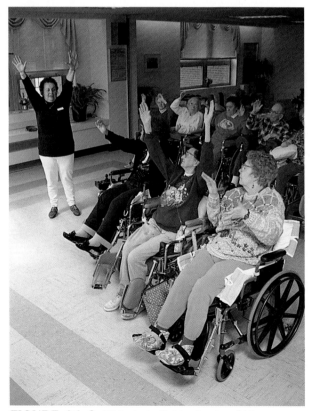

FIGURE 11-6 Elderly individuals should be encouraged to exercise as much as their physical condition permits.

CIRCULATORY SYSTEM

In the circulatory system, the heart muscle becomes less efficient at pushing blood into the arteries, and cardiac output decreases with aging. The blood vessels narrow and become less elastic. Blood flow to the brain and other vital organs may decrease. Blood pressure may increase or decrease.

Many elderly individuals do not notice any changes while at rest. They are more aware of changes when exercise, stress, excitement, illness, and other similar events call for increases in the body's need for oxygen and nutrients. During these periods, they experience weakness, dizziness, numbness in the hands and/or feet, and a rapid heart rate.

Elderly individuals who experience circulatory changes should avoid strenuous exercise or overexertion. They need periods of rest during the day. Moderate exercise, according to the individual's ability to tolerate it, does stimulate circulation and help prevent the formation of a **thrombus,** or blood clot. Support stockings, antiembolism hose, and not using garters or tight bands around the legs also help prevent blood clots. If an individual is confined to bed, range-of-motion exercises help circulation. If high blood pressure is present, a diet low in salt or sodium and, in some cases, fat may be recommended. Individuals with circulatory system disease should follow the diet and exercise plans recommended by their doctors.

RESPIRATORY SYSTEM

Respiratory muscles become weaker with age. The rib cage becomes more rigid. The alveoli, or air sacs in the lungs, become thinner and less elastic, which decreases the exchange of gases between the lungs and bloodstream. The bronchioles, or air tubes in the lungs, also lose elasticity. Changes in the larynx lead to a higher-pitched and weaker voice. Chronic conditions such as **emphysema,** in which the alveoli lose their elasticity, or **bronchitis,** in which the bronchioles become inflamed, decrease the efficiency of the respiratory system even more severely.

These changes frequently cause the elderly individual to experience *dyspnea,* or difficult breathing. Breathing becomes more rapid, and they have difficulty coughing up secretions from the lungs. This makes them more susceptible to respiratory infections such as colds and pneumonia.

Learning to alternate activity with periods of rest is important to avoid dyspnea. Proper body alignment and positioning can also ease breathing difficulties. The elderly individual with respiratory problems frequently sleeps in a semi-Fowler's position with two or three pillows elevating the upper body to make breathing easier. Avoiding polluted air, such as that in smoke-filled rooms, is essential. Breathing deeply and coughing at frequent intervals helps clear the lung passages and increase lung capacity. Elderly individuals with chronic respiratory problems often use oxygen on a continuous basis. Portable oxygen units allow many individuals to continue to lead active lives.

NERVOUS SYSTEM

Physical changes in the nervous system affect many body functions. Blood flow to the brain decreases, and there is a progressive loss of brain cells. This interferes with thinking, reacting, interpreting, and remembering. The senses of taste, smell, vision, and hearing diminish. Nerve endings are less sensitive, and there is a decreased ability to respond to pain and other stimuli.

As these physical changes occur, the elderly individual may experience memory loss. Short-term memory is usually affected. For example, an individual may not remember what he or she ate for breakfast, but does remember the entire menu from his or her retirement party. Long-term memory and intelligence do not always decrease. It may take elderly individuals longer to react, but given enough time, they can think and react appropriately. Individuals who remain mentally active and involved in current events usually show fewer mental changes (figure 11-7).

Changes in vision cause problems in reading small print or seeing objects at a distance. There is a decrease in peripheral (side) vision and night vision. The eyes take longer to adjust from light to dark, and there is an increased sensitivity to glare. Elderly individuals are also more prone to the development of **cataracts,** where the normally transparent lens of the eye becomes cloudy or opaque. **Glaucoma,** a condition in which the intraocular pressure of the eye increases and

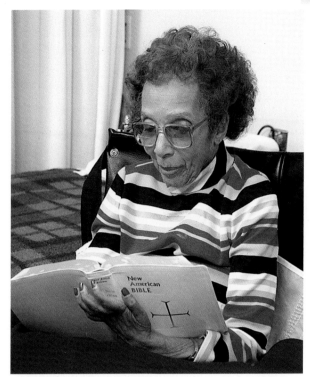

FIGURE 11-7 Individuals who remain mentally active usually show fewer mental changes.

interferes with vision, is also more common in the elderly. Proper eye care, prescription glasses/lenses, medical treatment of cataract or glaucoma, and proper lighting can all improve vision (figure 11-8).

Hearing loss usually occurs gradually in the elderly. The individual may speak more loudly than usual, ask for words to be repeated, and not hear high-frequency sounds such as the ringing of a telephone. Problems may be more apparent when there is a lot of background noise. For example, an elderly person may not hear well in a crowded restaurant where music is playing and many other people are talking. A hearing aid can help resolve some hearing problems. However, in cases of severe nerve damage, a hearing aid will not eliminate the problem. In addition, many individuals resist using hearing aids. If a person wears a hearing aid, it is important to keep the aid in good working condition by changing batteries, keeping the aid clean, and checking to make sure the individual is wearing it correctly. When a person has a hearing impairment, it is important to talk slowly and clearly. Avoid yelling or speaking excessively loud. Facing individuals while talking to them also helps in many situations. Eliminating background noise, such as that

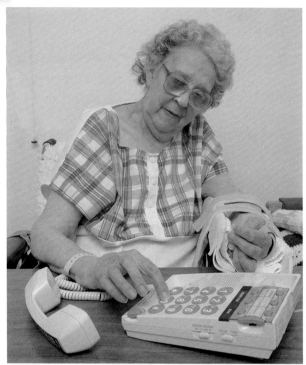

FIGURE 11-8 Good lighting and large numbers on a telephone can help improve vision.

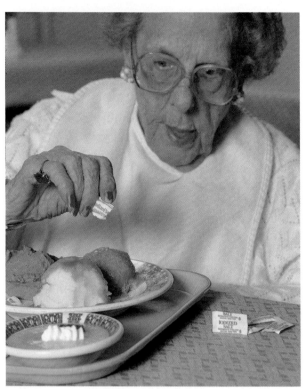

FIGURE 11-9 Elderly individuals may want to add salt to food because of their decreased sense of taste.

produced by a radio or television, also increases the ability to hear.

The decrease in the sense of taste and smell frequently affects the appetite. Elderly individuals often complain that food is tasteless and add sugar, salt, or pepper (figure 11-9). Attractive foods with a variety of textures and tastes may help stimulate the appetite. The decrease in the sense of smell may also make the elderly individual less sensitive to the smell of gas, chemicals, smoke, and other dangerous odors. A smoke detector, chemical detectors, and careful monitoring of the environment can help eliminate this danger.

Decreased sensation of pain and other stimuli can lead to injuries. The elderly are more susceptible to burns, frostbite, cuts, fractures, muscle strain, and many other injuries. At times, elderly people are not even aware of injury or disease because they do not sense pain. It is important for elderly individuals to handle hot or cold items with extreme care, and to be aware of dangers in the environment.

Changes in the nervous system usually occur gradually over a long period of time. This allows an individual time to adapt to the changes and learn to accommodate them. However, it is sometimes necessary for someone else to assist when the changes become severe. For example, many elderly individuals continue to drive cars. Because of slower reaction times, however, these individuals may be more prone to having automobile accidents. When an elderly person shows impaired driving ability, it often becomes necessary for a family member or the law to prevent the individual from driving.

DIGESTIVE SYSTEM

Physical changes in the digestive system occur when fewer digestive juices and enzymes are produced, muscle action becomes slower and peristalsis decreases, teeth are lost, and liver function decreases.

Dysphagia, or difficult swallowing, is a frequent complaint of the elderly. Less saliva and a slower gag reflex contribute to this problem. In addition, the loss of teeth or use of poor-fitting dentures makes it more difficult to chew food properly. Another common complaint is indigestion, which results from slower digestion of foods caused by decreased digestive juices. Flatulence (gas) and constipation are common because of decreased peristalsis and poor diet. The decreased sensation of taste also contributes to a poor appetite and diet.

Good oral hygiene, repair or replacement of damaged teeth, and a relaxed eating atmosphere can contribute to better chewing and digestion of food. Most elderly people find it is best to avoid dry, fried, and/or fatty foods because such foods are difficult to chew and digest. High-fiber and high-protein foods with different tastes and textures are recommended. Careful use of seasonings and herbs to improve taste also increases appetite. It is important to avoid excessive seasonings because they can cause indigestion. Increasing fluid intake makes swallowing easier, helps prevent constipation, and aids kidney function.

URINARY SYSTEM

With aging, the kidneys decrease in size and become less efficient at producing urine. Poor circulation to the kidneys and a decrease in the number of nephrons result in a loss of ability to concentrate the urine, which causes a loss of electrolytes and fluids. The ability of the bladder to hold urine decreases. Sometimes the bladder does not empty completely and urine is retained in the bladder, a major cause of bladder infections.

The elderly person may find it necessary to urinate more frequently. **Nocturia,** or urination at night, is common and disrupts the sleep pattern. Retention of urine in the bladder causes bladder infections. Men frequently experience enlargement of the prostate gland, which makes urination difficult and causes urinary retention. Loss of muscle tone results in **incontinence,** or the inability to control urination. Incontinence may also result from treatment for prostatic hypertrophy (enlargement) or cancer.

Many elderly individuals decrease fluid intake to cut down on the frequent need to urinate. This can cause dehydration, kidney disease, and infection. Elderly individuals should be encouraged to increase fluid intake to improve kidney function. To decrease incidents of nocturia, most fluids should be taken before evening. Regular trips to the bathroom, wearing easy-to-remove clothing, and using absorbent pads as needed can help the individual who has mild incontinence. Bladder training programs can also help increase bladder capacity and lead to more control over urination in incontinent persons. An indwelling catheter may be needed if all urinary control is lost.

When changes in the urinary system cause poor functioning of the kidneys, waste substances can build up in the bloodstream and cause serious illness. Therefore, it is important to keep the kidneys functioning as efficiently as possible.

ENDOCRINE SYSTEM

Changes in the endocrine system result in increased production of some hormones, such as parathormone and thyroid-stimulating hormone, and decreased production of other hormones, such as thyroxin, estrogen, progesterone, and insulin. The actions of these hormones are listed in Chapter 7:13 of this text.

Because hormones affect many body functions, several physical changes may occur. The immune system of the body is less effective, and elderly individuals are more prone to disease. The basal metabolic rate decreases, resulting in complaints of feeling cold, tired, and less alert (figure 11-10). Intolerance to glucose can develop, resulting in increased blood glucose levels.

As with the other body systems, changes in the endocrine system occur slowly over a long period of time. Many elderly individuals are not as aware of changes in this system. Proper exercise, adequate rest, medical care for illness, a

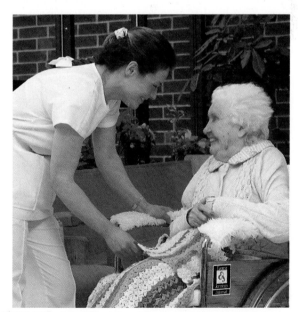

FIGURE 11-10 A lap blanket can help when an elderly person complains of feeling cold.

balanced diet, and a healthy lifestyle all help decrease the effects caused by changes in hormone activity.

REPRODUCTIVE SYSTEM

In the reproductive system, the decrease of estrogen and progesterone in women causes a thinning of the vaginal walls and a decrease in vaginal secretions. Vaginal infections or inflammations become more common. In some cases, a weakness in its supporting tissues causes the uterus to sag downward, a condition known as *prolapsed uterus*. The breasts sag when fat is redistributed.

Slowly decreasing levels of testosterone in men slow the production of sperm. Response to sexual stimulation of the penis is slower, and ejaculation may take longer. The testes become smaller and less firm. The seminal fluid becomes thinner, and smaller amounts are produced.

Sexual desire and need do not necessarily diminish with age (figure 11-11). Many elderly individuals are sexually active. Studies have shown that sex improves muscle tone and circulation. Even pain from arthritis seems to decrease after sexual activity, probably because of increased hormone levels. When elderly individuals are in long-term care facilities, it is important for the health care worker to understand both the physical and psychological sexual needs of the resident. Long-term care facilities now allow married couples to live together in the same room. The health care worker must respect the privacy of these residents and allow them to meet their sexual needs (figure 11-12).

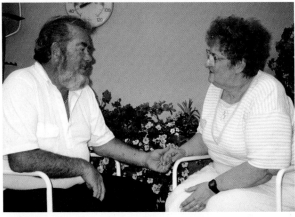

FIGURE 11-11 Elderly individuals still experience a need for companionship and sexuality.

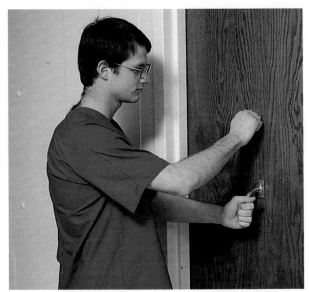

FIGURE 11-12 To respect the right to privacy, always knock before entering a resident's room.

SUMMARY

Aging causes many physical changes in all body systems. The rate and degree of the changes vary in different individuals, but all elderly individuals experience some degree of change. Providing means of adapting to and coping with changes allows elderly people to enjoy life even with physical limitations. It is important for all health care workers to learn to recognize changes and provide methods for dealing with them. Tolerance, patience, and empathy are essential.

STUDENT: *Go to the workbook and complete the assignment sheet for 11:2, Physical Changes of Aging.*

11:3 INFORMATION

Psychosocial Changes of Aging

In addition to physical changes, elderly individuals also experience psychological and social changes. Some individuals cope with these changes effectively, but others experience extreme frustration and mental distress. It is important for the health care worker to be aware of the psychosocial changes and stresses experienced by the elderly.

WORK AND RETIREMENT

Most adults spend a large portion of their days working. Many associate their feelings of self-worth with the jobs they perform. They are proud to state that they are nurses, electricians, teachers, lawyers, or secretaries. In addition, social contact while working is a major form of interaction with others.

Retirement is often viewed as an end to the working years. Many individuals are able to enjoy retirement and find other activities to replace job roles. Some individuals find part-time or consultant-type jobs after retirement from their primary jobs. Other individuals become active in volunteer work or take part in community or club activities. These individuals find satisfactory replacements for the feelings of self-worth once provided by their jobs.

However, some elderly individuals feel a major sense of loss upon retirement. They lose social contacts, develop feelings of uselessness, and in some cases, experience financial difficulties. This causes them to experience stress, and they frequently become depressed. Until other sources of restoring the individual's sense of self-worth are found, these elderly individuals can have difficulty coping with life.

SOCIAL RELATIONSHIPS

Social relationships change throughout life. Among the elderly, these changes may occur more frequently. Often, children marry and move away. This brings about a loss of contact with the family. If a spouse dies, the "couple" image is replaced by one of "widow" or "widower." As a person ages, more friends and relatives die, and social contacts decrease.

Some elderly individuals are able to adjust to these changes by making new friends and establishing new social contacts (figure 11-13). Church and community groups provide many social activities for the elderly. By taking part in these activities, individuals who made friends readily throughout their lives can continue to do so as they grow older.

Some elderly individuals cannot cope with the continuous loss of friends and relatives. They become withdrawn and depressed. They avoid

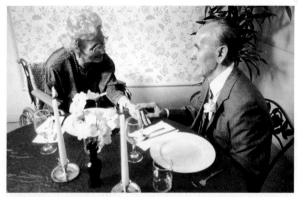

FIGURE 11-13 After the death of a spouse, the elderly individual sometimes may adjust by making new social contacts.

social events and isolate themselves from others. The death of a spouse is frequently devastating to an elderly individual, especially when a couple has had a close relationship for many years. A surviving spouse may even attempt suicide. Psychological help is essential in these cases.

LIVING ENVIRONMENTS

Changes in living environments create psychosocial changes. Most elderly individuals prefer to remain in their own homes. They feel secure surrounded by familiar environments. Many elderly individuals express fear at the thought of losing their homes.

Some elderly people leave their homes by personal choice. They find the burden of maintaining their homes too great and move to apartments or retirement communities. The elderly individual may even move to another state with a better climate. These individuals often cope well with the change in living environment and feel the change is beneficial.

Financial problems or physical disabilities may force some people to move from their homes, sometimes to retirement communities or apartments. If they can maintain their independence, coping is usually good. In other cases, an elderly individual may be forced to move in with a son or daughter. This move creates a change in roles, where the child becomes the caretaker of the parent. If the elderly person feels secure in this situation, coping occurs. However, if the elderly person feels unwanted or useless, conflicts and tension may develop.

Moving to a long-term care facility often creates stress in elderly individuals. They feel a loss of independence and become frightened by their lack of control over environment. Many elderly individuals view long-term care facilities as "places to die," even when they may require the use of the facility for only a short period. For this reason, it is important to allow individuals to create their own "home" environments in the facility (figure 11-14). Most long-term care facilities refer to the individuals as "residents." They allow the residents to bring favorite pieces of furniture, pictures, televisions, radios, and personal items. By being allowed choices in the arrangement of their items, residents are able to create comfortable, homelike environments. Factors such as these allow the elderly individual to adjust to the new environment and to cope with the changes it brings.

INDEPENDENCE

Most individuals want to be independent and self-sufficient. Even 2-year-olds begin to assert their right to choose and strive to be independent. Just as children learn that there are limits to independence, the elderly learn that independence can be threatened with age. Physical disability, illness, decreased mental ability, and other factors can all lead to a loss of independence in the elderly.

Individuals who once took care of themselves find it necessary to ask others for assistance. After driving for a lifetime, elderly individuals might find that they can no longer drive safely. They have to depend on others to take them where they need to go. Physical limitations prevent them from mowing lawns, cooking meals, washing, cleaning, and in some cases, even taking care of themselves. Frustration, anger, and depression can develop.

Any care provided to elderly individuals should allow as much independence as possible. Assistance should be provided as needed for the individual's safety, but the individual should be allowed to do as much as possible. For example, a health care worker should encourage elderly persons to choose their clothing and dress themselves, even if this takes longer (figure 11-15). Self-stick strips can replace buttons to make the task of dressing easier and to provide more independence. This helps the elderly individual adapt to the situation and maintain a sense of self-worth. At all times, elderly individuals should be allowed as much choice as possible to help them maintain their individuality.

DISEASE AND DISABILITY

Elderly people are more prone to disease and disability. **Disease** is usually defined as any condition that interferes with the normal function of the body. Common examples in the elderly include diabetes, heart disease, emphysema,

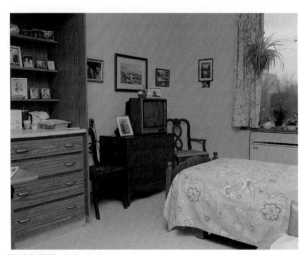

FIGURE 11-14 It is important to allow residents to create their own "home" environments in the long-term care facility.

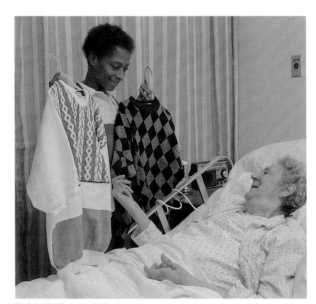

FIGURE 11-15 To promote independence, encourage elderly individuals to make as many decisions as possible.

arthritis, and osteoporosis. A **disability** is defined as a physical or mental defect or handicap that interferes with normal functions. Hearing impairments, visual defects, or the inability to walk caused by a fractured hip are examples. Diseases sometimes cause permanent disabilities. For example, a cerebrovascular accident, or stroke, can result in permanent paralysis of one side of the body, or *hemiplegia.*

When disease or disability affects the functioning of the body, an individual may experience psychological problems. When this occurs in an elderly individual already stressed by other changes or circumstances, it can be traumatic. A fractured hip can cause an elderly individual who had been living independently in his or her own home to be admitted to a long-term care facility. Disease or disability frequently occurs suddenly and does not allow for gradual adjustment to and coping with change.

Sick people often have fears of death, chronic illness, loss of function, and pain. These are normal fears, and these individuals need time to adjust to their situations. Listen to them as they express these fears and be patient and understanding. If they cannot discuss their feelings, accept this and provide supportive care (figure 11-16).

SUMMARY

Psychosocial changes can be major sources of stress in the elderly. As changes occur, the individual must learn to accommodate the changes and function in new situations. It is important to remember that older adults have survived many crises in their lives and have learned many different coping methods. These individuals must be encouraged to use their existing strengths and coping skills. With support, understanding, and patience, the health care worker can assist elderly individuals as they learn to adapt.

STUDENT: *Go to the workbook and complete the assignment sheet for 11:3, Psychosocial Changes of Aging.*

11:4 INFORMATION

Confusion and Disorientation in the Elderly

Although most elderly individuals remain mentally alert until death, some experience periods of confusion and disorientation. Signs of confusion or disorientation include talking incoherently, not knowing their own names, not recognizing others, wandering aimlessly, lacking awareness of time or place, displaying hostile and combative behavior (figure 11-17), hallucinating, regress-

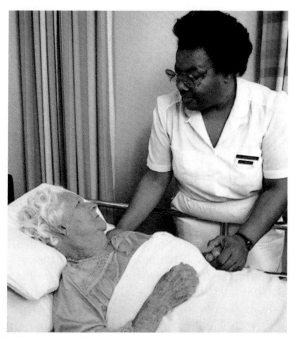

FIGURE 11-16 Provide supportive care and listen to sick individuals as they express their fears.

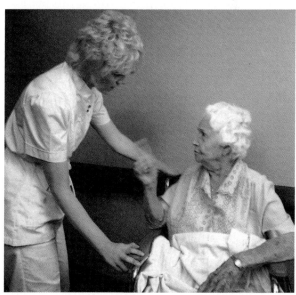

FIGURE 11-17 Hostile or combative behavior often signals feelings of frustration or confusion.

ing in behavior, paying less attention to personal hygiene, and being unable to respond to simple commands or follow instructions.

CAUSES OF CONFUSION AND DISORIENTATION

Delirium is the term used when confusion or disorientation is a temporary condition caused by a treatable condition. Stress and/or depression caused by physical or psychosocial changes is one possible cause. Use of alcohol or chemicals is another. Kidney disease, which interferes with electrolyte balance; respiratory disease, which decreases oxygen; or liver disease, which interferes with metabolism, are other causes. Elderly individuals are also more sensitive to medications, and drugs can sometimes accumulate in the body and cause confusion and disorientation. Even poor nutrition or lack of fluid intake can interfere with mental ability. Frequently, identification and treatment of any of these conditions decreases and even eliminates the confusion and disorientation. For example, changing a medication or giving it in smaller doses may restore normal function.

Disease and/or damage to the brain can sometimes result in chronic confusion or disorientation. A **cerebrovascular accident,** or stroke, which damages brain cells, is one possible cause. A blood clot can obstruct blood flow to the brain, or a vessel can rupture and cause hemorrhaging in the brain. **Arteriosclerosis,** a condition in which the walls of blood vessels become thick and lose their elasticity, is common in elderly individuals. If the vessels become narrow because of deposits of fat and minerals, such as calcium, the condition is called **atherosclerosis.** These conditions can cause **transient ischemic attacks (TIAs),** or ministrokes, which result in temporary periods of diminished blood flow to the brain. Each time an attack occurs, more damage to brain cells results.

Dementia, also called *brain syndrome,* is a loss of mental ability characterized by a decrease in intellectual ability, loss of memory, impaired judgment, personality change, and disorientation. When the symptoms are caused by high fever, kidney infection, dehydration, hypoxia (lack of oxygen), drug toxicity, or other treatable conditions, the condition is called *delirium* or, in some cases, *acute dementia.* When the symptoms are caused by permanent, irreversible damage to brain cells, the condition is called *chronic dementia.* Cerebrovascular accidents, arteriosclerosis, and TIAs can be contributing causes to chronic dementia. One modern theory suggests that chronic dementia is caused by either a complete lack or an inadequate amount of an enzyme. Whatever the cause, chronic dementia is usually regarded as a progressive, irreversible disease.

Alzheimer's disease (AD) is a form of dementia that causes progressive changes in brain cells. Individuals with AD lack a neurotransmitter, or chemical, that allows messages to pass between nerve cells in the brain. This results in the death of neurons and the development of neuritic plaques (deposits of protein) and neurofibrillary tangles. Alzheimer's disease can occur in individuals as young as 40 years of age, but frequently occurs in those in their 60s and 70s. The cause is unknown, but there are many theories currently being researched. A genetic defect, a missing enzyme, toxic effects of aluminum, a virus, and the faulty metabolism of glucose have all been implicated as possible causes. Whatever the cause, AD is viewed as a terminal, incurable brain disease usually lasting from 3 to 10 years.

In the early stages, the individual exhibits self-centeredness, a decreased interest in social activities, memory loss, mood and personality changes, anxiety, agitation, depression, poor judgment, confusion regarding time and place, and an inability to plan and follow through with many activities of daily living (figure 11-18). As the disease progresses, nighttime restlessness and wandering occur, mood swings become frequent, personal hygiene is ignored, confusion and forgetfulness become severe, perseveration or repetitive behavior occurs, the ability to understand others and/or speak coherently decreases, weight fluctuates, paranoia and hallucinations increase, and full-time supervision becomes necessary. In the terminal stages, the individual experiences total disorientation regarding person, time, and place; becomes incoherent and is unable to communicate with words; loses control of bladder and bowel functions; develops seizures; loses weight despite eating a balanced diet; becomes totally dependent; and finally, lapses into a coma and dies. Death is frequently caused by pneumonia, infections, and kidney failure. Progress through the various stages of this disease varies among individuals.

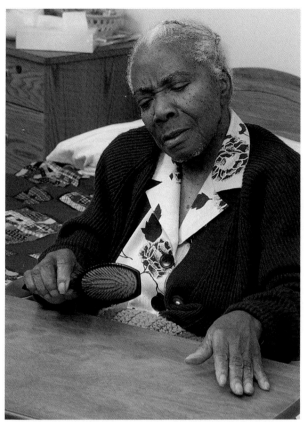

FIGURE 11-18 A patient with Alzheimer's disease may forget how common objects are used and have problems with normal activities of daily living.

CARING FOR CONFUSED OR DISORIENTED INDIVIDUALS

Whatever the cause of confusion or disorientation, certain courses of care should be followed. A primary concern is to provide a safe and secure environment. Dangerous objects such as drugs, poisons, scissors, knives, razors, guns, power tools, cleaning solutions, and matches and lighters should be kept out of reach and in a locked area. If the individual tends to wander, doors and windows should be secure. In severe cases, special sensors may be attached to the leg or wrist of the disoriented individual (figure 11-19). The sensors alert others if the individual starts to leave a specific area.

Following the same routine is also important. Meals, baths, dressing, walks, and bedtime should each occur at approximately the same time each day. Any change in routine can cause stress and confusion. Even though the individual should be encouraged to be as active as possible, activities should be kept simple and last for short periods of time (figure 11-20). A calm, quiet environment is also important. Loud noises, crowded rooms,

Diagnosing AD is difficult because there is no specific test that can be used. Currently, diagnosis is confirmed when neuritic plaques are found during an autopsy after death. However, researchers are currently evaluating two new high-technology brain scans that may assist in identifying AD in early stages. One scan checks for low levels of glucose metabolism in the hippocampus, a key memory center in the brain, because hippocampus shrinking is an indication of AD. A second scan uses magnetic resonance spectroscopy (MRS) to examine the biochemical activity in the brain of two neurochemicals typically altered in AD. Research is also being conducted to develop a blood test that checks for low levels of a protein called beta-amyloid 40 because low levels of this protein appear to indicate a high risk for developing AD. Although there is no cure for AD, several different medications have shown promise in improving memory and thinking skills in the earlier stages of the disease. For this reason, early diagnosis and intervention is essential.

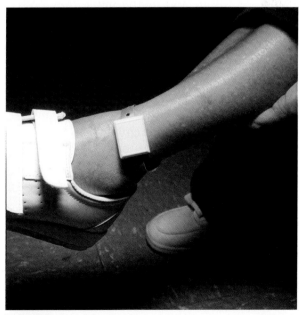

FIGURE 11-19 Special sensors may be attached to the leg or wrist of a wandering or disoriented individual.

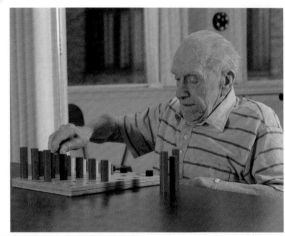

FIGURE 11-20 Activities for an individual who is confused or disoriented should be kept simple and last for short periods of time.

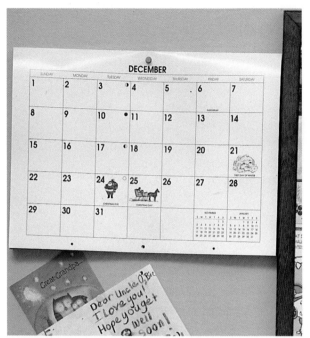

FIGURE 11-21 A large calendar may help orient a person to days and special events.

and excessive commotion can cause the individual to become agitated and even more disoriented.

Reality orientation (RO) consists of activities that help promote awareness of person, time, and place. The activities can be followed by anyone caring for the confused individual, whether the care is in the home or in a long-term care facility. Some aspects of reality orientation are the following:

♦ Be calm and gentle when approaching the individual.

♦ Address the person by the name they prefer, for example, "Mr. Smith" or "Mike."

♦ Avoid terms such as "sweetie," "baby," and "honey."

♦ State your name and correct the person if he or she calls you a wrong name. For example, if a patient thinks you are his or her daughter, say, "I am not your daughter Lisa. I am Mrs. Simmers, your nurse for today."

♦ Make constant references to day, time, and place. "It is 8:00 Tuesday morning and time for breakfast."

♦ Use clocks, calendars, and information boards to point out time, day, and activities (figure 11-21).

♦ Maintain a constant, limited routine.

♦ Keep the individual oriented to day night cycles. During the day, encourage the person to wear regular clothes. Also, open the curtains and point out the sunshine. At night, close the curtains, use night lights if necessary, and promote quiet and rest.

♦ Speak slowly and clearly and ask clear and simple questions.

♦ Never rush or hurry the individual.

♦ Repeat instructions patiently. Allow time for the individual to respond.

♦ Encourage conversations about familiar things or current events.

♦ Allow the person to reminisce or remember past experiences.

♦ Encourage the use of a television or radio, but avoid overstimulating the individual.

♦ Make sure the individual uses sensory aids such as glasses and hearing aids (if needed), and that the devices are in good working order.

♦ Keep familiar objects and pictures within view. Avoid moving the person's furniture or belongings.

♦ Do not argue with incorrect statements. Gently provide correct information if the person is able to accept the information without agitation. For example, when a person states it is time to dress for work, say, "You don't have to go to work today. You retired seven years ago."

- Do not hesitate to use touch, if culturally appropriate, to communicate with the person, unless this causes agitation (figure 11-22).

- Avoid arguments or recriminations. When you find an elderly resident in the wrong area, do not say, "You know you are not supposed to be here." Instead, say, "Let me show you how to get to your room."

- Encourage independence and self-help whenever possible.

- Always treat the person with respect and dignity.

Reality orientation is usually effective during the early stages of confusion or disorientation. In later stages, when the individual is not able to respond, it can cause increased anxiety and agitation. When patient assessment shows that this is occurring, avoid confronting the patient with reality. For example, do not tell a patient who wants to see her husband that her husband died 10 years ago. Instead, ask her to tell you about her husband and allow her to reminisce. Provide supportive care to allow the patient to maintain dignity and express feelings.

Caring for a confused or disoriented individual can be frustrating and even frightening at

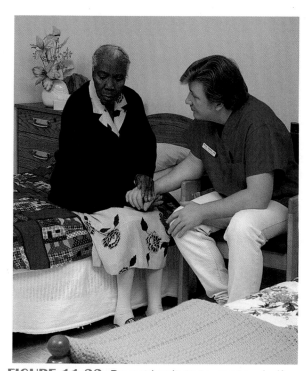

FIGURE 11-22 Do not hesitate to use touch, if culturally appropriate, to communicate with an individual who is disoriented.

times. Continual assessment of the individual's abilities and problems is needed to design a health care program that will allow the individual to function within the level of his or her ability. Patience, consistency, and sincere caring are essential on the part of the health care provider.

STUDENT: *Go to the workbook and complete the assignment sheet for 11:4, Confusion and Disorientation in the Elderly.*

11:5 INFORMATION

Meeting the Needs of the Elderly

Providing care to the elderly can be a challenging but rewarding experience. It is important to remember that the needs of the elderly do not differ greatly from the needs of any other individual. They have the same physical and psychological needs as any person at any age. However, these needs are sometimes intensified by physical or psychosocial changes that disrupt the normal life pattern. When this occurs, the elderly individual needs understanding, acceptance, and the knowledge that someone cares.

A few other factors must be considered when caring for elderly individuals. One is the importance of meeting cultural needs. **Culture** can be defined as the values, beliefs, ideas, customs, and characteristics that are passed from one generation to the next. An individual's culture can affect language, food habits, dress, work, leisure activities, and health care. Culture creates differences in individuals. For example, a person may speak a different language or have specific likes or dislikes about food or dress. It is important for the health care worker to learn about a person's culture, and about the person's likes, dislikes, and beliefs. This allows the health care worker to provide care that shows a respect and acceptance of the cultural differences. (Cultural diversity is discussed in greater detail in Chapter 10 of this text.)

Religious needs are another important aspect of care. **Religion** can be defined as the spiritual beliefs and practices of an individual. Like culture, religious or spiritual beliefs can affect the lifestyle of an individual. Diet, days of worship, practices relating to birth and death, and even acceptance of medical care can be affected. The beliefs of specific religions are discussed in table 10-2 in Chapter 10:3 of this text. It is important to accept an individual's beliefs without bias. It is equally important that health care workers do not force their own religious beliefs on the individuals for whom they provide care. For example, if a patient asks, "Do you believe in life after death?" a health care worker may respond by saying, "How do you feel?" or "You have been thinking about the meaning of life." This allows patients to express their own feelings and thoughts. Other ways the health care worker can show respect and consideration for a person's religious beliefs include proper treatment of religious articles, such as a Bible or Koran; allowing a person to practice religion with prayer, observance of religious holidays, or participation in religious services; honoring a patient's requests for special foods; and providing privacy during clergy visits (figure 11-23).

Freedom from abuse is another important aspect of care. Abuse of the elderly can be physical, verbal, psychological, or sexual. Handling the individual roughly; denying food, water, or medication; yelling or screaming at the person; or causing fear are all forms of abuse. Abuse is sometimes difficult to prove. Frequently, the abuser is a family member or caretaker. Elderly individuals may want to protect the abuser or may even feel that they deserve the abuse. All states have laws requiring the reporting of any suspected abuse. It is important for any health care worker who sees or suspects abuse of the elderly to report it to the proper agency.

A final aspect of meeting the needs of the elderly is to respect and follow the patient's rights. Patients' rights are discussed in Chapter 5:3 of this textbook. These rights assure the elderly individual of "kind and considerate care," and provide for meeting individual needs. One program that exists to ensure the rights of the elderly is the Ombudsman Program. It was developed by the federal government in its Older Americans Act. Each state has its own program designed to meet federal standards. Basically, an **ombudsman** is a specially trained individual who works with the elderly and their families, health care providers, and other concerned individuals to improve quality of care and quality of life. The ombudsman may investigate and try to resolve complaints, suggest improvements for health care, monitor and enforce state and/or federal regulations, report problems to the correct agency, and provide education for individuals involved in the care of the elderly. Although the role of the ombudsman may vary from state to state, it is important for the health care worker to cooperate and work effectively with the ombudsman to ensure that the needs of the elderly are met.

STUDENT: *Go to the workbook and complete the assignment sheet for 11:5, Meeting the Needs of the Elderly.*

CHAPTER 11 SUMMARY

Geriatric care is care provided to elderly individuals. Because this age group uses health care services frequently, and many individuals are now living longer, it is important for the health care worker to understand the special needs of the elderly population.

Many myths, or false beliefs, exist regarding elderly individuals. Examples include the belief that most elderly individuals are cared for in long-term care facilities, are incompetent and incapable of making decisions, live in poverty, do not want to work, and are unhappy and lonely. Although these beliefs may be true for some elderly individuals, they are not true for the majority.

Physical changes occur in all individuals as a normal part of the aging process. It is important to remember that most of the changes are grad-

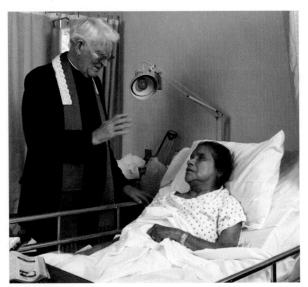

FIGURE 11-23 Respect religious needs and provide privacy while a resident is visiting with a member of the clergy.

TODAY'S RESEARCH: TOMORROW'S HEALTH CARE

People living to 200 years of age?

Aging has always been considered a normal deterioration of the human body. This concept changed when Cynthia Kenyon, a geneticist at the University of California, discovered a set of genes in worms that seemed to regulate aging. By suppressing the action of one of the genes, Kenyon was able to increase a worm's life span by six times and keep it young.

Research started with a mutant tiny nematode worm, about 1 millimeter long, that appeared to live about 50 percent longer than other nematode worms. By looking for mutant genes, Kenyon discovered the *daf-2* gene, a gene that controls the aging process. Further research showed that the *daf-2* gene is a protein that allows body tissues to respond to hormones. The mutant *daf-2* gene reduced this activity, making the tissue less responsive to hormones and allowing it to delay the aging process. A second gene, the *daf-16* gene, was identified as the fountain of youth gene because it promotes youthfulness. These genes allowed the mutant worms not only to delay the aging process, but also to remain youthful, similar to a 95-year-old functioning like a 45-year-old. The research showed that aging is regulated by hormones and the endocrine system. By slowing the action of the hormones, aging can be postponed and age-related diseases can be prevented. This is because age is the largest risk factor for many diseases. An individual is much more likely to experience development of a cancerous tumor at age 70 than at age 30.

Other researchers using this information are extending the life span of mice by more than 30 percent and are continuing to experiment with other mammals that have genes similar to those of humans. Their goal is to develop drugs that mimic the effects of the genes in the long-lived animals. If they succeed, many of the age-related diseases may be preventable, and individuals may remain youthful and productive throughout their life spans.

ual and occur over a long period of time. The physical changes may impose some limitations on the activities of the individual. If the health care worker is aware of these changes and is able to provide individuals with ways to adapt to and cope with the changes, many elderly individuals can enjoy life even with physical limitations.

Psychosocial changes also create special needs in the elderly. Retirement, death of a spouse and of friends, changes in social relationships, new living environments, loss of independence, and disease and disability can all cause stress and crisis for an individual. With support, understanding, and patience, health care workers can assist elderly individuals as they learn to accommodate the changes and to function in new situations.

Although most elderly individuals remain mentally alert until death, some have periods of confusion and disorientation. This is sometimes a temporary condition that can be corrected. Other times, disease and/or damage to the brain results in chronic confusion or disorientation. Special techniques should be used in dealing with these individuals. Providing a safe and secure environment, following a set routine, promoting reality orientation, and giving supportive care can allow individuals to function to the best of their abilities.

Meeting the cultural and religious needs of the elderly is also essential. In addition, it is important for health care workers to respect and follow the "rights" of elderly individuals and to protect the elderly from abuse.

INTERNET SEARCHES

Use the suggested search engines in Chapter 17:4 of this textbook to search the Internet for additional information on the following topics:

1. *Gerontology:* search words such as gerontology, geriatrics, and geriatric assistant for additional information on aging

2. *Long-term care facilities:* search for information on assisted-living, independent living, extended-care, and adult daycare facilities;

meals on wheels; and other resources for the elderly

3. *Diseases*: search for additional information on senile lentigines, osteoporosis, arthritis, emphysema, bronchitis, cerebrovascular accident, arteriosclerosis, atherosclerosis, transient ischemic attack, dementia, and Alzheimer's disease

4. *Disabilities*: search for information on different types of assistive devices for individuals with disabilities

5. *Federal government programs*: search for information on the Older American Act, Omnibus Budget Reconciliation Act of 1987, and an ombudsman

REVIEW QUESTIONS

1. Define *gerontology*.

2. Why is it important for a health care worker to differentiate between myths and facts of aging?

3. Identify factors that can decrease the speed and degree of physical changes of aging. Identify factors that can cause an increase.

4. What measures can be taken to help an individual adapt or cope with the following physical changes of aging?

   a. dry, itching skin

   b. increased sensitivity to cold

   c. hearing loss and the inability to hear high-frequency sounds

   d. difficulty in chewing and a decreased sense of taste

   e. indigestion, flatulence, and constipation

   f. weakness, dizziness, and dyspnea while exercising

5. Differentiate between disease and disability.

6. List four (4) factors that cause psychosocial changes in aging. For each factor, provide at least two (2) examples of ways an individual can be helped to adapt or cope with the change.

7. Differentiate between acute dementia (delirium) and chronic dementia. Identify four (4) causes for each type of dementia.

8. Why is it important to respect an individual's cultural and religious beliefs?

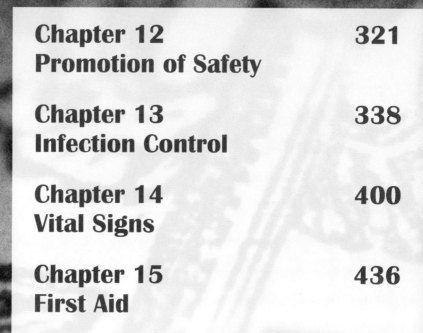

PART 4

Basics of Health Care

CHAPTER 12

Promotion of Safety

Observe Standard Precautions

Instructor's Check—Call Instructor at This Point

Safety—Proceed with Caution

OBRA Requirement—Based on Federal Law

Math Skill

Legal Responsibility

Science Skill

Career Information

Communications Skill

Technology

Chapter Objectives

After completing this chapter, you should be able to:

◆ Define *body mechanics*
◆ Use correct body mechanics while performing procedures in the laboratory or clinical area
◆ Observe all safety standards established by OSHA, especially the Occupational Exposure to Hazardous Chemicals Standard and the Bloodborne Pathogen Standard
◆ Follow safety regulations stated while performing in the laboratory area
◆ Observe all regulations for patient safety while performing procedures on a student partner in the laboratory or clinical area, or on a patient in any area
◆ List the four main classes of fire extinguishers
◆ Relate each class of fire extinguisher to the specific fire(s) for which it is used
◆ Simulate the operation of a fire extinguisher by following the directions on the extinguisher and specific measures for observing fire safety
◆ Locate and describe the operation of the nearest fire alarm
◆ Describe in detail the evacuation plan for the laboratory area according to established school policy
◆ Define, pronounce, and spell all key terms

KEY TERMS

base of support
Bloodborne Pathogen
    Standard
body mechanics
ergonomics
fire extinguishers

Material Safety Data Sheet
    (MSDS)
Occupational Exposure to
    Hazardous Chemicals
    Standard

Occupational Safety and
    Health Administration
    (OSHA)
safety standards

12:1 INFORMATION

Using Body Mechanics

To prevent injury to yourself and others while working in the health field, it is important that you observe good body mechanics.

Body mechanics refers to the way in which the body moves and maintains balance while making the most efficient use of all its parts. Basic rules for body mechanics are provided as guidelines to prevent strain and help maintain muscle strength.

There are four main reasons for using good body mechanics:

◆ Muscles work best when used correctly.

◆ Correct use of muscles makes lifting, pulling, and pushing easier.

◆ Correct application of body mechanics prevents unnecessary fatigue and strain, and saves energy.

◆ Correct application of body mechanics prevents injury to self and others.

Eight basic rules of good body mechanics include:

◆ Maintain a broad **base of support** by keeping the feet 8–10 inches apart, placing one foot slightly forward, balancing weight on both feet, and pointing the toes in the direction of movement (figure 12-1).

◆ Bend from the hips and knees to get close to an object, and keep your back straight (figure 12-2). Do not bend at the waist.

◆ Use the strongest muscles to do the job. The larger and stronger muscles are located in the shoulders, upper arms, hips, and thighs. Back muscles are weak.

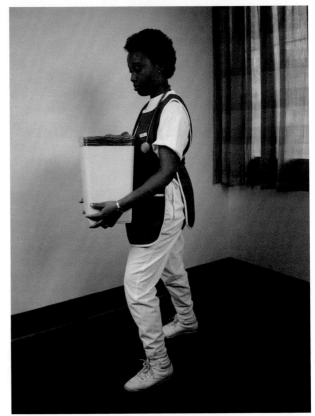

FIGURE 12-1 Maintain a broad base of support by keeping the feet 8–10 inches apart.

◆ Use the weight of your body to help push or pull an object. Whenever possible, push, slide, or pull rather than lift.

◆ Carry heavy objects close to the body. Also, stand close to any object or person being moved.

◆ Avoid twisting your body as you work. Turn with your feet and entire body when you change direction of movement.

◆ Avoid bending for long periods.

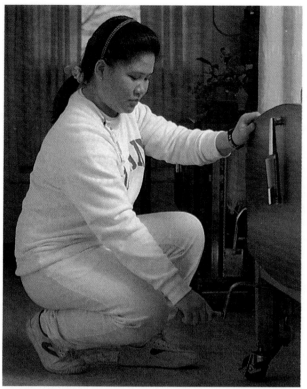

FIGURE 12-2 Bend from the hips and knees to get close to an object.

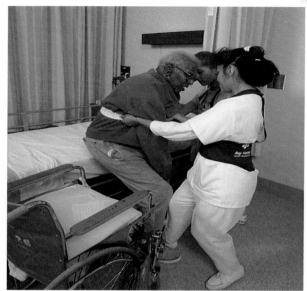

FIGURE 12-3 Some health care facilities now require workers to wear back supports while lifting or moving patients.

♦ If a patient or object is too heavy for you to lift alone, always get help. Mechanical lifts, transfer (gait) belts, wheelchairs, and other similar types of equipment are also available to help lift and move patients.

Some health care facilities now require health care workers to wear back supports while lifting or moving patients (figure 12-3). The supports are supposed to help prevent back injuries, but their use is controversial. Back supports may provide a false sense of security as an individual tries to lift heavier loads. It is important to remember that a back brace does not increase strength. Back sup-

ports may also cause sweating, skin irritation, and increased abdominal pressure. They do remind the wearer to use good body mechanics. If a back support is used, it should be the correct size to provide the maximum benefit. When the worker is performing strenuous tasks, the support should fit snugly. At other times, it should be loosened to decrease abdominal pressure.

STUDENT: *Go to the workbook and complete the assignment sheet for 12:1, Using Body Mechanics. Then return and continue with the procedure.*

PROCEDURE 12:1

Using Body Mechanics

Equipment and Supplies

Heavy book, bedside stand, bed with wheel locks

Procedure

1. Assemble equipment.

2. Compare using a narrow base of support to using a broad base of support. Stand on your toes, with your feet close

PROCEDURE 12:1

together. Next, stand on your toes with your feet farther apart. Then, stand with your feet flat on the floor but close together. Finally, stand with your feet flat on the floor but approximately 8–10 inches apart and with one foot slightly forward. Balance your weight on both feet. You should feel the best support in the final position because the broad base supports your body weight.

3. Place the book on the floor. Bend from the hips and knees (not the waist) and keep your back straight to pick up the book. Return to the standing position.

4. Place the book between your thumb and fingers, but not touching the palm of your hand, and hold your hand straight out in front of your body. Slowly move your hand toward your body, stopping several times to feel the weight of the book in different positions. Finally, hold the book with your entire hand and bring your hand close to your body. The final position should be the most comfortable.

    NOTE: This illustrates the need to carry heavy objects close to your body and to use the strongest muscles to do the job.

5. Stand at either end of the bed. Release the wheel locks on the bed. Position your feet to provide a broad base of sup-

port. Get close to the bed. Use the weight of your body to push the bed forward.

6. Place the book on the bed. Pick up the book and place it on the bedside stand. Avoid twisting your body. Turn with your feet to place the book on the stand.

    NOTE: Remember that holding the book close to your body allows you to use the strongest muscles.

7. Practice the rules of body mechanics by setting up situations similar to those listed in the previous steps. Continue until the movements feel natural to you.

8. Replace all equipment used.

Practice

Use the evaluation sheet for 12:1, Using Body Mechanics, to practice this procedure. When you believe you have mastered this skill, sign the sheet and give it to your instructor for further action.

 Final Checkpoint Using the criteria listed on the evaluation sheet, your instructor will grade your performance.

12:2 INFORMATION

Preventing Accidents and Injuries

The **Occupational Safety and Health Administration (OSHA),** a division of the Department of Labor, establishes and enforces **safety standards** for the workplace. Two main standards affect health care workers:

♦ The Occupational Exposure to Hazardous Chemicals Standard

♦ The Bloodborne Pathogen Standard

CHEMICAL HAZARDS

The **Occupational Exposure to Hazardous Chemicals Standard** requires that employers inform employees of all chemicals and hazards in the workplace. In addition, all manufacturers must provide **Material Safety Data Sheets (MSDSs)** with any hazardous products they sell (figure 12-4). The MSDSs must provide the following information:

The Clorox Company
1221 Broadway
Oakland, CA 94612
Tel. (510) 271-7000

Material Safety Data Sheet

I Product:	CLOROX REGULAR-BLEACH
Description:	CLEAR, LIGHT YELLOW LIQUID WITH A CHARACTERISTIC CHLORINE ODOR

Other Designations	Distributor	Emergency Telephone Nos.
Clorox Bleach EPA Reg. No. 5813-50	Clorox Sales Company 1221 Broadway Oakland, CA 94612	For Medical Emergencies call: (800) 446-1014 For Transportation Emergencies Chemtrec (800) 424-9300

II Health Hazard Data

DANGER: CORROSIVE. May cause severe irritation or damage to eyes and skin. Vapor or mist may irritate. Harmful if swallowed. Keep out of reach of children.

Some clinical reports suggest a low potential for sensitization upon exaggerated exposure to sodium hypochlorite if skin damage (e.g., irritation) occurs during exposure. Under normal consumer use conditions the likelihood of any adverse health effects are low.

Medical conditions that may be aggravated by exposure to high concentrations of vapor or mist: heart conditions or chronic respiratory problems such as asthma, emphysema, chronic bronchitis or obstructive lung disease.

FIRST AID:

Eye Contact: Hold eye open and rinse with water for 15-20 minutes. Remove contact lenses, after first 5 minutes. Continue rinsing eye. Call a physician.

Skin Contact: Wash skin with water for 15-20 minutes. If irritation develops, call a physician.

Ingestion: Do not induce vomiting. Drink a glassful of water. If irritation develops, call a physician. Do not give anything by mouth to an unconscious person.

Inhalation: Remove to fresh air. If breathing is affected, call a physician.

III Hazardous Ingredients

Ingredient	Concentration	Exposure Limit
Sodium hypochlorite CAS# 7681-52-9	6.15%	Not established
Sodium hydroxide CAS# 1310-73-2	<1%	2 mg/m³; [1] 2 mg/m³; [2]

[1] ACGIH Threshold Limit Value (TLV) - Ceiling

[2] OHSA Permissible Exposure Limit (PEL) – Time Weighted Average (TWA)

None of the ingredients in this product are on the IARC, NTP or OSHA carcinogen lists.

IV Special Protection and Precautions

No special protection or precautions have been identified for using this product under directed consumer use conditions. The following recommendations are given for production facilities and for other conditions and situations where there is increased potential for accidental, large-scale or prolonged exposure.

Hygienic Practices: Avoid contact with eyes, skin and clothing. Wash hands after direct contact. Do not wear product-contaminated clothing for prolonged periods.

Engineering Controls: Use general ventilation to minimize exposure to vapor or mist.

Personal Protective Equipment: Wear safety glasses. Use rubber or nitrile gloves if in contact liquid, especially for prolonged periods.

KEEP OUT OF REACH OF CHILDREN

V Transportation and Regulatory Data

DOT/IMDG/IATA - Not restricted.

EPA - SARA TITLE III/CERCLA: Bottled product is not reportable under Sections 311/312 and contains no chemicals reportable under Section 313. This product does contain chemicals (sodium hydroxide <0.2% and sodium hypochlorite <7.35%) that are regulated under Section 304/CERCLA.

TSCA/DSL STATUS: All components of this product are on the U.S. TSCA Inventory and Canadian DSL.

VI Spill Procedures/Waste Disposal

Spill Procedures: Control spill. Containerize liquid and use absorbents on residual liquid; dispose appropriately. Wash area and let dry. For spills of multiple products, responders should evaluate the MSDS's of the products for incompatibility with sodium hypochlorite. Breathing protection should be worn in enclosed, and/or poorly ventilated areas until hazard assessment is complete.

Waste Disposal: Dispose of in accordance with all applicable federal, state, and local regulations.

VII Reactivity Data

Stable under normal use and storage conditions. Strong oxidizing agent. Reacts with other household chemicals such as toilet bowl cleaners, rust removers, vinegar, acids or ammonia containing products to produce hazardous gases, such as chlorine and other chlorinated species. Prolonged contact with metal may cause pitting or discoloration.

VIII Fire and Explosion Data

Flash Point: None

Special Firefighting Procedures: None

Unusual Fire/Explosion Hazards: None. Not flammable or explosive. Product does not ignite when exposed to open flame.

IX Physical Data

Boiling point...°F/100°C approx. 212
Specific Gravity (H₂0=1) ....°F~ 1.1 at 70
Solubility in Water .... complete
pH ....~11.4

DATA SUPPLIED IS FOR USE ONLY IN CONNECTION WITH OCCUPATIONAL SAFETY AND HEALTH   DATE PREPARED 05/05

FIGURE 12-4 Read the Material Safety Data Sheet (MSDS) before using any chemical product. *(Courtesy of the Clorox Company, Oakland, CA)*

♦ Product identification information about the chemical

♦ Protection or precautions that should be used while handling the chemical (for example, wearing protective equipment or using only in a well-ventilated area)

♦ Instructions for the safe use of the chemical

♦ Procedures for handling spills, cleanup, and disposal of the product

♦ Emergency first-aid procedures to use if injury occurs

The Occupational Exposure to Hazardous Chemicals Standard also mandates that all employers train employees on the proper procedures or policies to follow with regard to:

♦ Identifying the types and locations of all chemicals or hazards

♦ Locating and using the MSDS manual containing all of the safety data sheets

♦ Reading and interpreting chemical labels and hazard signs

♦ Using personal protective equipment (PPE) such as masks, gowns, gloves, and goggles

♦ Locating cleaning equipment and following correct methods for managing spills and/or disposal of chemicals

♦ Reporting accidents or exposures and documenting any incidents that occur

BLOODBORNE PATHOGEN STANDARD

The **Bloodborne Pathogen Standard** has mandates to protect health care providers from diseases caused by exposure to body fluids. Examples of body fluids include blood and blood components, urine, stool, semen, vaginal secretions, cerebrospinal fluid, saliva, mucus, and other similar fluids. Three diseases that can be contracted by exposure to body fluids include hepatitis B, caused by the hepatitis B virus, hepatitis C, caused by the hepatitis C virus, and acquired immune deficiency syndrome (AIDS), caused by the human immunodeficiency virus. The mandates of this standard are discussed in detail in Chapter 13:4.

ENVIRONMENTAL SAFETY

Ergonomics is an applied science used to promote the safety and well-being of a person by adapting the environment and using techniques to prevent injuries. Ergonomics includes the correct placement of furniture and equipment, training in required muscle movements, efforts to avoid repetitive motions, and an awareness of the environment to prevent injuries. The prevention of accidents and injury centers around people and the immediate environment. The health worker must be conscious of personal and patient/resident safety at all times. In addition, every health care worker must be alert to unsafe situations and report them immediately. Examples include burned-out lightbulbs, frayed electrical cords, scalding water in a sink or bath area, missing floor tiles or torn carpet, and other similar hazards.

In addition, every health care worker must accept the responsibility for using good judgment in all situations, asking questions when in doubt, and following approved policies and procedures to create a safe environment. Always remember that a health care worker has a legal responsibility to protect the patient from harm and injury.

Equipment and Solutions Safety

Basic rules that must be followed when working with equipment and solutions include:

♦ Do *not* operate or use any equipment until you have been instructed on how to use it.

♦ Read and follow the operating instructions for all major pieces of equipment. If you do not understand the instructions, ask for assistance.

♦ Do *not* operate any equipment if your instructor/immediate supervisor is not in the room.

♦ Report any damaged or malfunctioning equipment immediately. Make no attempt to use it. Some facilities use a lockout tag system for damaged electrical or mechanical equipment. A locking device is placed on the equipment to prevent the equipment from being used (figure 12-5).

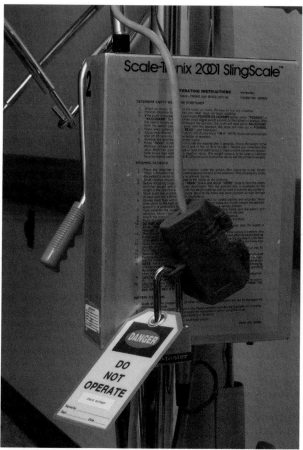

FIGURE 12-5 Some facilities use a lockout tag system for damaged equipment to prevent anyone from using the equipment.

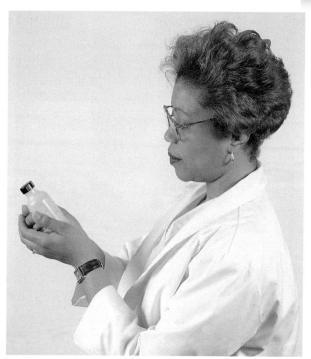

FIGURE 12-6 Read the label on a solution bottle at least three times to be sure you have the correct solution.

♦ Do not use frayed or damaged electrical cords. Do not use a plug if the third prong for grounding has been broken off. Never use excessive force to insert a plug into an outlet.

♦ Never handle any electrical equipment with wet hands or around water.

♦ Store all equipment in its proper place. Unused equipment should not be left in a patient's room, a hallway, or a doorway.

♦ When handling any equipment, observe all safety precautions that have been taught.

♦ Read MSDSs before using any hazardous chemical solutions.

♦ Never use solutions from bottles that are not labeled.

♦ Read the labels of solution bottles at least three times during use to be sure you have the correct solution (figure 12-6).

♦ Do *not* mix any solutions together unless instructed to do so by your instructor/imme-

diate supervisor or you can verify that they are compatible.

♦ Some solutions can be injurious or poisonous. Avoid contact with your eyes and skin. Avoid inhaling any fumes displaced by a solution. Use only as directed.

♦ Store all chemical solutions in a locked cabinet or closet following the manufacturer's recommendations. For example, some solutions must be kept at room temperature, while others must be stored in a cool area.

♦ Dispose of chemical solutions according to the instructions provided on the MSDS for the solution.

♦ If you break any equipment or spill any solutions, immediately report the incident to your instructor/immediate supervisor. You will be told how to dispose of the equipment or how to remove the spilled solution (figure 12-7).

Patient/Resident Safety

Basic rules that must be followed to protect a patient or resident include:

♦ Do *not* perform any procedure on patients unless you have been instructed to do so.

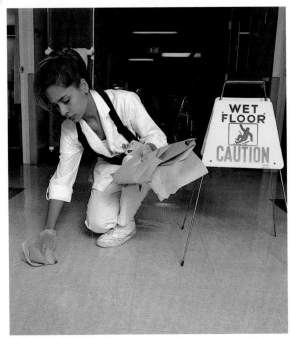

FIGURE 12-7 Follow proper procedure to clean up spilled solutions.

Make sure you have the proper authorization. Follow instructions carefully. Ask questions if you do not understand. Use correct or approved methods while performing any procedure. Avoid shortcuts or incorrect techniques.

♦ Provide privacy for all patients. Knock on the door before entering any room (figure 12-8A). Speak to the patient and identify yourself. Ask for permission to enter before going behind closed privacy curtains. Close the door and/or draw curtains for privacy before beginning a procedure on the patient (figure 12-8B).

♦ Always identify your patient. Be absolutely positive that you have the correct patient. Check the identification wristband, if present. Ask the patient to state his or her name. Repeat the patient's name at least twice. Check the name on the patient's bed and on the patient's record.

♦ Always explain the procedure so the patient knows what you are going to do (figure 12-8C). Answer any questions and make sure you have the patient's consent before performing any procedure. Never perform a procedure if a patient refuses to allow you to do so.

♦ Observe the patient closely during any procedure. If you notice any change, immediately report this. Be alert to the patient's condition at all times.

♦ Frequently check the patient area, waiting room, office rooms, bed areas, or home environment for safety hazards. Report all unsafe situations immediately to the proper person or correct the safety hazard.

♦ Before leaving a patient/resident in a bed, observe all safety checkpoints. Make sure the patient is in a comfortable position. Check the bed to be sure that the side rails are elevated, if indicated; the bed is at the lowest level to the floor; and the wheels on the bed are locked to prevent movement of the bed. Place the call

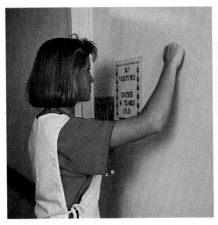

FIGURE 12-8A Always knock on the door or speak before entering a patient's room.

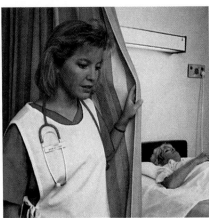

FIGURE 12-8B Close the door and draw curtains for privacy before beginning a procedure.

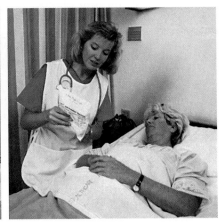

FIGURE 12-8C Explain the procedure and answer any questions to make sure you have the patient's consent.

signal (a bell can be used in a home situation) (figure 12-9A) and other supplies such as the telephone, television remote control, fresh water, and tissues within easy reach of the patient/resident (figure 12-9B). Open the privacy curtains if they were closed. Leave the area neat and clean, and make sure no safety hazards are present.

Personal Safety

Basic rules that must be followed to protect yourself and others include:

♦ Remember, it is your responsibility to protect yourself and others from injury.

♦ Use correct body mechanics while performing any procedure.

♦ Wear the required uniform.

♦ Walk—do *not* run—in the laboratory area or clinical area, in hallways, and especially on stairs. Keep to the right and watch carefully at intersections to avoid collisions. Use handrails on stairways.

♦ Promptly report any personal injury or accident, no matter how minor, to your instructor/immediate supervisor.

♦ If you see an unsafe situation or a violation of a safety practice, report it to your instructor/immediate supervisor promptly.

♦ Keep all areas clean and neat with all equipment and supplies in their proper locations at all times.

♦ Wash your hands frequently. Hands should always be washed before and after any procedure, and any time they become contaminated during a procedure (figure 12-10).

♦ Keep your hands away from your face, eyes, mouth, and hair.

♦ Dry your hands thoroughly before handling any electrical equipment.

♦ Wear safety glasses when instructed to do so and in situations that might result in possible eye injury.

♦ While working with your partner in patient simulations, observe all safety precautions taught in caring for a patient. Review the role each of you will have before you begin practicing a procedure so each person knows his or her responsibilities. Avoid horseplay and practical jokes; they cause accidents.

♦ If any solutions come in contact with your skin or eyes, immediately flush the area with cool water. Inform your instructor/immediate supervisor.

♦ If a particle gets in your eye, inform your instructor/immediate supervisor. Do *not* try to remove the particle or rub your eye.

STUDENT: *Go to the workbook and complete the assignment sheet for 12:2, Preventing Accidents and Injuries. Then return and continue with the procedure.*

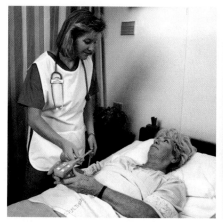

FIGURE 12-9A Lower the bed and place the call signal within easy reach of the patient before leaving a patient.

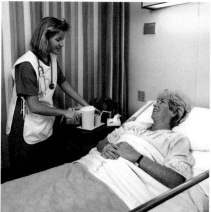

FIGURE 12-9B Make sure other supplies and equipment are conveniently placed within the patient's reach.

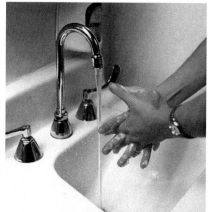

FIGURE 12-10 Wash your hands before and after any procedure, and any time they become contaminated during a procedure.

PROCEDURE 12:2

Preventing Accidents and Injuries

Equipment and Supplies

Information section on Preventing Accidents and Injuries, several bottles of solutions, laboratory area with equipment

Procedure

1. Assemble equipment.

2. Review the safety standards in the information section for Preventing Accidents and Injuries. Note standards that are not clear and ask your instructor for an explanation.

3. Examine several bottles of solutions. Read the labels carefully. Read the safety or danger warnings on the bottles. Read MSDSs provided with hazardous chemicals.

4. Practice reading the label three times to be sure you have the correct solution. Read the label before taking the bottle off the shelf, before pouring from the bottle, and after you have poured from the bottle.

5. Look at major pieces of equipment in the laboratory. Read the operating instructions for the equipment. Do *not* operate the equipment until you are taught how to do it correctly.

6. Role-play the following situations by using another student as a patient.

   • Show ways to provide privacy for the patient.

   • Identify the patient.

   • Explain a procedure to the patient.

   • Check various patient areas in the laboratory. Note any safety hazards that may be present. Discuss how you can correct the problems. Report your findings to your instructor.

   • Observe the patient during a procedure. List points you should observe to note a change in the patient's condition.

7. Discuss the following situations with another student and decide how you would handle them:

   • You see an unsafe situation or a violation of a safety practice

   • You see a wet area on the laboratory counter

   • You get a small cut on your hand while using a glass slide

   • A solution splashes on your arm

   • A particle gets in your eye

   • A piece of equipment is not working correctly

   • A bottle of solution does not have a label

   • You break a glass thermometer.

8. Observe and practice all of the safety regulations as you work in the laboratory.

9. Study the regulations in preparation for the safety examination. You must pass the safety examination.

10. Replace all equipment used.

Practice

Use the evaluation sheet for 12:2, Preventing Accidents and Injuries, to practice this procedure. When you believe you have mastered this skill, sign the sheet and give it to your instructor for further action.

 Final Checkpoint Using the criteria listed on the evaluation sheet, your instructor will grade your performance.

12:3 INFORMATION

Observing Fire Safety

This information section provides you with basic facts about fires, how they start, and how to prevent them. This information is important for fire safety in the laboratory and work environment.

Fires need three things in order to start (figure 12-11):

♦ *Oxygen*: present in the air

♦ *Fuel*: any material that will burn

♦ *Heat*: sparks, matches, flames

The major cause of fires is carelessness with smoking and with matches. Other causes include misuse of electricity (overloaded circuits, frayed electrical wires, and/or improperly grounded plugs), defects in heating systems, spontaneous ignition, improper rubbish disposal, and arson.

FIRE EXTINGUISHERS

Fire extinguishers are classified and labeled according to the kind of fire they extinguish. The main classes are:

♦ *Class A*: used on fires involving combustibles such as paper, cloth, plastic, and wood

♦ *Class B*: used on flammable or combustible liquids such as gasoline, oil, paint, grease, and cooking fat fires

♦ *Class C*: used on electrical fires such as fuse boxes, appliances, wiring, and electrical outlets; the *C* stands for nonconductive; if possible, the electricity should be turned off before using an extinguisher on an electrical fire

♦ *Class D*: used on burning or combustible metals; often specific for the type of metal being used and are not used on any other types of fires

Many different types of fire extinguishers are available. The main types include:

♦ *Water*: contains pressurized water and should only be used on Class A fires

♦ *Carbon dioxide*: contains carbon dioxide gas that provides a smothering action on the fire by forming a cloud of cool ice or snow that displaces the air and oxygen; does leave a powdery, snowlike residue that irritates the skin and eyes and can be dangerous if inhaled; most effective on Class B or C fires

♦ *Dry chemical*: contains a chemical that acts to smother a fire; type BC extinguishers contain potassium bicarbonate or sodium bicarbonate, which leaves a mildly corrosive residue that must be cleaned up as soon as possible; type ABC extinguishers contain monoammonium phosphate, a yellow powder that leaves a sticky residue that can damage electrical appliances such as computers; both residues can irritate the skin and eyes; used on Class A, B, or C fires

♦ *Halon*: contains a gas that interferes with the chemical reaction that occurs when fuels burn; used on electrical equipment because it does not leave a residue and will not damage appliances such as computers; most effective on Class C fires

Most fire extinguishers are labeled with a diagram and/or a letter showing the type of fire for which they are effective (figure 12-12). Many extinguishers are used on different types of fires and will be labeled with more than one diagram and/or letter. In addition, some extinguishers put all of the diagrams on the label; however, a diagonal red line is drawn through any diagram that depicts a fire for which the extinguisher should not be used. For example, if a diagonal red line is drawn through the diagram for electrical fires, it means the extinguisher should *not* be used on any electrical fire. Health care workers must

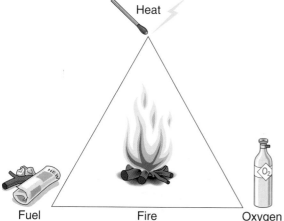

FIGURE 12-11 The fire triangle shows the three things needed to start a fire.

CLASSES OF FIRE EXTINGUISHERS

Ordinary Combustibles

CLASS A

Used for fires of ordinary combustibles such as wood, paper, cloth, and plastics

Flammable Liquids

CLASS B

Used for fires of flammable liquids and gases such as paint, gasoline, oil, grease, and cooking fats

Electrical Equipment

CLASS C

Used for electrical fires such as fuse boxes, wiring, electrical outlets, and appliances; if possible, turn off the electricity before using an extinguisher on this type of fire

Combustible Metals

CLASS D

Used on burning or combustible metals such as magnesium, titanium, and sodium; specific for the type of metal; not used on other types of fires

FIGURE 12-12 Fire extinguishers contain diagrams and/or letters to show the type of fire on which they should be used.

become familiar with the types and locations of fire extinguishers in their place of employment before a fire occurs so they are prepared to act when faced with this type of situation.

In case of fire, the main rule is to remain calm. If your personal safety is endangered, evacuate the area according to the stated method and sound the alarm. If the fire is small, confined to one area, and your safety is not endangered, determine what type of fire it is and use the proper extinguisher.

FIRE EMERGENCY PLAN

While working in a health care facility, know and follow the fire emergency plan established by the facility (figure 12-13). The plan usually states that all patients and personnel in immediate danger should be moved from the area. The alarm should be activated as quickly as possible. All doors and windows should be closed, if possible, to prevent drafts, which cause fire to spread more rapidly.

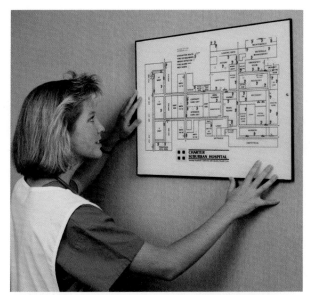

FIGURE 12-13 All personnel must be familiar with the fire emergency plan established by the facility in which they work.

Electrical equipment and oxygen should be shut off. Elevators should never be used during a fire. The acronym *RACE* is frequently used to remember the important steps. RACE stands for:

♦ *R* = Rescue anyone in immediate danger. Move patients to a safe area. If the patient can walk, escort him or her to a safe area. At times it may be necessary to move a patient in a bed or use the bed sheets as lift sheets to carry a patient to a safe area.

♦ *A* = Activate the alarm. Sound the alarm and give the location and type of fire.

♦ *C* = Contain the fire. Close windows and doors to prevent drafts. Shut off electrical equipment and oxygen if your safety is not endangered.

♦ *E* = Extinguish the fire or evacuate the area. If the fire is small and contained, and you are not in danger, locate the correct fire extinguisher to extinguish the fire. If the fire is large or spreading rapidly, or you or a patient/resident is in danger, evacuate the area.

By following the fire emergency plan, knowing the location of fire extinguishers and exit doors, and remaining calm, the health care worker can help prevent loss of life or serious injury during a fire.

Preventing fires is everyone's job. Constantly be alert to causes of fires, and correct all sit-uations that can lead to fires. Some rules for preventing fires are:

♦ Obey all "No Smoking" signs. Most health care facilities are now "smoke-free" environments and do not permit smoking anywhere on the premises.

♦ Extinguish matches, cigarettes, and any other flammable items completely. Do not empty ashtrays into trash cans or plastic bags that can burn. Always empty ashtrays into separate metal cans or containers partially filled with sand or water.

♦ Dispose of all waste materials in proper containers.

♦ Before using electrical equipment, check for damaged cords or improper grounding. Avoid overloading electrical outlets.

♦ Store flammable materials such as kerosene or gasoline in proper containers and in a safe area. If you spill a flammable liquid, wipe it up immediately.

♦ Do not allow clutter to accumulate in rooms, closets, doorways, or traffic areas. Make sure no equipment or supplies block any fire exits.

♦ When oxygen is in use, observe special precautions. Post a "No Smoking—Oxygen in Use" sign. Remove all smoking materials, candles, lighters, and matches from the room. Avoid the use of electrically operated equipment whenever possible. Do not use flammable liquids such as alcohol, nail polish, and oils. Avoid static electricity by using cotton blankets, sheets, and gowns.

DISASTER PLANS

In addition to fires, other types of disasters may occur. Examples include tornadoes, hurricanes, earthquakes, floods, and bomb threats. In any type of disaster, stay calm, follow the policy of the health care facility, and provide for the safety of yourself and the patient. It is important to note that health care workers are legally responsible for familiarizing themselves with disaster policies so appropriate action can be taken when a disaster strikes.

STUDENT: *Go to the workbook and complete the assignment sheet for 12:3, Observing Fire Safety. Then return and continue with the procedure.*

PROCEDURE 12:3

Observing Fire Safety

Equipment and Supplies

Fire alarm box, fire extinguishers

Procedure

1. Read the information section on Observing Fire Safety.

2. Learn the four classes of fire extinguishers and know for which kind of fire each type is used.

3. Locate the nearest fire alarm box. Read the instructions on how to operate the alarm. Be sure you could set off the alarm in case of a fire.

4. Locate any fire extinguishers in the laboratory area. Look for extinguishers in both the room and surrounding building. Identify each extinguisher and the kind of fire for which it is meant to be used.

5. Learn how to operate a fire extinguisher. Read the manufacturer's operating instructions carefully. Work with a practice extinguisher or do a mock demonstration.

   ▽ **CAUTION:** Do *not* discharge a real extinguisher in the laboratory.

   a. Check the extinguisher type to be sure it is the proper one to use for the mock fire (figure 12-14A).

   b. Locate the lock or pin at the top handle. Release the lock following the manufacturer's instructions (figure 12-14B).

      NOTE: During a mock demonstration, only pretend to release the lock.

   c. Grasp the handle to hold the extinguisher firmly in an upright position.

   d. Stand approximately 6–10 feet from the near edge of the fire.

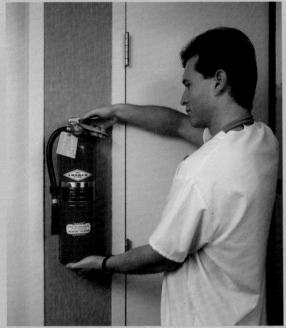

FIGURE 12-14A Check the extinguisher type to make sure it is the correct one to use.

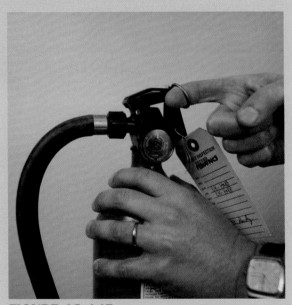

FIGURE 12-14B Release the pin.

   e. Aim the nozzle at the fire (figure 12-14C).

   f. Discharge the extinguisher. Use a side-to-side motion. Spray toward the near edge of the fire at the bottom of the fire.

PROCEDURE 12:3

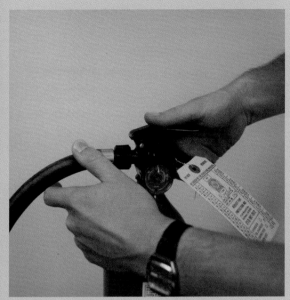

FIGURE 12-14C Aim the nozzle at the near edge of the fire, and push the handle to discharge the extinguisher.

▽ **CAUTION:** Do not spray into the center or top of the fire, because this will cause the fire to spread in an outward direction.

g. Continue with the same side-to-side motion until the fire is extinguished.

NOTE: The word *PASS* can help you remember the correct steps:

P = Pull the pin.

A = Aim the extinguisher at the near edge and bottom of the fire.

S = Squeeze the handle to discharge the extinguisher.

S = Sweep the extinguisher from side to side at the base of the fire.

h. At all times, stay a safe distance from the fire to avoid personal injury.

▽ **CAUTION:** Avoid contact with residues from chemical extinguishers.

i. After an extinguisher has been used, it must be recharged or replaced. Another usable extinguisher must be put in position when the extinguisher is removed.

6. Check the policy in your area for evacuating the laboratory area during a fire. Practice the method and know the locations of all exits.

NOTE: Remember to remain calm and avoid panic.

7. Replace all equipment used.

Practice

Use the evaluation sheet for 12:3, Observing Fire Safety, to practice this procedure. When you believe you have mastered this skill, sign the sheet and give it to your instructor for further action.

Practice

Study the safety regulations throughout Chapter 12 in preparation for the safety examination.

✔ **Final Checkpoint** Using the criteria listed on the evaluation sheet, your instructor will grade your performance.

✔ **Final Checkpoint** Take the safety examination and obtain a passing grade to demonstrate your knowledge of safety.

TODAY'S RESEARCH: TOMORROW'S HEALTH CARE

Draino for blood vessels?

Cardiovascular (heart and blood vessel) disease is the leading cause of death in the United States. Fatty plaques, caused mainly by an accumulation of LDL (low-density lipoprotein, or "bad" cholesterol), block the flow of blood in arterial walls, triggering a heart attack or stroke. HDL (high-density lipoprotein, or "good" cholesterol) helps protect the body from cardiovascular disease. HDL carries fats to the liver for disposal, helps prevent clots, and decreases inflammation in the blood vessels. For years, researchers have tried to find ways to increase the level of HDL while decreasing the level of LDL in the blood.

Scientists may have found the key to solve this problem in a small village in Italy. They discovered that residents of this village seemed to be immune to heart disease. Research showed that these individuals have a mutant gene that produces a powerful version of HDL. Scientists have produced a synthetic version of this HDL called *apo A-1 Milano*. When it was injected into a small group of volunteer heart patients, plaque in blood vessels was reduced by 4 percent and no new plaque buildup occurred. Scientists called it a miracle "blood vessel Draino." However, apo A-1 Milano is expensive to produce because it is a protein. It also must be injected into the body by an intravenous infusion, making it even more costly and inconvenient. Research is now directed toward gene therapy where the codes for the apo A-1 Milano protein are transferred into the body so the body can produce its own powerful version of HDL.

Scientists are also evaluating other methods to increase levels of HDL. They have discovered an enzyme called *cholesteryl ester transfer protein* that appears to reduce HDL levels and increase the levels of harmful LDL. Research is being conducted on new drugs that will block this enzyme. Who knows which approach will be most successful, but scientists will find the answer.

CHAPTER 12 SUMMARY

Safety is the responsibility of every health care worker. It is essential that established safety standards be observed by everyone. This protects the worker, the employer, and the patient.

One important aspect of safety is the correct use of body mechanics. Body mechanics refer to the way the body moves and maintains balance while making the most efficient use of all of its parts. Practicing basic principles of good body mechanics prevents strain and maintains muscle strength. In addition, correct body mechanics make lifting, pulling, and pushing easier.

Knowing and following basic safety standards is also important. In this unit, basic standards are listed in regard to the use of equipment and solutions, patient safety, and personal safety. It is important for everyone to learn and follow the established standards at all times.

An awareness of the causes and prevention of fires is essential. Every health care worker should be familiar with the types and use of fire extinguishers. In addition, every facility has a fire emergency plan. By following the fire emergency plan, knowing the location of fire extinguishers and exit doors, and remaining calm, the health care worker can help prevent loss of life or serious injury during a fire and/or a disaster.

INTERNET SEARCHES

Use the suggested search engines in Chapter 17:4 of this textbook to search the Internet for additional information on the following topics:

1. *Federal regulations*: obtain more information on federal safety regulations by searching sites of the Occupational Safety and Health Administration (OSHA), Occupational Exposure to

Hazardous Chemicals Standard, Bloodborne Pathogen Standard, and Material Safety Data Sheets (MSDSs)

2. *Ergonomics*: search for additional information on ergonomics and environmental safety

3. *Diseases*: obtain information on the causative agents and methods of transmission for hepatitis B and C and acquired immune deficiency syndrome (AIDS)

4. *Fire safety*: search for information on fire prevention and fire safety

5. *Fire extinguishers*: search for various manufacturers of fire extinguishers and obtain information on the types of extinguishers, their main uses, precautions for handling, and safety rules that must be observed while using extinguishers

6. *Disasters*: obtain information on safety procedures that must be followed for tornadoes, floods, hurricanes, earthquakes, bomb threats, or explosions

REVIEW QUESTIONS

1. Define *body mechanics* and list four (4) reasons why it is important to use good body mechanics.

2. You are using an electrical microhematocrit centrifuge to spin blood. You see smoke coming from the back of the machine. What should you do?

3. List four (4) safety precautions that must be followed while using solutions.

4. Identify three (3) things that must be done before performing any procedure on a patient.

5. State five (5) checkpoints that must be observed before leaving a patient/resident in bed.

6. List five (5) rules that must be followed while oxygen is in use.

7. What does the acronym *RACE* stand for?

8. Create a chart showing the four (4) main types of fire extinguishers and the type of fire for which each is effective.

9. What does the acronyn *PASS* stand for?

CHAPTER 13 | Infection Control

Chapter Objectives

After completing this chapter,
you should be able to:

- Identify five classes of microorganisms by describing the characteristics of each class
- List the 6 components of the chain of infection
- Differentiate between antisepsis, disinfection, and sterilization
- Define bioterrorism and identify at least four ways to prepare for a bioterrorism attack
- Wash hands following aseptic technique
- Observe standard precautions while working in the laboratory or clinical area
- Wash, wrap, and autoclave instruments, linen, and equipment
- Operate an autoclave with accuracy and safety
- Follow basic principles on chemical disinfection
- Clean instruments with an ultrasonic unit
- Open sterile packages with no contamination
- Don sterile gloves with no contamination
- Prepare a sterile dressing tray with no contamination
- Change a sterile dressing with no contamination
- Don and remove a transmission-based isolation mask, gloves, and gown
- Relate specific basic tasks to the care of a patient in a transmission-based isolation unit
- Define, pronounce, and spell all key terms

Observe Standard Precautions

Instructor's Check—Call Instructor at This Point

Safety—Proceed with Caution

OBRA Requirement—Based on Federal Law

Math Skill

Legal Responsibility

Science Skill

Career Information

Communications Skill

Technology

KEY TERMS

acquired immune deficiency
   syndrome (AIDS)
aerobic
airborne precautions
anaerobic
antisepsis *(ant"-ih-sep'-sis)*
asepsis *(a-sep'-sis)*
autoclave
bacteria
bioterrorism
causative agent
cavitation
   (kav"-ih-tay'-shun)
chain of infection
chemical disinfection
clean
communicable disease
contact precautions

contaminated
disinfection
droplet precautions
endogenous
epidemic
exogenous
fomites
fungi *(fun'-guy)*
helminths
hepatitis B
hepatitis C
microorganism *(my-crow-
   or'-gan-izm)*
mode of transmission
nonpathogens
nosocomial
opportunistic
pandemic

pathogens *(path'-oh-jenz")*
personal protective
   equipment (PPE)
portal of entry
portal of exit
protective (reverse) isolation
protozoa *(pro-toe-zo'-ah)*
reservoir
rickettsiae *(rik-et'-z-ah)*
standard precautions
sterile
sterile field
sterilization
susceptible host
transmission-based
   isolation precautions
ultrasonic
viruses

13:1 INFORMATION

Understanding the Principles of Infection Control

 Understanding the basic principles of infection control is essential for any health care worker in any field of health care. The principles described in this unit provide a basic knowledge of how disease is transmitted and the main ways to prevent disease transmission.

A **microorganism,** or microbe, is a small, living organism that is not visible to the naked eye. It must be viewed under a microscope. Microorganisms are found everywhere in the environment, including on and in the human body. Many microorganisms are part of the normal flora (plant life adapted for living in a specific environment) of the body and are beneficial in maintaining certain body processes. These are called **nonpathogens.** Other microorganisms cause infection and disease and are called **pathogens,** or germs. At times, a microorganism that is beneficial in one body system can become pathogenic when it is present in another body system.

For example, a bacterium called *Escherichia coli (E. coli)* is part of the natural flora of the large intestine. If *E. coli* enters the urinary system, however, it causes an infection.

To grow and reproduce, microorganisms need certain things. Most microorganisms prefer a warm environment, and body temperature is ideal. Darkness is also preferred by most microorganisms, and many are killed quickly by sunlight. In addition, a source of food and moisture is needed. Some microorganisms, called **aerobic** organisms, require oxygen to live. Others, called **anaerobic** organisms, live and reproduce in the absence of oxygen. The human body is the ideal supplier of all the requirements of microorganisms.

CLASSES OF MICROORGANISMS

There are many different classes of microorganisms. In each class, some of the microorganisms are pathogenic to humans. The main classes include:

◆ **Bacteria:** These are simple, one-celled organisms that multiply rapidly. They are classified by shape and arrangement. *Cocci* are round or spherical in shape (figure 13-1). If cocci occur in pairs, they are diplococci. Diplococci bacteria cause diseases such as gonorrhea, meningitis, and pneumonia. If cocci occur in chains, they are streptococci. A common streptococcus causes a severe sore throat (strep throat) and rheumatic fever. If cocci occur in clusters or groups, they are staphylococci. These are the most common pyogenic (pus-producing) microorganisms. Staphylococci cause infections such as boils, urinary tract infections, wound infections, and toxic shock. Rod-shaped bacteria are called *bacilli* (figure 13-2). They can occur singly, in pairs, or in chains. Many bacilli contain flagella, which are thread-like projections that are similar to tails and allow the organisms to move. Bacilli also have the ability to form spores, or thick-walled capsules, when conditions for growth are poor. In the spore form, bacilli are extremely difficult to kill. Diseases caused by different types of bacilli include tuberculosis, tetanus, pertussis, (whooping cough), botulism, diphtheria, and typhoid. Bacteria that are spiral or corkscrew in shape are called *spirilla* (figure 13-3). These include the comma-shaped vibrio and the corkscrew-shaped spirochete. Diseases caused by spirilla include syphilis and cholera. Antibiotics are used to kill bacteria. However, some strains of bacteria have become antibiotic-

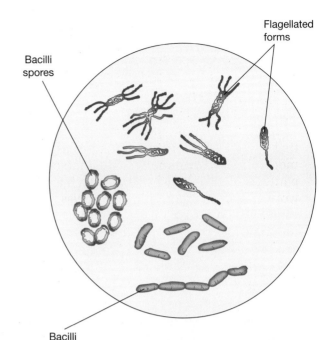

FIGURE 13-2 Bacilli bacteria.

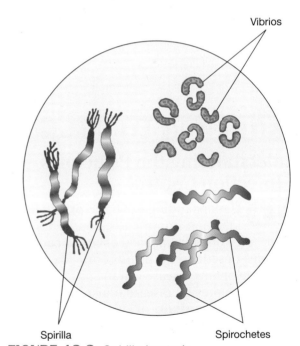

FIGURE 13-3 Spirilla bacteria.

resistant, which means that the antibiotic is no longer effective against the bacteria. Methicillin-resistant staphylococcus is an example. It causes a severe Staph infection that is difficult to treat because it is resistant to many different antibiotics.

◆ **Protozoa:** These are one-celled animal-like organisms often found in decayed materials, animal or bird feces, insect bites, and con-

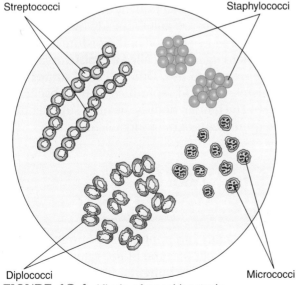

FIGURE 13-1 Kinds of cocci bacteria.

taminated water (figure 13-4). Many contain flagella, which allow them to move freely. Some protozoa are pathogenic and cause diseases such as malaria, amebic dysentery (intestinal infection), trichomonas, and African sleeping sickness.

♦ **Fungi:** These are simple, plantlike organisms that live on dead organic matter. Yeasts and molds are two common forms that can be pathogenic. They cause diseases such as ringworm, athlete's foot, histoplasmosis, yeast vaginitis, and thrush (figure 13-5). Antibiotics do not kill fungi. Antifungal medications are available for many of the pathogenic fungi, but they are expensive, must be taken internally for a long period, and may cause liver damage.

♦ **Rickettsiae:** These are parasitic microorganisms, which means they cannot live outside the cells of another living organism. They are commonly found in fleas, lice, ticks, and mites, and are transmitted to humans by the bites of

these insects. Rickettsiae cause diseases such as typhus fever and Rocky Mountain spotted fever. Antibiotics are effective against many different rickettsiae.

♦ ✪ **Viruses:** These are the smallest microorganisms, visible only using an electron microscope (figure 13-6A and B). They cannot reproduce unless they are inside another living cell. They are spread from human to human by blood and other body secretions. It is important to note that viruses are more difficult to kill because they are resistant to many disinfectants and are not affected by antibiotics. Viruses cause many diseases including the common cold, measles, mumps, chicken pox, herpes, warts, influenza, and polio. New and different viruses emerge constantly because viruses are prone to mutating and changing genetic information. In addition, viruses that infect animals can mutate to infect humans, often with lethal results. There are many examples of these viruses. *Severe acute respi-*

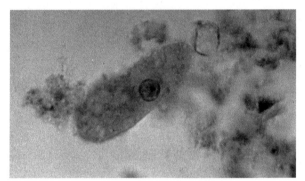

FIGURE 13-4 An intestinal protozoan, *Entamoeba coli. (Courtesy of the Centers for Disease Control and Prevention, Atlanta, GA)*

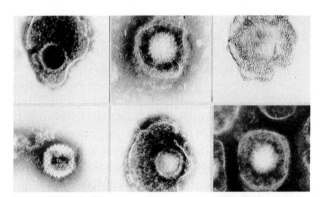

FIGURE 13-6A Electron micrographs of the various types of herpes simplex virus. *(Courtesy of the Centers for Disease Control and Prevention, Atlanta, GA)*

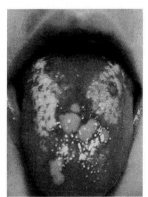

FIGURE 13-5 The yeast (fungus) called *thrush* causes these characteristic white patches on the tongue.

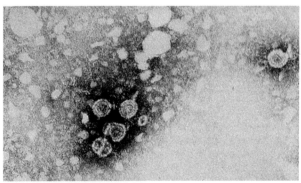

FIGURE 13-6B Electron micrograph of the hepatitis B virus. *(Courtesy of the Centers for Disease Control and Prevention, Atlanta, GA)*

ratory syndrome (SARS) is caused by a variant of the coronavirus family that causes the common cold. It is characterized by flu-like symptoms that can lead to respiratory failure and death. *West Nile virus (WNV)* is a mosquito-borne flavivirus that first infected birds but now infects humans. In some individuals, it causes only a mile febrile illness. In other individuals who are older or have poor immune systems, it can cause severe neurologic illnesses such as encephalitis or meningitis, which can lead to death. *Monkeypox*, a hantavirus that affects monkeys, other primates, and rodents, mutated and spread to humans. Infection usually occurs after contacting body secretions or excretions (urine and stool) of infected animals or ingesting food that has been contaminated by fluids from infected animals. A major outbreak occurred in the American southwest when infected prairie dogs contaminated food with fecal material. Monkeypox is similar to smallpox. It causes severe flu-like symptoms, lymphadenopathy (disease of the lymph nodes), and pustules that cause severe scarring of the skin. If the eyes are infected, blindness can occur. It can be prevented and/or treated with a smallpox vaccination. Filoviruses such as *Ebola* and *Marburg* first affected primates and then spread to humans. These viruses cause hemorrhagic fever, a disease that begins with fever, chills, headache, myalgia (muscle pain), and a skin rash. It quickly progresses to jaundice, pancreatitis, liver failure, massive hemorrhaging throughout the body, delirium, shock, and death. Most outbreaks of hemorrhagic fever have been in Africa, but isolated cases have appeared in other parts of the world when individuals were in contact with infected primates. A new *H5N1* virus that causes avian or bird flu has devastated bird flocks in many countries. The infection has appeared in humans, but most cases have resulted from contact with infected poultry or contaminated surfaces. The spread from one person to another has been reported only rarely. However, because the death rate for bird flu is between 50 and 60 percent, a major concern is that the *H5N1* virus will mutate and spread more readily. In addition to these viruses, there are three other viral diseases of major concern to the health care worker: hepatitis B, hepatitis C, and acquired immune deficiency syndrome (AIDS). **Hepatitis B,** or serum hepatitis, is caused by the HBV virus and is transmitted by blood, serum, and other body secretions. It affects the liver and can lead to the destruction and scarring of liver cells. A vaccine has been developed to protect individuals from this disease. The vaccine is expensive and involves a series of three injections. Under federal law, employers must provide the vaccination at no cost to any health care worker with occupational exposure to blood or other body secretions that may carry the HBV virus. An individual does have the right to refuse the vaccination, but a written record must be kept proving that the vaccine was offered. **Hepatitis C** is caused by the hepatitis C virus, or HCV, and is transmitted by blood and blood-containing body fluids. Many individuals who contract the disease are asymptomatic (display no symptoms); others have mild symptoms that are often diagnosed as influenza or flu. In either case, HCV can cause serious liver damage. At present, there is no preventive immunization, but a vaccine is being developed. Both HBV and HCV are extremely difficult to destroy. These viruses can even remain active for several days in dried blood. Health care workers must take every precaution to protect themselves from hepatitis viruses. **Acquired immune deficiency syndrome** is caused by the human immunodeficiency virus (HIV) and suppresses the immune system. An individual with AIDS cannot fight off many cancers and infections that would not affect a healthy person. Presently, there is no cure and no vaccine is available, so it is important for the health care worker to take precautions to prevent the spread of this disease.

- ◆ **Helminths:** These are multicellular parasitic organisms commonly called *worms* or *flukes*. They are transmitted to humans when humans ingest the eggs or larvae in contaminated food, ingest meat contaminated with the worms, or get bitten by infected insects. Some worms can also penetrate the skin to enter the body. Examples of helminths include: hookworms, which attach to the small intestine and can infect the heart and lungs; ascariasis, which live in the small intestine and can cause an obstruction of the intestine; trichinella spiralis, which causes trichinosis and is contracted by eating raw or inadequately cooked pork products; enterobiasis, which is commonly called *pinworm* and affects mainly young children; and taenia solium or pork tapeworm, which is contracted by eating inadequately cooked pork.

TYPES OF INFECTION

Pathogenic microorganisms cause infection and disease in different ways. Some pathogens produce poisons, called *toxins*, which harm the body. An example is the bacillus that causes tetanus, which produces toxins that damage the central nervous system. Some pathogens cause an allergic reaction in the body, resulting in a runny nose, watery eyes, and sneezing. Other pathogens attack and destroy the living cells they invade. An example is the protozoan that causes malaria. It invades red blood cells and causes them to rupture.

Infections and diseases are also classified as endogenous, exogenous, nosocomial, or opportunistic. **Endogenous** means the infection or disease originates within the body. These include metabolic disorders, congenital abnormalities, tumors, and infections caused by microorganisms within the body. **Exogenous** means the infection or disease originates outside the body. Examples include pathogenic organisms that invade the body, radiation, chemical agents, trauma, electric shock, and temperature extremes. A **nosocomial** infection is one acquired by an individual in a health care facility such as a hospital or long-term care facility. Nosocomial infections are usually present in the facility and transmitted by health care workers to the patient. Many of the pathogens transmitted in this manner are antibiotic-resistant and can cause serious and even life-threatening infections in patients. Common examples are staphylococcus, pseudomonas, and enterococci. Infection-control programs are used in health care facilities to prevent and deal with nosocomial infections. **Opportunistic** infections are those that occur when the body's defenses are weak. These diseases do not usually occur in individuals with intact immune systems. Examples include the development of Kaposi's sarcoma (a rare type of cancer) or *Pneumocystis carinii* pneumonia in individuals with AIDS.

CHAIN OF INFECTION

For disease to occur and spread from one individual to another, certain conditions must be met. These conditions are commonly called the **chain of infection** (figure 13-7). The parts of the chain include:

♦ **Causative agent:** a pathogen, such as a bacterium or virus that can cause a disease

♦ **Reservoir:** an area where the causative agent can live; some common reservoirs include the human body, animals, the environment, and **fomites,** or objects contaminated with infectious material that contains the pathogens. Common fomites include doorknobs, bedpans, urinals, linens, instruments, and specimen containers.

♦ **Portal of exit:** a way for the causative agent to escape from the reservoir in which it has been growing. In the human body, pathogens can leave the body through urine, feces, saliva, blood, tears, mucous discharge, sexual secretions, and draining wounds.

♦ **Mode of transmission:** a way that the causative agent can be transmitted to another reservoir or host where it can live. The pathogen can be transmitted in different ways. One way is by *direct contact*, which includes person-to-person contact (physical or sexual contact) or contact with a body secretion containing the pathogen. Contaminated hands are one of the most common sources of direct contact transmission. Another way is by *indirect contact*, when the pathogen is transmitted from contaminated substances such as food, air, soil, insects, feces, clothing, instruments, and equipment. Examples include touching contaminated equipment and spreading the pathogen on the hands, breathing in droplets carrying airborne infections, and contacting *vectors* (insects, rodents, or small animals), such as being bitten by an insect carrying a pathogen.

♦ **Portal of entry:** a way for the causative agent to enter a new reservoir or host. Some ways pathogens can enter the body are through breaks in the skin, breaks in the mucous membrane, the respiratory tract, the digestive tract, the genitourinary tract, and the circulatory system. If the defense mechanisms of the body

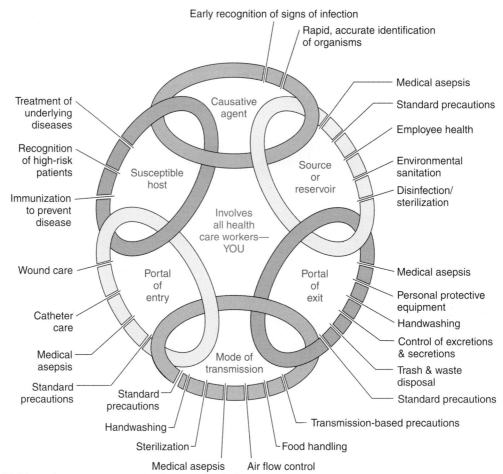

Early recognition of signs of infection

Rapid, accurate identification of organisms

Causative agent

Medical asepsis

Standard precautions

Employee health

Treatment of underlying diseases

Environmental sanitation

Recognition of high-risk patients

Susceptible host

Source or reservoir

Disinfection/ sterilization

Immunization to prevent disease

Involves all health care workers— YOU

Wound care

Portal of entry

Portal of exit

Medical asepsis

Catheter care

Personal protective equipment

Handwashing

Medical asepsis

Control of excretions & secretions

Standard precautions

Mode of transmission

Trash & waste disposal

Standard precautions

Standard precautions

Handwashing

Transmission-based precautions

Sterilization

Food handling

Medical asepsis

Air flow control

FIGURE 13-7 Note the components in the chain of infection and the ways in which the chain can be broken.

are intact and the immune system is functioning, a human can frequently fight off the causative agent and not contract the disease. Body defenses include:

mucous membrane: lines the respiratory, digestive, and reproductive tracts and traps pathogens

cilia: tiny, hairlike structures that line the respiratory tract and propel pathogens out of the body

coughing and sneezing

hydrochloric acid: destroys pathogens in the stomach

tears in the eye: contain bacteriocidal (bacteria-killing) chemicals

fever

inflammation: leukocytes, or white blood cells, destroy pathogens

immune response: body produces antibodies, protective proteins that combat pathogens, and protective chemicals secreted by cells, such as interferon and complement

♦ **Susceptible host:** a person likely to get an infection or disease, usually because body defenses are weak

Health care workers must constantly be aware of the parts in the chain of infection. If any part of the chain is eliminated, the spread of disease or infection will be stopped. A health care worker who is aware of this can follow practices to interrupt or break this chain and prevent the transmission of disease. It is important to remember that pathogens are everywhere and that preventing their transmission is a continuous process.

ASEPTIC TECHNIQUES

A major way to break the chain of infection is to use aseptic techniques while providing health care. **Asepsis** is defined as the absence of disease-producing microorganisms, or pathogens.

Sterile means free from all organisms, both pathogenic and nonpathogenic, including spores and viruses. **Contaminated** means that organisms and pathogens are present. Any object or area that may contain pathogens is considered to be contaminated. Aseptic techniques are directed toward maintaining cleanliness and eliminating or preventing contamination. Common aseptic techniques include handwashing, good personal hygiene, use of disposable gloves when contacting body secretions or contaminated objects, proper cleaning of instruments and equipment, and thorough cleaning of the environment.

Various levels of aseptic control are possible. These include:

♦ **Antisepsis:** Antiseptics prevent or inhibit growth of pathogenic organisms but are not effective against spores and viruses. They can usually be used on the skin. Common examples include alcohol and betadine.

♦ **Disinfection:** This is a process that destroys or kills pathogenic organisms. It is not always effective against spores and viruses. Chemical disinfectants are used in this process. Disinfectants can irritate or damage the skin and are used mainly on objects, not people. Some common disinfectants are bleach solutions and zephirin.

♦ **Sterilization:** This is a process that destroys all microorganisms, both pathogenic and nonpathogenic, including spores and viruses. Steam under pressure, gas, radiation, and chemicals can be used to sterilize objects. An autoclave is the most common piece of equipment used for sterilization.

In the sections that follow, correct methods of aseptic techniques are described. It is important for the health care worker to know and use these methods in every aspect of providing health care to prevent the spread and transmission of disease.

STUDENT: *Go to the workbook and complete the assignment sheet for 13:1, Understanding the Principles of Infection Control.*

13:2 INFORMATION

Bioterrorism

INTRODUCTION

Bioterrorism is the use of microorganisms, or biologic agents, as weapons to infect humans, animals, or plants. Throughout history, microor-ganisms have been used in biologic warfare. Some examples include:

♦ The Tartar army throwing bodies of dead plague victims over the walls of a city called Caffa in 1346, causing an epidemic of plague in the city

♦ The British army providing Delaware Indians with blankets and handkerchiefs contaminated with smallpox in 1763, resulting in a major outbreak of smallpox among the Indian population

♦ The Germans using a variety of animal and human pathogens in World War I

♦ The Japanese military using prisoners of war to experiment with many different pathogens in World War II

♦ The United States, Canada, the Soviet Union, and the United Kingdom developing biologic weapons programs until the late 1960s

♦ The release of sarin gas in Tokyo in 1995

♦ The mail attack with anthrax by an unknown individual or individuals in the United States in 2001

Today, there is a major concern that these biologic agents will be used not only in wars, but also against unsuspecting civilians.

BIOLOGIC AGENTS

Many different microorganisms can cause diseases in humans, animals, and plants. However, only a limited number are considered to be ideal for bioterrorism. Six characteristics of the "ideal" microorganism include:

♦ Inexpensive and readily available or easy to produce

♦ Spread through the air by winds or ventilation systems and inhaled into the lungs of potential victims, or spread by ingesting contaminated food or water

♦ Survives sunlight, drying, and heat

♦ Causes death or severe disability

♦ Easily transmitted from person to person

♦ Difficult to prevent and/or has no effective treatment

The Centers for Disease Control and Prevention (CDC) has identified and classified major bioterrorism agents. High-priority agents that have been identified include:

♦ *Smallpox*: Smallpox is a highly contagious infectious disease that is caused by a variola virus. A smallpox vaccination can provide protection against some types of smallpox, but one type, hemorrhagic smallpox, is usually fatal. Until the 1970s, people were vaccinated against smallpox. However, after many years with no reported cases, the vaccinations were no longer required. Now, with the threat of a smallpox bioterrorism attack, the U.S. government has started a new vaccination program. The program encourages first responders, police, fire department, and health care personnel to be vaccinated.

♦ *Anthrax*: Anthrax is an infectious disease caused by the spores of bacteria called *Bacillus anthracis*. The spores are highly resistant to destruction and can live in soil for years. Grazing animals such as cattle, sheep, and goats eat the contaminated soil and become infected. Humans develop anthrax by exposure through the skin (cutaneous) (figure 13-8), by eating undercooked or raw infected meat (gastrointestinal), or by inhaling the spores (pulmonary). Cutaneous and gastrointestinal anthrax are usually treated successfully with antibiotics, but some victims die. Inhalation anthrax causes death in more than 80 percent of its victims. An anthrax vaccine is available for prevention. The military has an active vaccination program.

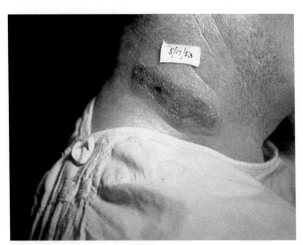

FIGURE 13-8 Cutaneous (skin) anthrax is usually treated successfully with antibiotics. *(Courtesy of the Centers for Disease Control Public Image Library)*

♦ *Plague*: This is an infectious disease that is caused by bacteria called *Yersinia pestis*. Usually plague is transmitted by the bites of infected fleas. In some cases, the organism enters the body through a break in the skin or by contact with tissue of an infected animal. Rats, rock squirrels, prairie dogs, and chipmunks are the most common sources for plague in the United States. If the disease is not treated immediately with antibiotics, the infection spreads to the blood and lungs, and causes death. No vaccine for plague is available in the United States.

♦ *Botulism*: Botulism is a paralytic illness caused by a nerve toxin produced by bacteria called *Clostridium botulinum*. Three main types of botulism exist. One type is caused by eating foods that contain the toxin. A second type is caused by the presence of the toxin in a wound or injury to the skin. A third type occurs in infants who eat the spores that then grow in the intestine and release the toxin. The toxin rapidly causes muscle paralysis. If it is not treated with an antitoxin, the paralysis spreads to the respiratory muscles and causes death.

♦ *Tularemia*: This is an infectious disease caused by bacteria called *Francisella tularensis*. This bacteria is commonly found in animals such as rats, rabbits, and insects (ticks and deerflies). Humans get the disease through the bite of an infected animal or insect, by eating contaminated food, by drinking contaminated water, or by breathing in the bacteria. The disease causes death if it is not treated with appropriate antibiotics. Currently, the Food and Drug Administration (FDA) is reviewing a vaccine, but it is not available in the United States.

♦ *Filoviruses*: A filovirus is an infectious disease that causes severe hemorrhagic fever. Two filoviruses have been identified. They are the Ebola viruses and the Marburg virus. The source of the viruses is still being researched, but the common belief is that the viruses are transmitted from animals such as bats. Once the viruses affect a human, the disease is spread rapidly from person to person by contact with body fluids. No effective treatment exists, and 50–90 percent of infected individuals die.

Many other pathogenic microorganisms can be used in a bioterrorism attack. In fact, any pathogenic organism could be used in a bioterrorism attack. For this reason, health care workers must be constantly alert to the threat of infection with a biologic agent.

PREPARING FOR BIOTERRORISM

A bioterrorism attack could cause an epidemic and public health emergency. Large numbers of infected people would place a major stress on health care facilities. Fear and panic could lead to riots, social disorder, and disregard for authority. For these reasons, the Bioterrorism Act of 2002 was passed by Congress and signed into law in June 2002. This act requires the development of a comprehensive plan against bioterrorism to increase security in the United States.

Preparing for bioterrorism will involve government at all levels—local, regional, state, and national. Some of the major aspects of preparation include:

♦ Community-based surveillance to detect early indications of a bioterrorism attack

♦ Notification of the public when a high-risk situation is detected

♦ Strict infection-control measures and public education about the measures

♦ Funding for studying pathogenic organisms, developing vaccines, researching treatments, and determining preventive actions

♦ Strict guidelines and restrictions for purchasing and transporting pathologic microorganisms

♦ Mass immunization, especially for military, first responders, police, fire department, and health care personnel

♦ Increased protection of food and water supplies

♦ Training personnel to properly diagnose and treat infectious diseases

♦ Establishing emergency management policies

♦ Criminal investigation of possible threats

♦ Improving the ability of health care facilities to deal with an attack by increasing emergency department space, preparing decontamination areas, and establishing isolation facilities

♦ Improving communications so information on bioterrorism is transmitted quickly and efficiently

Every health care worker must constantly be alert to the threat of bioterrorism. In today's world, it is likely that an attack will occur. Careful preparation and thorough training can limit the effect of the attack and save the lives of many people.

STUDENT: *Go to the workbook and complete the assignment sheet for 13:2, Bioterrorism.*

13:3 INFORMATION

Washing Hands

Handwashing is a basic task required in any health occupation. The method described in this unit has been developed to ensure that a thorough cleansing occurs. An aseptic technique is a method followed to prevent the spread of germs or pathogens. *Handwashing is the most important method used to practice aseptic technique.* Handwashing is also the most effective way to prevent the spread of infection.

The hands are a perfect medium for the spread of pathogens. Thoroughly washing the hands helps prevent and control the spread of pathogens from one person to another. It also helps protect the health worker from disease and illness.

The Centers for Disease Control and Prevention (CDC) published the results of handwashing research and new recommendations for hand hygiene in 2002. The recommendations call for regular handwashing using plain soap and water, antiseptic handwashing using an antimicrobial soap and water, and antiseptic hand rubs (waterless handwashing) using alcohol-based hand cleaners. Regular handwashing is recommended for routine cleansing of the hands when the hands are visibly dirty or soiled with blood or other body fluids. Antiseptic handwashing is recommended before invasive procedures, in critical care units, while caring for patients on specific organism transmission-based precautions, and in specific circumstances defined by the infection-control program of the health care facility. Antiseptic hand rubs are recommended if the hands are not visibly dirty or are not soiled with blood or body fluids.

Handwashing should be performed frequently. It should be done:

♦ When you arrive at the facility and immediately before leaving the facility

♦ Before and after every patient contact

♦ After contact with a patient's intact skin (for example, after taking a blood pressure)

♦ Before moving from a contaminated body site to a clean body site during patient care (for example, before washing the patient's hands after removing a bedpan)

♦ Any time the hands become contaminated during a procedure

♦ Before applying and immediately after removing gloves

♦ Any time gloves are torn or punctured

♦ Before and after handling any specimen

♦ After contact with any soiled or contaminated item

♦ After picking up any item off the floor

♦ After personal use of the bathroom

♦ After you cough, sneeze, or use a tissue

♦ Before and after any contact with your mouth or mucous membrane, such as eating, drinking, smoking, applying lip balm, or inserting or removing contact lenses

The recommended method for handwashing is based on the following principles; they should be observed whenever hands are washed:

♦ Soap is used as a cleansing agent because it aids in the removal of germs through its sudsy action and alkali content. Pathogens are trapped in the soapsuds and rinsed away. Liquid soap from a dispenser should be used whenever possible because bar soap can contain microorganisms.

♦ Warm water should be used. This is less damaging to the skin than hot water. It also creates a better lather with soap than does cold water.

♦ Friction must be used in addition to soap and water. This action helps rub off pathogens from the surface of the skin.

♦ All surfaces on the hands must be cleaned. This includes the palms, the backs/tops of the hands, and the areas between the fingers.

♦ Fingertips must be pointed downward. The downward direction prevents water from getting on the forearms and then running down to contaminate the clean hands.

♦ Dry paper towels must be used to turn the faucet on and off. This action prevents contamination of the hands from pathogens on the faucet. A dry towel must be used because pathogens can travel more readily through a wet towel.

Nails also harbor dirt and pathogens, and must be cleaned during the handwashing process. An orange/cuticle stick can be used. Care must be taken to use the blunt end of the stick because the pointed end can injure the nailbeds. A brush can also be used to clean the nails. If a brush or orange stick is not available or the nails are not visibly dirty, the nails can be rubbed against the palm of the opposite hand to get soap under the nails. Most health care facilities prohibit the use of artificial nails and require that nails be kept short, usually less than 1/4-inch long. Artificial or long nails can harbor organisms and increase the risk for infection for both the patient and health care worker. In addition, long nails can puncture or tear gloves.

Waterless hand cleaning with an alcohol-based gel, lotion, or foam has been proved safe for

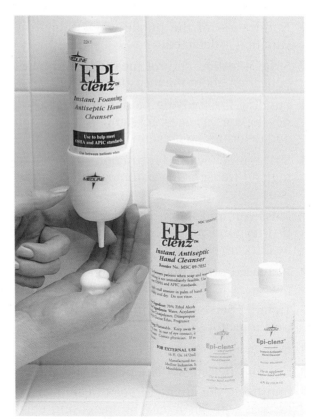

FIGURE 13-9 Waterless handwashing using an alcohol-based hand cleaner is an effective way of cleaning hands that are not visibly soiled. *(Courtesy of Medline Industries Inc., 1-860-MEDLINE)*

use during routine patient care. Its use is recommended when the hands are not visibly dirty and are not contaminated with blood or body fluids (figure 13-9). Most waterless hand cleaning products contain alcohol to provide antisepsis and a moisturizer to prevent drying of the skin. It is important to read the manufacturer's instructions before using any product. Usually a small amount of the alcohol-based cleaner is applied to the palm of the hands. The hands are then rubbed vigorously so the solution is applied to all surfaces of the hands, fingers, nails, and wrists. The hands should be rubbed until they are dry, usually at least 15 seconds. Most manufacturers recommend that the hands be washed with soap and water after 6–10 cleanings with the alcohol-based product. In addition, if the hands are visibly soiled, or if there has been contact with blood or body fluid, the hands must be washed with soap and water.

Every health care facility has written policies for hand hygiene as a part of their standard precautions manual. Health care workers must become familiar with and follow these policies to prevent the spread of infection.

STUDENT: *Go to the workbook and complete the assignment sheet for 13:3, Washing Hands. Then return and continue with the procedure.*

PROCEDURE 13:3

Washing Hands

Equipment and Supplies

Paper towels, running water, waste container, hand brush or orange/cuticle stick, soap

Procedure

1. Assemble all equipment. Stand back slightly from the sink so you do not contaminate your uniform or clothing. Avoid touching the inside of the sink with your hands since it is considered contaminated. Remove any rings and push your wristwatch up above your wrist.

2. Turn the faucet on by holding a paper towel between your hand and the faucet (figure 13-10A). Regulate the temperature of the water and let water flow over your hands. Discard the towel in the waste container.

   NOTE: Water should be warm.

   ▽ **CAUTION:** Hot water will burn your hands.

3. With your fingertips pointing downward, wet your hands.

   NOTE: Washing in a downward direction prevents water from getting on the forearms and then running back down to contaminate hands.

4. Use soap to get a lather on your hands.

5. Put the palms of your hands together and rub them using friction and a circular motion for at least 15 seconds.

6. Put the palm of one hand on the back of the other hand. Rub together several times. Repeat this after reversing position of hands (figure 13-10B).

7. Interlace the fingers on both hands and rub them back and forth (figure 13-10C).

8. Encircle your wrist with the palm and fingers of the opposite hand. Use a circular motion to clean the front, back, and sides of the wrist. Repeat for the opposite wrist.

9. Clean the nails with an orange/cuticle stick and/or hand brush if they are visibly dirty or if this is the first hand cleaning of the day (figures 13-10D and E). If the nails are not visibly dirty, they can be cleaned by rubbing them against the palm of the opposite hand.

   ▽ **CAUTION:** Use the blunt end of orange/cuticle stick to avoid injury.

   NOTE: Steps 3 through 9 ensure that all parts of both hands are clean.

PROCEDURE 13:3

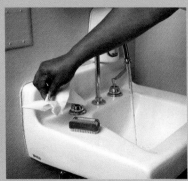

FIGURE 13-10A Use a dry towel to turn the faucet on.

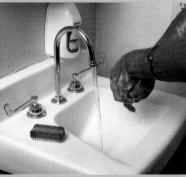

FIGURE 13-10B Point the fingertips downward and use the palm of one hand to clean the back of the other hand.

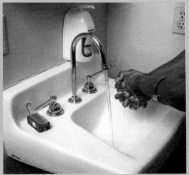

FIGURE 13-10C Interlace the fingers to clean between the fingers.

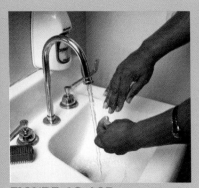

FIGURE 13-10D The blunt end of an orange stick can be used to clean the nails.

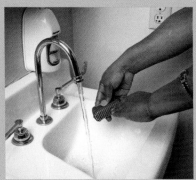

FIGURE 13-10E A hand brush can also be used to clean the nails.

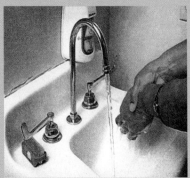

FIGURE 13-10F With the fingertips pointing downward, rinse the hands thoroughly.

10. Rinse your hands from the forearms down to the fingertips, keeping fingertips pointed downward (figure 13-10F).

11. Use a clean paper towel to dry hands thoroughly, from tips of fingers to wrist. Discard the towel in the waste container.

12. Use another dry paper towel to turn off the faucet.

   ▽ **CAUTION:** Wet towels allow passage of pathogens.

13. Discard all used towels in the waste container. Leave the area neat and clean.

14. Apply a water-based hand lotion if desired.

Practice

Go to the workbook and use the evaluation sheet for 13:3, Washing Hands, to practice this procedure. When you believe you have mastered this skill, sign the sheet and give it to your instructor for further action.

 Final Checkpoint Using the criteria listed on the evaluation sheet, your instructor will grade your performance.

13:4 Information

Observing Standard Precautions

To prevent the spread of pathogens and disease, the chain of infection must be broken. The standard precautions discussed in this unit are an important way health care workers can break this chain.

BLOODBORNE PATHOGENS STANDARD

One of the main ways that pathogens are spread is by blood and body fluids. Three pathogens of major concern are the hepatitis B virus (HBV), the hepatitis C virus (HCV), and the human immunodeficiency virus (HIV), which causes AIDS. Consequently, extreme care must be taken at all times when an area, object, or person is contaminated with blood or body fluids. In 1991, the Occupational Safety and Health Administration (OSHA) established *Bloodborne Pathogen Standards* that must be followed by all health care facilities. The employer faces civil penalties if the regulations are not implemented by the employer and followed by the employees. These regulations require all health care facility employers to:

♦ Develop a written exposure control plan, and update it annually, to minimize or eliminate employee exposure to bloodborne pathogens.

♦ Identify all employees who have occupational exposure to blood or potentially infectious materials such as semen, vaginal secretions, and other body fluids.

♦ Provide hepatitis B vaccine free of charge to all employees who have occupational exposure, and obtain a written release form signed by any employee who does not want the vaccine.

♦ Provide **personal protective equipment (PPE)** such as gloves, gowns, lab coats, masks, and face shields in appropriate sizes and in accessible locations.

♦ Provide adequate handwashing facilities and supplies.

♦ Ensure that the worksite is maintained in a clean and sanitary condition, follow measures for immediate decontamination of any sur-

face that comes in contact with blood or infectious materials, and dispose of infectious waste correctly.

♦ Enforce rules of no eating, drinking, smoking, applying cosmetics or lip balm, handling contact lenses, and mouth pipetting or suctioning in any area that can be potentially contaminated by blood or other body fluids.

♦ Provide appropriate containers that are color coded (fluorescent orange or orange-red) and labeled for contaminated sharps (needles, scalpels) and other infectious or biohazard wastes.

♦ Post signs at the entrance to work areas where there is occupational exposure to biohazardous materials. Label any item that is biohazardous with the red biohazard symbol (figure 13-11). The label must show both the symbol and the word "biohazard."

♦ Provide a confidential medical evaluation and follow-up for any employee who has an exposure incident. Examples might include an accidental needlestick or the splashing of blood or body fluids on the skin, eyes, or mucous membranes.

♦ Provide training about the regulations and all potential biohazards to all employees at no cost during working hours, and provide additional education as needed when procedures or working conditions are changed or modified.

NEEDLESTICK SAFETY ACT

In 2001, OSHA revised its Bloodborne Pathogen Standards in response to Congress passing the *Needlestick Safety and Prevention Act* in Novem-

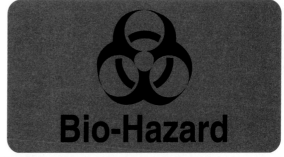

FIGURE 13-11 The universal biohazard symbol indicates a potential source of infection.

ber 2000. This act was passed after the Centers for Disease Control and Prevention (CDC) estimated that 600,000 to 800,000 needlesticks occur each year, exposing health care workers to bloodborne pathogens. Employers are required to:

♦ *Identify and use effective and safer medical devices.* OSHA defines safer devices as sharps with engineered injury protections and includes, but is not limited to, devices such as syringes with a sliding sheath that shields the needle after use, needles that retract into a syringe after use, shielded or retracting catheters that can be used to administer intravenous medications or fluids, and intravenous systems that administer medication or fluids through a catheter port or connector site using a needle housed in a protective covering (figure 13-12). OSHA also encourages the use of needleless systems, which include, but are not limited to, intravenous medication delivery systems that administer medication or fluids through a catheter port or connector site using a blunt cannula or other non-needle connection, and jet injection systems that deliver subcutaneous or intramuscular injections through the skin without using a needle.

♦ *Incorporate changes in annual update of exposure control plan.* Employers must include changes in technology that eliminate or reduce exposure to bloodborne pathogens in the annual update and document the implementation of any safer medical devices.

♦ *Solicit input from nonmanagerial employees who are responsible for direct patient care.* Employees who provide patient care, and are exposed to injuries from contaminated sharps, must be included in a multidisciplinary team that identifies, evaluates, and selects safer medical devices, and determines safer work practice controls.

♦ *Maintain a sharps injury log.* Employers with more than 11 employees must maintain a sharps injury log to help identify high-risk areas and evaluate ways of decreasing injuries. Each injury recorded must protect the confidentiality of the injured employee, but must state the type and brand of device involved in the incident, the work area or department where the exposure injury occurred, and a description of how the incident occurred.

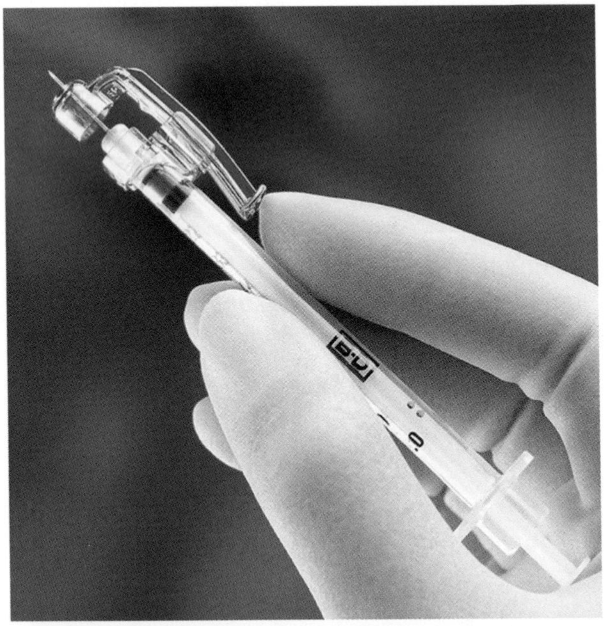

STANDARD PRECAUTIONS

Employers are also required to make sure that every employee uses standard precautions at all times to prevent contact with blood or other potentially infectious materials. **Standard precautions** (figure 13-13) are rules developed by the CDC. According to standard precautions, every body fluid must be considered a potentially infectious material, and all patients must be considered potential sources of infection, regardless of their disease or diagnosis. Standard precautions must be used in any situation where health care providers may contact:

♦ Blood or any fluid that may contain blood

♦ Body fluids, secretions, and excretions, such as mucus, sputum, saliva, cerebrospinal fluid, urine, feces, vomitus, amniotic fluid (surrounding a fetus), synovial (joint) fluid, pleural (lung) fluid, pericardial (heart) fluid, peritoneal (abdominal cavity) fluid, semen, and vaginal secretions

FIGURE 13-12 The Safety-Glide syringe is one example of a safer device to prevent needlesticks. *(Photo reprinted courtesy of BD [Becton Dickinson and Company])*

STANDARD PRECAUTIONS

FOR INFECTION CONTROL

Wash Hands (Plain soap)
Wash after touching **blood**, **body fluids**, **secretions**, **excretions**, and **contaminated items**. Wash immediately **after gloves are removed** and **between patient contacts**.
Avoid transfer of microorganisms to other patients or environments.

Wear Gloves
Wear when touching **blood**, **body fluids**, **secretions**, **excretions**, and **contaminated items**.
Put on **clean** gloves just **before touching mucous membranes** and **nonintact skin**.
Change gloves between tasks and procedures on the same patient after contact with material that may contain high concentrations of microorganisms. Remove gloves promptly after use, before touching noncontaminated items and environmental surfaces, and before going to another patient, and wash hands immediately to avoid transfer of microorganisms to other patients or environments.

Wear Mask and Eye Protection or Face Shield
Protect mucous membranes of the eyes, nose and mouth during procedures and patient–care activities that are likely to generate **splashes** or **sprays** of **blood**, **body fluids**, **secretions**, or **excretions**.

Wear Gown
Protect skin and prevent soiling of clothing during procedures that are likely to generate **splashes** or **sprays** of **blood**, **body fluids**, **secretions**, or **excretions**. Remove a soiled gown as promptly as possible and wash hands to avoid transfer of microorganisms to other patients or environments.

Patient-Care Equipment
Handle used patient–care equipment soiled with **blood**, **body fluids**, **secretions**, or **excretions** in a manner that prevents skin and mucous membrane exposures, contamination of clothing, and transfer of microorganisms to other patients and environments. Ensure that reusable equipment is not used for the care of another patient until it has been appropriately cleaned and reprocessed and single use items are properly discarded.

Environmental Control
Follow hospital procedures for routine care, cleaning, and disinfection of environmental surfaces, beds, bedrails, bedside equipment and other frequently touched surfaces.

Linen
Handle, transport, and process used linen soiled with **blood**, **body fluids**, **secretions**, or **excretions** in a manner that prevents exposures and contamination of clothing, and avoids transfer of microorganisms to other patients and environments.

Occupational Health and Bloodborne Pathogens
Prevent injuries when using needles, scalpels, and other sharp instruments or devices; when handling sharp instruments after procedures; when cleaning used instruments; and when disposing of used needles.

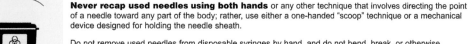

Never recap used needles using both hands or any other technique that involves directing the point of a needle toward any part of the body; rather, use either a one-handed "scoop" technique or a mechanical device designed for holding the needle sheath.

Do not remove used needles from disposable syringes by hand, and do not bend, break, or otherwise manipulate used needles by hand. Place used disposable syringes and needles, scalpel blades, and other sharp items in puncture–resistant sharps containers located as close as practical to the area in which the items were used, and place reusable syringes and needles in a puncture–resistant container for transport to the reprocessing area.

Use **resuscitation devices** as an alternative to mouth–to–mouth resuscitation.

Patient Placement
Use a **private room** for a patient who contaminates the environment or who does not (or cannot be expected to) assist in maintaining appropriate hygiene or environmental control. Consult Infection Control if a private room is not available.

The information on this sign is abbreviated from the HICPAC Recommendations for Isolation Precautions in Hospitals.

Form No. **SPR**   BREVIS CORP., 3310 S 2700 E, SLC, UT 84109   © 1996 Brevis Corp.

FIGURE 13-13 Standard precautions must be observed while working with all patients. *(Courtesy of Brevis Corporation)*

♦ Mucous membranes

♦ Nonintact skin

♦ Tissue or cell specimens

The basic rules of standard precautions include:

♦ *Handwashing*: Hands must be washed before and after contact with any patient. If hands or other skin surfaces are contaminated with blood, body fluids, secretions, or excretions, they must be washed immediately and thoroughly with soap and water. Hands must always be washed immediately before donning and immediately after removal of gloves.

♦ *Gloves*: Gloves (figure 13-14) must be worn whenever contact with blood, body fluids, secretions, excretions, mucous membranes, tissue specimens, or nonintact skin is possible; when handling or cleaning any contaminated items or surfaces; when performing any invasive (entering the body) procedure; and when performing venipuncture or blood tests. Rings must be removed before putting on gloves to avoid puncturing the gloves. Gloves must be changed after contact with each patient and even between tasks or procedures on the same patient if there is any chance the gloves are contaminated. Hands must be washed immediately after removal of gloves.

Care must be taken while removing gloves to avoid contamination of the skin. Gloves must *not* be washed or disinfected for reuse because washing may allow penetration of liquids through undetected holes, and disinfecting agents may cause deterioration of gloves.

♦ *Gowns*: Gowns must be worn during any procedure that is likely to cause splashing or spraying of blood, body fluids, secretions, or excretions. This helps prevent contamination of clothing or uniforms. Contaminated gowns must be handled according to agency policy and local and state laws. Wash hands immediately after removing a gown.

♦ *Masks and Eye Protection*: Masks and protective eyewear or face shields (figure 13-15) must be worn during procedures that may produce splashes or sprays of blood, body fluids, secretions, or excretions. Examples include irriga-

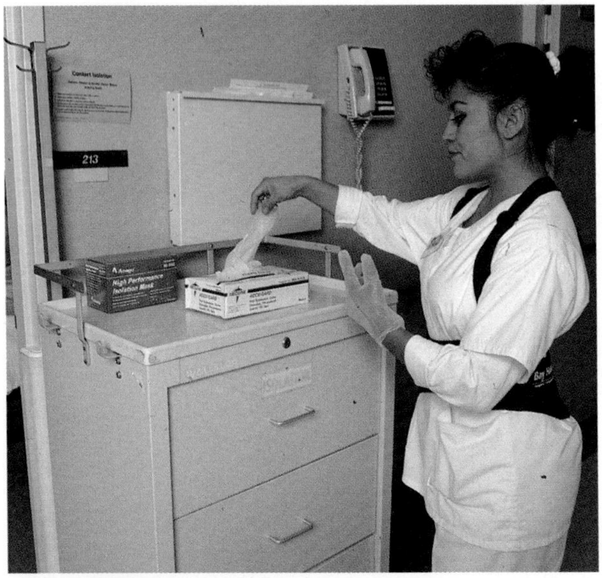

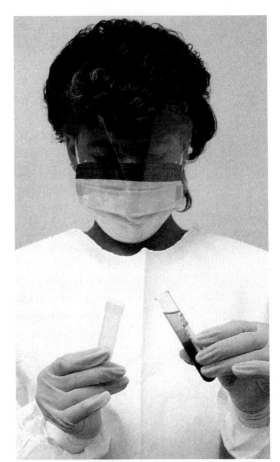

FIGURE 13-15 Gloves, a gown, a mask, and protective eyewear must be worn during any procedure that may produce droplets or cause splashing of blood, body fluids, secretions, or excretions.

FIGURE 13-14 Gloves must be worn whenever contact with blood, body fluids, secretions, excretions, mucous membranes, or nonintact skin is possible.

tion of wounds, suctioning, dental procedures, delivery of a baby, and surgical procedures. This prevents exposure of the mucous membranes of the mouth, nose, and eyes to any pathogens.

Masks must be used once and then discarded. In addition, masks should be changed every 30 minutes or anytime they become moist or wet. They should be removed by grasping the ties or elastic strap. Hands must be washed immediately after the mask is removed. Protective eyewear or face shields should provide protection for the front, top, bottom, and sides of the eyes. If eyewear is not disposable, it must be cleaned and disinfected before it is reused.

♦ *Sharps*: To avoid accidental cuts or punctures, extreme care must be taken while handling sharp objects. Whenever possible, safe needles or needleless devices must be used. Disposable needles must never be bent or broken after use. They must be left uncapped and attached to the syringe and placed in a leakproof puncture-resistant sharps container (figure 13-16). The sharps container must be labeled with a red biohazard symbol. Surgical blades, razors, and other sharp objects must also be discarded in the sharps container.

The sharps containers must *not* be emptied or reused. Federal, state, and local laws establish regulations for the disposal of sharps containers. In some areas, the filled container is placed in a special oven and melted. The material remaining is packaged as biohazard or infectious waste and disposed of according to legal requirements for infectious waste.

♦ *Spills or Splashes*: Spills or splashes of blood, body fluids, secretions, or excretions must be wiped up immediately (figure 13-17). Gloves must be worn while wiping up the area with disposable cleaning cloths. The area must then be cleaned with a disinfectant solution such as a 10-percent bleach solution. Furniture or equipment contaminated by the spill or splash must be cleaned and disinfected immediately. For large spills, an absorbent powder may be used to soak up the fluid. After the fluid is absorbed, it is swept up and placed in an infectious waste container.

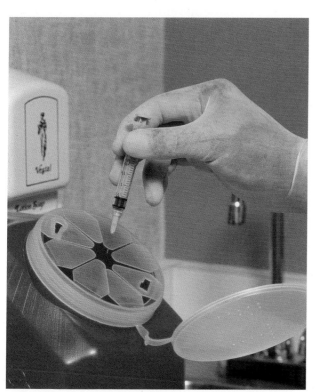

FIGURE 13-16 All needles and sharp objects must be discarded immediately in a leakproof puncture-resistant sharps container.

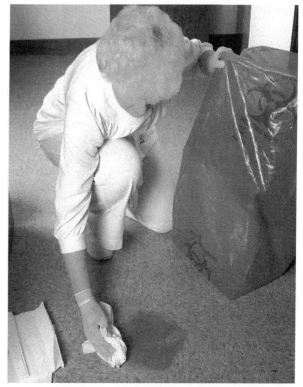

FIGURE 13-17 Gloves must be worn while wiping up any spills of blood, body fluids, secretions, or excretions.

◆ *Resuscitation Devices*: Whenever possible, mouthpieces or resuscitation devices should be used to avoid the need for mouth-to-mouth resuscitation. These devices should be placed in convenient locations and be readily accessible for use.

◆ *Waste and Linen Disposal*: Health care workers must wear gloves and follow the agency policy developed according to law to dispose of waste and soiled linen. Infectious wastes such as contaminated dressings; gloves; urinary drainage bags; incontinent pads; vaginal pads; disposable emesis basins, bedpans, and/or urinals; and body tissues must be placed in special infectious waste or biohazardous material bags (figure 13-18) according to law. Other trash is frequently placed in plastic bags and incinerated. The health care worker must dispose of waste in the proper container (figure 13-19) and know the requirements for disposal. Soiled linen should be placed in laundry bags to prevent any contamination. Linen soiled with blood, body fluids, or excretions is placed in a special bag for contaminated linen and is usually soaked in a disinfectant prior to being laundered. Gloves must be worn while handling any contaminated linen, and any bag containing contaminated linen must be clearly labeled and color coded.

◆ *Injuries*: Any cut, injury, needlestick, or splashing of blood or body fluids must be reported immediately. Agency policy must be followed to deal with the injury or contamination. Every health care facility must have a policy for stating actions that must be taken immediately when exposure or injury occurs, reporting any incident, documenting any exposure incident, recording the care given, noting follow-up to the exposure incident, and identifying ways to prevent a similar incident.

Standard precautions must be followed at all times by all health care workers. By observing these precautions, health care workers can help break the chain of infection and protect themselves, their patients, and all other individuals.

STUDENT: *Go to the workbook and complete the assignment sheet for 13:4, Observing Standard Precautions. Then return and continue with the procedure.*

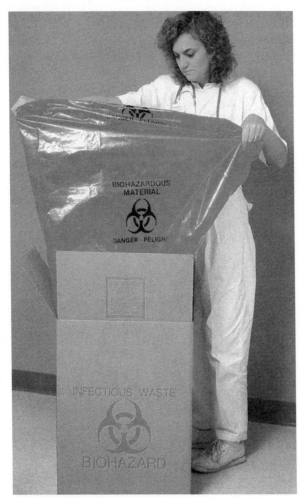

FIGURE 13-18 All infectious wastes must be placed in special infectious waste or biohazardous material bags.

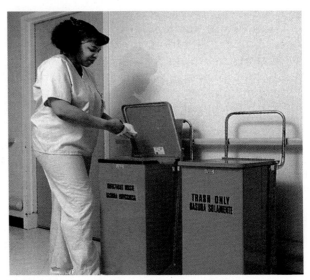

FIGURE 13-19 The health care worker must know the requirements for disposal of waste materials and dispose of wastes in the proper containers.

PROCEDURE 13:4

Observing Standard Precautions

Equipment and Supplies

Disposable gloves, infectious waste bags, needle and syringe, sharps container, gown, masks, protective eyewear, resuscitation devices

⊞ **NOTE:** This procedure will help you learn standard precautions. It is important for you to observe these precautions at all times while working in the laboratory or clinical area.

Procedure

1. Assemble equipment.

2. Review the precautions in the information section for Observing Standard Precautions. Note points that are not clear, and ask your instructor for an explanation.

3. Practice handwashing according to Procedure 13:3. Identify at least six times that hands must be washed according to standard precautions.

4. Name four instances when gloves must be worn to observe standard precautions. Put on a pair of disposable gloves. Practice removing the gloves without contaminating the skin. With a gloved hand, grasp the cuff of the glove on the opposite hand, handling only the outside of the glove (figure 13-20A). Pull the glove down and turn it inside out while removing it. Take care not to touch the skin with the gloved hand. Using the ungloved hand, slip the fingers under the cuff of the glove on the opposite hand (figure 13-20B). Touching only the inside of the glove and taking care not to touch the skin, pull the glove down and turn it inside out while removing it. Place the gloves in an infectious waste container. Wash your hands immediately.

5. Practice putting on a gown. State when a gown is to be worn. To remove the gown, touch only the inside. Fold the contaminated gown so the outside is folded inward. Roll it into a bundle and place it in an infectious waste container if it is disposable, or in a bag for contaminated linen if it is not disposable.

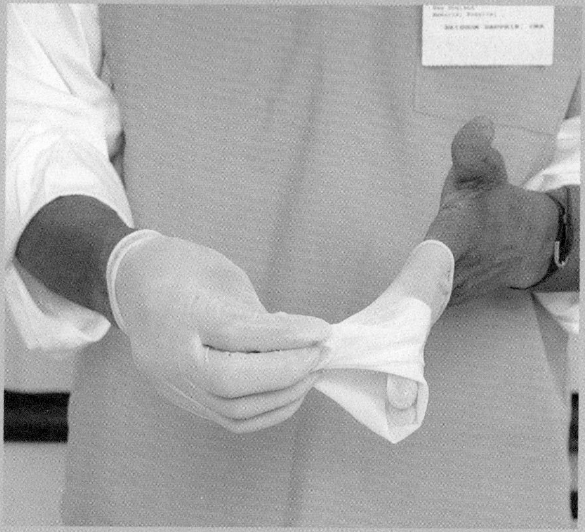

FIGURE 13-20A To remove the first glove, use a gloved hand to grasp the outside of the glove on the opposite hand. Pull the glove down and turn it inside out while removing it.

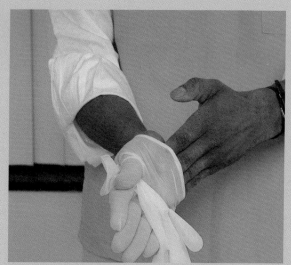

FIGURE 13-20B To remove the second glove, slip the fingers of the ungloved hand inside the cuff of the glove. Touch only the inside of the glove while pulling it down and turning it inside out.

PROCEDURE 13:4

▽ **CAUTION:** If a gown is contaminated, gloves should be worn while removing the gown.

NOTE: Folding the gown and rolling it prevents transmission of pathogens.

6. Practice putting on a mask and protective eyewear. To remove the mask, handle it by the ties only. Clean and disinfect protective eyewear after use.

7. Practice proper disposal of sharps. Uncap a needle attached to a syringe, taking care not to stick yourself with the needle. Place the entire needle and syringe in a sharps container. State the rules regarding disposal of the sharps container.

8. Spill a small amount of water on a counter. Pretend that it is blood. Put on gloves and use disposable cloths or gauze to wipe up the spill. Put the contaminated cloths or gauze in an infectious waste bag. Use clean disposable cloths or gauze to wipe the area thoroughly with a disinfectant agent. Put the cloths or gauze in the infectious waste bag, remove your gloves, and wash your hands.

9. Practice handling an infectious waste bag. Fold down the top edge of the bag to form a cuff at the top of the bag. Wear gloves to close the bag after contaminated wastes have been placed in it. Put your hands under the folded cuff (figure 13-21A) and gently expel excess air from the bag. Twist the top of the bag shut and fold down the top edges to seal the bag. Secure the fold with tape or a tie according to agency policy (figure 13-21B).

10. Examine mouthpieces and resuscitation devices that can be used in place of mouth-to-mouth resuscitation. You will be taught to use these devices when you learn cardiopulmonary resuscitation (CPR).

11. Discuss the following situations with another student and determine which standard precautions should be observed:

    • A patient has an open sore on the skin and pus is seeping from the area. You are going to bathe the patient.

    • You are cleaning a tray of instruments that contains a disposable surgical blade and needle with syringe.

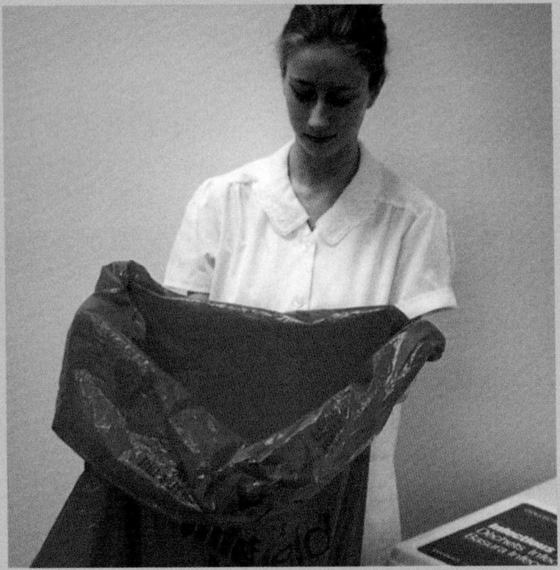

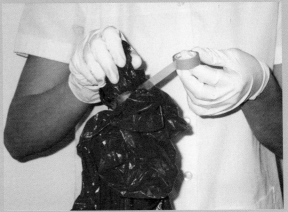

FIGURE 13-21A To close an infectious waste bag, wear gloves and place your hands under the cuff to gently expel excess air.

FIGURE 13-21B After folding down the top edge of the infectious waste bag, tie or tape it securely.

PROCEDURE 13:4

- A tube of blood drops to the floor and breaks, spilling the blood on the floor.

- Drainage from dressings on an infected wound has soiled the linen on the bed you are changing.

- You work in a dental office and are assisting a dentist while a tooth is being extracted (removed).

12. Replace all equipment used.

Practice

Go to the workbook and use the evaluation sheet for 13:4, Observing Standard Precautions. When you believe you have mastered this skill, sign the sheet and give it to your instructor for further action.

✓ **Final Checkpoint** Using the criteria listed on the evaluation sheet, your instructor will grade your performance.

13:5 Information

Sterilizing with an Autoclave

Sterilization of instruments and equipment is essential in preventing the spread of infection. In any of the health fields, you may be responsible for proper sterilization. The following basic principles relate to sterilization methods. The autoclave is the safest, most efficient sterilization method.

An **autoclave** is a piece of equipment that uses steam under pressure or gas to sterilize equipment and supplies (figure 13-22). It is the most efficient method of sterilizing most articles,

and it will destroy all microorganisms, both pathogenic and nonpathogenic, including spores and viruses.

Autoclaves are available in various sizes and types. Offices and health clinics usually have smaller units, and hospitals or surgical areas have large floor model units. A pressure cooker can be used in home situations.

Before any equipment or supplies are sterilized in an autoclave, they must be prepared properly. All items must be washed thoroughly and then rinsed. Oily substances can often be removed with alcohol or ether. Any residue left on articles will tend to bake and stick to the article during the autoclaving process.

Items that are to remain sterile must be wrapped before they are autoclaved. A wide variety of wraps are available. The wrap must be a material that will allow for the penetration of steam during the autoclaving process. Samples of wraps include muslin, autoclave paper, special plastic or paper bags, and autoclave containers (figure 13-23).

Autoclave indicators are used to ensure that articles have been sterilized (figure 13-24). Examples of indicators include autoclave tape, sensitivity marks on bags or wraps, and indicator capsules. The indicator is usually placed on or near the article when the article is put into the autoclave. Indicators can also be placed in the center of a package, such as a tray of instruments, to show that sterilization of the entire package has occurred. The indicator will change appear-

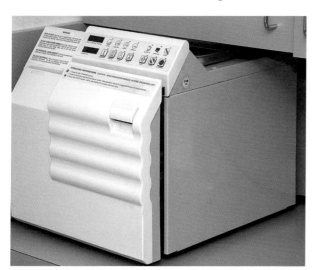

FIGURE 13-22 An autoclave uses steam under pressure to sterilize items.

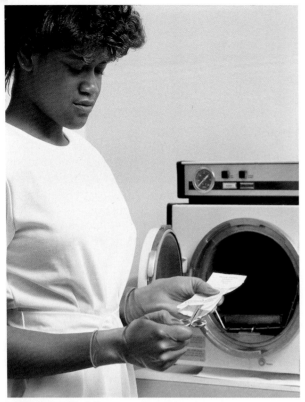

FIGURE 13-23 Special plastic or paper autoclave bags can be used to sterilize instruments.

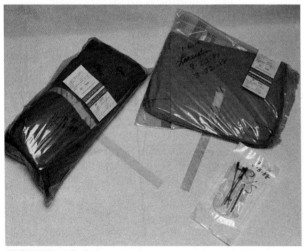

FIGURE 13-24 Autoclave indicators change color to show that sterilization has occurred. The strips below each package show how the indicators looked before sterilization.

ance during the autoclaving process because of time and temperature, which leads to sterilization. Learn how to recognize that an article is sterile by reading the directions provided with indicators.

The autoclave must be loaded correctly for all parts of an article to be sterilized. Steam builds at the top of the chamber and moves downward. As it moves down, it pushes cool, dry air out of the bottom of the chamber. Therefore, materials must be placed so the steam can penetrate along the natural planes between the packages of articles in the autoclave. Place the articles in such a way that there is space between all pieces. Packages should be placed on the sides, not flat. Jars, basins, and cans should be placed on their sides, not flat, so that steam can enter and air can flow out. No articles should come in contact with the sides, top, or door of the autoclave.

The length of time and amount of pressure required to sterilize different items varies (figure 13-25). *It is important to check the directions that come with the autoclave.* Because different types of articles require different times and pressures, it is important to separate loads so that all articles sterilized at one time require the same time and pressure. For example, rubber tubings usually require a relatively short period of time and can

Articles	Time at 250° to 254°F (121° to 123°C)
Glassware: empty, inverted Instruments: metal in covered or open, padded or unpadded tray Needles, unwrapped Syringes: unassembled, unwrapped Instruments, metal combined with other materials in covered and/or padded tray	15 minutes
Instruments wrapped in double-thickness muslin Flasked solutions, 75–250 mL Needles, individually packaged in glass tubes or paper	20 minutes
Syringes: unassembled, individually packed in muslin or paper Dressings wrapped in paper or muslin (small packs only) Flasked solutions, 500–1,000 mL Sutures: silk, cotton, or nylon; wrapped in paper or muslin Treatment trays wrapped in muslin or paper	30 minutes

FIGURE 13-25 The length of time required to sterilize different items varies.

be damaged by long exposure. Certain instruments and needles require a longer period of time to ensure sterilization; therefore, items of this type should not be sterilized in the same load as are rubber tubings.

Wet surfaces permit rapid infiltration of organisms, so it is important that all items are thoroughly dry before being removed from the autoclave. The length of time for drying varies. Follow the manufacturer's instructions.

Sterilized items must be stored in clean, dust-proof areas. Items usually remain sterile for 30 days after autoclaving. However, if the wraps loosen or tear, if they become wet, or if any chance of contamination occurs, the items should be rewrapped and autoclaved again.

NOTE: At the end of the 30-day sterile period—providing that the wrap has not loosened, been torn, or gotten wet—remove the old autoclave tape from the package, replace with a new, dated tape, and resterilize according to correct procedure.

Some autoclaves are equipped with a special door that allows the autoclave to be used as a dry-heat sterilizer. Dry heat involves the use of a high temperature for a long period of time. The temperature is usually a minimum of 320–350°F (160–177°C). The minimum time is usually 60 minutes. Dry-heat sterilization is a good method for sterilizing instruments that may corrode, such as knife blades, or items that would be destroyed by the moisture in steam sterilization, such as powders. Dry heat should never be used on soft rubber goods because the heat will destroy the rubber. Some types of plastic will also melt in dry heat. An oven can be used for dry-heat sterilization in home situations.

Procedures 13:5A and 13:5B describe wrapping articles for autoclaving and autoclaving techniques. These procedures vary in different agencies and areas, but the same principles apply. In some facilities, many supplies are purchased as sterile, disposable items; needles and syringes are purchased in sterilized wraps, used once, and then destroyed. In other facilities, however, special treatment trays are sterilized and used more than one time.

It is important that you follow the directions specific to the autoclave with which you are working as well as the agency policy for sterile supplies. Careless autoclaving permits the transmission of disease-producing organisms. Infection control is everyone's responsibility.

STUDENT: *Go to the workbook and complete the assignment sheet for 13:5, Sterilizing with an Autoclave. Then return and continue with the procedures.*

PROCEDURE 13:5A

Wrapping Items for Autoclaving

Equipment and Supplies

Items to wrap: instrument, towel, bowl; autoclave wrap: paper, muslin, plastic or paper bag; autoclave tape or indicator; disposable or utility gloves; pen or autoclave marker; masking tape (if autoclave tape is not used)

Procedure

1. Assemble equipment.
2. Wash hands. Put on gloves.

CAUTION: If the items to be autoclaved are contaminated with blood, body fluids, or tissues, gloves must be worn while cleaning the items.

3. Sanitize the items to be sterilized. Instruments, bowls, and similar items should be cleaned thoroughly in soapy water (figure 13-26). Rinse the items well in cool water to remove any soapy residue. Then rinse well with hot water. Dry the items with a towel. After the items are sanitized and dry, remove the gloves and wash hands.

NOTE: If stubborn stains are present, it may be necessary to soak the items.

PROCEDURE 13:5A

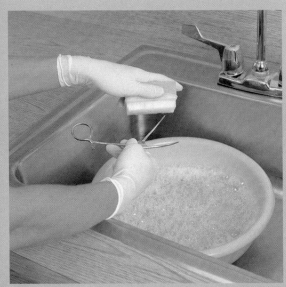

FIGURE 13-26 Wear gloves to scrub instruments thoroughly with soapy water.

NOTE: Check the teeth on serrated (notched like a saw) instruments. Scrub with a brush as necessary.

4. To prepare linen for wrapping, check first to make sure it is clean and dry. Fold the linen in half lengthwise. If it is very wide, fold lengthwise again. Fanfold or accordion pleat the linen from end to end until a compact package is formed (figure 13-27A). All folds should be the same size. Fold back one corner on the top fold (figure 13-27B). This provides a piece to grab when opening the linen.

NOTE: Fanfolding linens allows for easy handling after sterilization.

5. Select the correct wrap for the item. Make sure the wrap is large enough to enclose the item to be wrapped.

NOTE: Double-thickness muslin, disposable paper wraps, and plastic or paper bags are the most common wraps.

6. With the wrap positioned at a diagonal angle and one corner pointing toward you, place the item to be sterilized in the center of the wrap.

NOTE: Make sure that hinged instruments are open so the steam can sterilize all edges.

7. Fold up the bottom corner to the center (figure 13-28A). Double back a small corner (figure 13-28B).

8. Fold a side corner over to the center. Make sure the edges are sealed and that there are no air pockets. Bring back a small corner (figure 13-28C).

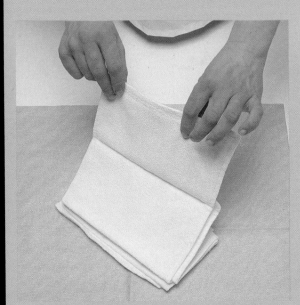

FIGURE 13-27A Fanfold clean, dry linen so all the folds are the same size.

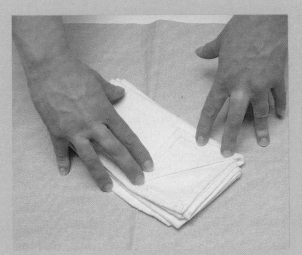

FIGURE 13-27B Fold back one corner on the top fold of the linen.

PROCEDURE 13:5A

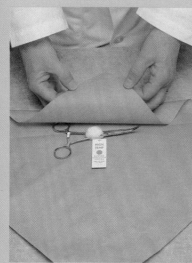

FIGURE 13-28A Place the instrument in the center of the wrap. Fold the bottom corner in to the center.

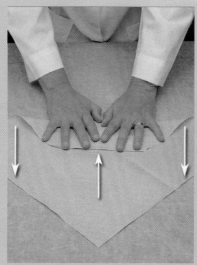

FIGURE 13-28B Turn a small corner back to form a tab.

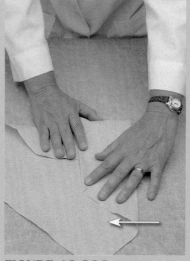

FIGURE 13-28C Fold in one side and fold back a tab.

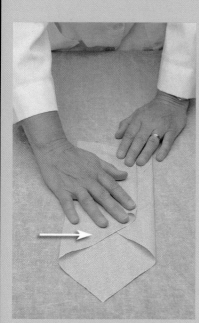

FIGURE 13-28D Fold in the opposite side and fold back a tab.

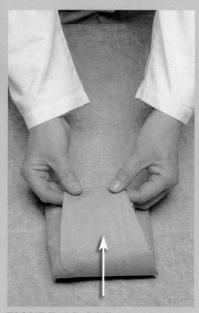

FIGURE 13-28E Bring the final corner up and over the top of the pack and tuck it in, leaving a small corner exposed.

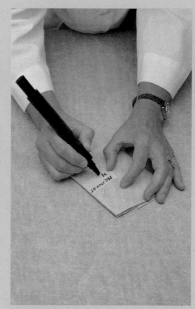

FIGURE 13-28F Secure the package with autoclave tape. Label it with the date, contents, and your initials.

PROCEDURE 13:5A

 CAUTION: Any open areas at corners will allow pathogens to enter.

9. Fold in the other side corner. Again, watch for and avoid open edges. Bring back a small corner (figure 13-28D).

10. Bring the final corner up and over the top of the package. Check the two edges to be sure they are sealed and tight. Tuck this under the pocket created by the previous folds. Leave a small corner exposed so it can be used when unwrapping the package (figure 13-28E).

   NOTE: This is frequently called an "envelope" wrap, because the final corner is tucked into the wrap similar to the way the flap is tucked into an envelope.

11. Secure with autoclave or pressure-sensitive indicator tape.

   NOTE: If regular masking tape is used, attach an autoclave indicator to reflect when contents are sterilized.

12. Label the package by marking the tape with the date and contents (figure 13-28F). Some health care agencies may require you to initial the label.

   NOTE: For certain items, the type or size of item should be noted, for example, curved hemostat or mosquito hemostat, hand towel or bath towel, small bowl or large bowl.

   NOTE: Contents will not be sterile after 30 days, so the date of sterilization must be noted on the package.

13. Check the package. It should be firm enough for handling but loose enough for proper circulation of steam.

14. To use a plastic or paper autoclave bag (refer to figure 13-23), select or cut the correct size for the item to be sterilized. Place the clean item inside the bag. Double fold the open end(s) and tape or secure with autoclave tape. Check the package to make sure it is secure.

   NOTE: In some agencies, the ends are sealed with heat prior to autoclaving.

   NOTE: If the bag has an autoclave indicator, regular masking tape can be used to seal the ends.

15. Replace all equipment used.

16. Wash hands.

Practice

Go to the workbook and use the evaluation sheet for 13:5A, Wrapping Items for Autoclaving, to practice this procedure. When you believe you have mastered this skill, sign the sheet and give it to your instructor for further action.

 Final Checkpoint Using the criteria listed on the evaluation sheet, your instructor will grade your performance.

PROCEDURE 13:5B

Loading and Operating an Autoclave

NOTE: Follow the operating instructions for your autoclave. The basic principles of loading apply to all autoclaves. Basic controls for one autoclave are shown in figure 13-29.

Equipment and Supplies

Autoclave, distilled water, small pitcher or measuring cup, items wrapped or prepared for autoclaving, time chart for autoclave, 13:5 Information section

Procedure

Review the Information section for 13:5, Sterilizing with an Autoclave. Then proceed with the following activities. You should read through the procedure first, checking against the diagram. Then practice with an autoclave.

1. Assemble equipment.

2. Wash and dry hands thoroughly.

3. Check the three-prong plug and the electrical cord. If either is damaged or prongs are missing, do not use the autoclave. If no problems are present, plug the cord into a wall outlet.

4. Use distilled water to fill the reservoir to within 2 1/2 inches below the opening or to the level indicated on the autoclave.

    NOTE: Distilled water prevents the collection of mineral deposits and prolongs the life and effectiveness of the autoclave.

5. Check the pressure gauge to make sure it is at zero.

    CAUTION: Never open the door unless the pressure is zero.

6. Open the safety door by following the manufacturer's instructions. Some door handles require an upward and inward pressure; others require a side-pressure technique.

7. Load the autoclave. Make sure all articles have been prepared correctly. Check for autoclave indicators, secure wraps, and correct labels. Separate loads so all items require the same time, temperature, and pressure. Place packages on their sides. Place bowls or basins on their sides so air and steam can flow in and out of the container (figure 13-30). Make sure there is space between the packages so the steam can circulate.

    NOTE: Check to make sure no large packages block the steam flow to smaller packages. Place large packages on the bottom.

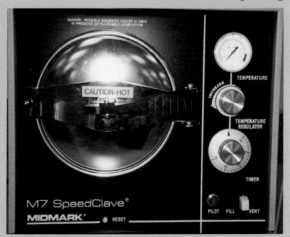

FIGURE 13-29 Autoclave control valves vary, but most contain the same basic controls.

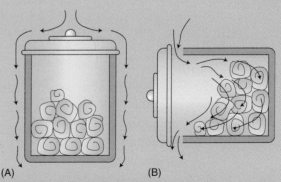

(A)   (B)

FIGURE 13-30 Bowls or basins should be placed on their sides in the autoclave so air and steam can flow in and out of the container: (A) incorrect placement; (B) correct placement.

PROCEDURE 13:5B

▽ **CAUTION:** Make sure no item comes in contact with the sides, top, or door of the autoclave chamber.

8. Follow the instructions for filling the chamber with the correct amount of water. Most autoclaves have a "Fill" setting on the control. Allow water to enter the chamber until the water covers the fill plate inside the chamber.

9. When the correct amount of water is in the chamber, follow the instructions for stopping the flow of water. In many autoclaves, turning the control valve to "Sterilize" stops the flow of water from the reservoir.

10. Check the load in the chamber to be sure it is properly spaced. The chamber can also be loaded at this point, if this has not been done previously.

11. Close and lock the door.

▽ **CAUTION:** Be sure the door is securely locked; check by pulling slightly.

12. Read the time chart for the specific time and temperature required for sterilization of items that were placed in the autoclave.

13. After referring to the chart provided with the autoclave or reviewing figure 13-25, set the control valves to allow the temperature and pressure to increase in the autoclave.

14. When the desired temperature (usually 250–254°F or 121–123°C) and pressure (usually 15 pounds) have been reached, set the controls to maintain the desired temperature during the sterilization process. Follow the manufacturer's instructions.

15. Based on the information in the time chart, set the timer to the correct time.

NOTE: Many autoclaves require you to rotate the timer past 10 (minutes) before setting the time.

16. Check the pressure and temperature gauges at intervals to make sure they remain as originally set.

NOTE: Most autoclaves automatically shut off when pressure reaches 35 pounds.

17. When the required time has passed, set the controls so the autoclave will vent the steam from the chamber.

18. Put on safety glasses.

▽ **CAUTION:** Never open the door without glasses. The escaping steam can burn the eyes.

19. Check the pressure and temperature gauges. When the pressure gauge is at zero, and the temperature gauge is at or below 212°F, open the door about 1/2 to 1 inch to permit thorough drying of contents.

▽ **CAUTION:** Do not open the door until pressure is zero.

NOTE: Most autoclaves have a safety lock on the door that does not release until the pressure is at zero.

20. After the autoclaved items are completely dry, remove and store them in a dry, dust-free area.

▽ **CAUTION:** Handle supplies and equipment carefully. They may be hot.

21. If there are additional loads to run, leave the main valve in the vent position. This will keep the autoclave ready for immediate use.

22. If this is the final load, turn the autoclave off. Unplug the cord from the wall outlet; do not pull on the cord.

NOTE: The autoclave must be cleaned on a regular basis. Follow manufacturer's instructions.

23. Replace all equipment used.

24. Wash hands.

Practice

Go to the workbook and use the evaluation sheet for 13:5B, Loading and Operating an Autoclave, to practice this procedure. When you believe you have mastered this skill, sign the sheet and give it to your instructor for further action.

 Final Checkpoint Using the criteria listed on the evaluation sheet, your instructor will grade your performance.

13:6 Information

Using Chemicals for Disinfection

Many health fields require the use of chemicals for aseptic control. Certain points that must be observed while using the chemicals are discussed in the following section.

Chemicals are frequently used for aseptic control. Many chemicals do not kill spores and viruses; therefore, chemicals are not a method of sterilization. Because sterilization does not occur, **chemical disinfection** is the appropriate term (rather than cold sterilization, a term sometimes used). A few chemicals will kill spores and viruses, but these chemicals frequently require that instruments be submerged in the chemical for 10 or more hours. It is essential to read an entire label to determine the effectiveness of the product before using any chemical.

Chemicals are used to disinfect instruments that do not penetrate body tissue. Many dental instruments, percussion hammers, scissors, and similar items are examples. In addition, chemicals are used to disinfect thermometers and other items that would be destroyed by the high heat used in the autoclave.

Proper cleaning of all instruments or articles is essential. Particles or debris on items may contaminate the chemicals and reduce their effectiveness. In addition, all items must be rinsed thoroughly because the presence of soap can also reduce the effectiveness of chemicals. The articles must be dry before being placed in the disinfectant to keep the chemical at its most effective strength.

Some chemical solutions used as disinfectants are 90-percent isopropyl alcohol, formaldehyde–alcohol, 2-percent phenolic germicide, 10-percent bleach (sodium hypochlorite) solution, glutaraldehyde, iodophor, Lysol, Cidex, and benzalkonium (zephiran). The manufacturer's directions should be read completely before using any solution. Some solutions must be diluted or mixed before use. The directions will also specify the recommended time for the most thorough disinfection.

Chemical solutions can cause rust to form on certain instruments, so antirust tablets or solutions are frequently added to the chemicals. Again, it is important to read the directions provided with the tablets or solution. If improperly used, antirust substances may cause a chemical reaction with a solution and reduce the effectiveness of the chemical disinfectant.

The container used for chemical disinfection must be large enough to accommodate the items. In addition, the items should be separate so each one will come in contact with the chemical. A tight-fitting lid must be placed on the container while the articles are in the solution to prevent evaporation that could affect the strength of the solution. The lid also decreases the chance of dust and airborne particles from falling into the solution.

The chemical disinfectant must completely cover the article. This is the only way to be sure that all parts of the article will be disinfected.

Before removing items from solutions, health workers must wash their hands. Sterile gloves or sterile pick-ups or transfer forceps may be used to remove the instruments from the solution. The items should be rinsed with sterile water to remove any remaining chemical solution. After rinsing, the instruments are placed on a sterile or clean towel to dry, and then stored in a drawer or dust-free closet.

Solutions must be changed frequently. Some solutions can be used over a period of time, but others must be discarded after one use. Follow the manufacturer's instructions. However, any time contamination occurs or dirt is present in the solution, discard it. A fresh solution must be used.

STUDENT: *Go to the Workbook and complete the assignment sheet for 13:6, Using Chemicals for Disinfection. Then return and continue with the procedure.*

PROCEDURE 13:6

Using Chemicals for Disinfection

Equipment and Supplies

Chemicals, container with tight-fitting lid, basin, soap, water, instruments, brush, sterile pick-ups or transfer forceps, sterile towel, sterile gloves, eye protection, disposable gloves

Procedure

1. Assemble equipment.

2. Wash hands. Put on disposable or heavy-duty utility gloves and eye protection.

   NOTE: Wear gloves if any of the instruments or equipment are contaminated with blood or body fluids. Wear eye protection if there is any chance splashing will occur.

3. Wash all instruments or equipment thoroughly. Use warm soapy water. Use the brush on serrated edges of instruments.

   NOTE: All tissue and debris must be removed from the instrument or item or it will not be disinfected.

4. Rinse in cool water to remove soapy residue. Then rinse well with hot water. Dry all instruments or equipment thoroughly.

   NOTE: Water on the instruments or equipment will dilute the chemical disinfectant.

5. Check container. Make sure lid fits securely.

   NOTE: A loose cover will permit entrance of pathogens and/or evaporation of the chemical solution.

6. Place instruments in the container. Make sure there is a space between instruments. Leave hinged edges open so the solution can flow between the surfaces.

7. Carefully read label instructions about the chemical solution. Some solutions must be diluted. Check the manufacturer's recommended soaking time.

   CAUTION: Reread instructions to be sure solution is safe to use on instruments.

   NOTE: An antirust substance must be added to some solutions.

8. Pour solution into the container slowly to avoid splashing. Make sure that all instruments are covered (figure 13-31). Close the lid of the container.

   NOTE: Read label three times: before pouring, while pouring, and after pouring.

   CAUTION: Avoid splashing the chemical on your skin. Improper handling of chemicals may cause burns and/or injuries.

9. Remove gloves. Wash hands.

10. Leave the instruments in the solution for the length of time recommended by the manufacturer.

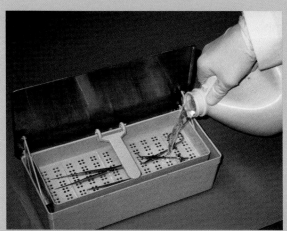

FIGURE 13-31 Pour the chemical disinfectant into the container until all instruments are covered with solution.

PROCEDURE 13:6

NOTE: Twenty to 30 minutes is the usual soaking time.

NOTE: If the solution requires a long period (for example, 10–12 hours) for disinfecting, label the container with the date and time the process began, ending date and time, and your initials.

11. When instruments have soaked the correct amount of time, use sterile gloves or sterile pick-ups or transfer forceps to remove the instruments from the solution. Hold the instruments over a sink or basin and pour sterile water over them to rinse them thoroughly. Place them on a sterile towel to dry. A second sterile towel is sometimes used to dry the instruments or to cover the instruments while they are drying. Store the instruments in special drawers, containers, or dust-free closets.

NOTE: Some contamination occurs when instruments are exposed to the air. In some cases, such as with external instruments, this minimal contamination will not affect usage.

12. Replace all equipment used.

 CAUTION: If the disinfectant solution can be used again, label the container with the name of the disinfectant, date, and number of days it can be used according to manufacturer's instructions. When solutions cannot be reused, dispose of the solution according to manufacturer's instructions.

13. Remove gloves. Wash hands.

Practice

Go to the workbook and use the evaluation sheet for 13:6, Using Chemicals for Disinfection, to practice this procedure. When you believe you have mastered this skill, sign the sheet and give it to your instructor for further action.

✔ **Final Checkpoint** Using the criteria listed on the evaluation sheet, your instructor will grade your performance.

13:7 Information

Cleaning with an Ultrasonic Unit

Ultrasonic units are used in many dental and medical offices and other health agencies to remove dirt, debris, blood, saliva, and tissue from a large variety of instruments prior to sterilizing them. **Ultrasonic** cleaning uses sound waves to clean. When the ultrasonic unit is turned on, the sound waves produce millions of microscopic bubbles in a cleaning solution. When the bubbles strike the items being cleaned, they explode, a process known as **cavitation,** and drive the cleaning solution onto the article. Accumulated dirt and residue are easily and gently removed from the article.

Ultrasonic cleaning is not sterilization because spores and viruses remain on the articles. If sterilization is desired, other methods must be used after the ultrasonic cleaning.

Only ultrasonic solutions should be used in the unit. Different solutions are available for different materials. A general, all-purpose cleaning solution is usually used in the permanent tank and to clean many items. There are other specific solutions for alginate, plaster and stone removal, and tartar removal. The solution chart provided with the ultrasonic unit will state which solution should be used. It is important to read labels carefully before using any solutions. Some solutions must be diluted before use. Some can be used only on specific materials. All solutions are toxic. They can also cause skin irritation, so contact with the skin and eyes should be avoided. Solutions should be discarded when they become cloudy or contaminated, or if cleaning results are poor.

The permanent tank of the ultrasonic unit (figure 13-32) must contain a solution at all times. A general, all-purpose cleaning solution is used most of the time. Glass beakers or auxiliary pans or baskets can then be placed in the permanent tank. The items to be cleaned and the proper cleaning solution are then put in the beakers or pans. The bottoms of the beakers or pans must always be positioned below the level of the solution present in the permanent tank. In this way, cavitation can be transmitted from the main tank and through the solution to the items being cleaned in the beakers or pans. The ultrasonic unit should never be operated without solutions in both containers. In addition, the items being cleaned must be submerged in the cleaning solution.

Many different items can be cleaned in an ultrasonic unit. Examples include instruments, impression trays, glass products, and most jewelry. The ultrasonic unit should not be used on jewelry with pearls or pasted stones. The sound waves can destroy the pearls or the paste holding the stones. Prior to cleaning, most of the dirt or particles should be brushed off the items being cleaned. It is better to clean a few articles at a time and avoid overloading the unit. If items are close together, the process of cavitation is poor because the bubbles cannot strike all parts of the items being cleaned.

The glass beakers used in the ultrasonic unit are made of a type of glass that allows the passage of sound waves. After continual use, the sound waves etch the bottom of the beakers. A white, opaque coating forms. The beakers must be discarded and replaced when this occurs. After each use, the beakers should be washed with soap and water and rinsed thoroughly to remove any soapy residue. They must be dry before being filled with solution because water in the beaker can dilute the solution.

The permanent tank of the unit must be drained and cleaned at intervals based on tank use or appearance of the solution in the tank. A drain valve on the side of the tank is opened to allow the solution to drain. The tank is then wiped with a damp cloth or disinfectant. Another damp cloth or disinfectant is used to wipe off the outside of the unit. The unit should never be submerged in water to clean it. After cleaning, a fresh solution should be placed in the permanent tank.

The manufacturer's instructions must be read carefully before using any ultrasonic unit. Most manufacturers provide cleaning charts that state the type of solution and time required for a variety of cleaning problems. Each time an item is cleaned in an ultrasonic unit, the chart should be used to determine the correct cleaning solution and time required.

STUDENT: *Go to the workbook and complete the assignment sheet for 13:7, Cleaning with an Ultrasonic Unit. Then return and continue with the procedure.*

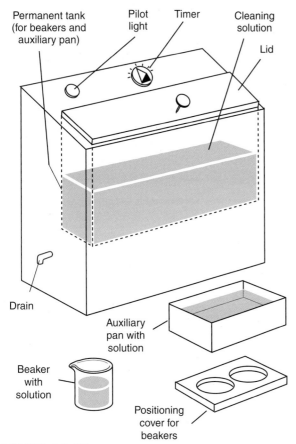

FIGURE 13-32 Parts of an ultrasonic cleaning unit.

PROCEDURE 13:7

Cleaning with an Ultrasonic Unit

Equipment and Supplies

Ultrasonic unit, permanent tank with solution, beakers, auxiliary pan or basket with covers, beaker bands, cleaning solutions, transfer forceps or pick-ups, paper towels, gloves, brush, soap, water for rinsing, articles for cleaning, solution chart

Procedure

1. Assemble all equipment.

2. Wash hands. Put on gloves if any items are contaminated with blood, body fluids, secretions, or excretions.

   NOTE: Use heavy-duty utility gloves if instruments are sharp.

3. Use a brush and soap and water to remove any large particles of dirt from articles to be cleaned. Rinse articles thoroughly. Dry items.

   NOTE: Rinsing is important because soap may interact with the cleaning solution.

4. Check the permanent tank to be sure it has enough cleaning solution. An all-purpose cleaning solution is usually used in this tank.

   CAUTION: Never run the unit without solution in the permanent tank.

   NOTE: Many solutions must be diluted before use; if new solution is needed, read the instructions on the bottle.

5. Pour the proper cleaning solution into the auxiliary pan or beakers.

   NOTE: Use the cleaning chart to determine which solution to use.

   CAUTION: Read label before using.

   CAUTION: Handle solutions carefully. Avoid contact with skin and eyes.

6. Place the beakers, basket, or auxiliary pan into the permanent tank (figures 13-33A and B). Use beaker positioning covers and beaker bands. Beaker bands are large bands that circle the beakers to hold them in position and keep them from hitting the bottom of the permanent tank.

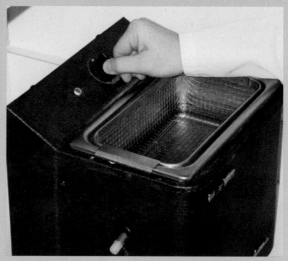

FIGURE 13-33A The auxiliary basket can be used to clean larger items in an ultrasonic unit.

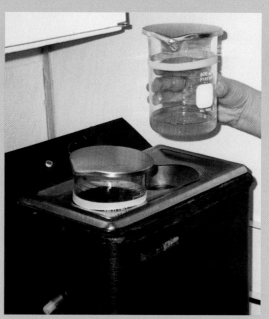

FIGURE 13-33B Glass beakers can be used to clean smaller items in an ultrasonic unit.

PROCEDURE 13:7

7. Check to be sure that the bottoms of the beakers, basket, or pan are below the level of solution in the permanent tank.

   NOTE: For sonic waves to flow through solutions in the beakers, basket, or pan, the two solution levels must overlap.

8. Place articles to be cleaned in the beakers, basket, or pan. Be sure the solution completely covers the articles. Do not get solution on your hands.

   NOTE: Remember that pearls or pasted stones cannot be cleaned in an ultrasonic unit.

9. Turn the timer past 5 (minutes) and then set the proper cleaning time. Use the cleaning chart to determine the correct amount of time required for the items. Most articles are cleaned in 2–5 minutes.

10. Check that the unit is working. You should see a series of bubbles in both solutions. This is called *cavitation*.

    CAUTION: Do not get too close. Solution can spray into your face and eyes. Use beaker lids to prevent spray.

11. When the timer stops, cleaning is complete. Use transfer forceps or pick-ups to lift articles from the basket, pan, or beakers. Place the articles on paper towels. Then rinse articles thoroughly under running water.

    CAUTION: Avoid contact with skin. Solutions are toxic.

12. Allow articles to air-dry or dry them with paper towels. Inspect the articles for cleanliness. If they are not clean, repeat the process.

13. Periodically change solutions in the permanent tank and auxiliary containers. Do this when solutions become cloudy or cleaning has not been effective. To clean the permanent tank, place a container under the side drain to collect the solution. Then open the valve and drain solution from the tank. Wash the inside with a damp cloth or disinfectant. To clean the auxiliary pans or beakers, discard the solution. (It can be poured down the sink, but allow water to run for a time after disposing of the solution.) Then wash the containers and rinse thoroughly.

    NOTE: If the bottoms of beakers are etched and white, the beakers must be discarded and replaced.

14. Clean and replace all equipment used. Make sure all beakers are covered with lids.

15. Wash hands.

Practice

Go to the workbook and use the evaluation sheet for 13:7, Cleaning with an Ultrasonic Unit, to practice this procedure. When you believe you have mastered this skill, sign the sheet and give it to your instructor for further action.

 Final Checkpoint Using the criteria listed on the evaluation sheet, your instructor will grade your performance.

13:8 INFORMATION

Using Sterile Techniques

Many procedures require the use of sterile techniques to protect the patient from further infection. *Surgical asepsis* refers to procedures that keep an object or area free from living organisms. The main facts are presented here.

Sterile means "free from all organisms," including spores and viruses. **Contaminated** means that organisms and pathogens are present. While working with sterile supplies, it is important that correct techniques be followed to maintain sterility and avoid contamination. It is also important that you are able to recognize sterile surfaces and contaminated surfaces.

A clean, uncluttered working area is required when working with sterile supplies. A sterile object must never touch a nonsterile object. If other objects are in the way, it is easy to contaminate sterile articles. If sterile articles touch the skin or any part of your clothing, they are no longer sterile. Because any area below the waist is considered contaminated, sterile articles must be held away from and in front of the body and above the waist.

Once a **sterile field** has been set up (for example, a sterile towel has been placed on a tray), never reach across the top of the field. Microorganisms can drop from your arm or clothing and contaminate the field. Always reach in from either side to place additional articles on the field. Keep the sterile field in constant view. Never turn your back to a sterile field. Avoid coughing, sneezing, or talking over the sterile field because airborne particles can fall on the field and contaminate it.

The 2-inch border around the sterile field (towel-covered tray) is considered contaminated. Therefore, 2 inches around the outside of the field must not be used when sterile articles are placed on the sterile field.

All sterile items must be checked carefully before they are used. If the item was autoclaved and dated, most health care facilities believe the date should not be more than 30 days from autoclaving. Follow agency guidelines for time limits. If tears or stains are present on the package, the item should *not* be used because it could be contaminated. If there are any signs of moisture on the package, it has been contaminated and should *not* be used.

Organisms and pathogens travel quickly through a wet surface, so the sterile field must be kept dry. If a sterile towel or article gets wet, contamination has occurred. It is very important to use care when pouring solutions into sterile bowls or using solutions around a sterile field.

Various techniques can be used to remove articles from sterile wraps, depending on the article being unwrapped. Some common techniques are the drop, mitten, and transfer-forceps techniques:

♦ *Drop technique*: This technique is used for gauze pads, dressings, and small items. The wrapper is partially opened and then held upside down over the sterile field. The item drops out of the wrapper and onto the sterile field (figure 13-34A). It is important to keep fingers back so the article does not touch the skin as it falls out of the wrapper. It is also important to avoid touching the inside of the wrapper.

♦ *Mitten technique*: This technique is used for bowls, drapes, linen, and other similar items. The wrapper is opened and its loose ends are grasped around the wrist with the opposite hand (figure 13-34B). In this way, a mitten is formed around the hand that is still holding the item (for example, a bowl). With the mitten hand, the item can be placed on the sterile tray.

♦ *Transfer forceps*: These are used for cotton balls, small items, or articles that cannot be removed by the drop or mitten techniques. Either sterile gloves or sterile transfer forceps (pick-ups) are used. Sterile transfer forceps or pick-ups are removed from their container of disinfectant solution and used to grasp the

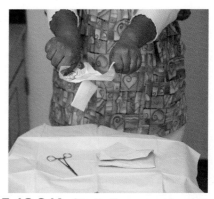

FIGURE 13-34A Sterile items can be dropped from the wrapper onto the sterile field.

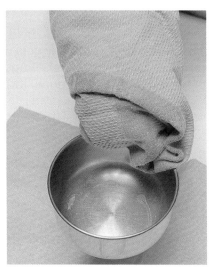

FIGURE 13-34B By using the wrap as a mitten, sterile supplies can be placed on a sterile field.

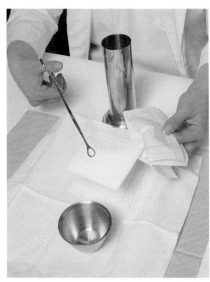

FIGURE 13-34C Sterile transfer forceps or pick-ups can be used to grasp sterile items and place them on a sterile field.

article from the opened package. The item is removed from the opened, sterile wrap and placed on the sterile field (figure 13-34C). The transfer forceps must be pointed in a downward direction. If they are pointed upward, the solution will flow back to the handle, become contaminated, and return to contaminate the sterile tips when they are being used to pick up items. In addition, care must be taken not to touch the sides or rim of the forceps container while removing or inserting the transfer forceps. Also, the transfer forceps must be shaken gently to get rid of excess disinfectant solution before they are used.

Make sure the sterile tray is open and you are ready to do the sterile procedure *before* putting the sterile gloves on your hands. Sterile gloves are considered sterile on the outside and contaminated on the inside (side against the skin). Once they have been placed on the hands, it is impor-

tant to hold the hands away from the body and above the waist to avoid contamination. Handle only sterile objects while wearing sterile gloves.

If at any time during a procedure there is any suspicion that you have contaminated any article, start over. Never take a chance on using contaminated equipment or supplies.

A wide variety of commercially prepared sterile supplies is available. Packaged units are often set up for special procedures, such as changing dressings. Many agencies use these units instead of setting up special trays. Observe all sterile principles while using these units and read any directions provided with the units.

STUDENT: *Go to the workbook and complete the assignment sheet for 13:8, Using Sterile Techniques. Then return and continue with the procedures.*

PROCEDURE 13:8A

Opening Sterile Packages

Equipment and Supplies

Sterile package of equipment or supplies, a table or other flat surface, sterile field (tray with sterile towel)

Procedure

1. Assemble equipment.

2. Wash hands.

3. Take equipment to the area where it will be used. Check the autoclave indicator and date on the package. Check the package for stains, tears, moisture, or

PROCEDURE 13:8A

evidence of contamination. Do *not* use the package if there is any evidence of contamination.

NOTE: Contents are not considered sterile if 30 days have elapsed since autoclaving.

4. Pick up the package with the tab or sealed edge pointing toward you. If the item is small, it can be held in the hand while being unwrapped. If it is large, place it on a table or other flat surface.

5. Loosen the wrapper fastener (usually tape).

6. Check to be sure the package is away from your body. If it is on a table, make sure it is not close to other objects.

NOTE: Avoid possible contamination by keeping sterile supplies away from other objects.

7. Open the distal (furthest) flap of the wrapper by grasping the outside of the wrapper and pulling it away from you (figure 13-35A).

▽ **CAUTION:** Do not reach across the top of the package. Reach around the package to open it.

8. With one hand, raise a side flap and pull laterally (sideways) away from the package (figure 13-35B).

▽ **CAUTION:** Do not touch the inside of the wrapper at any time.

9. With the opposite hand, open the other side flap by pulling the tab to the side (figure 13-35C).

NOTE: Always reach in from the side. Never reach across the top of the sterile field or across any opened edges.

10. Open the proximal (closest) flap by lifting the flap up and toward you. Then drop it over the front of your hand (or the table) (figure 13-35D).

▽ **CAUTION:** Be careful not to touch the inside of the package or the contents of the package.

11. Transfer the contents of the sterile package using one of the following techniques:

a. *Drop*: Separate the ends of the wrap and pull apart gently (figure 13-36). Avoid touching the inside of the wrap. Secure the loose ends of the wrap and hold the package upside down over

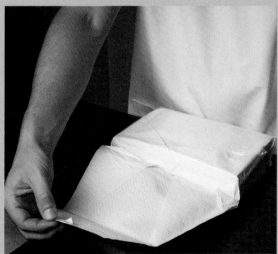

FIGURE 13-35A To open a sterile package, open the top flap away from you, handling only the outside of the wrap.

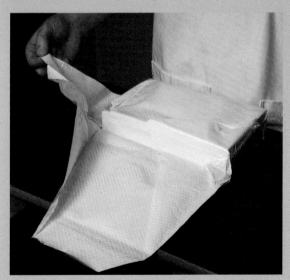

FIGURE 13-35B Open one side by pulling the wrap out to the side.

PROCEDURE 13:8A

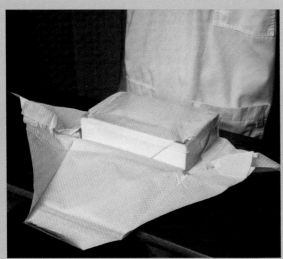

FIGURE 13-35C Open the opposite side by pulling the wrap out to the opposite side.

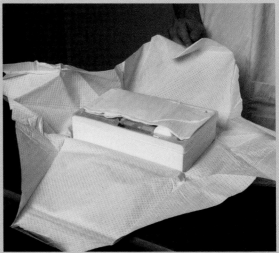

FIGURE 13-35D Open the side nearest to you by pulling back on the wrap.

the sterile field. Allow the contents to drop onto the sterile tray (refer to figure 13-34A).

b. *Mitten*: Grasp the contents securely by holding on to the outside of the wrapper as you unwrap it. With your free hand, gather the loose edges of the wrapper together and hold them

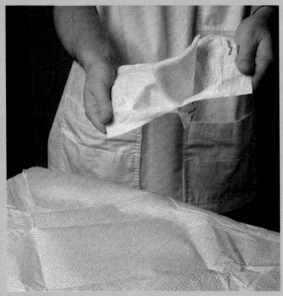

FIGURE 13-36 Separate the ends of the wrap and pull the edges apart gently without touching the contents.

securely around your wrist. This can be compared to making a mitten of the wrapper (with the sterile equipment on the outside of the mitten). Place the item on the sterile tray or hand it to someone who is wearing sterile gloves (refer to figure 13-34B).

c. *Transfer forceps*: Remove forceps from their sterile container, taking care not to touch the side or rim of the container with the forceps (figure 13-37). Hold the forceps pointed downward. Shake them gently to remove excess disinfectant solution. Take care not to touch anything with the forceps. Use the forceps to grasp the item in the package and then place the item on the sterile tray.

NOTE: The method of transfer depends on the sterile item being transferred.

NOTE: If at any time during the procedure there is any suspicion that you have contaminated any article, start over. Never take a chance on using equipment for a sterile procedure if there is any possibility that the equipment is contaminated.

12. Replace all equipment used.

13. Wash hands.

PROCEDURE 13:8A

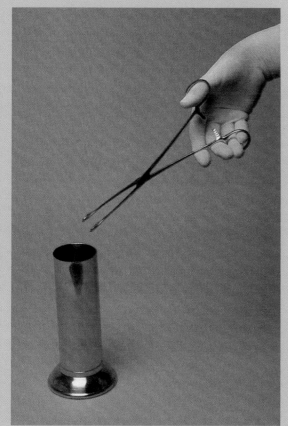

FIGURE 13-37 Remove the transfer or pick-up forceps without touching the sides or rim of the container and point them in a downward direction.

Practice

Go to the workbook and use the evaluation sheet for 13:8A, Opening Sterile Packages, to practice this procedure. When you believe you have mastered this skill, sign the sheet and give it to your instructor for further action.

✓ **Final Checkpoint** Using the criteria listed on the evaluation sheet, your instructor will grade your performance.

PROCEDURE 13:8B

Preparing a Sterile Dressing Tray

Equipment and Supplies

Tray or Mayo stand, sterile towels, sterile basin, sterile cotton balls or gauze sponges, sterile dressings (different sizes), antiseptic solution, forceps in disinfectant solution

Procedure

1. Assemble all equipment.

2. Wash hands.

3. Check the date and autoclave indicator for sterility. If more than 30 days have elapsed, use another package with a more recent date. Put the unsterile package aside for resterilization. Check the package for stains, tears, moisture, or evidence of contamination. Do not use the package if there is any evidence of contamination.

4. Place the tray on a flat surface or a Mayo stand.

    NOTE: Make sure the work area is clean and dry, and there is sufficient room to work.

PROCEDURE 13:8B

5. Open the package that contains the sterile towel. Be sure it is held away from your body. Place the wrapper on a surface away from the tray or work area. Touch only the outside of the towel. Pick up the towel at its outer edge. Allow it to open by releasing the fanfolds (figure 13-38A). Place the towel with the outer side (side you have touched) on the tray or Mayo stand (figure 13-38B). The untouched, or sterile, side will be facing

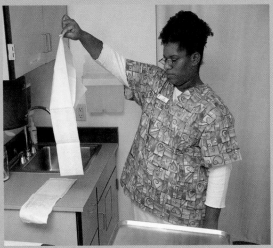

FIGURE 13-38A Pick up the sterile towel at its outer edge and allow it to open by releasing the fanfolds.

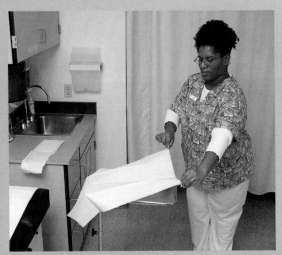

FIGURE 13-38B Place the towel on the Mayo stand without reaching across the top of the towel.

up to create a sterile field. Holding on to the outside edges of the towel, fanfold the back of the towel so the towel can be used later to cover the supplies.

▽ **CAUTION:** Do not reach across the top of the sterile field. Reach in from either side.

NOTE: If you are setting up a relatively large work area, one towel may not be large enough when fanfolded to cover the supplies. In such a case, you will need a second sterile towel (later) to cover your sterile field.

▽ **CAUTION:** At all times, make sure that you do *not* touch the sterile side of the towel. Avoid letting the towel come in contact with your uniform, other objects, or contaminated areas.

6. Correctly unwrap the package containing the sterile basin. Place the basin on the sterile field. Do not place it close to the edge.

NOTE: A 2-inch border around the outside edges of the sterile field is considered to be contaminated. No equipment should come in contact with this border.

▽ **CAUTION:** Make sure that the wrapper does *not* touch the towel while placing the basin in position.

7. Unwrap the package containing the sterile cotton balls or gauze sponges. Use a dropping motion to place them in the basin. Do not touch the basin with the wrapper.

8. Unwrap the package containing the larger dressing. Use the sterile forceps to remove the dressing from the package and place it on the sterile field. Make sure the dressing is not too close to the edge of the sterile field.

NOTE: The larger, outside dressing is placed on the sterile field first (before other dressings). In this way, the supplies will be in the order of use. For

PROCEDURE 13:8B

example, gauze dressings placed directly on the skin will be on top of the pile, and a thick abdominal pad used on top of the gauze pads will be on the bottom of the pile.

NOTE: The forceps must be lifted straight up out of the container and must *not* touch the side or rim of the container. Keep the tips pointed down and above the waist at all times. Shake off excess disinfectant solution.

9. Unwrap the inner dressings correctly. Use the sterile forceps to place them on top of the other dressings on the sterile field, or use a drop technique.

NOTE: Dressings are now in a pile; the dressing that will be used first is on the top of the pile.

NOTE: The number and type of dressings needed is determined by checking the patient being treated.

10. Open the bottle containing the correct antiseptic solution. Place the cap on the table, with the inside of the cap facing up. Pour a small amount of the solution into the sink to clean the lip of the bottle. Then hold the bottle over the basin and pour a sufficient amount of solution into the basin (figure 13-39).

▽ CAUTION: Make sure that no part of the bottle touches the basin or the sterile field. Pour carefully to avoid splashing. If the sterile field gets wet, the entire tray will be contaminated, and you must begin again.

11. Check the tray to make sure all needed equipment is on it.

12. Pick up the fanfolded edge of the towel by placing one hand on each side edge of the towel on the underside, or contaminated side. Do not touch the sterile side. Keep your hands and arms to the side of the tray, and bring the towel forward to cover the supplies.

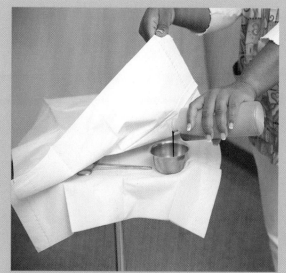

FIGURE 13-39 Avoid splashing the solution onto the sterile field while pouring it into the basin.

NOTE: A second sterile towel may be used to cover the supplies if the sterile field area is too large to be covered by the one fanfolded towel (figure 13-40).

▽ CAUTION: Never reach across the top of the sterile tray.

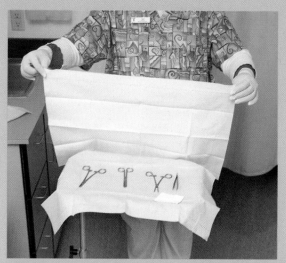

FIGURE 13-40 Use a second sterile towel to cover the sterile towel to cover the sterile field, taking care not to reach across the field.

PROCEDURE 13:8B

13. Once the sterile tray is ready, never allow it out of your sight. Take it to the patient area and use it immediately. If you need more equipment, you must take the tray with you. This is the only way to be completely positive that the tray does not become contaminated.

14. Replace equipment.

15. Wash hands.

Practice

Go to the workbook and use the evaluation sheet for 13:8B, Preparing a Sterile Dressing Tray, to practice this procedure. When you believe you have mastered this skill, sign the sheet and give it to your instructor for further action.

✔ **Final Checkpoint** Using the criteria listed on the evaluation sheet, your instructor will grade your performance.

PROCEDURE 13:8C

Donning and Removing Sterile Gloves

Equipment and Supplies

Sterile gloves

Procedure

1. Assemble equipment and take it to the area where it is to be used. Check the package for stains, tears, moisture, or evidence of contamination. Do *not* use the package if there is any evidence of contamination.

2. Remove rings. Wash hands. Dry hands thoroughly.

3. Open the package of gloves, taking care not to touch the inside of the inner wrapper. The inner wrapper contains the gloves. Reach in from the sides to open the inner package and expose the sterile gloves (figure 13-41A). The folded cuffs will be nearest you.

 CAUTION: If you touch the *inside* of the package (where the gloves are), get a new package and start again.

4. The glove for the right hand will be on the right side and the glove for the left hand will be on the left side of the package. With the thumb and forefinger of the nondominant hand, pick up the top edge of the folded-down cuff (inside of glove) of the glove for the dominant hand. Remove the glove carefully (figure 13-41B).

▽ **CAUTION:** Do *not* touch the outside of the glove. This is sterile. Only the part that will be next to the skin can be touched. Remember, unsterile touches unsterile and sterile touches sterile.

5. Hold the glove by the inside cuff and slip the fingers and thumb of your other hand into the glove. Pull it on carefully (figure 13-41C).

NOTE: Hold the glove away from the body. Pull gently to avoid tearing the glove.

PROCEDURE 13:8C

6. Insert your gloved hand under the cuff (outside) of the other glove and lift the glove from the package (figure 13-41D). Do not touch any other area with your gloved hand while removing the glove from the package.

▽ **CAUTION:** If contamination occurs, discard the gloves and start again.

7. Holding your gloved hand under the cuff of the glove, insert your other hand into the glove (figure 13-41E). Keep the thumb of your gloved hand tucked in to avoid possible contamination.

8. Turn the cuffs up by manipulating only the sterile surface of the gloves (sterile touches sterile). Go up under the folded cuffs, pull out slightly, and turn cuffs over and up (figure 13-41F.) Do not touch the inside of the gloves or the skin with your gloved hand.

9. Interlace the fingers to position the gloves correctly, taking care not to touch the skin with the gloved hands (figure 13-41G).

▽ **CAUTION:** If contamination occurs, start again with a new pair of gloves.

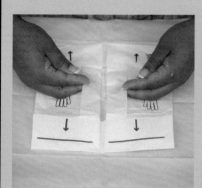

FIGURE 13-41A Reach in from the sides to open the inner package and expose the sterile gloves.

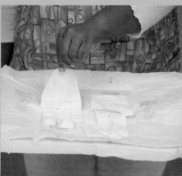

FIGURE 13-41B Pick up the first glove by grasping the glove on the top edge of the folded-down cuff.

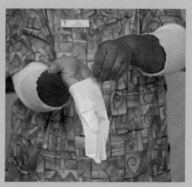

FIGURE 13-41C Hold the glove securely by the cuff and slip the opposite hand into the glove.

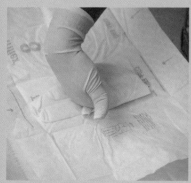

FIGURE 13-41D Slip the gloved fingers under the cuff of the second glove to lift it from the package.

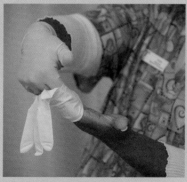

FIGURE 13-41E Hold the gloved hand under the cuff while inserting the other hand into the glove.

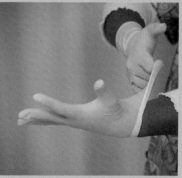

FIGURE 13-41F Insert the gloved fingers under the cuff, pull out slightly, and turn the cuffs over and up without touching the inside of the gloves or the skin.

PROCEDURE 13:8C

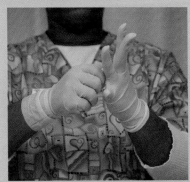

FIGURE 13-41G Interlace the fingers to position the gloves correctly, taking care not to touch the skin with the gloved hands.

10. Do not touch anything that is not sterile once the gloves are in place. Gloves are applied for the purpose of performing procedures requiring sterile technique. During the procedure, they will become contaminated with organisms related to the patient's condition, for example, wound drainage, blood, or other body discharges. Even a clean, dry wound may contaminate gloves.

    NOTE: Gloved hands should remain in position above the waist. Do *not* allow them to fall below waist.

11. After the procedure requiring sterile gloves is completed, dispose of all contaminated supplies before removing gloves.

    NOTE: This reduces the danger of cross-infection caused by handling contaminated supplies without glove protection.

12. To remove the gloves, use one gloved hand to grasp the other glove by the outside of the cuff. Taking care not to touch the skin, remove the glove by pulling it down over the hand. It will be wrong side out when removed.

    NOTE: This prevents contamination of your hands by organisms picked up dur-

ing performance of the procedure. Now you must consider the outside of the gloves contaminated, and the area inside, next to your skin, clean.

13. Insert your bare fingers on the inside of the second glove. Remove the glove by pulling it down gently, taking care not to touch the outside of the glove with your bare fingers. It will be wrong side out when removed.

     CAUTION: Avoid touching your uniform or any other object with the contaminated gloves.

14. Put the contaminated gloves in an infectious waste container immediately after removal.

15. Wash your hands immediately and thoroughly after removing gloves.

16. Once the gloves have been removed, do not handle any contaminated equipment or supplies such as soiled dressings or drainage basins. Protect yourself.

17. Replace equipment if necessary.

18. Wash hands thoroughly.

Practice

Go to the workbook and use the evaluation sheet for 13:8C, Donning and Removing Sterile Gloves, to practice this procedure. When you believe you have mastered this skill, sign the sheet and give it to your instructor for further action.

✔ **Final Checkpoint** Using the criteria listed on the evaluation sheet, your instructor will grade your performance.

PROCEDURE 13:8D

Changing a Sterile Dressing

Equipment and Supplies

Sterile tray with basin, solution, gauze sponges and pads (or a prepared sterile dressing package); sterile gloves; adhesive or non-allergic tape; disposable gloves; infectious waste bag

Procedure

1. Check doctor's written orders or obtain orders from immediate supervisor.

   NOTE: Dressings should *not* be changed without orders.

   NOTE: The policy of your agency will determine how you obtain orders for procedures.

2. Assemble equipment. Check autoclave indicator and date on all equipment. If more than 30 days have elapsed, use another package with a more recent date. Put the unsterile package aside for resterilization.

3. Wash hands thoroughly.

4. Prepare a sterile tray as previously taught in Procedure 13:8B or obtain a commercially prepared sterile dressing package.

   NOTE: Prepared packages are used in some agencies.

   CAUTION: Never let the tray out of your sight once it has been prepared.

5. Take all necessary equipment to the patient area. Place it where it will be convenient for use yet free from possible contamination by other equipment.

6. Introduce yourself. Identify the patient. Explain the procedure. Close the door and/or windows to avoid drafts and flow of organisms into the room.

7. Screen the unit or draw curtains to provide privacy for the patient. If the patient is in a bed, elevate the bed to a comfortable working height and lower the siderail. Expose the body area needing the dressing change. Use sheets or drapes as necessary to prevent unnecessary exposure of the patient.

8. Fold down a 2- to 3-inch cuff on the top of the infectious waste bag. Position it in a convenient location. Tear off the tape you will need later to secure the clean dressing. Place it in an area where it will be available for easy access.

9. Put on disposable, nonsterile gloves. Gently but firmly remove the tape from the soiled dressing. Discard it in the infectious waste bag. Hold the skin taut and then lift the dressing carefully, taking care not to pull on any surgical drains. Note the type, color, and amount of drainage on the dressing. Discard dressing in the infectious waste bag.

   NOTE: Surgical drains are placed in some surgical incisions to aid in the removal of secretions. Care must be taken to avoid moving the drains when the dressing is removed.

10. Check the incision site. Observe the type and amount of remaining drainage, color of drainage, and degree of healing.

    CAUTION: Report any unusual observations immediately to your supervisor. Examples are bright red blood, pus, swelling, or abnormal discharges at the wound site or patient complaints of pain or dizziness.

11. Remove disposable gloves and place in infectious waste bag. Immediately wash your hands.

    CAUTION: Nonsterile disposable gloves should be worn while removing dressings to avoid contamination of the hands or skin by blood or body discharge.

PROCEDURE 13:8D

12. Fanfold the top cover back to uncover the sterile field.

   ▽ **CAUTION:** Handle only the contaminated (outside) side of the towel. The side in contact with the tray's contents is the sterile side.

   NOTE: If a prepared package is used, open it at this time.

13. Don sterile gloves as previously taught in Procedure 13:8C.

14. Using thumb and forefinger, pick up a gauze sponge from the basin. Squeeze it slightly to remove any excess solution. Warn the patient that the solution may be cool.

15. Cleanse the wound. Use a circular motion (figure 13-42).

   NOTE: Begin near the center of the wound and move outward or away from the wound. Make an ever-widening circle. Discard the wet gauze sponge after use. Never go back over the same area with the same gauze sponge. Repeat this procedure until the area is clean, using a new gauze sponge each time.

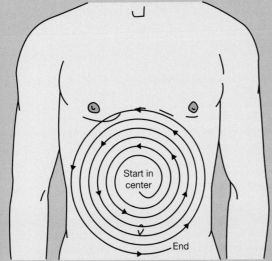

FIGURE 13-42 Use a circular motion to clean the wound, starting at the center of the wound and moving in an outward direction.

16. Do not cleanse directly over the wound unless there is a great deal of drainage or it is specifically ordered by the physician. If this is to be done, use sterile gauze and wipe with a single stroke from the top to the bottom. Discard the soiled gauze. Repeat as necessary, using a new sterile gauze sponge each time.

17. The wound is now ready for clean dressings. Lift the sterile dressings from the tray and place them lightly on the wound. Make sure they are centered over the wound.

   NOTE: The inner dressing is usually made up of 4-by-4-inch gauze sponges.

18. Apply outer dressings until the wound is sufficiently protected.

   NOTE: Heavier dressings such as abdominal pads are usually used.

   NOTE: The number and size of dressings needed to dress the wound will depend on the amount of drainage and the size of the wound.

19. Remove the sterile gloves as previously taught. Discard them in the infectious waste bag. Immediately wash your hands.

20. Place the precut tape over the dressing at the proper angle. Check to make sure that the dressing is secure and the ends are closed.

   NOTE: Tape should be applied so it runs opposite from body action or movement (figure 13-43). It should be the correct width for the dressing. It should be long enough to support the dressing, but it should not be too long because it will irritate the patient's skin.

21. Check to be sure the patient is comfortable and that safety precautions have been observed before leaving the area.

22. Put on disposable, nonsterile gloves. Clean and replace all equipment used.

PROCEDURE 13:8D

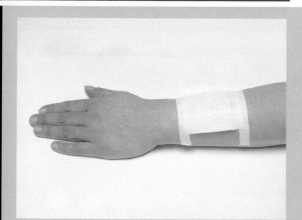

FIGURE 13-43 Tape should be applied so that it runs opposite to body action or movement.

Tie or tape the infectious waste bag securely. Dispose of it according to agency policy.

 CAUTION: Disposable, nonsterile gloves should be worn to provide a protective barrier while cleaning equipment or supplies that may be contaminated by blood or body fluids.

23. Remove disposable gloves. Wash hands thoroughly. Protect yourself from possible contamination.

24. Record the following information on the patient's chart or agency form: date, time, dressing change, amount and type of drainage, and any other pertinent information, or tell this information to your immediate supervisor.

Example: 1/8/—, 9:00 A.M. Dressing changed on right abdominal area. Small amount of thick, light-yellow discharge noted on dressings. No swelling or inflammation apparent at incision site. Sterile dressing applied. Your signature and title.

NOTE: Report any unusual observations immediately.

Practice

Go to the workbook and use the evaluation sheet for 13:8D, Changing a Sterile Dressing, to practice this procedure. When you believe you have mastered this skill, sign the sheet and give it to your instructor for further action.

✓ **Final Checkpoint** Using the criteria listed on the evaluation sheet, your instructor will grade your performance.

13:9 INFORMATION

Maintaining Transmission-Based Isolation Precautions

INTRODUCTION

 In health occupations, you will deal with many different diseases/disorders. Some diseases are communicable and require isolation. A **communicable disease** is caused by a pathogenic organism that can be easily transmitted to others. An **epidemic** occurs when the communicable disease spreads rapidly from person to person and affects a large number of people at the same time. A **pandemic** exists when the outbreak of disease occurs over a wide geographic area and affects a high proportion of the population. Because individuals can travel readily throughout the world, a major concern is that worldwide pandemics will become more and more frequent.

Transmission-based isolation precautions are a method or technique of caring for patients who have communicable diseases. Examples of communicable diseases are tuberculosis, wound infections, and pertussis (whooping cough). Standard precautions, discussed in Information section 13:4, do not eliminate the need for specific transmission-based isolation precautions. Standard precautions are used on all patients. Transmission-based isolation techniques are used to provide extra protection against specific diseases or pathogens to prevent their spread.

Communicable diseases are spread in many ways. Some examples include direct contact with the patient; contact with dirty linen, equipment, and/or supplies; and contact with blood, body fluids, secretions, and excretions such as urine, feces, droplets (from sneezing, coughing, or spitting), and discharges from wounds. Transmission-based isolation precautions are used to limit contact with pathogenic organisms. These techniques help prevent the spread of the disease to other people and protect patients, their families, and health care providers.

The type of transmission-based isolation used depends on the causative organism of the disease, the way the organism is transmitted, and whether the pathogen is antibiotic resistant (not affected by antibiotics). Personal protective equipment (PPE) is used to provide protection from the pathogen. Some transmission-based isolation precautions require the use of gowns, gloves, face shields, and masks (figure 13-44), while others only require the use of a mask.

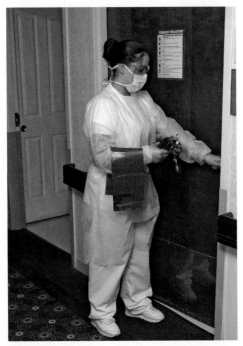

FIGURE 13-44 Some transmission-based isolation precautions require the use of gowns, gloves, and a mask, while others only require the use of a mask.

Two terms are extensively used in transmission-based isolation: contaminated and clean. These words refer to the presence of organisms on objects.

♦ **Contaminated,** or dirty, means that objects contain disease-producing organisms. These objects must not be touched, unless the health worker is protected by gloves, gown, and other required items.

NOTE: The outside and waist ties of the gown, protective gloves, and mask are considered contaminated.

♦ **Clean** means that objects or parts of objects do *not* contain disease-producing organisms and therefore have minimal chance of spreading the disease. Every effort must be made to prevent contamination of these objects or parts of objects.

NOTE: The insides of the gloves and gown are clean, as are the neckband, its ties, and the mask ties.

The Centers for Disease Control and Prevention (CDC) in conjunction with the National Center for Infectious Diseases (NCID) and the Hospital Infection Control Practices Advisory Committee (HICPAC) has recommended four main classifications of precautions that must be followed: standard, airborne, droplet, and contact. Health care facilities are provided with a list of infections/conditions that shows the type and duration of precautions needed for each specific disease. In this way, facilities can follow the guidelines to determine the type of transmission-based isolation that should be used along with the specific precautions that must be followed.

STANDARD PRECAUTIONS

Standard precautions (discussed in Information section 13:4) are used on all patients. In addition, a patient must be placed in a private room if the patient contaminates the environment or does not (or cannot be expected to) assist in maintaining appropriate hygiene. Every health care worker must be well informed about standard precautions and follow the recommendations for the use of gloves, gowns, and face masks when conditions indicate their use.

AIRBORNE PRECAUTIONS

Airborne precautions (figure 13-45) are used for patients known or suspected to be infected with pathogens transmitted by airborne droplet nuclei. These are small particles of evaporated droplets that contain microorganisms and remain suspended in the air or on dust particles. Examples of diseases requiring these isolation precautions are rubella (measles), varicella (chicken pox), tuberculosis, and shingles or herpes zoster (varicella zoster). Standard precautions are used at all times. In addition, the following precautions must be taken:

♦ The patient must be placed in a private room, and the door should be kept closed.

♦ Air in the room must be discharged to outdoor air or filtered before being circulated to other areas.

♦ Each person who enters the room must wear respiratory protection in the form of an N95, P100 or more powerful filtering mask such as

a high-efficiency particulate air (HEPA) mask (figures 13-46A, B). These masks contain special filters to prevent the entrance of the small airborne pathogens. The masks must be fit tested to make sure they create a tight seal each time they are worn by a health care provider. Men with facial hair cannot wear a standard filtering mask because a beard prevents an airtight seal. Men with facial hair can use a special HEPA-filtered hood.

♦ People susceptible to measles or chicken pox should not enter the room.

♦ If at all possible, the patient should not be moved from the room. If transport is essential, however, the patient must wear a surgical mask during transport to minimize the release of droplets into the air.

DROPLET PRECAUTIONS

Droplet precautions (figure 13-47) must be followed for a patient known or suspected to be infected with pathogens transmitted by large-particle droplets expelled during coughing, sneez-

AIRBORNE PRECAUTIONS
In Addition to Standard Precautions
Visitors - Report to Nurses' Station Before Entering Room

BEFORE CARE

1. Private room and closed door with monitored negative air pressure, frequent air exchanges, and high-efficiency filtration.
2. Wash hands.
3. Wear respiratory protection appropriate for disease.

DURING CARE

1. Limit transport of patient/resident to essential purposes only. Patient resident must wear mask appropriate for disease.
2. Limit use of noncritical care equipment to a single patient/resident.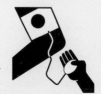

AFTER CARE

1. Bag linen to prevent contamination of self, environment, or outside of bag.
2. Discard infectious trash to prevent contamination of self, environment, or outside of bag.
3. Wash hands.

FIGURE 13-45 Airborne precautions. *(Courtesy of Brevis Corporation)*

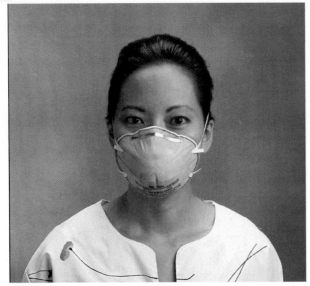

FIGURE 13-46A The N95 respirator mask. *(Courtesy of 3M Company, St. Paul, MN)*

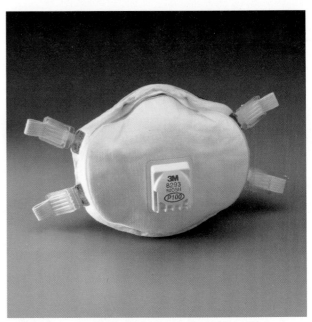

FIGURE 13-46B The P100 respirator mask. *(Courtesy of 3M Company, St. Paul, MN)*

ing, talking, or laughing. Examples of diseases requiring these isolation precautions include *Haemophilus influenzae* meningitis and pneumonia; *Neisseria* meningitis and pneumonia; multidrug-resistant *Streptococcus* meningitis,

pneumonia, sinusitis, and otitis media; diphtheria; *Mycoplasma* pneumonia; pertussis; adenovirus; mumps; and severe viral influenza. Standard precautions are used at all times. In addition, the following precautions must be taken:

DROPLET PRECAUTIONS
In Addition to Standard Precautions

Visitors - Report to Nurses' Station Before Entering Room

BEFORE CARE

1. Private room. Maintain 3 feet of spacing between patient/resident and visitors.

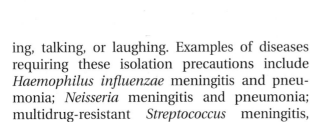

2. Mask/face shield for staff and visitors within 3 feet of patient/resident.

DURING CARE

1. Limit transport of patient/resident to essential purposes only. Patient/resident must wear mask appropriate for disease.

2. Limit use of noncritical care equipment to a single patient/resident.

AFTER CARE

1. Bag linen to prevent contamination of self, environment, or outside of bag.

2. Discard infectious trash to prevent contamination of self, environment, or outside of bag.

3. Wash hands.

FIGURE 13-47 Droplet precautions. *(Courtesy of Brevis Corporation)*

♦ The patient should be placed in a private room. If a private room is not available and the patient cannot be placed in a room with a patient who has the same infection, a distance of at least 3 feet should separate the infected patient and other patients or visitors.

♦ Masks must be worn when working within 3 feet of the patient, and the use of masks anywhere in the room is strongly recommended

♦ If transport or movement of the patient is essential, the patient must wear a surgical mask.

CONTACT PRECAUTIONS

Contact precautions (figure 13-48) must be followed for any patients known or suspected to be infected with *epidemiologically* (capable of spreading rapidly from person to person, an epidemic) microorganisms that can be transmitted by either direct or indirect contact. Examples of diseases requiring these precautions include any gastrointestinal, respiratory, skin, or wound infections caused by multidrug-resistant organisms; diapered or incontinent patients with enterohemorrhagic *E. coli*, *Shigella*, hepatitis A, or rotavirus; viral or hemorrhagic conjunctivitis or fevers; and any skin infections that are highly contagious or that may occur on dry skin, such as diphtheria, herpes simplex virus, impetigo, pediculosis (head or body lice), scabies, and staphylococcal infections. Standard precautions are used at all times. In addition, the following precautions must be taken:

♦ The patient should be placed in a private room or, if a private room is not available, in a room with a patient who has an active infection caused by the same organism.

♦ Gloves must be worn when entering the room.

♦ Gloves must be changed after having contact with any material that may contain high concentrations of the microorganism, such as wound drainage or fecal material.

♦ Gloves must be removed before leaving the room, and the hands must be washed with an antimicrobial agent.

♦ A gown must be worn in the room if there is any chance of contact with the patient, environmental surfaces, or items in the room. The

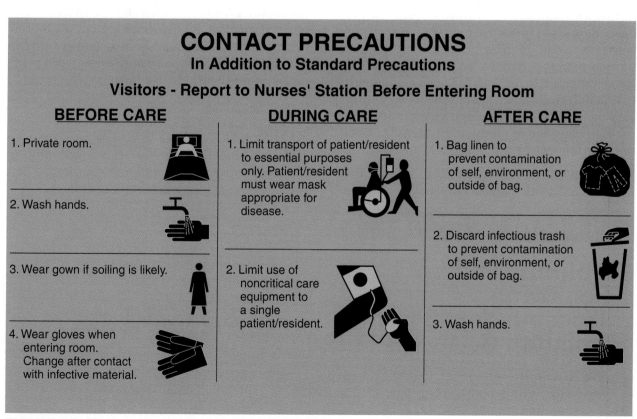

CONTACT PRECAUTIONS
In Addition to Standard Precautions

Visitors - Report to Nurses' Station Before Entering Room

BEFORE CARE

1. Private room.

2. Wash hands.

3. Wear gown if soiling is likely.

4. Wear gloves when entering room. Change after contact with infective material.

DURING CARE

1. Limit transport of patient/resident to essential purposes only. Patient/resident must wear mask appropriate for disease.

2. Limit use of noncritical care equipment to a single patient/resident.

AFTER CARE

1. Bag linen to prevent contamination of self, environment, or outside of bag.

2. Discard infectious trash to prevent contamination of self, environment, or outside of bag.

3. Wash hands.

FIGURE 13-48 Contact precautions. *(Courtesy of Brevis Corporation)*

gown must be removed before leaving the room and care must be taken to ensure that clothing is not contaminated after gown removal.

♦ Movement and transport of the patient from the room should be for essential purposes only.

♦ The room and items in it must receive daily cleaning and disinfection as needed.

♦ If possible, patient-care equipment (bedside commode, stethoscope, sphygmomanometer, thermometer) should be left in the room and used only for this patient. If this is not possible, all equipment must be cleaned and disinfected before being used on another patient.

PROTECTIVE OR REVERSE ISOLATION

Protective or **reverse isolation** refers to methods used to protect certain patients from organisms present in the environment. Protective isolation is used mainly for *immunocompromised* patients, or those whose body defenses are not capable of protecting them from infections and disease. Examples of patients requiring this protection are patients whose immune systems have been depressed prior to receiving transplants (such as bone marrow transplants), severely burned patients, patients receiving chemotherapy or radiation treatments for cancer, or patients whose immune systems have failed. Precautions vary depending on the patient's condition. Standard precautions are used at all times. In addition, the following precautions may be taken:

♦ The patient is usually placed in a room that has been cleaned and disinfected

♦ Frequent disinfection occurs while the patient occupies the room

♦ Anyone entering the room must wear clean or sterile gowns, gloves, and masks

♦ All equipment or supplies brought into the room are clean, disinfected, and/or sterile

♦ Special filters may be used to purify air that enters the room

♦ Every effort is made to protect the patient from microorganisms that cause infection or disease

SUMMARY

Exact procedures for maintaining transmission-based isolation precautions vary from one facility to another. The procedures used depend on the type of units provided for isolation patients, and on the kind of supplies or special isolation equipment available. Most facilities convert a regular patient room into an isolation room, but some facilities use special, two-room isolation units. Most facilities use disposable supplies such as gloves, gowns, and treatment packages. Therefore, it is essential that you learn the isolation procedure followed by your agency. However, the basic principles for maintaining transmission-based isolation are the same regardless of the facility. Therefore, if you know these basic principles, you will be able to adjust to any setting.

STUDENT: *Go to the workbook and complete the assignment sheet for 13:9, Maintaining Transmission-Based Isolation Precautions. Then return and continue with the procedures.*

PROCEDURE 13:9A

Donning and Removing Transmission-Based Isolation Garments

 NOTE: The following procedure deals with contact transmission-based isolation precautions. For other types of transmission-based isolation, follow only the steps that apply.

Equipment and Supplies

Isolation gown, surgical mask, gloves, small plastic bag, linen cart or container, infectious waste container, paper towels, sink with running water

PROCEDURE 13:9A

Procedure

1. Assemble equipment.

   NOTE: In many agencies, clean isolation garments and supplies are kept available on a cart outside the isolation unit, or in the outer room of a two-room unit. A waste container should be positioned just inside the door.

2. Wash hands.

3. Remove rings and place them in your pocket or pin them to your uniform.

4. Remove your watch and place it in a small plastic bag or centered on a clean paper towel. If placed on a towel, handle only the bottom part of the towel; do not touch the top.

   NOTE: The watch will be taken into the room and placed on the bedside stand for taking vital signs. Because it cannot be sterilized, it must be kept clean.

   NOTE: In some agencies, a plastic-covered watch is left in the isolation room.

5. Put on the mask. Secure it under your chin. Make sure to cover your mouth and nose. Handle the mask as little as possible. Tie the mask securely behind your head and neck. Tie the top ties first and the bottom ties second (figure 13-49A).

NOTE: The tie bands on the mask are considered clean. The mask is considered contaminated.

NOTE: The mask is considered to be contaminated after 30 minutes in isolation or anytime it gets wet. If you remain in isolation longer than 30 minutes, or if the mask gets wet, you must wash your hands, and remove and discard the old mask. Then wash your hands again, and put on a clean mask.

6. If uniform sleeves are long, roll them up above the elbows before putting on the gown.

7. Lift the gown by placing your hands inside the shoulders.

   NOTE: The inside of the gown and the ties at the neck are considered clean.

   NOTE: Most agencies use disposable gowns that are discarded after use.

8. Work your arms into the sleeves of the gown by gently twisting (figure 13-49B). Take care not to touch your face with the sleeves of the gown.

9. Place your hands *inside* the neckband, adjust until it is in position, and then tie the bands at the back of your neck (figure 13-49C).

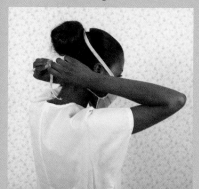
FIGURE 13-49A Put on the mask, tying the top ties before the bottom ties.

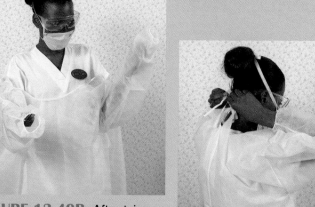
FIGURE 13-49B After tying the mask in place, put on the gown by placing your hands inside the shoulders to ease your arms into the sleeves.

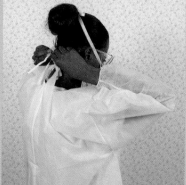
FIGURE 13-49C Slip your fingers inside the neckband to tie the gown at the neck.

PROCEDURE 13:9A

10. Reach behind and fold the edges of the gown over so that the uniform is completely covered. Tie the waistbands (figure 13-49D). Some waistbands are long enough to wrap around your body before tying.

11. If gloves are to be worn, put them on. Make sure that the cuff of the glove comes over the top of the cuff of the gown (figure 13-49E). In this way, there are no open areas for entrance of organisms.

12. You are now ready to enter the isolation room. Double-check to be sure you have all equipment and supplies that you will need for patient care before you enter the room.

13. When patient care is complete, you will be ready to remove isolation garments. In a two-room isolation unit, go to the outer room. In a one-room unit, remove garments while you are standing close to the inside of the door. Take care to avoid touching the room's contaminated articles.

14. Untie the waist ties (figure 13-50A). Loosen the gown at the waist.

NOTE: The waist ties are considered contaminated.

15. If gloves are worn, remove the first glove by grasping the outside of the cuff with the opposite gloved hand. Pull the glove over the hand so that the glove is inside out (figure 13-50B). Remove the second glove by placing the bare hand inside the cuff. Pull the glove off so it is inside out. Place the disposable gloves in the infectious waste container.

16. To avoid unnecessary transmission of organisms, use paper towels to turn on the water faucet. Wash and dry your hands thoroughly. When they are dry, use a clean, dry paper towel to turn off the faucet.

▽ **CAUTION:** Organisms travel rapidly through wet towels.

17. Untie the bottom ties of the mask first followed by the top ties. Holding the mask by the top ties only, drop it into the infectious waste container (figure 13-50C).

NOTE: The ties of the mask are considered clean. Do not touch any other part of the mask, because it is considered contaminated.

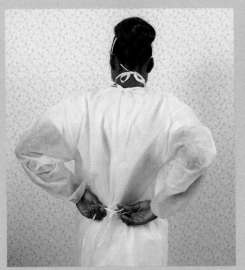

FIGURE 13-49D Overlap the back edges of the gown so your uniform is completely covered before tying the waist ties.

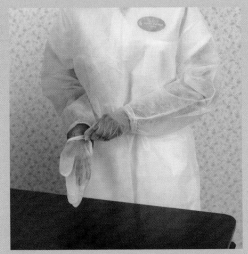

FIGURE 13-49E Put on gloves making sure that the cuff of the glove is over the top of the cuff on the gown.

PROCEDURE 13:9A

18. Untie the neck ties. Loosen the gown at the shoulders, handling only the inside of the gown.

   NOTE: The neck ties are considered clean.

19. Slip the fingers of one hand inside the opposite cuff. Do *not* touch the outside. Pull the sleeve down over the hand (figure 13-50D).

   ▽ **CAUTION:** The outside of the gown is considered contaminated and should not be touched.

20. Using the gown-covered hand, pull the sleeve down over the opposite hand (figure 13-50E).

21. Ease your arms and hands out of the gown. Keep the gown in front of your body and keep your hands away from the outside of the gown. Use as gentle a motion as possible.

   NOTE: Excessive flapping of the gown will spread organisms.

22. With your hands inside the gown at the shoulders, bring the shoulders together and turn the gown so that it is inside out (figure 13-50F). In this manner, the outside of the contaminated gown is on the inside. Fold the gown in half and then roll it together. Place it in the infectious waste container.

   NOTE: Avoid excess motion during this procedure because motion causes the spread of organisms.

23. Wash hands thoroughly. Use dry, clean paper towels to operate the faucets.

24. Touch only the inside of the plastic bag to remove your watch. Discard the bag in the waste container. If the watch is on a paper towel, handle only the "clean," top portion (if necessary). Discard the towel in the infectious waste container.

25. Use a clean paper towel to open the door. Discard the towel in the waste container before leaving the room.

   ▽ **CAUTION:** The inside of the door is considered contaminated.

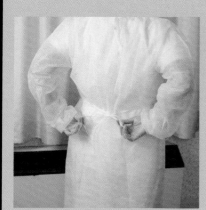

FIGURE 13-50A Untie the waist ties of the gown before removing the gloves.

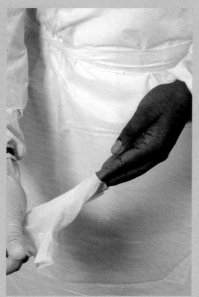

FIGURE 13-50B To remove the gloves, pull them over the hand so the glove is inside out.

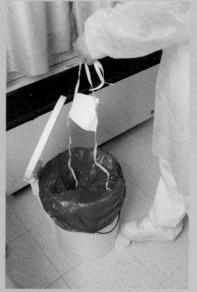

FIGURE 13-50C Remove the mask and hold only the top ties to drop it in an infectious waste container.

PROCEDURE 13:9A

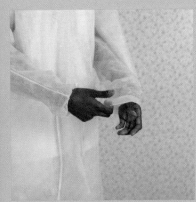

FIGURE 13-50D To remove the gown, slip the fingers of one hand under the cuff of the opposite arm to pull the gown down over the opposite hand.

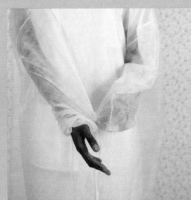

FIGURE 13-50E Using the gown-covered hand, grasp the outside of the gown on the opposite arm and pull the gown down over the hand.

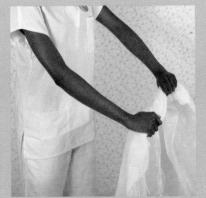

FIGURE 13-50F With your hands inside the gown at the shoulders, bring the shoulders together and turn the gown so that it is inside out, with the contaminated side on the inside.

NOTE: The waste container should be positioned just inside the door of the room.

26. After leaving the isolation room, wash hands thoroughly. This will help prevent spread of the disease. It also protects you from the illness.

✓ **Final Checkpoint** Using the criteria listed on the evaluation sheet, your instructor will grade your performance.

Practice

Go to the workbook and use the evaluation sheet for 13:9A, Donning and Removing Transmission-Based Isolation Garments, to practice this procedure. When you believe you have mastered this skill, sign the sheet and give it to your instructor for further action.

PROCEDURE 13:9B

Working in a Hospital Transmission-Based Isolation Unit

Equipment and Supplies

Clothes hamper, two laundry bags, two trays, dishes, cups, bowls, waste container lined with a plastic bag, infectious waste bags, bags, tape, pencil, pen, paper

Procedure

1. Assemble all equipment.

   NOTE: Any equipment or supplies to be used in the isolation room must be assembled prior to entering the room.

2. Wash hands.

3. Put on appropriate isolation garments as previously instructed.

PROCEDURE 13:9B

4. Tape paper to the outside of the isolation door. This will be used to record vital signs.

5. Enter the isolation room. Take all needed equipment into the room.

6. Introduce yourself. Greet and identify patient. Provide patient care as needed.

   NOTE: All care is provided in a routine manner. However, transmission-based isolation garments must be worn as ordered.

7. To record vital signs:

   a. Take vital signs using the watch in the plastic bag. (If the watch is not in a plastic bag, hold it with the bottom part of a paper towel.) Use other equipment in the room as needed.

   b. Open the door touching only the inside, or contaminated side.

   c. Using a pencil, record the vital signs on the paper taped to the door. Do *not* touch the outside of the door at any time.

   NOTE: The pencil remains in the room because it is contaminated.

8. To transfer food into the isolation unit:

   a. Transfer of food requires two people; one person must stay outside the unit and one inside.

   b. The person inside the isolation unit picks up the empty tray in the room and opens door, touching only the inside of the door.

   c. The person outside holds the tray while the dishes are being transferred (figure 13-51).

   d. When transferring food, the two people should handle the opposite sides of the dishes. In this manner, one person will not touch the other person.

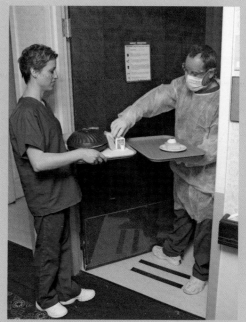

FIGURE 13-51 To transfer food into an isolation unit, a health care worker holds the tray so the worker in isolation can transfer the food onto the tray kept inside the unit.

   e. Glasses should be held near the top by the transfer person on the outside. The transfer person on the inside should receive the glasses by holding them on the bottom.

9. To dispose of leftover food or waste:

   a. Liquids can be poured down the sink or flushed down the toilet.

   b. Soft foods such as mashed potatoes or cooked vegetables can be flushed down the toilet.

   c. Hard particles of food, such as bone, should be placed in the plastic-lined trash container.

   d. Disposable utensils or dishes should be placed in the plastic-lined trash container.

   e. Metal utensils should be washed and kept in the isolation room to be used as needed for other meals. These

PROCEDURE 13:9B

utensils, however, are contaminated. When they are removed from the isolation room, they must be disinfected or double bagged and labeled before being sent for decontamination and reprocessing.

10. To transfer soiled linen from the unit, two people are required:

   a. All dirty linen should be folded and rolled.

   b. Place linen in the linen hamper.

   c. The person outside the unit should cuff the top of a clean infectious waste laundry bag and hold it. Hands should be kept on the inside of the bag's cuff to avoid contamination.

   d. The person in isolation should seal the isolation bag. The bag is then placed inside the outer bag, which is being held by the person outside.

   e. Outer bag should be folded over at the top and taped by the person outside. The bag should be labeled as "BIOHAZARDOUS LINEN."

   f. At all times, no direct contact should occur between the two people transferring linen.

   NOTE: Many agencies use special isolation linen bags. Hot water dissolves the bags during the washing process. Therefore, no other personnel handle the contaminated linen after it leaves the isolation unit.

11. To transfer trash from the isolation unit, two people are required:

   a. Any trash in the isolation room should be in plastic bags. Any trash or disposable items contaminated with blood, body fluids, secretions, or excretions should be placed in infectious waste bags.

   b. When the bag is full, expel excess air by pushing gently on the bag.

   c. Tie a knot at the top of the bag to seal it or fold the top edge twice and tape it securely.

   d. Place this bag inside a cuffed biohazardous waste bag held by a "clean" person outside the unit (figure 13-52).

   e. The outside person then ties the outer bag securely or tapes the outer bag shut.

   f. The double-bagged trash should then be burned. Double-bagged infectious waste is autoclaved prior to incineration or disposal as infectious waste according to legal requirements.

   g. At all times, direct contact between the two people transferring trash must be avoided.

12. To transfer equipment from the isolation unit two people are required:

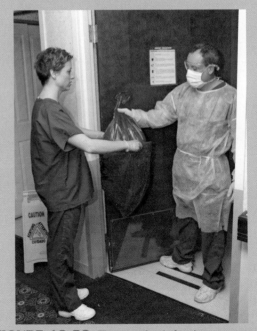

FIGURE 13-52 To transfer infectious waste from an isolation unit, the worker in the unit places the sealed infectious waste bag inside a second bag held by a "clean" worker outside the unit.

PROCEDURE 13:9B

a. Thoroughly clean and disinfect all equipment in the unit.

b. After cleaning, place equipment in a plastic bag or special isolation bag. Label the bag with the contents and the word "ISOLATION."

c. After folding the bag down twice at the top, tape the bag shut.

d. A second person outside the isolation room should hold a second, cuffed infectious waste bag.

e. The person in isolation places the sealed, contaminated bag inside the bag being held outside the unit. The person in isolation should have no direct contact with the clean bag.

f. The person outside the unit turns down the top of the infectious waste bag twice and securely tapes the bag. The outside person then labels the bag with the contents, for example, "ISOLATION DISHES."

g. The double-bagged material is then sent to Central Supply or another designated area for sterilization and/or decontamination.

13. The transmission-based isolation unit must be kept clean and neat at all times. Equipment no longer needed should be transferred out of the unit using the appropriate isolation technique.

14. Before leaving an isolation room, ask the patient whether a urinal or bedpan is needed. This will save time and energy by reducing the need to return to provide additional patient care shortly after leaving. Also, prior to leaving, check all safety and comfort points to make sure patient care is complete.

15. Remove isolation garments as previously instructed in Procedure 13:9A.

16. Wash hands thoroughly.

Practice

Go to the workbook and use the evaluation sheet for 13:9B, Working in a Hospital Transmission-Based Isolation Unit, to practice this procedure. When you believe you have mastered this skill, sign the sheet and give it to your instructor for further action.

 Final Checkpoint Using the criteria listed on the evaluation sheet, your instructor will grade your performance.

CHAPTER 13 SUMMARY

Understanding the basic principles of infection control is essential for any health care worker in any health care field. Disease is caused by a wide variety of pathogens, or germs. An understanding of the types of pathogens, methods of transmission, and the chain of infection allows health care workers to take precautions to prevent the spread of disease.

Bioterrorism is the use of microorganisms as weapons to infect humans, animals, or plants. The CDC has identified and classified agents that could be used for bioterrorism. In today's world, it is likely that an attack will occur. Every health care worker must constantly be alert to the threat of bioterrorism. Careful preparation of a comprehensive plan against bioterrorism and thorough training of all individuals can limit the effect of the attack and save the lives of many people.

Asepsis is defined as "the absence of disease-producing microorganisms, or pathogens." Various levels of aseptic control are possible. Antisepsis refers to methods that prevent or inhibit the growth of pathogenic organisms. Proper handwashing and using an ultrasonic unit to

TODAY'S RESEARCH: TOMORROW'S HEALTH CARE

Super water that kills germs?

Treating chronic wounds is a multibillion-dollar market worldwide. Any health product catalog advertises hundreds of antiseptics and disinfectants designed to kill germs. However, many of these products irritate the skin, and only a few can be used on open infected sores.

Now scientists have created a superoxygenated water, Microcyn, that appears to kill bacteria, viruses, fungi, mold, and spores. Microcyn is water mixed with salt that has been charged with an electric current to create superoxidized water. The highly oxidized water contains hydrogen ions that have been split. The ions surround and rupture the cell wall of a single-cell organism, such as a bacterium or virus, and cause the organism to lose its cytoplasm, effectively killing the cell. Multicellular organisms, such as humans, are not affected by the ions because their cells are packed closely together, forming an effective wall to prevent the superoxygenated water from surrounding the cells. Early tests show that chronic diabetic ulcers and burns heal quickly when this solution is used in place of other antiseptics.

In the United States, approximately 18.2 million people, or 6.3 percent of the population, have diabetes. As the disease progresses, many of these individuals experience development of chronic ulcers that do not heal. Statistics show that more than 60 percent of nontraumatic lower leg amputations occur in people with diabetes. Many amputations could be avoided if chronic ulcers could be healed. In addition, think of the many other uses for this superwater. It could be used as an effective handwashing agent. It could be used as a spray mist to disinfect a room. It might even prove to be an agent that can be used to stop a flu epidemic or a biologic terrorist attack. If this superwater can destroy many of the germs that cause disease, it will change health care.

clean instruments and supplies are examples. Disinfection is a process that destroys or kills pathogenic organisms, but is not always effective against spores and viruses. Chemical disinfectants are used for this purpose. Sterilization is a process that destroys all microorganisms, including spores and viruses. The use of an autoclave is an example. Instruments and equipment are properly prepared, and then processed in the autoclave to achieve sterilization.

Following the standard precautions established by the CDC helps prevent the spread of pathogens by way of blood, body fluids, secretions, and excretions. The standard precautions provide guidelines for handwashing; wearing gloves; using gowns, masks, and protective eyewear when splashing is likely; proper handling and disposal of contaminated sharp objects; proper disposal of contaminated waste; and proper methods to wipe up spills of blood, body fluids, secretions, and excretions. Every health care worker must be familiar with and follow the recommended standard precautions while working with all patients.

Sterile techniques are used in specific procedures, such as changing dressings. Health care workers must learn and follow sterile techniques when they are required to perform these procedures.

Transmission-based isolation precautions are used for patients who have communicable diseases, or diseases that are easily transmitted from one person to another. An awareness of the major types of transmission-based isolation presented in this unit will help the health care worker prevent the transmission of communicable diseases.

Infection control must be followed when performing any and every health care procedure. By learning and following the principles discussed in this unit, health care workers will protect themselves, patients, and others from disease.

INTERNET SEARCHES

Use the suggested search engines in Chapter 17:4 of this textbook to search the Internet for additional information on the following topics:

1. *Organizations regulating infection control*: find the organization sites for the Occupational Safety and Health Administration (OSHA), Centers for Disease Control and Prevention (CDC), National Center for Infectious Diseases (NCID), and the Hospital Infection Control Practices Advisory Committee (HICPAC) to obtain information on regulations governing infection control

2. *Microbiology*: search for specific information on bacteria (can also search for specific types such as *Escherichia coli*), protozoa, fungi, rickettsiae, and viruses

3. *Diseases*: obtain information on the method of transmission, signs and symptoms, treatment, and complications for diseases such as hepatitis B, hepatitis C, acquired immune deficiency syndrome, and specific diseases listed by the discussion on microorganisms in this unit

4. *Infections*: research endogenous infections, exogenous infections, nosocomial infections, and opportunistic infections

5. *Bioterrorism*: find information on pathogens that can be used as weapons, how they are spread, methods for prevention and/or treatment of diseases caused by the pathogens, and bioterrorism preparedness plans developed as a result of the Bioterrorism Act of 2002

6. *Foreign trip*: plan a trip to an exotic foreign country; research the Internet to determine specific health precautions that must be taken during your stay, and determine which immunizations you will need before the trip

7. *Infection control*: locate and read the Blood-borne Pathogen Standards, Needlestick Safety and Prevention Act, Standard Precautions, and Transmission-Based Isolation Precautions (airborne precautions, droplet precautions, and contact precautions)

8. *Medical supply companies*: search for names of specific medical supply companies to research products available such as autoclaves, chemical disinfectants, and spill clean-up kits

REVIEW QUESTIONS

1. List the classifications of bacteria by shape and give two (2) examples of diseases caused by each class.

2. Draw the chain of infection and identify three (3) ways to break each section of the chain.

3. Differentiate between antisepsis, disinfection, and sterilization.

4. Develop a plan showing at least five (5) ways you can protect yourself and your family from a bioterrorism attack.

5. List eight (8) times the hands must be washed.

6. Name the different types of personal protective equipment (PPE) and state when each type must be worn to meet the requirements of standard precautions.

7. What level of infection control is achieved by an ultrasonic cleaner? chemicals? an autoclave?

8. Name three (3) methods that can be used to place sterile items on a sterile field. Identify the types of items that can be transferred by each method.

9. List the three (3) types of transmission-based isolation precautions and the basic principles that must be followed for each type.

CHAPTER 14 Vital Signs

Chapter Objectives

After completing this chapter,
you should be able to:

- ◆ List the four main vital signs
- ◆ Convert Fahrenheit to Celsius, or vice versa
- ◆ Read a clinical thermometer to the nearest two-tenths of a degree
- ◆ Measure and record oral temperature accurately
- ◆ Measure and record rectal temperature accurately
- ◆ Measure and record axillary temperature accurately
- ◆ Measure and record tympanic (aural) temperature accurately
- ◆ Measure and record temporal temperature accurately
- ◆ Measure and record radial pulse to an accuracy within ± 2 beats per minute
- ◆ Count and record respirations to an accuracy within ± 1 respiration per minute
- ◆ Measure and record apical pulse to an accuracy within ± 2 beats per minute
- ◆ Measure and record blood pressure to an accuracy within ± 2 mm of actual reading
- ◆ State the normal range for oral, axillary, and rectal temperature; pulse; respirations; and systolic and diastolic pressure
- ◆ Define, pronounce, and spell all key terms

Observe Standard Precautions

Instructor's Check—Call Instructor at This Point

Safety—Proceed with Caution

OBRA Requirement—Based on Federal Law

Math Skill

Legal Responsibility

Science Skill

Career Information

Communications Skill

Technology

KEY TERMS

apical pulse *(ape'-ih-kal)*
apnea *(ap'-nee"-ah)*
arrhythmia *(ah-rith'-me-ah)*
aural temperature
axillary temperature
blood pressure
bradycardia
   (bray'-dee-car'-dee-ah)
bradypnea *(brad"-ip-nee'-ah)*
character
Cheyne–Stokes
   (chain' stokes")
clinical thermometers
cyanosis
diastolic *(die"-ah-stall'-ik)*
dyspnea *(dis(p)'-nee"-ah)*
electronic thermometers
fever

homeostasis
   (home"-ee-oh-stay'-sis)
hypertension
hyperthermia
   (high-pur-therm'-ee-ah)
hypotension
hypothermia
   (high-po-therm'-ee-ah)
oral temperature
orthopnea *(or"-thop-nee'-ah)*
pulse
pulse deficit
pulse pressure
pyrexia
rale *(rawl)*
rate
rectal temperature

respirations
rhythm
sphygmomanometer *(sfig"-
   moh-ma-nam'-eh-ter)*
stethoscope *(steth'-uh-scope)*
systolic *(sis"-tall'-ik)*
tachycardia
   (tack"-eh-car'-dee-ah)
tachypnea *(tack"-ip-nee'-ah)*
temperature
temporal scanning
   thermometer
temporal temperature
tympanic thermometers
vital signs
volume
wheezing

14:1 INFORMATION

Measuring and Recording Vital Signs

Vital signs are important indicators of health states of the body. This unit discusses all of the vital signs in detail. The basic information that follows serves as an introduction for this topic.

Vital signs are defined as various determinations that provide information about the basic body conditions of the patient. The four main vital signs are temperature, pulse, respirations, and blood pressure. Many health care professionals are now regarding the degree of pain as the fifth vital sign. Patients are asked to rate their level of pain on a scale of 1 to 10, with 1 being minimal pain and 10 being severe pain. Other important vital signs that provide information about the patient's condition include the color of the skin, the size of the pupils in the eyes and their reaction to light, the level of consciousness, and the patient's response to stimuli. As a health care worker, it will be your responsibility to measure and record the vital signs of patients. However, it is not in your realm of duties to reveal this information to the patient. The physician will decide if the patient should be given this information. It is essential that vital signs be accurate. They are often the first indication of a disease or abnormality in the patient.

Temperature is a measurement of the balance between heat lost and heat produced by the body. Temperature can be measured in the mouth (oral), rectum (rectal), armpit (axillary), ear (aural), or by the temporal artery in the forehead (temporal). A low or high reading can indicate disease. Most temperatures are measured in degrees on a thermometer that has a Fahrenheit scale. However, some health care facilities are now measuring temperature in degrees on a Celsius (centigrade) scale. A comparison of the two scales is shown in figure 14-1. At times, it may be necessary to convert Fahrenheit temperatures to Celsius, or Celsius to Fahrenheit. The formulas for the conversion are as follows:

♦ To convert Fahrenheit (F) temperatures to Celsius (C) temperatures, subtract 32 from the Fahrenheit temperature and then multiply the result by 5/9, or 0.5556. For exam-

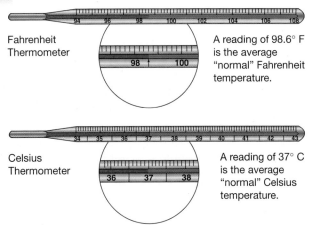

FIGURE 14-1 Normal oral body temperature on Fahrenheit and Celsius thermometers.

ple, to convert a Fahrenheit temperature of 212 to Celsius, subtract 32 from 212 to get 180. Then multiply 180 by 5/9, or 0.5556, to get the Celsius temperature of 100.0.

♦ To convert Celsius (C) temperatures to Fahrenheit (F) temperatures, multiply the Celsius temperature by 9/5, or 1.8, and then add 32 to the total. For example, to convert a Celsius temperature of 37 to Fahrenheit, multiply 37 by 9/5, or 1.8, to get 66.6. Then add 32 to 66.6 to get the Fahrenheit temperature of 98.6.

Pulse is the pressure of the blood felt against the wall of an artery as the heart contracts and relaxes, or beats. The rate, rhythm, and volume are recorded. **Rate** refers to the number of beats per minute, **rhythm** refers to regularity, and **volume** refers to strength. The pulse is usually taken over the radial artery, although it may be felt over any superficial artery that has a bone behind it. Any abnormality can indicate disease.

Respirations reflect the breathing rate of the patient. In addition to the respiration count, the rhythm (regularity) and character (type) of respirations are noted. Abnormal respirations usually indicate that a health problem or disease is present.

Blood pressure is the force exerted by the blood against the arterial walls when the heart contracts or relaxes. Two readings (systolic and diastolic) are noted to show the greatest pressure and the least pressure. Both are very important. Abnormal blood pressure is often the first indication of disease.

Another vital sign is the **apical pulse.** This pulse is taken with a stethoscope at the apex of the heart. The actual heartbeat is heard and counted. At times, because of illness, hardening of the arteries, a weak or very rapid radial pulse, or doctor's orders, you will be required to take an apical pulse. Also, because infants and small children have a very rapid radial pulse that is difficult to count, apical pulses are usually taken.

If you note any abnormality or change in any vital sign, it is your responsibility to report this immediately to your supervisor. If you have difficulty obtaining a correct reading, ask another individual to check the patient. Never guess or report an inaccurate reading.

STUDENT: *Go to the workbook and complete the assignment sheet for 14:1, Measuring and Recording Vital Signs.*

14:2 INFORMATION

Measuring and Recording Temperature

Body temperature is one of the main vital signs. This section provides the basic guidelines for taking and recording temperature.

Temperature is defined as "the balance between heat lost and heat produced by the body." Heat is lost through perspiration, respiration, and excretion (urine and feces). Heat is produced by the metabolism of food, and by muscle and gland activity. A constant state of fluid balance, known as **homeostasis,** is the ideal health state in the human body. The rates of chemical reactions in the body are regulated by body temperature. Therefore, if body temperature is too high or too low, the body's fluid balance is affected.

VARIATIONS IN BODY TEMPERATURE

The normal range for body temperature is 97–100° Fahrenheit, or 36.1–37.8° Celsius (sometimes called centigrade). However, variations in body temperature can occur. Some reasons for variations include:

♦ *Individual Differences*: some people have accelerated body processes and usually have higher temperatures; others have slower body processes and usually have lower temperatures

♦ *Time of Day*: body temperature is usually lower in the morning, after the body has rested and higher in the evening, after muscular activity and daily food intake have taken place

♦ *Body Sites*: parts of the body where temperatures are taken lead to variations; temperature variations by body site are shown in table 14-1.

Oral temperatures are taken in the mouth. The clinical thermometer is left in place for 3–5 minutes. This is usually the most common, convenient, and comfortable method of obtaining a temperature. Eating, drinking hot or cold liquids, and/or smoking can alter the temperature in the mouth. It is important to make sure the patient has *not* had anything to eat or drink, or has *not* smoked for at least 15 minutes prior to taking the patient's oral temperature. If the patient has done any of these things, explain why you cannot take the temperature and that you will return to do so.

Rectal temperatures are taken in the rectum. The clinical thermometer is left in place for 3–5 minutes. This is an internal measurement and is the most accurate of all methods. Rectal temperatures are frequently taken on infants and small children.

Axillary temperatures are taken in the armpit, under the upper arm. The arm is held close to the body, and the thermometer is inserted between the two folds of skin. A *groin* temperature is taken between the two folds of skin formed by the inner part of the thigh and the lower abdomen. Both axillary and groin are external temperatures and, thus, less accurate. The clinical thermometer is held in place for 10 minutes.

Aural temperatures are taken with a special tympanic thermometer that is placed in the ear or auditory canal. The thermometer detects and measures the thermal, infrared energy radiating from blood vessels in the tympanic membrane, or eardrum. Because this pro-

vides a measurement of body core temperature, there is no normal range. Instead, the temperature is calculated by the thermometer into an equivalent of one of four usual settings: equal mode, oral equivalent, rectal equivalent, or core equivalent. The equal mode provides no offset (adjustment) and is recommended for newborns, for whom axillary temperature is often taken. The oral equivalent is calculated with an offset; this mode is used for adults and children over 3 years of age, for whom oral readings are commonly used. The rectal mode is calculated with an offset and is used mainly for infants up to 3 years of age, for whom rectal temperatures are commonly taken. When the rectal mode is used on adults, the temperature may read higher than average. The core equivalent is calculated with an offset and measures core body temperatures such as those found in the bladder or pulmonary artery. The core equivalent mode should only be used where adult "core" temperatures are commonly used and should not be used for routine vital sign measurements. Most aural thermometers record temperature in less than 2 seconds; so this is a fast and convenient method for obtaining temperature. However, a drawback to using tympanic thermometers is that inaccurate results will be obtained if the thermometer is not inserted into the ear correctly or if an ear infection or wax buildup is present.

Temporal temperatures are a newer way to take temperature. A special temporal scanning thermometer is passed in a straight line across the forehead, midway between the eyebrows and upper hairline. The thermometer measures the temperature in the temporal artery to provide an accurate measurement of blood temperature. A normal temporal temperature is similar to a rectal temperature, because it measures the temperature inside the body or bloodstream. Research has shown that temporal thermometers are more accurate than other methods of taking temperature. Errors occur with clinical thermometers

TABLE 14-1 Temperature Variations by Body Site

	ORAL	RECTAL AND/OR TEMPORAL	AXILLARY AND/OR GROIN
Average Temperature	98.6°F (37°C)	99.6°F (37.6°C)	97.6°F (36.4°C)
Normal Range of Temperature	97.6–99.6°F (36.5–37.5°C)	98.6–100.6°F (37–38.1°C)	96.6–98.6°F (36–37°C)

because they are not inserted correctly, they are misread, or they are not left in place for the required period. Eating, drinking, smoking, and other actions alter or change an oral temperature. Perspiration or sweating alters or changes an axillary or groin temperature. These actions have no effect on a temporal temperature. Because a temporal scanning thermometer is easy to use and produces accurate results, it will become a common way to record body temperature.

♦ *Causes of increased body temperature*: illness, infection, exercise, excitement, and high temperatures in the environment

♦ *Causes of decreased body temperature*: starvation or fasting, sleep, decreased muscle activity, mouth breathing, exposure to cold temperatures in the environment, and certain diseases

Very low or very high body temperatures are indicative of abnormal conditions. **Hypothermia** is a low body temperature, below 95°F (35°C) measured rectally. It can be caused by prolonged exposure to cold. Death usually occurs if body temperature drops below 93°F (33.9°C) for a period of time. A **fever** is an elevated body temperature, usually above 101°F (38.3°C) measured rectally. **Pyrexia** is another term for fever. The term *febrile* means a fever is present; *afebrile* means no fever is present or the temperature is within the normal range. Fevers are usually caused by infection or injury. **Hyperthermia** occurs when the body temperature exceeds 104°F (40°C) measured rectally. It can be caused by prolonged exposure to hot temperatures, brain damage, and serious infections. Immediate actions must be taken to lower body temperature, because temperatures above 106°F (41.1°C) can quickly lead to convulsions, brain damage, and death.

TYPES OF THERMOMETERS

Clinical thermometers may be used to record temperatures. A clinical thermometer consists of a slender glass tube containing mercury or alcohol with red dye, which expands when exposed to heat. There are different types of clinical thermometers (figure 14-2). The glass oral thermometer has a long, slender bulb or a blue tip. A security oral thermometer has a shorter, rounder

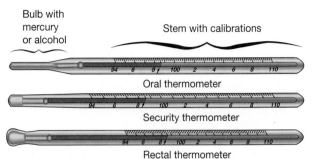

FIGURE 14-2 Types of clinical thermometers.

bulb and is usually marked with a blue tip. A rectal thermometer has a short, stubby, rounded bulb and may be marked with a red tip. In addition, some clinical thermometers have the word "oral" or "rectal" written on their stems. Disposable plastic sheaths may be used to cover the thermometer when it is used on a patient.

To avoid the chance of mercury contamination, the Occupational Health and Safety Administration (OSHA), the Environment Protection Agency (EPA), and the American Medical Association (AMA) recommend the use of alcohol-filled thermometers or digital thermometers. If a clinical thermometer containing mercury breaks, the mercury can evaporate and create a toxic vapor that can harm both humans and the environment. Mercury poisoning attacks the central nervous system in humans. Children, especially those under the age of six, are very susceptible. Mercury can contaminate water supplies and build up in the tissues of fish and animals. Therefore, proper cleanup of a broken clinical thermometer is essential. *Never* use a vacuum cleaner or broom to clean up mercury because this will break up the beads of mercury and allow them to vaporize more quickly. *Never* pour mercury down a drain or discard it in a toilet because this causes contamination of the water supply. If a clinical thermometer breaks, close doors to other indoor areas and open the windows in the room with the mercury spill to vent any vapors outside. Put on gloves and use two cards or stiff paper to push the droplets of mercury and broken glass into a plastic container with a tight-fitting lid. If necessary, use an eyedropper to pick up the balls of mercury. Shine a flashlight in the area of the spill because the light will reflect off the shiny mercury beads and make them easier to see. Wipe the entire area with a damp sponge. Then place all cleanup material, including the paper, eyedropper, gloves, and sponge, in the plastic container and label it "Mercury for Recycling." Seal the lid tightly and take the container to a mercury recycling center. Most waste disposal companies will accept mercury for recycling. To discard unbroken mercury thermometers, place the intact thermometer in a plastic container with a tight-fitting lid, label it, and take it to a mercury recycling center.

Electronic thermometers are used in many facilities. This type of thermometer registers the temperature on a viewer in a few seconds (figure 14-3). Electronic thermometers can be used to take oral, rectal, axillary, and/or groin temperatures. Most facilities have electronic thermometers with blue probes for oral use and red probes for axillary or rectal use. To prevent cross-contamination, a disposable cover is placed over the thermometer probe before the temperature is taken. By changing the disposable cover after each use, one unit can be used on many patients. Electronic digital thermometers are excellent for home use because they eliminate the hazard of a mercury spill that occurs when a clinical thermometer is broken (figure 14-4). The small battery-operated unit usually will register the temperature in about 60 seconds on a digital display screen. Disposable probe covers prevent contamination of the probe.

Tympanic thermometers are specialized electronic thermometers that record the aural temperature in the ear (figure 14-5). A disposable plastic cover is placed on the ear probe. By inserting the probe into the auditory canal and pushing a scan button, the temperature is recorded on the screen within 1–2 seconds. It is important to

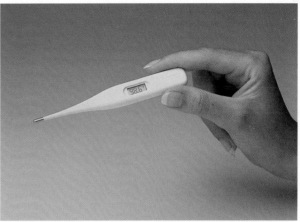

FIGURE 14-4 Electronic digital thermometers are excellent for home use. *(Courtesy of Omron Healthcare Inc., Vernon Hills, IL)*

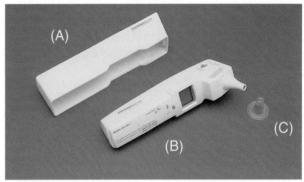

FIGURE 14-5 Tympanic thermometers record the aural temperature in the ear. Parts include: (A) holder, (B) thermometer, and (C) disposable cover.

read and follow instructions while using this thermometer to obtain an accurate reading.

Temporal scanning thermometers are specialized electronic thermometers that measure the temperature in the temporal artery of the forehead (figure 14-6). The thermometer probe is placed on the forehead and passed in a straight line across the forehead, midway between the eyebrows and upper hairline. In this area, the temporal artery is less than 2 millimeters (mm) below the skin surface and easy to find. The temperature registers on the screen in 1–2 seconds. This thermometer provides an accurate measurement of internal body temperature, is easy to use, and is noninvasive. It is important to make sure that the area of forehead scanned is not covered by hair, a wig, or a hat. If the person's head is lying on a pillow, the side of the forehead by the pillow should not be used for the measurement. Any type of head covering or a pillow prevents heat from dissipating and causes the reading to be falsely high.

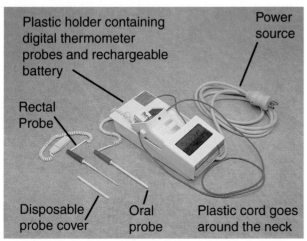

Plastic holder containing digital thermometer probes and rechargeable battery

Power source

Rectal Probe

Disposable probe cover

Oral probe

Plastic cord goes around the neck

FIGURE 14-3 An electronic thermometer registers the temperature in easy-to-read numbers on a viewer.

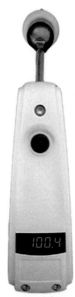

FIGURE 14-6 Temporal scanning thermometers measure the temperature in the temporal artery of the forehead. *(Courtesy of Exergen Corporation, Watertown, MA)*

Plastic or *paper disposable thermometers* are used in some health care facilities (figure 14-7). These thermometers contain special chemical dots or strips that change color when exposed to specific temperatures. Some types are placed on the forehead and skin temperature is recorded. Other types are used orally. Both types are used once and discarded.

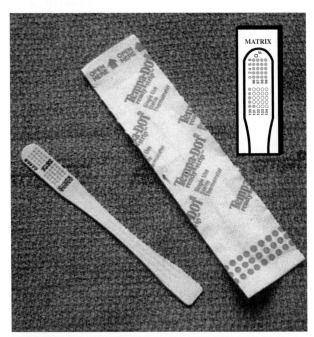

FIGURE 14-7 Plastic disposable thermometers have chemical dots that change color to register body temperature. The matrix shown reads 101°F.

READING AND RECORDING TEMPERATURE

Electronic and tympanic thermometers are easy to read because they have digital displays. Reading a glass clinical thermometer is a procedure that must be practiced. The thermometer should be held at eye level and rotated slowly to find the solid column of mercury or alcohol (figure 14-8). The thermometer is read at the point where the mercury or alcohol line ends. Each long line on a thermometer is read as 1 degree. An exception to this is the long line for 98.6°F (37°C), which is the normal oral body temperature. Each short line represents 0.2 (two-tenths) of a degree. Temperature is always recorded to the next nearest two-tenths of a degree. In figure 14-9, the line ends at 98.6°F (the inset explains the markings for each line).

To record the temperature, write 98[6] instead of 98.6. This reduces the possibility of making an error in reading. For example, a temperature of 100.2 could easily be read as 102. By writing 100[2], the chance of error decreases. If a temperature is taken orally, it is not necessary to indicate that it is an oral reading. If it is taken rectally, place an (R) beside the recording. If it is taken in the axillary area, place an (Ax) beside the record-

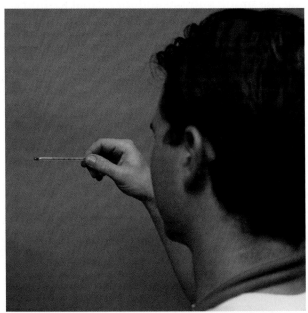

FIGURE 14-8 A clinical thermometer must be held at eye level to find the solid column of mercury or alcohol.

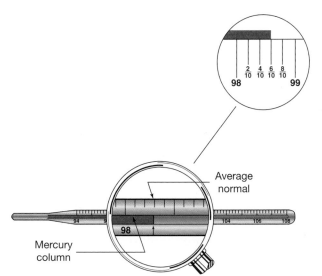

FIGURE 14-9 Each line on a thermometer equals two-tenths of a degree, so the thermometer shown reads 98.6°F.

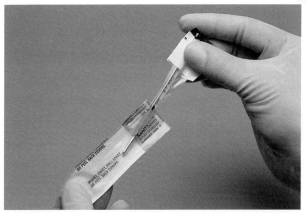

FIGURE 14-10 A clinical thermometer can be covered with a plastic sheath that is discarded after each use.

ing. If it is taken tympanically (aurally), place an (A) beside the recording. For example:

♦ 98⁶ is an oral reading

♦ 99⁶ (R) is a rectal reading

♦ 97⁶ (Ax) is an axillary reading

♦ 98⁶ (A) is an aural reading

CLEANING THERMOMETERS

Thermometers must be cleaned thoroughly after use. The procedure used varies with different agencies and types of thermometers. In some agencies, the glass clinical thermometer is washed and rinsed. Cool water is used to prevent breakage and to avoid destroying the column of mercury or alcohol. The thermometer is then soaked in a disinfectant solution (frequently 70 percent alcohol) for a minimum of 30 minutes before it is used again. Other agencies cover the clinical thermometer with a plastic sheath that is discarded after use (figure 14-10). The probe on electronic thermometers is covered with a plastic sheath that is discarded after each use. These covers prevent the thermometers from coming into contact with each patient's mouth or skin and prevent transmission of germs. Electronic thermometers all use disposable probes so contamination of the thermometer is limited. Some health care facilities do use disinfectants to wipe the outside of electronic thermometers. In most cases, it is best to follow the recommendations of the manufacturer for cleaning and proper care of electronic thermometers. Every health care worker should learn and follow the agency's policy for cleaning and care of thermometers.

STUDENT: *Go to the workbook and complete the assignment sheet for 14:2, Measuring and Recording Temperature. Then return and continue with the procedures.*

PROCEDURE 14:2A

Cleaning a Clinical Thermometer

Equipment and Supplies

Clinical thermometer, soapy cotton balls, small trash bag or waste can, running water, soaking basin with 70 percent alcohol, alcohol sponges or cotton balls, dry cotton balls or gauze pads, thermometer holder, disposable gloves

Procedure

1. Assemble equipment.

PROCEDURE 14:2A

2. Wash hands. Put on gloves if needed.

   ⊞ **CAUTION:** Follow standard precautions. Wear gloves if the thermometer was used for an oral or rectal temperature and was not covered with a plastic sheath.

3. After using the thermometer, use a soapy cotton ball or gauze pad to wipe the thermometer once from the top toward the tip or bulb (figure 14-11A). Discard the soiled cotton ball in trash bag or waste can.

   NOTE: Rotate the thermometer while wiping it to clean all sides and parts.

4. With the bulb pointed downward, hold the thermometer by the stem and rinse the thermometer in cool water.

   ▽ **CAUTION:** Hot water will break the thermometer or destroy the mercury column.

5. Shake the thermometer down to 96°F (35.6°C) or lower.

   ▽ **CAUTION:** Hold the thermometer securely between your thumb and index finger. Use a snapping motion of the wrist. Avoid countertops, tables, and other surfaces.

6. Place the thermometer in a small basin or container filled with disinfectant solution (usually 70 percent alcohol). Make sure the thermometer is completely covered by the solution (figure 14-11B).

   NOTE: Thirty minutes is usually the minimum time recommended for soaking.

7. Remove gloves and discard in an infectious waste container. Wash hands.

8. After 30 minutes, remove the thermometer from the soaking solution and use an alcohol cotton ball or alcohol sponge to wipe it from the stem toward the bulb. This removes any sediment from the thermometer.

9. Rinse the thermometer in cool water. Examine it carefully for any signs of breakage. Discard any broken thermometers according to the agency policy for disposal of mercury or mercury-containing items.

10. Read the thermometer to be sure it reads 96°F (35.6°C) or lower. Place it in a clean gauze-lined container. It is now ready for use.

    NOTE: Many health care agencies fill the container or thermometer holder with a disinfectant, usually 70 percent alcohol.

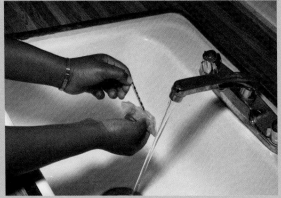

FIGURE 14-11A After each use, use a soapy cotton ball or gauze to wipe the thermometer in a circular motion from the stem to the bulb.

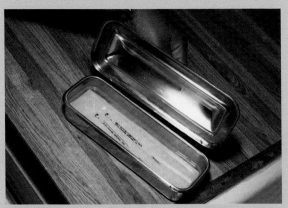

FIGURE 14-11B Soak the thermometer in a disinfectant solution for a minimum of 30 minutes.

PROCEDURE 14:2A

11. Replace all equipment used.

12. Wash hands.

    NOTE: This procedure may vary according to agency policy.

✔ **Final Checkpoint** Using the criteria listed on the evaluation sheet, your instructor will grade your performance.

Practice
Go to the workbook and use the evaluation sheet for 14:2A, Cleaning a Clinical Thermometer, to practice this procedure. When you believe you have mastered this skill, sign the sheet and give it to your instructor for further action.

PROCEDURE 14:2B

Measuring and Recording Oral Temperature

Equipment and Supplies

Oral thermometer, plastic sheath (if used), holder with disinfectant solution, tissues or dry cotton balls, container for used tissues, watch with second hand, soapy cotton balls, disposable gloves, notepaper, pencil/pen

Procedure

1. Assemble equipment.

2. Wash hands and put on gloves.

   CAUTION: Follow standard precautions for contact with saliva or the mucous membrane of the mouth.

3. Introduce yourself. Identify the patient. Explain the procedure.

4. Position the patient comfortably. Ask the patient if he/she has eaten, has had hot or cold fluids, or has smoked in the past 15 minutes.

   NOTE: Eating, drinking liquids, or smoking can affect the temperature in the mouth. Wait at least 15 minutes if the patient says "yes" to your question.

5. Remove the clean thermometer by the upper end. Use a clean tissue or dry cotton ball to wipe the thermometer from stem to bulb.

   NOTE: If the thermometer was soaking in a disinfectant, rinse first in cool water.

   CAUTION: Hold the thermometer securely to avoid breaking.

6. Read the thermometer to be sure it reads 96°F (35.6°C) or lower. Check carefully for chips or breaks.

   CAUTION: Never use a cracked thermometer because it may injure the patient.

7. If a plastic sheath is used, place it on the thermometer.

8. Insert the bulb under the patient's tongue, toward the side of the mouth (figure 14-12). Ask the patient to hold it in place with the lips, and caution against biting it.

   NOTE: Check to be sure patient's mouth is closed.

PROCEDURE 14:2B

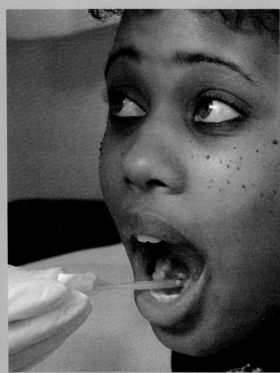

FIGURE 14-12 Insert the bulb of the thermometer under the patient's tongue (sublingually).

9. Leave the thermometer in place for 3–5 minutes.

   NOTE: Some agencies require that a clinical thermometer be left in place for 5–8 minutes. Follow your agency's policy.

   NOTE: If an electronic thermometer is used, hold the thermometer in place until the temperature registers on the screen.

10. Remove the thermometer. Hold it by the stem and use a tissue or cotton ball to wipe toward the bulb.

    NOTE: If a plastic sheath was used to cover the thermometer, there is no need to wipe the thermometer. Simply remove the sheath, taking care not to touch the part that was in the patient's mouth.

▽ **CAUTION:** Do *not* hold the bulb end. This could alter the reading because of the warmth of your hand.

11. Read the thermometer. Record the reading on notepaper.

    NOTE: Recheck the reading and your notation for accuracy.

    NOTE: If the reading is less than 97°F, reinsert the thermometer in the patient's mouth for 1–2 minutes.

12. Clean the thermometer as instructed. Shake down to 96°F (35.6°C) or lower for next use.

13. Check the patient for comfort and safety before leaving.

14. Replace all equipment.

15. Remove gloves and discard in infectious waste container. Wash hands.

16. Record required information on the patient's chart or agency form, for example, date and time, T 98⁶, your signature and title. Report any abnormal reading to your supervisor immediately.

Practice

Go to the workbook and use the evaluation sheet for 14:2B, Measuring and Recording Oral Temperature, to practice this procedure. When you believe you have mastered this skill, sign the sheet and give it to your instructor for further action.

✔ **Final Checkpoint** Using the criteria listed on the evaluation sheet, your instructor will grade your performance.

PROCEDURE 14:2C

Measuring and Recording Rectal Temperature

Equipment and Supplies

Rectal thermometer, plastic sheath (if used), lubricant, tissues/cotton balls, waste bag or container, watch with second hand, paper, pencil/pen, soapy cotton ball, disposable gloves

NOTE: A manikin is frequently used to practice this procedure.

Procedure

1. Assemble equipment.

2. Wash hands and put on gloves.

   ⊞ **CAUTION:** Follow standard precautions if contact with rectal discharge is possible.

3. Introduce yourself. Identify the patient. Explain the procedure. Screen unit, draw curtains, and/or close door to provide privacy for the patient.

4. Remove rectal thermometer from its container. If the thermometer was soaking in a disinfectant, hold it by the stem end and rinse in cool water. Use a dry tissue/cotton ball to wipe from stem to bulb. Check that the thermometer reads 96°F (35.6°C) or lower. Check condition of thermometer. If a plastic sheath is used, position it on the thermometer.

   ▽ **CAUTION:** Breaks in a thermometer can injure the patient. Never use a cracked thermometer.

5. Place a small amount of lubricant on the tissue. Roll the bulb end of the thermometer in the lubricant to coat it. Leave the lubricated thermometer on the tissue until the patient is properly positioned.

6. Turn the patient on his or her side. If possible, use Sims' position (lying on left side with right leg bent up near the abdomen). Infants are usually placed on their backs, with legs raised and held securely, or on their abdomens (figure 14-13).

7. Fold back covers just enough to expose the anal area.

   NOTE: Avoid exposing the patient unnecessarily.

8. With one hand, raise the upper buttock gently. With the other hand, insert the

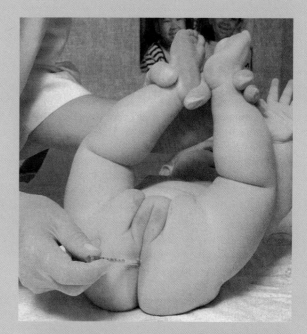

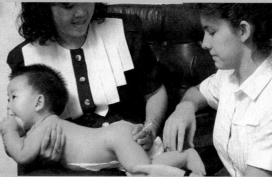

FIGURE 14-13 The infant can be positioned on the back or abdomen for a rectal temperature.

PROCEDURE 14:2C

lubricated thermometer approximately 1 to 1½ inches (½ to 1 inch for an infant) into the rectum. Tell the patient what you are doing.

NOTE: At times, rotating the thermometer slightly will make it easier to insert.

⚠ **CAUTION:** Never force the thermometer. It can break. If you are unable to insert it, obtain assistance.

9. Replace the covers. Keep your hand on the thermometer the entire time it is in place.

⚠ **CAUTION:** *Never* let go of the thermometer. It could slide further into the rectum or break.

10. Hold the thermometer in place for 3–5 minutes.

NOTE: If an electronic thermometer is used, hold the thermometer in place until the temperature registers on the screen.

11. Remove the thermometer gently. Tell the patient what you are doing.

12. Remove plastic sheath, if used, and discard it or use a tissue to remove excess lubricant from the thermometer. Wipe from stem to bulb. Hold by the stem area only. Discard the tissue into a waste container.

13. Read and record. Recheck your reading for accuracy. Remember to place an (R) next to the recording to indicate a rectal temperature was taken.

14. Reposition the patient. Observe all safety checkpoints before leaving the patient.

15. Clean the thermometer as instructed in Procedure 14:2A, Cleaning a Clinical Thermometer.

16. Replace all equipment.

17. Remove gloves and discard in infectious waste container. Wash hands.

18. Record required information on the patient's chart or agency form, for example, date and time, T 99⁶ (R), your signature and title. Report any abnormal reading immediately to your supervisor.

Practice

Go to the workbook and use the evaluation sheet for 14:2C, Measuring and Recording Rectal Temperature, to practice this procedure. When you believe you have mastered this skill, sign the sheet and give it to your instructor for further action.

 Final Checkpoint Using the criteria listed on the evaluation sheet, your instructor will grade your performance.

PROCEDURE 14:2D

Measuring and Recording Axillary Temperature

Equipment and Supplies

Oral thermometer, plastic sheath (if used), disposable gloves (if needed), tissues/cotton balls, towel, waste container, watch with sec-ond hand, paper, pencil/pen, soapy cotton ball

Procedure

1. Assemble equipment.

2. Wash hands. Put on gloves if necessary.

PROCEDURE 14:2D

⊞ **CAUTION:** Follow standard precautions if contact with open sores or body fluids is possible.

3. Introduce yourself. Identify the patient. Explain the procedure.

4. Remove oral thermometer from its container. Use a tissue to wipe from stem to bulb. Check thermometer for damaged areas. Read the thermometer to be sure it reads below 96°F (36.5°C). Place a plastic sheath on the thermometer, if used.

5. Expose the axilla and use a towel to pat the armpit dry (figure 14-14A).

    NOTE: Moisture can alter a temperature reading. Do not rub area hard because this too can alter the reading.

6. Raise the patient's arm and place the bulb end of the thermometer in the hollow of the axilla (figure 14-14B). Bring the arm over the chest and rest the hand on the opposite shoulder.

    NOTE: This position holds the thermometer in place.

7. Leave the thermometer in place for 10 minutes.

    NOTE: If an electronic thermometer is used, hold the thermometer in place until the temperature registers on the screen.

8. Remove the thermometer. Remove sheath, if used, and discard. Wipe from stem to bulb to remove moisture. Hold by the stem end only.

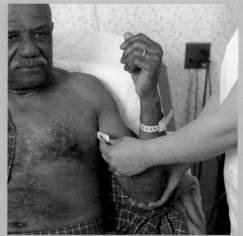

FIGURE 14-14B To take an axillary temperature, insert the bulb end of the thermometer in the hollow of the axilla or armpit.

▽ **CAUTION:** Holding the bulb end will change the reading.

9. Read and record. Check your reading for accuracy. Remember to mark (Ax) by the recording to indicate axillary temperature.

10. Reposition the patient. Be sure to check for safety and comfort before leaving.

11. Clean the thermometer as instructed.

12. Replace all equipment used.

13. Remove gloves if worn and discard in an infectious waste container. Wash hands.

14. Record required information on the patient's chart or agency form, for example, date and time, T 97⁶ (Ax), your signature and title. Report any abnormal reading immediately to your supervisor.

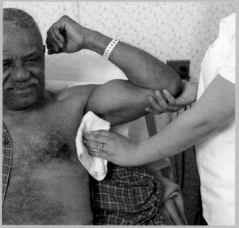

FIGURE 14-14A Before taking an axillary temperature, use a towel to pat the armpit dry.

Practice

Go to the workbook and use the evaluation sheet for 14:2D, Measuring and Recording Axillary Temperature, to practice this procedure. When you believe you have mastered this skill, sign the sheet and give it to your instructor for further action.

✔ **Final Checkpoint** Using the criteria listed on the evaluation sheet, your instructor will grade your performance.

PROCEDURE 14:2E

Measuring and Recording Tympanic (Aural) Temperature

Equipment and Supplies

Tympanic thermometer, probe cover, paper, pencil/pen, container for soiled probe cover

Procedure

1. Assemble equipment.

   NOTE: Read the operating instructions so you understand exactly how the thermometer must be used.

2. Wash hands. Put on gloves if needed.

   ⊞ **CAUTION:** Follow standard precautions if contact with open sores or body fluids is possible.

3. Introduce yourself. Identify the patient. Explain the procedure.

4. Remove the thermometer from its base. Set the thermometer on the proper mode according to operating instructions. The equal mode is usually used for newborn infants, the rectal mode for children under 3 years of age, and the oral mode for children over 3 years of age and all adults. In areas where core body temperatures are recorded, such as critical care units, the core mode may be used.

5. Install a probe cover according to instructions. This will usually activate the thermometer, showing the mode selected and the word *ready*, indicating the thermometer is ready for use.

   ▽ **CAUTION:** Do not use the thermometer until *ready* is displayed because inaccurate readings will result.

6. Position the patient. Infants under 1 year of age should be positioned lying flat with the head turned for easy access to the ear. Small children can be held on the parent's lap, with the head held against the parent's chest for support. Adults who can cooperate and hold the head steady can either sit or lie flat. Patients in bed should have the head turned to the side, and stabilized against the pillow.

7. Hold the thermometer in your right hand to take a temperature in the right ear, and in your left hand to take a temperature in the left ear. With your other hand, pull the ear pinna (external lobe) up and back on any child over 1 year of age and on adults (figure 14-15A). Pull the ear pinna straight back for infants under 1 year of age.

   NOTE: Pulling the pinna correctly straightens the auditory canal so the probe tip will point directly at the tympanic membrane.

8. Insert the covered probe into the ear canal as far as possible to seal the canal (figure 14-15B). Do not apply pressure.

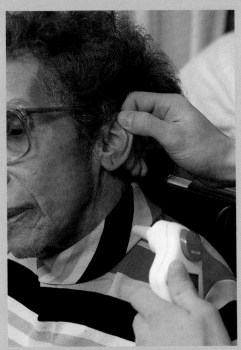

FIGURE 14-15A Before inserting the tympanic thermometer, pull the pinna up and back on adults and children older than 1 year.

PROCEDURE 14:2E

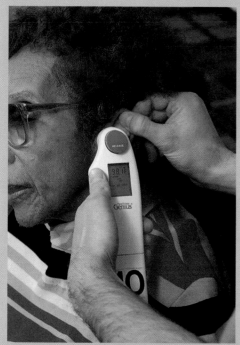

FIGURE 14-15B After inserting the covered probe of the tympanic thermometer into the ear canal, press the scan or activation button and hold the thermometer steady until the temperature reading is displayed.

9. Rotate the thermometer handle slightly until it is aligned with the patient's jaw. Hold the thermometer steady and press the scan or activation button. Hold it for the required amount of time, usually 1–2 seconds, until the reading is displayed on the screen.

10. Remove the thermometer from the patient's ear. Read and record the temperature. Place an (A) by the recording to indicate tympanic temperature.

   NOTE: The temperature will remain on the screen until the probe cover is removed.

CAUTION: If the temperature reading is low or does not appear to be accurate, change the probe cover and repeat the procedure. The opposite ear can be used for comparison.

11. Press the eject button on the thermometer to discard the probe cover into a waste container.

12. Return the thermometer to its base.

13. Reposition the patient. Observe all safety checkpoints before leaving the patient.

14. Remove gloves if worn and discard in an infectious waste container. Wash hands.

15. Record required information on the patient's chart or agency form, for example, date and time, T 98° (A), your signature and title. Report any abnormal reading immediately to your supervisor.

Practice

Go to the workbook and use the evaluation sheet for 14:2E, Measuring and Recording Tympanic (Aural) Temperature, to practice this procedure. When you believe you have mastered this skill, sign the sheet and give it to your instructor for further action.

Final Checkpoint Using the criteria listed on the evaluation sheet, your instructor will grade your performance.

PROCEDURE 14:2F

Measuring Temperature with an Electronic Thermometer

Equipment and Supplies

Electronic thermometer with probe, sheath (probe cover), paper, pen/pencil, container for soiled sheath

Procedure

1. Assemble equipment.

   NOTE: Read the operating instructions for the electronic thermometer so you understand how the particular model operates.

2. Wash hands. Put on gloves if needed.

   CAUTION: Follow standard precautions. Always wear gloves if you are taking a rectal temperature.

   NOTE: Many health care facilities do not require gloves for an oral temperature taken with an electronic thermometer because there is usually no contact with oral fluids. Follow agency policy.

3. Introduce yourself. Identify the patient. Explain the procedure.

4. Position the patient comfortably and correctly.

   NOTE: For an oral temperature, ask the patient if he/she has eaten, has had hot or cold fluids, or has smoked in the past 15 minutes. Wait at least 15 minutes if the patient answers "yes."

   NOTE: For a rectal temperature, position the patient in Sims' position if possible.

5. If the probe has to be connected to the thermometer unit, insert the probe into the correct receptacle. If the thermometer has an "on" or "activate" button,
push the button to turn on the thermometer.

6. Cover the probe with the sheath or probe cover.

   NOTE: For a rectal temperature, the sheath must be lubricated.

7. Insert the covered probe into the desired location. Most probes are heavy, so it is usually necessary to hold the probe in position (figure 14-16A).

   CAUTION: Hold on to the probe at all times for a rectal temperature.

8. When the unit signals that the temperature has been recorded, remove the probe.

   NOTE: Many electronic thermometers have an audible "beep." Others indicate that temperature has been recorded

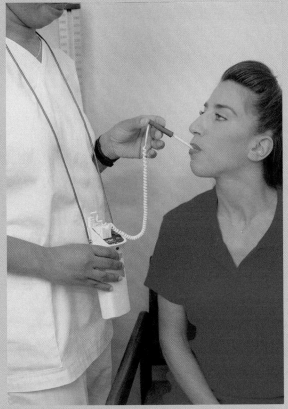

FIGURE 14-16A While taking a temperature, hold the probe of the electronic thermometer in place.

PROCEDURE 14:2F

when the numbers stop flashing and become stationary.

9. Read and record the temperature. Recheck your reading for accuracy.

   NOTE: Remember to place an (R) next to rectal readings or an (Ax) next to axillary readings.

10. Without touching the sheath or probe cover, discard the sheath in an infectious waste container (figure 14-16B). Most thermometers have an eject but-

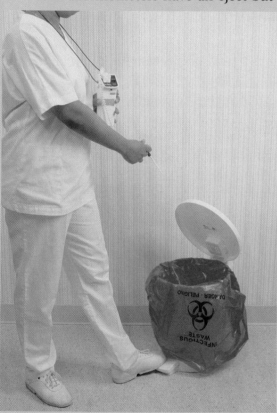

FIGURE 14-16B Discard the probe cover in an infectious waste container without touching the cover.

ton that is pushed to remove the sheath.

11. Reposition the patient. Observe all safety checkpoints before leaving the patient.

12. Return the probe to the correct storage position in the thermometer unit. Turn off the unit if this is necessary. Place the unit in the charging stand if the model has a charging unit.

13. Replace all equipment.

14. Remove gloves if worn and discard in an infectious waste container. Wash hands.

15. Record required information on the patient's chart or agency form, for example, date and time, T 98⁸, your signature and title. Report any abnormal reading immediately to your supervisor.

Practice

Go to the workbook and use the evaluation sheet for 14:2F, Measuring Temperature with an Electronic Thermometer, to practice this procedure. When you believe you have mastered this skill, sign the sheet and give it to your instructor for further action.

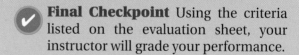

Final Checkpoint Using the criteria listed on the evaluation sheet, your instructor will grade your performance.

PROCEDURE 14:2G

Measuring and Recording Temporal Temperature

Equipment and Supplies

Temporal scanning thermometer, paper, pen/pencil

Procedure

1. Assemble equipment.

   NOTE: Read the operating instructions for the temporal scanning thermometer so you understand how the particular model works.

2. Wash hands.

3. Introduce yourself. Identify the patient. Explain the procedure.

4. Remove the protective cap on the lens of the thermometer. Hold the thermometer upside down to clean the lens with an alcohol wipe and allow it to dry. Check the lens for cleanliness after it has dried.

   NOTE: Holding the thermometer upside down prevents excess moisture from entering the sensor area. The moisture will not harm the sensor, but a temperature cannot be taken until the sensor lens is dry.

5. Position the patient comfortably. Adults who can cooperate and hold the head steady can either sit or lie flat. Infants younger than 1 year should be positioned lying flat on the back. Small children can be held on the parent's lap, with the head held against the parent's chest for support, or lying flat.

6. Check the forehead to make sure there is no sign of perspiration. If perspiration is present, use a towel to pat the forehead dry. Make sure no covering, such as a hat, wig, or hair, is on the forehead.

If the patient was lying on a pillow, do not use the side of the forehead that was on the pillow.

▽ **CAUTION:** Head coverings or a pillow prevent heat from dissipating from the forehead and cause a falsely high temperature reading.

7. Gently position the probe flat on the center of the forehead, midway between the eyebrow and hairline. Press and hold the *scan* button.

8. Slide the thermometer across the forehead lightly and slowly (figure 14-17). Keep the sensor flat and in contact with the skin until you reach the hairline on the side of the face.

   NOTE: The thermometer will emit a beeping sound and a red light will blink to indicate that a measurement is taking place.

9. Release the *scan* button and remove the thermometer from the head.

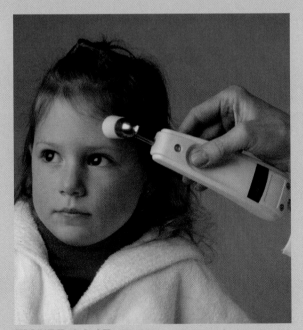

FIGURE 14-17 To take a temporal temperature, hold the scan button while lightly sliding the thermometer across the forehead midway between the eyebrow and hairline. *(Courtesy of Exergen Corporation, Watertown, MA)*

PROCEDURE 14:2G

NOTE: If sweating is profuse and you are not able to dry the forehead completely, scan the temperature as normal but keep the scan button depressed when the thermometer is removed from the forehead. Immediately nestle the thermometer on the neck directly behind the earlobe. Release the button and read the temperature.

10. Read and record the temperature that is displayed on the thermometer. Double-check your reading.

11. Press and release the activation button quickly to turn off the thermometer. Put the protective cap on the lens to protect the lens.

NOTE: Most thermometers will turn off automatically after 30 seconds to 1 minute.

12. Reposition the patient. Observe all safety checkpoints before leaving the patient.

13. Replace all equipment. Wipe the outside of the thermometer with an alcohol wipe or disinfectant.

14. Wash hands.

15. Record required information on the patient's chart or agency form, for example, date and time, T 99^8, your signature, and your title. Report any abnormal reading immediately to your supervisor.

Practice

Go to the workbook and use the evaluation sheet for 14:2G, Measuring and Recording Temporal Temperature, to practice this procedure. When you believe you have mastered this skill, sign the sheet and give it to your instructor for further action.

✓ **Final Checkpoint** Using the criteria listed on the evaluation sheet, your instructor will grade your performance.

14:3 INFORMATION

Measuring and Recording Pulse

Pulse is a vital sign that you will be required to take. There are certain facts you must know when you take this measurement. This section provides the main information.

Pulse refers to the pressure of the blood pushing against the wall of an artery as the heart beats and rests. In other words, it is a throbbing of the arteries that is caused by the contractions of the heart. The pulse is more easily felt in arteries that lie fairly close to the skin and can be pressed against a bone by the fingers.

The pulse can be felt at different arterial sites on the body. Some of the major sites are shown in figure 14-18 and include:

♦ *Temporal*: on either side of the forehead

♦ *Carotid*: at the neck on either side of the trachea

♦ *Brachial*: inner aspect of forearm at the antecubital space (crease of the elbow)

♦ *Radial*: at the inner aspect of the wrist, above the thumb

♦ *Femoral*: at the inner aspect of the upper thigh where the thigh joins with the trunk of the body

♦ *Popliteal*: behind the knee

♦ *Dorsalis pedis*: at the top of the foot arch

NOTE: Pulse is usually taken over the radial artery.

Each time a pulse is measured, three different facts must be noted: the rate, the rhythm, and the volume of the pulse. These facts are important to

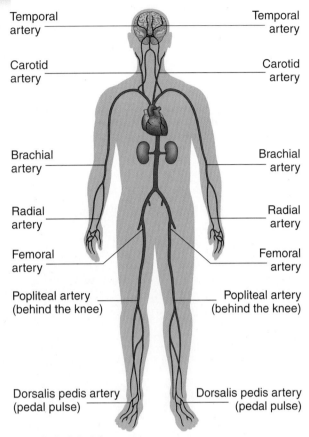

Temporal artery

Temporal artery

Carotid artery

Carotid artery

Brachial artery

Brachial artery

Radial artery

Radial artery

Femoral artery

Femoral artery

Popliteal artery (behind the knee)

Popliteal artery (behind the knee)

Dorsalis pedis artery (pedal pulse)

Dorsalis pedis artery (pedal pulse)

FIGURE 14-18 Major pulse sites.

provide complete information about the pulse. For example, a pulse of 82, strong and regular, is much different than a pulse of 82, weak and very irregular.

The **rate** of the pulse is measured as the number of beats per minute. Pulse rates vary among individuals, depending on age, sex, and body size:

♦ *Adults*: general range of 60–100 beats per minute

♦ *Adult men*: 60–70 beats per minute

♦ *Adult women*: 65–80 beats per minute

♦ *Children aged over 7*: 70–100 beats per minute

♦ *Children aged from 1–7*: range of 80–110 beats per minute

♦ *Infants*: 100–160 beats per minute

♦ **Bradycardia:** a pulse rate under 60 beats per minute

♦ **Tachycardia:** a pulse rate over 100 beats per minute (except in children)

NOTE: Any variations or extremes in pulse rates should be reported immediately.

Rhythm of the pulse is also noted. Rhythm refers to the regularity of the pulse, or the spacing of the beats. It is described as *regular* or *irregular*. An **arrhythmia** is an irregular or abnormal rhythm, usually caused by a defect in the electrical conduction pattern of the heart.

Volume, or the strength or intensity of the pulse, is also noted. It is described by words such as *strong, weak, thready*, or *bounding*.

Various factors will change pulse rate. Increased, or accelerated, rates can be caused by exercise, stimulant drugs, excitement, fever, shock, nervous tension, and other similar factors. Decreased, or slower, rates can be caused by sleep, depressant drugs, heart disease, coma, physical training, and other similar factors.

STUDENT: *Go to the workbook and complete the assignment sheet for 14:3, Measuring and Recording Pulse. Then return and continue with the procedure.*

PROCEDURE 14:3

Measuring and Recording Radial Pulse

Equipment and Supplies

Watch with second hand, paper, pencil/pen

Procedure

1. Assemble equipment.

2. Wash hands.

3. Introduce yourself. Identify the patient. Explain the procedure.

4. Place the patient in a comfortable position, with the arm supported and the palm of the hand turned downward.

    NOTE: If the forearm rests on the chest, it will be easier to count respirations after taking the pulse.

PROCEDURE 14:3

5. With the tips of your first two or three fingers, locate the pulse on the thumb side of the patient's wrist (figure 14-19).

   NOTE: Do not use your thumb; use your fingers. The thumb contains a pulse that you may confuse with the patient's pulse.

6. When the pulse is felt, exert slight pressure and start counting. Use the second hand of the watch and count for 1 full minute.

   NOTE: In some agencies, the pulse is counted for 30 seconds and the final number multiplied by 2. To detect irregularities, it is better to count for 1 full minute.

7. While counting the pulse, also note the volume (character or strength) and the rhythm (regularity).

8. Record the following information: date, time, rate, rhythm, and volume. Follow your agency's policy for recording.

9. Check the patient before leaving. Observe all safety precautions to protect the patient.

10. Replace all equipment used.

11. Wash hands.

12. Record all required information on the patient's chart or agency form, for example, date, time, P 82 strong and regular, your signature and title. Report any unusual observations immediately to your supervisor.

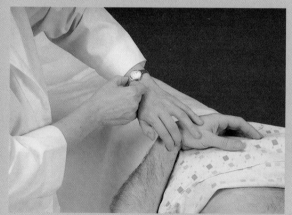

FIGURE 14-19 To count a radial pulse, put the tips of two or three fingers on the thumb side of the patient's wrist.

Practice

Go to the workbook and use the evaluation sheet for 14:3, Measuring and Recording Radial Pulse, to practice this procedure. When you believe you have mastered this skill, sign the sheet and give it to your instructor for further action.

✓ **Final Checkpoint** Using the criteria listed on the evaluation sheet, your instructor will grade your performance.

14:4 INFORMATION

Measuring and Recording Respirations

Respirations are another vital sign that you must observe, count, and record correctly. This section provides the main points you must note when counting and recording the quality of respirations.

Respiration is the process of taking in oxygen (O_2) and expelling carbon dioxide (CO_2) from the lungs and respiratory tract. One respiration consists of one inspiration (breathing in) and one expiration (breathing out).

Each time respiration is measured, three different facts must be noted: the rate, the character, and the rhythm of respirations. These three facts provide complete information about how the patient is breathing. For example, a respiration measurement of 18, deep and regular, is much different than a measurement of 18, very shallow and irregular.

Rate of respirations counts the numbers of breaths per minute. The normal rate for respirations in adults is a range of 12–20 breaths per minute. In children, respirations are slightly faster than those for adults and average 16–30 per minute. In infants, the rate may be 30–50 per minute.

In addition to rate, the character and rhythm of respirations should be noted. **Character** refers to the depth and quality of respirations. Words used to describe character include *deep, shallow, labored, difficult, stertorous* (abnormal sounds like snoring), and *moist.* Rhythm refers to the regularity of respirations, or equal spacing between breaths. It is described as *regular* or *irregular.*

The following terminology is used to describe abnormal respirations:

♦ **Dyspnea:** difficult or labored breathing

♦ **Apnea:** absence of respirations, usually a temporary period of no respirations

♦ **Tachypnea:** rapid, shallow respiratory rate above 25 respirations per minute

♦ **Bradypnea:** slow respiratory rate, usually below 10 respirations per minute

♦ **Orthopnea:** severe dyspnea in which breathing is very difficult in any position other than sitting erect or standing

♦ **Cheyne–Stokes:** abnormal breathing pattern characterized by periods of dyspnea followed by periods of apnea; frequently noted in the dying patient

♦ **Rales:** bubbling or noisy sounds caused by fluids or mucus in the air passages

♦ **Wheezing:** difficult breathing with a high-pitched whistling or sighing sound during expiration; caused by a narrowing of bronchioles (as seen in asthma) and/or an obstruction or mucus accumulation in the bronchi

♦ **Cyanosis:** a dusky, bluish discoloration of the skin, lips, and/or nail beds as a result of decreased oxygen and increased carbon dioxide in the bloodstream

Respirations must be counted in such a way that the patient is unaware of the procedure. Because respirations are partially under voluntary control, patients may breathe more quickly or more slowly when they become aware of the fact that respirations are being counted. Do not tell the patient you are counting respirations. Also, leave your hand on the pulse site while counting respirations. The patient will think you are still counting pulse and will not be likely to alter the respiratory rate.

STUDENT: *Go to the workbook and complete the assignment sheet for 14:4, Measuring and Recording Respirations. Then return and continue with the procedure.*

PROCEDURE 14:4

Measuring and Recording Respirations

Equipment and Supplies

Watch with second hand, paper, pen/pencil

Procedure

1. Assemble equipment.

2. Wash hands.

3. Introduce yourself. Identify the patient.

4. After the pulse rate has been counted, leave your hand in position on the pulse site and count the number of times the chest rises and falls during 1 minute (figure 14-20).

   NOTE: This is done so the patient is not aware that respirations are being counted. If patients are aware, they can alter their rate of breathing.

5. Count each expiration and inspiration as one respiration.

PROCEDURE 14:4

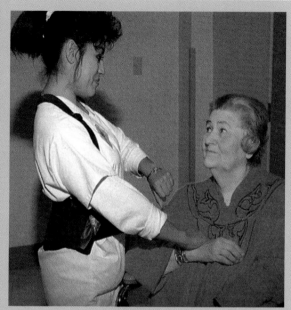

FIGURE 14-20 Positioning the patient's hand on his or her chest makes it easier to count pulse and respiration.

6. Note the depth (character) and rhythm (regularity) of the respirations.

7. Record the following information: date, time, rate, character, and rhythm.

8. Check the patient before leaving the area. Observe all safety precautions to protect the patient.

9. Replace all equipment.

10. Wash hands.

11. Record all required information on the patient's chart or agency form, for example, date, time, R 16 deep and regular (or even), your signature and title. Report any unusual observations immediately to your supervisor.

Practice

Go to the workbook and use the evaluation sheet for 14:4, Measuring and Recording Respirations, to practice this procedure. When you believe you have mastered this skill, sign the sheet and give it to your instructor for further action.

✔ **Final Checkpoint** Using the criteria listed on the evaluation sheet, your instructor will grade your performance.

14:5 INFORMATION

Graphing TPR

In some agencies, you may be required to chart temperature, pulse, and respirations (TPR) on graphic records. This section provides basic information about these records.

Graphic sheets are special records used for recording temperature, pulse, and respirations. The forms vary in different health care facilities, but all contain the same basic information. The graphic chart presents a visual diagram of variations in a patient's vital signs. The progress is easier to follow than a list of numbers that give the same information. Graphic charts are used most often in hospitals and long-term-care facilities. However, similar records may be kept in medical offices or other health care facilities. Patients are sometimes taught how to maintain these records.

Some charts make use of color coding. For example, temperature is recorded in blue ink, pulse is recorded in red ink, and respirations are recorded in green ink. Other agencies use blue ink for 7 A.M. to 7 P.M. (days) and red ink for 7 P.M. to 7 A.M. (nights). Follow the policy of your institution.

Factors that affect vital signs are often included on the graph. Examples include surgery, medications that lower temperature (such as aspirin), and antibiotics.

The graph is a medical record, so it must be neat, legible, and accurate. Double-check all information recorded on the graph. If an error occurs, it should be crossed out carefully with red ink and initialed. Correct information should then be inserted on the graph.

STUDENT: *Read the complete procedure for 14:5, Graphing TPR. Then go back and start doing the procedure. Your assignment will follow the procedure.*

PROCEDURE 14:5

Graphing TPR

Equipment and Supplies

Blank TPR graphic sheets in the workbook, TPR sample graph, assignment sheets on graphing in the workbook, pen, ruler

Procedure

1. Assemble equipment.

2. Examine the sample graphic sheet (figure 14-21). This will vary, depending on the agency. However, most graphic sheets contain time blocks across the top and number blocks for TPRs on the side. Note areas for recording temperature, pulse, and respirations. Refer to the example while completing the procedure steps.

3. Using a blank graphic sheet, fill in patient information in the spaces provided at the top. Write last name first in most cases. Be sure patient identification, hospital, and room number are accurate.

NOTE: Forms vary. Follow directions as they apply to your form.

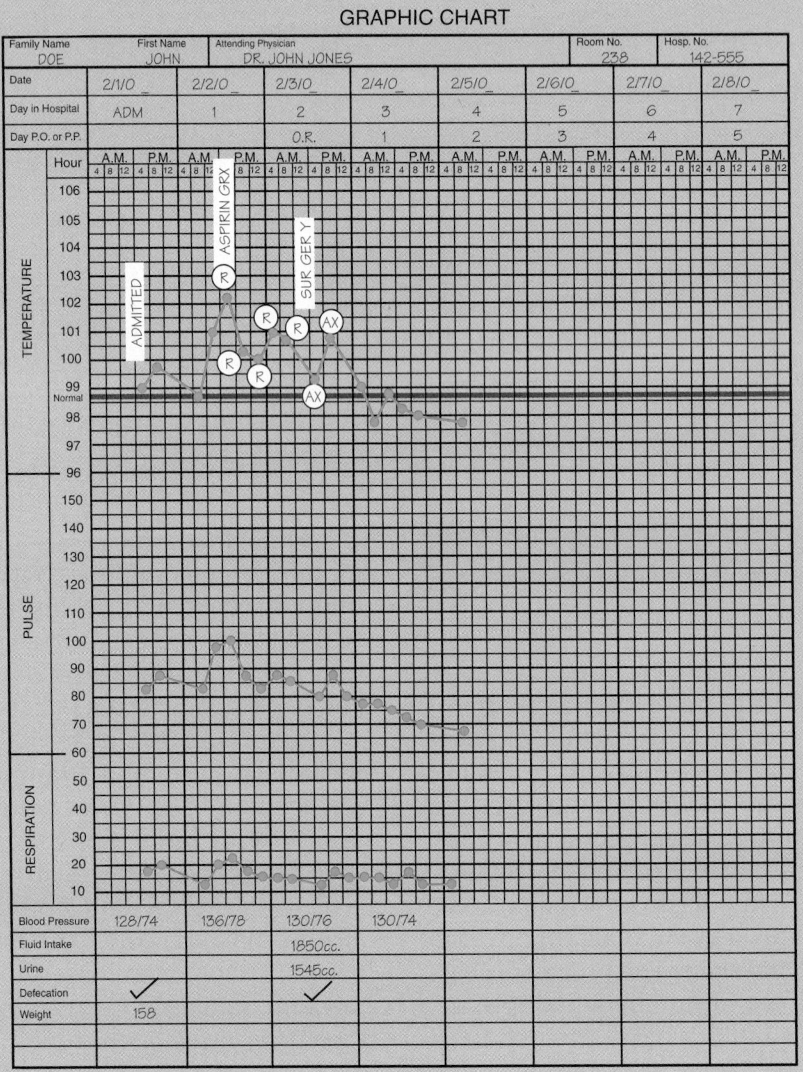

GRAPHIC CHART

FIGURE 14-21 A sample graphic sheet.

PROCEDURE 14:5

4. Fill in the dates in the spaces provided after DATE.

   NOTE: A graphic chart provides a day-to-day visual representation of the variations in a patient's TPRs.

5. If your chart calls for DAY IN HOSPITAL below the dates, enter *Adm* under the first date. This stands for day of admission. The second date would then be day *1*, or first full day in the hospital. The third date would be day *2*, and so forth.

6. Some graphs contain a third line, DAYS PO or PP, which means days post-op (after surgery) or postpartum (after delivery of a baby). The day of surgery would be shown as *OR* or *Surgery*. The next day would be day *1*, or first day after surgery. The day of delivery of a baby is shown as *Del*, with the next day as day *1*, or first day after delivery. Numbers continue in sequence for each following day.

7. Go to the Assignment Sheet #1. Note the TPRs. On the graphic sheet, find the correct *Date and Time* column. Move down the column until the correct temperature number is found on the side of the chart. Mark this with a dot (•) in the box. Do the same for the pulse and respirations.

   ▽ CAUTION: Double-check your notations. Be sure they are accurate.

   ✔ CHECKPOINT: Your instructor will check your notations.

8. Repeat step 7 for the next TPR. Check to be sure you are in the correct time column. Mark the dots clearly under the time column and at the correct temperature measurement, pulse rate, or respiration rate.

9. Use a straight paper edge or ruler to connect the dots for temperature. Do the same with the dots for pulse and, finally, with the dots for respiration.

   NOTE: A ruler makes the line straight and neat, and the readings are more legible.

10. Continue to graph the remaining TPRs from Assignment Sheet #1. Double-check all entries for accuracy. Use a ruler to connect all dots for each of the vital signs.

11. Any drug that might alter or change temperature or other vital sign is usually noted on the graph in the time column closest to the time when the drug was first given. Turn the paper sideways and write the name of the drug in the correct time column. Aspirin is often recorded in this column because it lowers temperature. A rapid drop in body temperature would be readily explained by the word *aspirin* in the time column. Antibiotics and medications that alter heart rate are also noted in many cases.

12. Other events in a patient's hospitalization are also recorded in the time column. Examples include surgery and discharge. In some hospitals, if the patient is placed in isolation, this is also noted on the graph.

13. Blood pressure, weight, height, defecation (bowel movements), and other similar kinds of information are often recorded in special areas at the bottom of the graphic record. Record any information required in the correct areas on your form.

14. Recheck your graph for neatness, accuracy, and completeness of information.

Practice

Go to the workbook and complete Assignment Sheet #1 for Graphing TPR. Give it to your instructor for grading. Note all changes. Then complete Assignment Sheet #2 for Graphing TPR in the workbook. Repeat this process by completing Graphing TPR assignments #3 to #5 until you have mastered graphic records.

 Final Checkpoint Your instructor will grade your performance on this skill according to the accuracy of the completed assignments.

14:6 INFORMATION

Measuring and Recording Apical Pulse

An **apical pulse** is a pulse count taken with a stethoscope at the apex of the heart. The actual heartbeat is heard and counted. A **stethoscope** is an instrument used to listen to internal body sounds. The stethoscope amplifies the sounds so they are easier to hear. Parts of the stethoscope include the earpieces, tubing, and bell or thin, flexible disk called a *diaphragm* (figure 14-22). The tips of the earpieces should be bent forward when they are placed in the ears. The earpieces should fit snugly but should not cause pain or discomfort. To prevent the spread of microorganisms, the earpieces and bell/diaphragm of the stethoscope should be cleaned with a disinfectant such as alcohol before and after every use.

Usually, a physician orders an apical pulse. It is frequently ordered for patients with irregular heartbeats, hardening of the arteries, or weak or rapid radial pulses. Because children and infants have very rapid radial pulse counts, apical pulse counts are usually taken (figure 14-23). It is generally easier to count a rapid pulse while listening to it through a stethoscope than by feeling it with your fingers.

It is important that you protect the patient's privacy when counting an apical pulse. Avoid exposing the patient during this procedure.

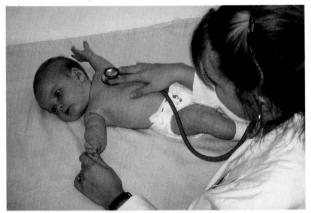

FIGURE 14-23 An apical pulse is frequently taken on infants and small children because their pulses are more rapid.

Two separate heart sounds are heard while listening to the heartbeat. The sounds resemble a "lubb-dupp." Each lubb-dupp counts as one heartbeat. The sounds are caused by the closing of the heart valves as blood flows through the chambers of the heart. Any abnormal sounds or beats should be reported immediately to your supervisor.

A **pulse deficit** is a condition that occurs with some heart conditions. In some cases, the heart is weak and does not pump enough blood to produce a pulse. In other cases, the heart beats too fast (tachycardia), and there is not enough time for the heart to fill with blood; there-

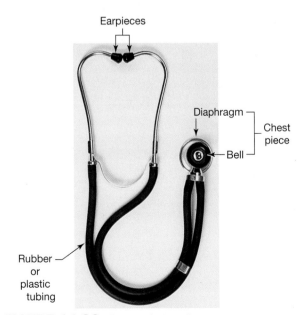

FIGURE 14-22 Parts of a stethoscope.

Earpieces

Diaphragm

Chest piece

Bell

Rubber or plastic tubing

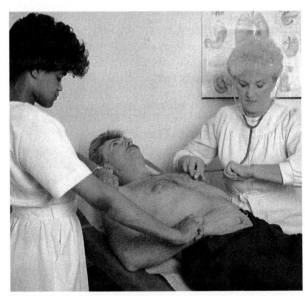

FIGURE 14-24 To determine a pulse deficit, one person should count an apical pulse while another person is counting a radial pulse.

fore, the heart does not produce a pulse during each beat. In such cases, the apical pulse rate is higher than the pulse rate at other pulse sites on the body. For the most accurate determination of a pulse deficit, one person should check the apical pulse while a second person checks another pulse site, usually the radial pulse (figure 14-24). If this is not possible, one person should first check the apical pulse and then immediately check the radial pulse. Then, subtract the rate of the radial pulse from the rate of the apical pulse. The difference is the pulse deficit. For example, if the apical pulse is 130 and the radial pulse is 92, the pulse deficit would be 38 (130 – 92 = 38).

STUDENT: *Go to the workbook and complete the assignment sheet for 14:6, Measuring and Recording Apical Pulse. Then return and continue with the procedure.*

PROCEDURE 14:6

Measuring and Recording Apical Pulse

Equipment and Supplies

Stethoscope, watch with second hand, paper, pencil/pen, alcohol or disinfectant swab

Procedure

1. Assemble equipment. Use alcohol or a disinfectant to wipe the earpieces and the bell/diaphragm of the stethoscope.

2. Wash hands.

3. Introduce yourself. Identify the patient and explain the procedure. If the patient is an infant or child, explain the procedure to the parent(s).

   NOTE: It is usually best to say, "I am going to listen to your heartbeat." Some patients do not know what an apical pulse is.

4. Close the door to the room. Screen the unit or draw curtains around the bed to provide privacy.

5. Uncover the left side of the patient's chest. The stethoscope must be placed directly against the skin.

   NOTE: If the diaphragm of the stethoscope is cold, warm it by placing it in the palm of your hand before placing it on the patient's chest.

6. Place the stethoscope tips in your ears. Locate the apex of the heart, 2–3 inches to the left of the breastbone. Use your index finger to locate the fifth intercostal (between the ribs) space at the midclavicular (collarbone) line (figure 14-25). Place the bell/diaphragm over the apical region and listen for heart sounds.

   ▽ **CAUTION:** Be sure the tips of the stethoscope are facing forward before placing them in your ears.

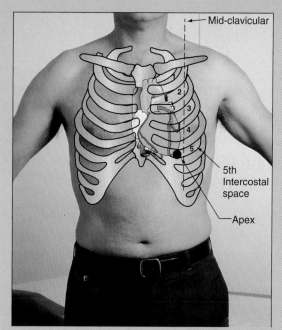

FIGURE 14-25 Locate the apex of the heart at the fifth intercostal (between the ribs) space by the midclavicular (middle of the collarbone) line.

CHAPTER 14 — 428

PROCEDURE 14:6

7. Count the apical pulse for 1 full minute. Note the rate, rhythm, and volume.

   NOTE: Remember to count each lubb-dupp as one beat.

8. If you doubt your count, recheck your count for another minute.

9. Record your reading. Note date, time, rate, rhythm, and volume. Chart according to the agency policy. Some use an *A* and others use an *AP* to denote apical pulse.

   NOTE: If both a radial and apical pulse are taken, it may be recorded as A82/R82. If a pulse deficit exists, it should be noted. For example, with A80/R64, there is a pulse deficit of 16 (that is, 80 − 64 = 16). This would be recorded as A80/R64 Pulse deficit: 16.

10. Check all safety and comfort points before leaving the patient.

11. Use an alcohol or disinfectant swab to clean the earpieces and the bell/diaphragm of the stethoscope. If the tubing contacted the patient's skin, wipe the tubing with a disinfectant. Replace all equipment.

12. Wash hands.

13. Record all required information on the patient's chart or agency form. For example: date, time, AP 86 strong and regular, your signature and title. If any abnormalities or changes were observed, note and report these immediately.

Practice

Go to the workbook and use the evaluation sheet for 14:6, Measuring and Recording Apical Pulse, to practice this procedure. When you believe you have mastered this skill, sign the sheet and give it to your instructor for further action.

Final Checkpoint Using the criteria listed on the evaluation sheet, your instructor will grade your performance.

14:7 INFORMATION

Measuring and Recording Blood Pressure

Blood pressure (BP) is one of the vital signs you will be required to take. It is important that your recording be accurate and that you understand what the blood pressure reading means.

Blood pressure is a measurement of the pressure that the blood exerts on the walls of the arteries during the various stages of heart activity. Blood pressure is read in millimeters (mm) of mercury (Hg) on an instrument known as a *sphygmomanometer*.

There are two types of blood pressure measurements: systolic and diastolic. **Systolic** pressure occurs in the walls of the arteries when the left ventricle of the heart is contracting and pushing blood into the arteries. **Diastolic** pressure is the constant pressure in the walls of the arteries when the left ventricle of the heart is at rest, or between contractions. Blood has moved forward into the capillaries and veins, so the volume of blood in the arteries has decreased.

Normal values and classifications for diastolic and systolic pressure are shown in table 14-2.

Blood pressure is recorded as a fraction. The systolic reading is the top number, or numerator. The diastolic reading is the bottom number, or denominator. For example, a systolic reading of 120 and a diastolic reading of 80 is recorded as 120/80.

Pulse pressure is the difference between systolic and diastolic pressure. The pulse

TABLE 14-2 Classifications of Blood Pressure in Adults

Category	Blood Pressure Level Millimeters of Mercury (mm Hg)		
	Systolic		Diastolic
Normal blood pressure	<120	and	<80
Normal range	100–120	and	60–80
Prehypertension	120–139	or	80–89
Hypertension			
Stage 1 Hypertension	140–159	or	90–99
Stage 2 Hypertension	≥160	or	≥100

Legend: < less than; ≥ greater than or equal to

pressure is an important indicator of the health and tone of arterial walls. A normal range for pulse pressure in adults is 30 to 50 mm Hg. For example, if the systolic pressure is 120 mm Hg and the diastolic pressure is 80 mm Hg, the pulse pressure is 40 mm Hg (120 − 80 = 40). The pulse pressure should be approximately one third of the systolic reading. A high pulse pressure can be caused by an increase in blood volume or heart rate, or a decrease in the ability of the arteries to expand.

Prehypertension is indicated when pressures are between 120 and 139 mm Hg systolic or 80 and 89 mm Hg diastolic. Prehypertension is a warning that high blood pressure will develop unless steps are taken to prevent it. Research has proven that prehypertension can harden arteries, dislodge plaque, and block vessels that nourish the heart. Proper nutrition and a regular exercise program are the main treatments for prehypertension.

Hypertension, or high blood pressure, is indicated when pressures are greater than 140 mm Hg systolic and 90 mm Hg diastolic. Common causes include stress, anxiety, obesity, high salt intake, aging, kidney disease, thyroid deficiency, and vascular conditions such as arteriosclerosis. Hypertension is often called a "silent killer" because most individuals do not have any signs or symptoms of the disease. If hypertension is not treated, it can lead to stroke, kidney disease, and/or heart disease.

Hypotension, or low blood pressure, is indicated when pressures are less than 90 mm Hg

systolic and 60 mm Hg diastolic. Hypotension may occur with heart failure, dehydration, depression, severe burns, hemorrhage, and shock. *Orthostatic*, or postural, hypotension occurs when there is a sudden drop in both systolic and diastolic pressure when an individual moves from a lying to a sitting or standing position. It is caused by the inability of blood vessels to compensate quickly to the change in position. The individual becomes lightheaded and dizzy, and may experience blurred vision. The symptoms last a few seconds until the blood vessels compensate and more blood is pushed to the brain.

Many factors can influence blood pressure readings. These factors can cause blood pressure to be high or low. Some examples include:

♦ *Factors causing changes in readings*: force of the heartbeat, resistance of the arterial system, elasticity of the arteries, volume of blood in the arteries, and position of the patient (lying down, sitting, or standing)

♦ *Factors that may increase blood pressure*: excitement, anxiety, nervous tension, exercise, eating, pain, obesity, smoking, and/or stimulant drugs

♦ *Factors that may decrease blood pressure*: rest or sleep, depressant drugs, shock, dehydration, hemorrhage (excessive loss of blood), and fasting (not eating)

A **sphygmomanometer** is an instrument used to measure blood pressure in millimeters of mercury (mm Hg). There are three main types of sphygmomanometers: mercury, aneroid, and electronic. The mercury sphygmomanometer has a long column of mercury (figure 14-26). Each mark on the gauge represents 2 mm Hg. The mercury sphygmomanometer must always be placed on a flat, level surface or mounted on a wall. If it is calibrated correctly, the level of mercury should be at zero when viewed at eye level. Even though the mercury sphygmomanometer has proven to be the most accurate instrument for measuring blood pressure, the Occupational Health and Safety Administration (OSHA) discourages its use because of the possibility of a mercury spill and contamination. The aneroid sphygmomanometer does not have a mercury column (figure 14-27A). However, it is calibrated in mm Hg. Each line represents 2 mm Hg pressure. When the cuff is deflated, the needle must be on zero (figure

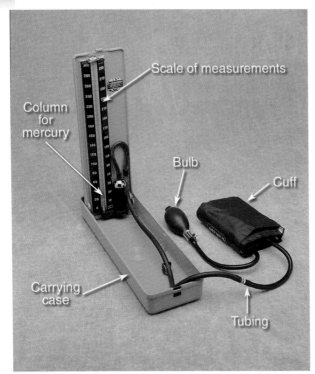

FIGURE 14-26 The gauge on a mercury sphygmomanometer has a column of mercury.

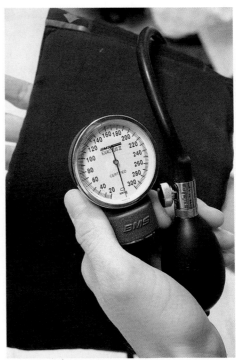

FIGURE 14-27B If the needle is not on zero when the aneroid cuff is deflated, the sphygmomanometer should not be used until it is recalibrated.

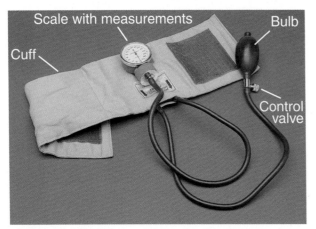

FIGURE 14-27A The gauge on an aneroid sphygmomanometer does not contain a column of mercury.

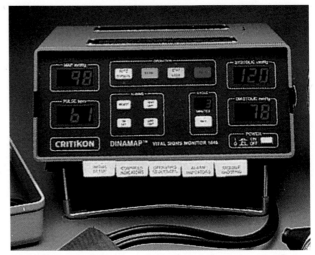

FIGURE 14-28 Electronic sphygmomanometers provide a digital display of blood pressure and pulse readings.

14-27B). If the needle is not on zero, the sphygmomanometer should not be used until it is recalibrated. Electronic sphygmomanometers are used in many health care facilities (figure 14-28). Blood pressure and pulse readings are shown on a digital display after a cuff is placed on the patient.

In order to obtain accurate blood pressure readings, it is important to observe several factors. The American Heart Association (AHA) recommends that the patient sit quietly for at least 5 minutes before blood pressure is taken. The AHA also recommends that two separate readings be taken and averaged, with a minimum wait of 30 seconds between readings.

The size and placement of the sphygmomanometer cuff is also important (figure 14-29). The cuff contains a rubber bladder that fills with air to apply pressure to the arteries. Cuffs that are too wide or too narrow give inaccurate readings. A

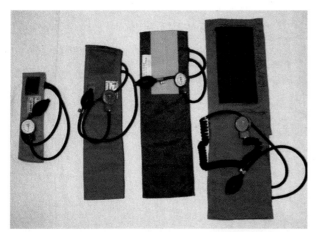

FIGURE 14-29 It is important to use the correct size cuff because cuffs that are too wide or too narrow will result in inaccurate readings.

cuff that is too small will give an artificially high reading; if it is too large it will give an artificially low reading. To ensure the greatest degree of accuracy, the width of the cuff should be approximately 40 percent of the circumference (distance around) of the patient's upper arm. The length of the bladder should be approximately 80 percent of the circumference of the patient's upper arm. The patient should be seated or lying comfortably and have the forearm supported on a flat surface. The area of the arm covered by the cuff should be at heart level. The arm must be free of any constrictive clothing. The deflated cuff should be placed on the arm with the center of the bladder in the cuff directly over the brachial artery, and the lower edge of the cuff 1 to 1½ inches above the antecubital area (bend of the elbow).

A final point relating to accuracy is placement of the stethoscope bell/diaphragm. The bell/diaphragm should be placed directly over the brachial artery at the antecubital area and held securely but with as little pressure as possible.

For a health care worker, a major responsibility is accuracy in taking and recording blood pressure. You should *not* discuss the reading with the patient. This is the responsibility of the physician because the information may cause a personal reaction that can affect the treatment. Only the physician should determine whether an abnormal blood pressure is an indication for treatment.

STUDENT: *Go to the workbook and complete the assignment sheets for 14:7, Measuring and Recording Blood Pressure, Reading a Mercury Sphygmomanometer, and Reading an Aneroid Sphygmomanometer. Then return and continue with the procedure.*

PROCEDURE 14:7

Measuring and Recording Blood Pressure

Equipment and Supplies

Stethoscope, sphygmomanometer, alcohol swab or disinfectant, paper, pencil/pen

Procedure

1. Assemble equipment. Use an alcohol swab or disinfectant to clean the earpieces and bell/diaphragm of the stethoscope.

2. Wash hands.

3. Introduce yourself. Identify the patient. Explain the procedure.

NOTE: If possible, allow the patient to sit quietly for 5 minutes before taking the blood pressure.

NOTE: Reassure the patient as needed. Nervous tension and excitement can alter or elevate blood pressure.

4. Roll up the patient's sleeve to approximately 5 inches above the elbow. Position the arm so that it is supported, comfortable, and close to the level of the heart. The palm should be up.

NOTE: If the sleeve constricts the arm, remove the garment. The arm must be bare and unconstricted for an accurate reading.

5. Wrap the deflated cuff around the upper arm 1 to inches above the elbow and over the brachial artery. The center of

PROCEDURE 14:7
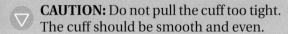

the bladder inside the cuff should be over the brachial artery.

⚠ **CAUTION:** Do not pull the cuff too tight. The cuff should be smooth and even.

6. Determine the palpatory systolic pressure (figure 14-30A). To do this, find the radial pulse and keep your fingers on it. Inflate the cuff until the radial pulse disappears. Inflate the cuff 30 mm Hg above this point. Slowly release the pressure on the cuff while watching the gauge. When the pulse is felt again, note the reading on the gauge. This is the palpatory systolic pressure.

7. Deflate the cuff completely. Ask the patient to raise the arm and flex the fingers to promote blood flow. Wait 30–60 seconds to allow blood flow to resume completely.

8. Use your fingertips to locate the brachial artery (figure 14-30B). The brachial

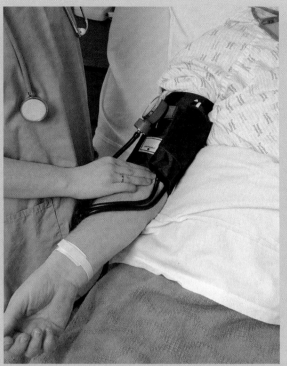

FIGURE 14-30B Locate the brachial artery on the inner part of the arm at the antecubital space.

artery is located on the inner part of the arm at the antecubital space (area where the elbow bends). Place the stethoscope over the artery (figure 14-30C). Put the earpieces in your ears.

NOTE: Earpieces should be pointed forward.

9. Check to make sure the tubings are separate and not tangled together.

10. Gently close the valve on the rubber bulb by turning it in a clockwise direction. Inflate the cuff to 30 mm Hg above the palpatory systolic pressure.

NOTE: Make sure the sphygmomanometer gauge is at eye level.

11. Open the bulb valve slowly and let the air escape gradually at a rate of 2–3 mm Hg per second (or per heartbeat if the heart rate is very slow).

NOTE: Deflating the cuff too rapidly will cause an inaccurate reading.

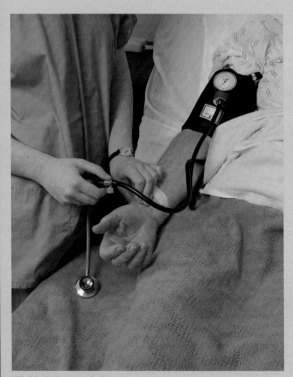

FIGURE 14-30A Determine the palpatory systolic pressure by checking the radial pulse as you inflate the cuff.

PROCEDURE 14:7

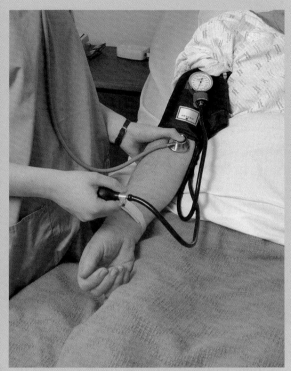

FIGURE 14-30C Place the stethoscope over the brachial artery as you listen for the blood pressure sounds.

12. When the first sound is heard, note the reading on the manometer. This is the systolic pressure.

13. Continue to release the air until there is an abrupt change of the sound, usually soft or muffled. Note the reading on the manometer. Continue to release the air until the sound changes again, becoming first faint and then no longer heard. Note the reading on the manometer. The point at which the first change in sound occurs is the diastolic pressure in children. The diastolic pressure in adults is the point at which the sound becomes very faint or stops.

NOTE: If you still hear sound, continue to the zero mark. Record both readings (the change of sound and the zero reading). For a systolic of 122 and a continued diastolic of 78, this can be written as 122/78/0.

14. Continue to listen for sounds for 10–20 mm Hg below the last sound. If no further sounds are heard, rapidly deflate the cuff.

15. If you need to repeat the procedure to recheck your reading, completely deflate the cuff, wait 1 minute, and repeat the procedure. Ask the patient to raise the arm and flex the fingers to promote blood flow.

▽ **CAUTION:** If you cannot obtain a reading, report to your supervisor promptly.

16. Record the time and your reading. The reading is written as a fraction, with systolic over diastolic. For example, BP 124/72 (or 124/80/72 if the change in sound is noted).

17. Remove the cuff. Expel any remaining air by squeezing the cuff. Use alcohol or a disinfectant to clean the stethoscope earpieces and diaphragm/bell. Replace all equipment.

18. Check patient for safety and comfort before leaving.

19. Wash hands.

20. Record all required information on the patient's chart or agency form, for example, date, time, BP 126/74, your signature and title. Report any abnormal readings immediately to your supervisor.

Practice

Go to the workbook and use the evaluation sheet for 14:7, Measuring and Recording Blood Pressure, to practice this procedure. When you believe you have mastered this skill, sign the sheet and give it to your instructor for further action.

 Final Checkpoint Using the criteria listed on the evaluation sheet, your instructor will grade your performance.

TODAY'S RESEARCH: TOMORROW'S HEALTH CARE

An artificial heart that eliminates the need for heart transplants?

Artificial hearts have been in use for many years. They are used to keep a patient alive until a heart transplant can be found. The first artificial heart was used on Barney Clark, a Seattle dentist, in 1982. It was implanted by Dr. William DeVries. This heart, the Jarvik-7, was connected to an electrical generator the size of a refrigerator. Wires connected the heart with the generator. Barney Clark lived for 112 days connected to this device.

Now researchers have developed a new type of artificial heart. By using miniaturized electronics and high-capacity lithium batteries, scientists have created a heart that allows a patient to wear a battery pack on his or her waist. Electrical energy passes through the patient's skin to power the implanted heart. This allows the patient to resume many normal daily activities. The patient is no longer attached by wires to a power source. Patients have lived for many months with this type of heart while waiting for a suitable transplant.

Researchers are now working on an artificial heart that will work with or in place of a patient's damaged heart. This heart will have computerized intelligence to understand when additional blood is needed by the body. It will be able to respond to the demands of the body, and increase or decrease the heart rate as needed. It will be created from materials that will not cause a rejection reaction in the body. And finally, it will last for many years.

CHAPTER 14 SUMMARY

Vital signs are important indicators of health states of the body. The four main vital signs are temperature, pulse, respiration, and blood pressure.

Temperature is a measurement of the balance between heat lost and heat produced by the body. It can be measured orally, rectally, aurally (by way of the ear), temporally, and between folds of skin. An abnormal body temperature can indicate disease.

Pulse is the pressure of the blood felt against the wall of an artery as the heart contracts or beats. Pulse can be measured at various body sites, but the most common site is the radial pulse, which is at the wrist. The rate, rhythm, and volume (strength) should be noted each time a pulse is taken. An apical pulse is taken with a stethoscope at the apex of the heart. The stethoscope is used to listen to the heartbeat. Apical pulse is frequently taken on infants and small children with rapid pulse rates.

Respiration refers to the breathing process. Each respiration consists of an inspiration (breathing in) and an expiration (breathing out). The rate, rhythm, and character, or type, of respirations should always be noted.

Blood pressure is the force exerted by the blood against the arterial walls when the heart contracts or relaxes. Two measurements are noted: systolic and diastolic. An abnormal blood pressure can indicate disease.

Vital signs are major indications of body function. The health care worker must use precise methods to measure vital signs so results are as accurate as possible. A thorough understanding of vital signs and what they indicate will allow the health care worker to be alert to any abnormalities so they can be immediately reported to the correct individual.

INTERNET SEARCHES

Use the suggested search engines in Chapter 17:4 of this textbook to search the Internet for additional information on the following topics:

1. *Organization*: find the American Heart Association Web site to obtain information on the heart, pulse, arrhythmias, and blood pressure

2. *Vital signs*: research body temperature, pulse, respiration, blood pressure, and apical pulse

3. *Temperature scales*: research Celcius (Centigrade) versus Fahrenheit temperatures: try to

locate conversion charts that can be used to compare the two scales

4. *Diseases*: research hypothermia, fever or pyrexia, hypertension, hypotension, and heart arrhythmias.

REVIEW QUESTIONS

1. List the four (4) main vital signs.

2. State the normal value or range for an adult for each of the following:
a. oral temperature
b. rectal or temporal temperature
c. axillary or groin temperature
d. pulse
e. respiration

3. What three (3) factors must be noted about every pulse?

4. Why is an apical pulse taken?

5. What is the pulse deficit if an apical pulse is 112 and the radial pulse is 88?

6. Differentiate between hypertension and hypotension, and list the basic causes of each.

7. How does systolic pressure differ from diastolic pressure? What are the normal ranges for each?

8. Define each of the following:
a. bradycardia
b. arrhythmia
c. dyspnea
d. tachypnea
e. rales

CHAPTER 15 | First Aid

Chapter Objectives

After completing this chapter,
you should be able to:

◆ Demonstrate cardiopulmonary resuscitation
for one-person rescue, two-person rescue,
infants, children, and obstructed-airway
victims

◆ Describe first aid for
—bleeding and wounds
—shock
—poisoning
—burns
—heat exposure
—cold exposure
—bone and joint injuries, including fractures
—specific injuries to the eyes, head, nose, ears,
    chest, abdomen, and genital organs
—sudden illness including heart attack, stroke,
    fainting, convulsions, and diabetic reactions

◆ Apply dressings and bandages, observing all
safety precautions and using the circular,
spiral, figure-eight, and recurrent, or finger
wrap

◆ Define, pronounce, and spell all key terms

Observe Standard
Precautions

Instructor's Check—Call
Instructor at This Point

Safety—Proceed with
Caution

OBRA Requirement—Based
on Federal Law

Math Skill

Legal Responsibility

Science Skill

Career Information

Communications Skill

Technology

KEY TERMS

abrasion *(ah"-bray'-shun)*
amputation
avulsion *(ay"-vul'-shun)*
bandages
burn
cardiopulmonary
   resuscitation *(car'-dee-oh-
   pull'-meh-nah-ree ree"-
   suh-sih-tay'-shun)*
cerebrovascular accident
   *(seh-ree'-bro-vass"-ku-lehr
   ax'-ih-dent)*
convulsion
diabetic coma

diaphoresis
   (dy"-ah-feh-ree'-sis)
dislocation
dressing
fainting
first aid
fracture
frostbite
heart attack
heat cramps
heat exhaustion
heat stroke
hemorrhage

hypothermia
incision
infection
insulin shock
laceration
poisoning
puncture
shock
sprain
strain
triage *(tree'-ahj)*
wound

15:1 INFORMATION

Providing First Aid

INTRODUCTION

In every health care career you may have experiences that require a knowledge of first aid. This section provides basic guidelines for all the first aid topics discussed in the remaining sections of this unit. All students are strongly encouraged to take the First Aid Certification Course through their local Red Cross divisions to become proficient in providing first aid.

First aid is not full and complete treatment. Rather, **first aid** is best defined as "immediate care that is given to the victim of an injury or illness to minimize the effect of the injury or illness until experts can take over." Application of correct first aid can often mean the difference between life and death, or recovery versus permanent disability. In addition, by knowing the proper first aid measures, you can help yourself and others in a time of emergency.

BASIC PRINCIPLES OF FIRST AID

 In any situation where first aid treatment is necessary, it is essential that you remain calm. Avoid panic. Evaluate the situation thoroughly. Always have a reason for anything you do. The treatment you provide will vary depending on the type of injury or illness, the environment, others present, equipment or supplies on hand, and the availability of medical help. Therefore, it is important for you to think about all these factors and determine what action is necessary.

The first step of first aid is to recognize that an emergency exists. Many senses can alert you to an emergency. Listen for unusual sounds such as screams, calls for help, breaking glass, screeching tires, or changes in machinery or equipment noises. Look for unusual sights such as an empty medicine container, damaged electrical wires, a stalled car, smoke or fire, a person lying motionless, blood, or spilled chemicals. Note any unusual, unfamiliar, or strange odors such as those of chemicals, natural gas, or pungent fumes. Watch for unusual appearances or behaviors in others such as difficulty in breathing, clutching of the chest or throat, abnormal skin colors, slurred or confused speech, unexplained confusion or drowsiness, excessive perspiration, signs of pain, and any symptoms of distress. Sometimes, signs of an emergency are clearly evident. An example is an automobile accident with victims in cars or on the street. Other times, signs are less obvious and require an alert individual to note that something is different or wrong. An empty medicine container and a small child with slurred speech, for example, are less obvious signs.

After determining that an emergency exists, the next step is to take appropriate action to help the victim or victims. Check the scene and make sure it is safe to approach. A quick glance at the area can provide information on what has occurred, dangers present, number of people involved, and other important factors. If live electrical wires are lying on the ground around an accident victim, for example, a rescuer could be electrocuted while trying to assist the victim. An infant thrown from a car during an automobile accident may be overlooked. A rescuer who pauses briefly to assess the situation will avoid such dangerous pitfalls and provide more efficient care. If the scene is not safe, call for medical help. Do not endanger your own life or the lives of other bystanders. Allow professionals to handle fires, dangerous chemicals, damaged electrical wires, and other life-threatening situations.

If the scene appears safe, approach the victim. Determine whether the victim is conscious (figure 15-1). If the victim shows no sign of consciousness, tap him gently and call to him. If the victim shows signs of consciousness, try to find out what happened and what is wrong. Never move an injured victim unless the victim is in a dangerous area such as an area filled with fire and/or smoke, flood waters, or carbon monoxide or poisonous fumes, or one with dangerous traffic, where vehicles cannot be stopped. If it is necessary to move the victim, do so as quickly and carefully as possible. Victims have been injured more severely by improper movement at the scenes of accidents, so avoid any unnecessary movement.

In an emergency, it is essential to call the emergency medical services (EMS) as soon as possible (figure 15-2). The time factor is critical. Early access to the EMS system and advanced medical care increases the victim's chance of survival. Use a telephone, cellular phone, or CB radio to contact the police, ambulance or rescue squad, fire department, utility company, or other resources. In most areas of the country, the emergency number 911 can be used to contact any of the emergency medical services. Sometimes, it may be necessary to instruct others to contact authorities while you are giving first aid. Make sure that complete, accurate information is given to the correct authority. Describe the situation, actions taken, exact location, telephone number from which you are calling, assistance required, number of people involved, and the condition of the victim(s). Do not hang up the receiver or end the CB radio call until the other party has all the necessary information. If you are alone, call EMS immediately before providing any care to:

♦ an unconscious adult

♦ an unconscious child who has reached puberty

♦ an unconscious infant or child with a high risk for heart problems

♦ any victim for whom you witness a sudden cardiac arrest

If you are alone, shout for help and start cardiopulmonary resuscitation (CPR) if needed for:

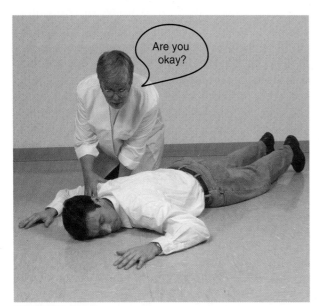

FIGURE 15-1 Determine whether the victim is conscious by gently tapping and by calling to him or her.

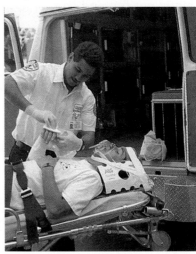

FIGURE 15-2 Call for emergency medical services (EMS) as soon as possible.

- an unconscious infant or child 1 year of age to puberty

- any victim of submersion or near drowning

- any victim with cardiac arrest caused by a drug overdose or trauma

If no one arrives to call EMS, continue providing care by giving five cycles of CPR (approximately 2 minutes). Then go to the nearest telephone, call for EMS, and return immediately to the victim.

After calling for help, provide care to the victim. If possible, obtain the victim's permission before providing any care. Introduce yourself and ask if you can help. If the victim can respond, he or she should give you permission before you provide care. If the victim is a child or minor, and a parent is present, obtain permission from the parent. If the victim is unconscious, confused, or seriously ill and unable to consent to care, and no other relative is available to give permission, you can assume that you have permission. It is important to remember that every individual has the right to refuse care. If a person refuses to give consent for care, do not proceed. If possible, have someone witness the refusal of care. If a life-threatening emergency exists, call EMS, alert them to the situation, and allow the professionals to take over.

At times it may be necessary to **triage** the situation. Triage is a method of prioritizing treatment. If a victim has more than one injury or illness, the most severe injury or illness must be treated first. If two or more people are involved, triage also determines which person is treated first. Life-threatening emergencies must be treated first. Examples include:

- no breathing or difficulty in breathing

- no pulse

- severe bleeding

- persistent pain in the chest or abdomen

- vomiting or passing blood

- poisoning

- head, neck, or spine injuries

- open chest or abdominal wounds

- shock

- severe partial-thickness and all full-thickness burns

Proper care for these emergencies is described in the sections that follow. If the victim is conscious, breathing, and able to talk, reassure the victim and try to determine what has happened. Examine the victim thoroughly. Always have a sound reason for anything you do. Examples include:

- Ask the victim about pain or discomfort

- Check the victim for other types of injuries such as fractures (broken bones), burns, shock, and specific injuries

- Note any abnormal signs or symptoms

- Check vital signs

- Note the temperature, color, and moistness of the skin

- Check and compare the pupils of the eyes

- Look for fluids or blood draining from the mouth, nose, or ears

- Gently examine the body for cuts, bruises, swelling, and painful areas

Report any abnormalities noted to emergency medical services when they arrive at the scene.

Obtain as much information regarding the accident, injury, or illness as possible. This information can then be given to the correct authorities. Information can be obtained from the victim, other persons present, or by examination of items present at the scene. Emergency medical identification contained in a bracelet, necklace, medical card, or Vial-of-Life is an important source of information. Empty medicine containers, bottles of chemicals or solutions, or similar items also can reveal important information. Be alert to all such sources of information. Use this information to determine how you may help the victim.

SUMMARY

Some general principles of care should be observed whenever first aid is necessary. Some of these principles are:

- Obtain qualified assistance as soon as possible. Report all information obtained, observations noted, treatment given, and other important facts to the correct authorities. It may sometimes be necessary to send someone at the scene to obtain help.

- Avoid any unnecessary movement of the victim. Keep the victim in a position that will allow for providing the best care for the type of injury or illness.

♦ Reassure the victim. A confident, calm attitude will help relieve the victim's anxiety.

♦ If the victim is unconscious or vomiting, do not give him or her anything to eat or drink. It is best to avoid giving a victim anything to eat or drink while providing first aid treatment, unless the specific treatment requires that fluids or food be given.

♦ Protect the victim from cold or chilling, but avoid overheating the victim.

♦ Work quickly, but in an organized and efficient manner.

♦ Do not make a diagnosis or discuss the victim's condition with observers at the scene. It is essential to maintain confidentiality and protect the victim's right to privacy while providing treatment.

♦ Make every attempt to avoid further injury.

CAUTION: Provide only the treatment that you are qualified to provide.

STUDENT: *Go to the workbook and complete the assignment sheet for 15:1, Providing First Aid.*

15:2 INFORMATION

Performing Cardiopulmonary Resuscitation

INTRODUCTION

At some time in your life, you may find an unconscious victim who is not breathing. This is an emergency situation. Correct action can save a life. Students are strongly encouraged to take certification courses in cardiopulmonary resuscitation (CPR) offered by the American Red Cross and American Heart Association. This section provides the basic facts about CPR for health care providers according to the 2005 American Heart Association standards. *The information provided is not intended to take the place of an approved certification course.*

The word parts of **cardiopulmonary resuscitation** provide a fairly clear description of the procedure: cardio (the heart) plus pulmonary (the lungs) plus resuscitation (to remove from

apparent death or unconsciousness). When you administer CPR, you breathe for the person *and* circulate the blood. The purpose is to keep oxygenated blood flowing to the brain and other vital body organs until the heart and lungs start working again, or until medical help is available.

Clinical death occurs when the heart stops beating and the victim stops breathing. *Biological death* refers to the death of the body cells. Biological death occurs 4–6 minutes after clinical death and can result in permanent brain damage, as well as damage to other vital organs. If CPR can be started immediately after clinical death occurs, the victim may be revived.

ABCDs OF CPR

Cardiopulmonary resuscitation is as simple as ABCD. In fact, the *ABCD*s serve as guides to lifesaving techniques for persons who have stopped breathing and have no pulse.

♦ *A stands for airway.* To open the victim's airway, use the *head-tilt/chin-lift* method (figure 15-3). Put one hand on the victim's forehead and put the fingertips of the other hand under the bony part of the jaw, near the chin. Tilt the head back without closing the victim's mouth. This action prevents the tongue from falling back and blocking the air passage. If the vic-

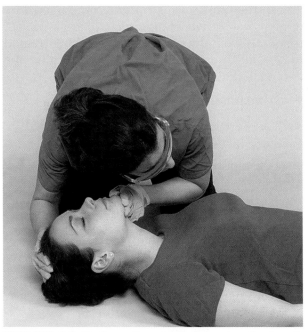

FIGURE 15-3 Open the airway by using the head-tilt/chin-lift method.

tim has a suspected neck or upper spinal cord injury, try to open the airway by lifting the chin without tilting the head back. If it is difficult to keep the jaw lifted with one hand, use a *jaw-thrust maneuver* to open the airway. Assume a position at the victim's head and rest your elbows on the surface on which the victim is lying. Grasp the angles of the victim's lower jaw by positioning one hand on each side. Lift with both hands to move the lower jaw forward, making every attempt to avoid excessive backward tilting or side-to-side movement of the head.

♦ *B stands for breathing.* Breathing means that you breathe into the victim's mouth or nose to supply needed oxygen or provide ventilations. To avoid loss of air when providing mouth-to-mouth breathing, it is important to pinch the victim's nose shut and make a tight seal around the victim's mouth with your mouth. Each breath should take about 1 second and the chest should rise. Rapid or forceful breaths should be avoided because they can force air into the esophagus and stomach, causing gastric distension. This can cause serious complications such as vomiting, aspiration of fluids into the lungs, and even pneumonia.

CAUTION: Follow standard precautions. If possible, use a CPR pocket face mask with a one-way valve to provide a barrier and prevent the transmission of disease (figure 15-4). Special training is required for the use of this mask. Other protective barrier face shields are also available.

♦ *C stands for circulation.* By applying pressure to a certain area of the sternum (breastbone), the heart is compressed between the sternum and vertebral column. Blood is squeezed out of the heart and into the blood vessels. In this way, oxygen is supplied to body cells.

♦ *D stands for defibrillation.* One of the most common causes of cardiac arrest is ventricular fibrillation, an arrhythmia, or abnormal electrical conduction pattern in the heart. When the heart is fibrillating, it does not pump blood effectively. A defibrillator is a machine that delivers an electric shock to the heart to try to restore the normal electrical pattern and rhythm. Automated external defibrillators (AEDs) are now available for use by trained first responders, emergency medical technicians, and even citizens (figure 15-5). After electrode pads are positioned on the victim's chest, the AED determines the heart rhythm, recognizes abnormal rhythms that may respond to defibrillation, and sounds an audible or visual warning telling the operator to push a "shock" button. Some AEDs are fully automatic and even administer the shock. Anytime a shock is administered with an AED, it is essential to make sure no one is touching the victim. The rescuer should state "Clear the victim," and look carefully to make sure no one is in contact with the victim before pushing the shock button. Serious injuries, such as cardiac arrest, could occur in other rescuers if they are shocked by the AED. Newer models of

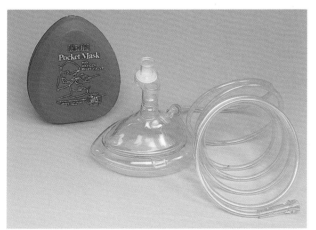

FIGURE 15-4 Whenever possible, use a CPR barrier mask to prevent transmission of disease while giving respirations. The tubing on the mask can be connected to an oxygen supply.

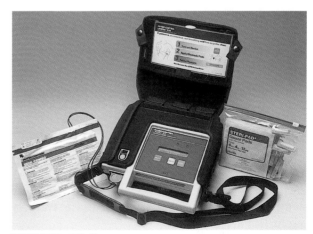

FIGURE 15-5 When cardiac arrest occurs, an automated external defibrillator (AED) can be used to analyze the electrical rhythm of the heart and to apply a shock to try to restore the normal heart rhythm.

AEDs allow the rescuer to deliver either adult or child defibrillator shocks. By using smaller pediatric electrodes and/or a switch on the AED, the rescuer can deliver a smaller electrical shock. The pediatric dose is recommended for any child from 1–8 years of age. The adult defibrillator dose and adult electrodes should be used for any child 8 years or older. In addition, if an AED does not have the option of a pediatric dosage, the adult dosage and electrodes should be used on the child. Currently, there is no recommendation for or against the use of AEDs in infants younger than 1 year. Studies have shown that the sooner defibrillation is provided, the greater the chances of survival are from a cardiac arrest caused by an arrhythmia. However, it is essential to remember that CPR is used until an AED is available. CPR will circulate the blood and prevent biological death.

It is important to know and follow the ABCDs in proper sequence while administering CPR.

BASIC PRINCIPLES OF CPR

Extreme care must be taken to evaluate the victim's condition before CPR is started. The first step is to determine whether the victim is conscious. Tap the victim gently and ask, "Are you OK?" If you know the victim, call the victim by name and speak loudly. If there is no response and the victim is unconscious, call for help. The American Heart Association and the American Red Cross recommend a "call first, call fast" priority. If you are alone, call first before providing any care to:

◆ an unconscious adult

◆ an unconscious child who has reached puberty as defined by the presence of secondary sex characteristics

◆ an unconscious infant or child with a high risk for heart problems

◆ any victim for whom you witness a sudden cardiac arrest

If you are alone, shout for help, and start CPR if needed for:

◆ an unconscious infant or child from 1 year of age to puberty

◆ any victim of submersion or near drowning

◆ any victim with cardiac arrest caused by a drug overdose or trauma

If no help arrives to call EMS, administer five cycles of CPR (about 2 minutes), and then *call fast* for EMS. Return to the victim immediately to continue providing care until EMS arrives.

After determining that a victim is unconscious, the second step is to check for breathing. Try not to move the victim while you check breathing. If the victim is breathing, leave the victim in the same position and proceed with other needed care. If the victim is not breathing, or you are unable to determine whether the victim is breathing, position the victim on his or her back. If you must turn the victim, support the victim's head and neck, and keep the victim's body in as straight a line as possible while turning (figure 15-6). Then, open the airway by using the head-tilt/chin-lift or, if a neck or spinal cord injury is suspected, the jaw-thrust maneuver. This step will sometimes start the victim breathing. To check for breathing, use a three-point evaluation for at least 5 but not more than 10 seconds. *Look* for chest movement. *Listen* for breathing through the nose or mouth. *Feel* for movement of air from the nose or mouth. If the victim is not breathing, give two breaths, each breath lasting approximately 1 second. Make sure the breaths are effective by watching for the victim's chest to rise. Do *not* give breaths too quickly or with too much

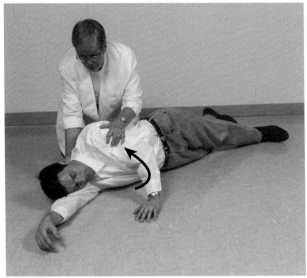

FIGURE 15-6 To turn a victim, support the victim's head and neck, and keep the victim's body in as straight a line as possible.

force because this can cause gastric distension. Pause very briefly between breaths to allow air flow back out of the lungs. In addition, take a breath between the two breaths to increase the oxygen content of the rescue breath.

After giving two breaths, check the carotid pulse in the neck to determine whether cardiac compression is needed. Take at least 5 but no more than 10 seconds to determine whether the pulse is absent before starting compressions.

▽ **CAUTION:** Cardiac compressions are not given if the pulse can be felt. If a person has stopped breathing but still has a pulse, it may be necessary to give only pulmonary respiration.

Correct hand placement is essential before performing chest compressions. For adults, the hand is placed on the lower half of the sternum between the nipples. While kneeling alongside the victim, find the correct position by using the middle finger of your hand that is closest to the victim's feet to follow the ribs up to where the ribs meet the sternum, at the substernal notch (figure 15-7A). Keep the middle finger on the notch and position the index finger above it so two fingers are on the sternum. Then place the heel of your opposite hand (the hand closest to the victim's head) on the sternum, next to the index finger (figure 15-7B). Measuring in this manner minimizes the danger of applying pressure to the tip of the sternum, called the *xiphoid process.*

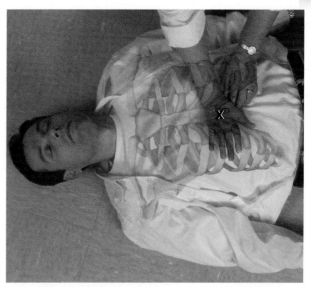

FIGURE 15-7B Place the heel of your opposite hand two fingers' width above the substernal notch. This should place the hand on the lower half of the sternum between the nipples.

▽ **CAUTION:** The xiphoid process can be broken off quite easily and therefore should not be pressed.

After positioning your hands on the sternum, straighten your arms and align your shoulders directly over your hands. To give compressions, push straight down on the victim's sternum with a hard, fast motion. On an adult, the sternum should be compressed 1½ to 2 inches. After each compression, allow the chest to recoil completely. Deliver compressions at a rate of 100 compressions per minute. Proper administration of compressions will produce adequate blood flow and improve the victim's chances of survival.

CPR FOR ADULTS, INFANTS, AND CHILDREN

Cardiopulmonary resuscitation can be performed on adults, children, and infants. In addition, it can be done by one person or two persons. Rates of ventilations and compressions vary according to the number of persons giving CPR and the age of the victim.

♦ *One-person adult rescue:* For adults, a lone rescuer should provide 30 compressions followed by 2 ventilations, for a cycle ratio of 30:2. Compressions should be hard, fast, and

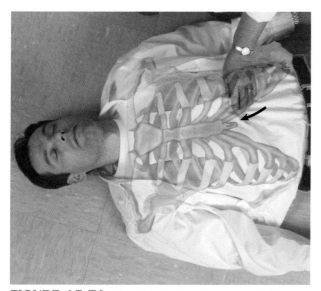

FIGURE 15-7A To position hands correctly for chest compressions, first use a finger to follow the ribs up to where they meet the sternum at the substernal notch.

deep, and given at the rate of approximately 100 per minute. Five 30:2 cycles should be completed every 2 minutes. The hands should be positioned correctly on the sternum. The two hands should be interlaced and only the heel of the palm should rest on the sternum. Pressure should be applied straight down to compress the sternum approximately 1½ to 2 inches, or 3.8 to 5.0 centimeters.

♦ *Two-person adult rescue*: Two people performing a rescue on an adult victim allows one person to give breaths while the second person provides compressions. During the rescue, the person giving breaths can check the effectiveness of the compressions by feeling for a carotid pulse while chest compressions are administered. One rescuer applies the compressions at the rate of 100 per minute. After every 30 compressions, the second rescuer provides 2 ventilations. Thus, there is a 30:2 ratio.

♦ *Infants*: Cardiopulmonary resuscitation for an infant is given to any infant from birth to 1 year of age. It is different than that for an adult because of the infant's size. To open the airway, use a head-tilt/chin-lift method, but the infant's head should not be tilted as far back as an adult's because this can obstruct the infant's airway. Ventilations are given by covering both the infant's nose and mouth; a seal is made by the mouth of the rescuer. Breaths are given until the infant's chest visibly rises. Extreme care must be taken to avoid overinflating the lungs and/or forcing air into the stomach. The brachial pulse site in the arm is used to check pulse (figure 15-8). Compressions are given by placing two fingers on the lower half of the sternum just below an imaginary line drawn between the nipples. The sternum should be compressed about ⅓ to ½ of the depth of the chest. Compressions are given at a rate of 100 per minute. A lone rescuer gives 30 compressions followed by 2 respirations for a 30:2 ratio. The infant's back must be supported at all times when giving compressions. If two rescuers are available to perform CPR on an infant, a two-thumb technique can be used by one rescuer to perform compressions while the second rescuer gives breaths. The rescuer providing compressions

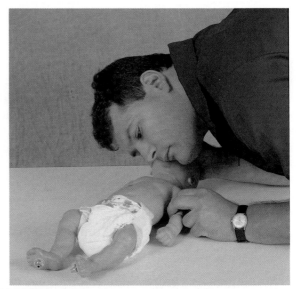

FIGURE 15-8 Use the brachial pulse site in the arm to check for a pulse in an infant.

stands at the infant's feet and places his or her thumbs next to each other on the lower half of the sternum just below the nipple line. The rescuer then wraps his or her hands around the infant to support the infant's back with the fingers. A ratio of 15 compressions to 2 ventilations is used by the two rescuers.

♦ *Children*: Cardiopulmonary resuscitation for children depends on the size of the child. Health care providers should use child CPR methods for any child from 1 year of age to puberty. If a child shows signs of puberty, as evidenced by secondary sex characteristics, adult CPR methods should be used. The initial steps of CPR for a child are the same steps used in adult CPR, except that the head is not tilted as far back when the airway is opened. The main differences relate to compressions. The heel of one hand (or two hands) is placed on the lower half of the sternum in the same position used for adult compressions. If only one hand is used, the other hand remains on the forehead to keep the airway open. The sternum is compressed ⅓ to ½ the depth of the chest. Compressions are given at a rate of 100 per minute. After each set of 30 compressions, 2 breaths are given until the chest visibly rises. This provides a 30:2 ratio. Approximately five cycles of CPR should be completed every 2 minutes.

CHOKING VICTIMS

★ A choking victim has an obstructed airway (an object blocking the airway). Special measures must be taken to clear this obstruction.

♦ If the victim is conscious, coughing, talking or making noise, and/or able to breathe, the airway is not completely obstructed. Remain calm and encourage the victim to remain calm. Encourage the victim to cough hard. Coughing is the most effective method of expelling the object from the airway.

♦ If the victim is conscious but not able to talk, make noise, breathe, or cough, the airway is completely obstructed. The victim usually grasps his or her throat and appears cyanotic (blue discoloration of the skin) (figure 15-9). Immediate action must be taken to clear the airway. Abdominal thrusts, as described in Procedure 15:2E, are given to provide a force of air to push the object out of the airway.

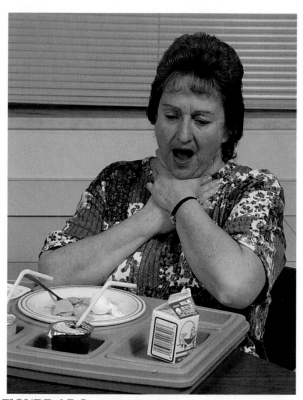

FIGURE 15-9 A choking victim usually grasps her throat and appears cyanotic.

♦ If the victim is unconscious and has an obstructed airway, administer adult CPR. The only change to the adult CPR method is that every time the airway is opened to give breaths, the rescuer should look in the victim's mouth for the object. If the object is visible, the rescuer should use a C-shaped or hooking motion to remove the object. If the object is not seen, the rescuer should try to administer breaths and then continue with chest compressions.

♦ If an infant (birth to 1 year old) has an obstructed airway, a different sequence of steps is used to remove the obstruction. The sequence includes five back blows; five chest thrusts; a check of the mouth; a finger sweep, if the object is seen; and an attempt to ventilate. The sequence, described in detail in Procedure 15:2F, is repeated until the object is expelled, ventilations are successful, or other qualified medical help arrives.

♦ If a child aged 1 to puberty has an obstructed airway, the same sequence of steps used for an adult is followed. A finger sweep of the mouth is *not* performed unless the object can be seen in the mouth.

Once CPR is started, it must be continued unless one of the following situations occur:

♦ The victim recovers and starts to breathe.

♦ Other qualified help arrives and takes over.

♦ A doctor or other legally qualified person orders you to discontinue the attempt.

♦ The rescuer is so physically exhausted, CPR can no longer be continued.

♦ The scene suddenly becomes unsafe.

♦ You are given a legally valid do not resuscitate (DNR) order.

STUDENT: *Go to the workbook and complete the assignment sheet for 15:2, Performing Cardiopulmonary Resuscitation. Then return and continue with the procedures.*

PROCEDURE 15:2A

Performing CPR—One-Person Adult Rescue

Equipment and Supplies

CPR manikin, alcohol or disinfecting solution, gauze sponges

Procedure

⚠ **CAUTION:** Only a CPR training manikin (figure 15-10) should be used to practice this procedure. *Never* practice CPR on another person.

1. Assemble equipment. Position the manikin on a firm surface, usually the floor.

2. *Check for consciousness.* Shake the "victim" by tapping the shoulder. Ask, "Are you OK?" If the victim does not respond, activate EMS immediately. Follow the "call first, call fast" priority. Get an AED if available.

3. *Open the airway.* Use the head-tilt/chin-lift method. Place one hand on the victim's forehead. Place the fingertips of the other hand under the bony part of the victim's jaw, near the chin. Tilt the head without closing the victim's mouth.

   NOTE: This action moves the tongue away from the back of the throat and prevents the tongue from blocking the airway.

   ⚠ **CAUTION:** If the victim has a suspected neck or upper spinal cord injury, use a jaw-thrust maneuver to open the airway. Assume a position on either side of the patient's head. Grasp the angles of the victim's lower jaw by positioning one hand on each side. Lift with both hands to move the lower jaw forward, making every attempt to avoid excessive backward tilting or side-to-side movement of the head.

4. *Check for breathing.* Put your ear close to the victim's nose and mouth while looking at the chest. Look, listen, and feel for respirations for at least 5 but not more than 10 seconds (figure 15-11A).

5. *If the victim is breathing*, keep the airway open and obtain medical help. *If the victim is not breathing*, administer mouth-to-mouth resuscitation as follows:

   a. Keep the airway open.

   b. Resting your hand on the victim's forehead, use your thumb and forefinger to pinch the victim's nose shut.

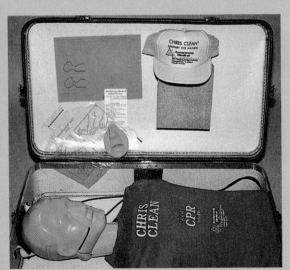

FIGURE 15-10 Use only training manikins while practicing CPR.

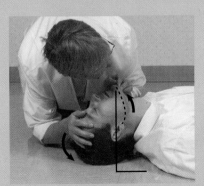

FIGURE 15-11A Open the airway and take at least 5 but no more than 10 seconds to look, listen, and feel for breathing.

PROCEDURE 15:2A

c. Seal the victim's mouth with your mouth or position your mouth on the barrier mask.

d. Give two breaths, each lasting approximately 1 second until the chest visibly rises (figure 15-11B). Pause slightly between breaths. This allows air to flow out and provides you with a chance to take a breath and increase the oxygen level for the second rescue breath.

e. Watch the chest for movement to be sure the air is entering the victim's lungs. Avoid overinflating the lungs and/or forcing air into the stomach.

CAUTION: Follow standard precautions. If possible, use a CPR pocket face mask with a one-way valve to provide a barrier and prevent the transmission of disease.

CAUTION: Giving breaths too quickly or with too much force can cause gastric distention. This can lead to serious complications such as vomiting, aspiration of fluids into the lungs, and pneumonia.

6. *Palpate the carotid pulse.* Kneeling at the victim's side, place the fingertips of your hand on the victim's voice box. Then slide the fingers toward you and into the groove at the side of the victim's neck, where you should find the carotid pulse. Take at least 5 seconds but not

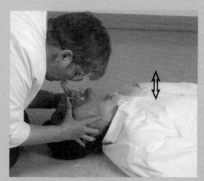

FIGURE 15-11B If the victim is not breathing, open the airway and give two breaths. Watch for the chest to visibly rise.

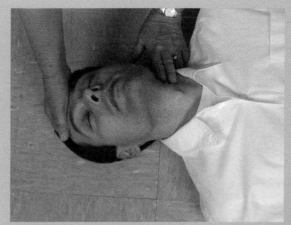

FIGURE 15-11C Palpate the carotid pulse for at least 5 but not more than 10 seconds to determine whether the heart is beating.

more than 10 seconds to feel for the pulse (figure 15-11C). At the same time, watch for breathing, signs of circulation, and/or movement.

NOTE: The pulse may be weak, so check carefully.

7. *If the victim has a pulse, continue providing mouth-to-mouth resuscitation.* Give one breath every 5–6 seconds. Count, "One, one thousand; two, one thousand; three, one thousand; four, one thousand; and breathe," to obtain the correct timing. Recheck the pulse every 2 minutes to make sure the heart is still beating.

8. *If the victim does not have a pulse, administer chest compressions* as follows:

a. Locate the correct place on the sternum. While kneeling alongside the victim, use the middle finger of your hand that is closest to the victim's feet to follow the ribs up to where the ribs meet the sternum, at the substernal notch. Keep the middle finger on the notch and position the index finger above it so two fingers are on the sternum. Then, place the heel of the opposite hand (the one closest to the victim's head) on the sternum, next to the index finger.

PROCEDURE 15:2A

▽ **CAUTION:** The heel of your hand should be on the lower half of the sternum at the nipple line.

b. Place your other hand on top of the hand that is correctly positioned. Keep your fingers off the victim's chest. It may help to interlock your fingers.

c. Rise up on your knees so that your shoulders are directly over the victim's sternum. Lock your elbows and keep your arms straight.

NOTE: This position will allow you to push straight down on the sternum and compress the heart, which lies between the sternum and vertebral column.

d. Push down hard and fast to compress the chest approximately 1½ to 2 inches, or 3.8 to 5.0 centimeters (figure 15-11D). Use a smooth, even motion.

e. Administer 30 compressions at the rate of 100 per minute. Count, "One, two, three," and so forth, to obtain the correct rate.

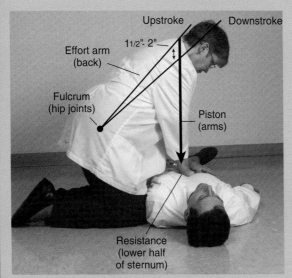

FIGURE 15-11D Use hard and fast motions to compress the chest straight down while giving 30 compressions.

f. Allow the chest to recoil or re-expand completely after each compression. Keep your hands on the sternum during the upstroke (chest relaxation period).

NOTE: When the chest recoils or re-expands completely, this allows more blood to refill the heart between compressions.

9. After administering 30 compressions, give the victim 2 ventilations, or respirations. Avoid excessive body movement while giving the ventilations. Keep your knees in the same position and swing your body upward to give the respirations.

NOTE: Make every effort to minimize any interruptions to chest compressions. There is no blood flow to the brain and heart when compressions are not being performed.

10. Continue the cycles of 30 compressions followed by 2 ventilations until EMS providers take over, an AED arrives, or the victim recovers.

11. If an automated external defibrillator (AED) is available, give five cycles of CPR and then use the AED. Even though AEDs have different manufacturers and models, they all operate in basically the same way.

a. Position the AED at the victim's side next to the rescuer who is using it. If another person arrives to help, the second person can activate EMS (if this has not already been done) and then administer cycles of CPR on the victim's other side.

b. Open the case on the AED and turn on the power control.

NOTE: Some AEDs power on automatically when the case is opened.

c. Expose the victim's chest and attach the chest electrodes to bare skin. If

PROCEDURE 15:2A

the chest is covered with sweat or water, quickly wipe it dry. Choose the correct size electrode pad. Use adult size pads for any victim 8 years and older. Peel the backing off of the electrode pad. Place one pad on the upper right side of the chest, below the clavicle (collarbone) and to the right of the sternum (breastbone). Place the second electrode pad on the left side of the chest to the left of the nipple and a few inches below the axillae (armpit).

d. If necessary, attach the connecting cables of the electrodes to the electrode pad and AED. Some types of electrodes are preconnected.

e. Clearly state "Clear the victim." Look carefully to make sure no one is touching the victim. Push the analyze control to allow the AED to evaluate the heart rhythm (figure 15–12). The analysis may take 5–15 seconds.

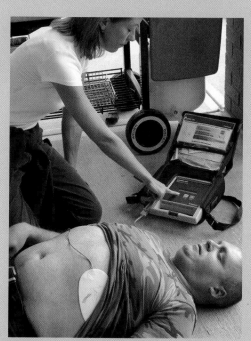

FIGURE 15-12 "Clear" the victim before pushing the control to allow the automated external defibrillator (AED) to analyze the victim's heart rhythm.

f. Follow the recommendations of the AED. If the AED says NO SHOCK, resume CPR by giving 30 compressions followed by 2 ventilations.

g. If the AED says SHOCK, make sure the victim is clear. Loudly state "Clear victim," and look to make sure no one is touching the victim. Push the shock button.

CAUTION: If another rescuer is touching the victim, the rescuer will also receive the shock. This can cause a serious injury and/or a cardiac arrest.

h. Begin cycles of CPR by starting with chest compressions immediately after the shock is delivered to the victim. After 2 minutes of CPR, most AEDs will prompt you to reanalyze the rhythm and deliver additional shocks if necessary.

12. After you begin CPR, do not stop unless

a. the victim recovers

b. help arrives to take over and give CPR and/or apply an AED

c. a physician or other legally qualified person orders you to discontinue the attempt

d. you are so physically exhausted, you cannot continue

e. the scene suddenly becomes unsafe

f. you are given a legally valid do not resuscitate (DNR) order

13. After the practice session, use a gauze pad saturated with 70-percent alcohol or a 10-percent bleach disinfecting solution to clean the manikin. Wipe the face and clean inside the mouth thoroughly. Saturate a clean gauze pad with the solution and lay it on the mouth area for at least 30 seconds. Use another gauze pad to wipe the area dry. Follow manufacturer's instructions for any additional cleaning required.

PROCEDURE 15:2A

NOTE: A 10-percent bleach solution is more effective than alcohol. Some manikins have disposable mouthpieces that are discarded after use. If the mouthpiece is discarded, the remainder of the face should still be disinfected.

14. Replace all equipment used. Wash hands.

✔ **Final Checkpoint** Using the criteria listed on the evaluation sheet, your instructor will grade your performance.

Practice
Go to the workbook and use the evaluation sheet for 15:2A, Performing CPR—One-Person Adult Rescue, to practice this procedure. When you believe you have mastered this skill, sign the sheet and give it to your instructor for further action.

PROCEDURE 15:2B

Performing CPR—Two-Person Adult Rescue

Equipment and Supplies

CPR manikin, alcohol or disinfecting solution, gauze sponges

Procedure

▽ CAUTION: Only a CPR training manikin should be used to practice this procedure. *Never* practice CPR on another person.

1. Assemble equipment. Position the manikin on a firm surface, usually the floor.

2. Shake the victim to check for consciousness. Ask, "Are you OK?"

3. If the victim is unconscious, one rescuer checks for breathing and begins CPR. The second rescuer activates emergency medical services and obtains an AED if available.

4. Use the head-tilt/chin-lift method to open the victim's airway. Place one hand on the victim's forehead. Place the fingertips of the other hand under the bony part of the victim's jaw, near the chin. Tilt the victim's head back without closing the victim's mouth.

5. Check for breathing. Look, listen, and feel for breathing for at least 5 but not more than 10 seconds.

6. *If the victim is not breathing,* give two breaths, each lasting approximately 1 second. Watch the chest for movement to be sure air is entering the victim's lungs. Avoid overinflating the lungs and/or forcing air into the stomach.

⊞ CAUTION: Follow standard precautions. If possible, use a CPR pocket face mask with a one-way valve to provide a barrier and prevent the transmission of disease.

7. Feel for the carotid pulse for at least 5 seconds and not more than 10 seconds. Watch for signs of breathing, circulation, and/or movement.

8. *If there is no pulse,* give chest compressions. Locate the correct hand position on the sternum. Until the second rescuer returns, provide compressions and respirations as for a one-person rescue. Give 30 hard, fast, and deep compressions followed by 2 respirations.

PROCEDURE 15:2B

9. When the second rescuer returns after calling for help, the first rescuer should complete the cycle of 30 compressions and 2 respirations.

10. The second rescuer should get into position for compressions and locate the correct hand placement while the first rescuer is giving the two breaths. The second rescuer should begin compressions at the rate of 100 per minute (figure 15-13A). The second rescuer should count out loud, "One, two, three, four, five . . ." After each set of 30 compressions, the second rescuer should pause very briefly to allow the first rescuer to give 2 breaths. Rescue then continues with 2 breaths after each 30 compressions.

11. After every five cycles of CPR (approximately 2 minutes) the rescuers should change positions. The person giving compressions can provide a clear signal to change positions, such as, "Change, two, three, four. . . ." The compressor should complete a cycle of 30 compressions. The ventilator should give 2 breaths at the end of the 30 compressions. The ventilator should then move to the chest and locate the correct hand placement

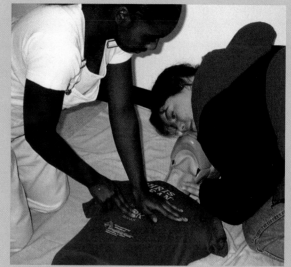

FIGURE 15-13B Rescuers should change positions after every five cycles of CPR because the person doing compressions gets tired, and compressions are not as effective.

for compressions (figure 15-13B). The compressor should move to the head and open the airway. The new compressor should then give 30 hard, fast, and deep compressions at the rate of 100 per minute. The rescue should continue with 2 ventilations after each 30 compressions.

12. If an AED is available, one rescuer should set up the AED while the other rescuer is giving cycles of CPR. When the AED is ready to analyze the heart rhythm, the rescuer operating the AED must make sure the other rescuer is clear of the victim. The steps for using the AED are discussed in detail in step 11 of Procedure 15:2A.

13. The rescuers should continue CPR until qualified medical help arrives, the victim recovers, a doctor or other legally qualified person orders CPR discontinued, the scene suddenly becomes unsafe, or they are presented with a legally valid do not resuscitate (DNR) order.

14. After the practice session, use a gauze pad saturated with 70-percent alcohol

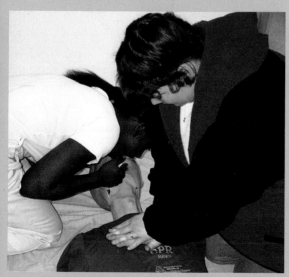

FIGURE 15-13A In a two-person rescue, two breaths are given after every 30 compressions.

PROCEDURE 15:2B

or a 10-percent bleach disinfecting solution to clean the manikin. Wipe the face and clean inside the mouth thoroughly. Saturate a clean gauze pad with the solution and lay it on the mouth area for at least 30 seconds. Use another gauze pad to wipe the area dry. Follow manufacturer's instructions for any additional cleaning required.

NOTE: A 10-percent bleach solution is more effective than alcohol. Some manikins have disposable mouthpieces that are discarded after use. If the mouthpiece is discarded, the remainder of the face should still be disinfected.

15. Replace all equipment used. Wash hands.

Practice
Go to the workbook and use the evaluation sheet for 15:2B, Performing CPR—Two-Person Adult Rescue, to practice this procedure. When you believe you have mastered this skill, sign the sheet and give it to your instructor for further action.

 Final Checkpoint Using the criteria listed on the evaluation sheet, your instructor will grade your performance.

PROCEDURE 15:2C

Performing CPR on Infants

Equipment and Supplies

CPR infant manikin, alcohol or disinfecting solution, gauze pads

Procedure

▽ **CAUTION:** Only a CPR training manikin should be used to practice this procedure. *Never* practice CPR on a human infant.

1. Assemble equipment.

2. Gently shake the infant or tap the infant's foot (for reflex action) to determine consciousness. Call to the infant.

   NOTE: For CPR techniques, infants are usually considered to be under 1 year old.

3. If the infant is unconscious, call aloud for help, and begin the steps of CPR. If no one arrives to call EMS, stop CPR after five cycles (approximately 2 minutes) to telephone for medical assistance. Resume CPR as quickly as possible.

   NOTE: If the infant is known to have a high risk for heart problems or a sudden collapse was witnessed, activate EMS and then begin CPR.

4. Use the head-tilt/chin-lift method to open the infant's airway. Tip the head back gently, taking care not to tip it as far back as you would an adult's head.

   ▽ **CAUTION:** Tipping the head too far will cause an obstruction of the infant's airway.

5. Look, listen, and feel for breathing (figure 15-14A). Check for at least 5 but not more than 10 seconds.

6. *If there is no breathing,* give two breaths, each breath lasting approximately 1 second. Cover the infant's nose and mouth with your mouth. Breathe until the chest

PROCEDURE 15:2C

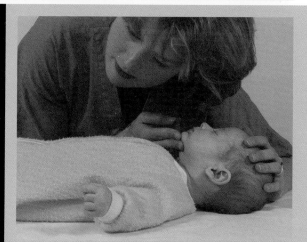

FIGURE 15-14A Look, listen, and feel for breathing for at least 5 but not more than 10 seconds.

rises visibly during each ventilation. Allow for chest deflation after each breath.

7. Check the pulse over the brachial artery. Place your fingertips on the inside of the upper arm and halfway between the elbow and shoulder (figure 15-14B). Put your thumb on the posterior (outside) of the arm. Squeeze your fingers gently toward your thumb. Feel for the pulse for at least 5 but not more than 10 seconds.

8. *If a pulse is present,* continue providing ventilations by giving the infant one ventilation every 3 seconds (approximately 20 breaths per minute). Recheck the pulse every 2 minutes.

9. *If no pulse is present or if the heart rate is below 60 beats per minute with signs of poor circulation such as cyanosis,* administer cardiac compressions. Locate the correct position for compressions by drawing an imaginary line between the nipples. Place two fingers on the sternum just below this imaginary line. Give compressions at the rate of 100 per minute (figure 15-14C). Make sure the infant is on a firm surface, or use one hand to support the infant's back while administering compressions. Press hard, fast, and deep enough to compress the infant's chest ⅓ to ½ the depth of the chest. Give 30 compressions at the rate of 100 per minute. Allow the chest to recoil or re-expand completely between compressions.

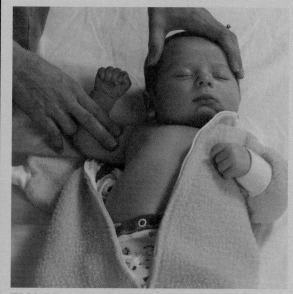

FIGURE 15-14B Check the pulse at the brachial artery in the upper arm.

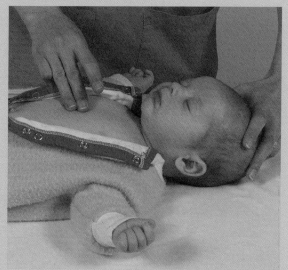

FIGURE 15-14C Use two fingers to give hard and fast compressions to the infant, at a rate of 100 compressions per minute.

PROCEDURE 15:2C

10. After every 30 compressions, give 2 breaths until the chest rises visibly.

11. Continue the cycle of 30 compressions followed by 2 ventilations. To establish the correct rate, count, "One, two, three, four, five."

12. If a second rescuer arrives to assist, the second rescuer should activate EMS if this has not been done. Then both rescuers can perform CPR on the infant.

 a. The first rescuer should finish a cycle of 30 compressions followed by 2 respirations.

 b. The second rescuer should stand at the infant's feet and place his or her thumbs next to each other on the lower half of the sternum just below the nipple line. The rescuer then wraps his or her hands around the infant to support the infant's back with the fingers, and uses the thumbs to administer 15 compressions.

 c. After 15 compressions, the person giving compressions pauses very briefly so the other rescuer can give 2 ventilations.

 NOTE: The ratio of compressions to ventilations is 15:2 for a two-person rescue on an infant.

 d. The rescuers should switch positions after every six to eight cycles (approximately 2 minutes) of CPR.

13. The rescuers should continue the cycles of CPR until qualified medical help arrives, the infant recovers, a doctor or other legally qualified person orders CPR discontinued, or they are presented with a legally valid do not resuscitate (DNR) order (very rare for infants).

14. After the practice session, use a gauze pad saturated with 70-percent alcohol or a 10-percent bleach disinfecting solution to clean the manikin. Wipe the face and clean inside the mouth thoroughly. Saturate a clean gauze pad with the solution and lay it on the mouth area for at least 30 seconds. Use another gauze pad to wipe the area dry. Follow manufacturer's instructions for specific cleaning.

NOTE: The 10-percent bleach solution is more effective than alcohol. Some manikins have disposable mouthpieces that are discarded after use. If the mouthpiece is discarded, the remainder of the face should still be disinfected.

15. Replace all equipment used. Wash hands.

Practice

Go to the workbook and use the evaluation sheet for 15:2C, Performing CPR on Infants to practice this procedure. When you believe you have mastered this skill, sign the sheet and give it to your instructor for further action.

 Final Checkpoint Using the criteria listed on the evaluation sheet, your instructor will grade your performance.

PROCEDURE 15:2D

Performing CPR on Children

Equipment and Supplies

CPR child manikin, alcohol or disinfecting solution, gauze pads

Procedure

△ **CAUTION:** Only a CPR training manikin should be used to practice this procedure. *Never* practice CPR on a human child.

1. Assemble equipment.

2. Gently shake the child to determine consciousness. Call to the child.

   NOTE: Health care providers should use child CPR techniques on any child from 1 year of age to puberty, as evidenced by the development of secondary sex characteristics.

3. If the child is unconscious, call aloud for help, and begin the steps of CPR. If no one arrives to call EMS, stop CPR after five cycles (approximately 2 minutes) to telephone for medical assistance and obtain an AED if available. Resume CPR as quickly as possible.

   NOTE: If the child is known to have a high risk for heart problems or a sudden collapse was witnessed, activate EMS first and then begin CPR.

4. Use the head-tilt/chin-lift method to open the child's airway. Tip the head back gently, taking care not to tip it as far back as you would an adult's head.

5. Look, listen, and feel for breathing. Check for at least 5 but not more than 10 seconds.

6. *If there is no breathing*, give two breaths, each breath lasting approximately 1 second. Cover the child's nose and mouth with your mouth, or pinch the child's nose and cover the child's mouth with your mouth. Breathe until the chest rises visibly during each ventilation. Allow for chest deflation after each breath.

7. Check the pulse at the carotid pulse site. Feel for the pulse for at least 5 but not more than 10 seconds.

8. *If a pulse is present*, continue providing ventilations by giving the child one ventilation every 3 seconds (approximately 20 breaths per minute). Recheck the pulse every 2 minutes.

9. *If no pulse is present or if the heart rate is below 60 beats per minute with signs of poor circulation such as cyanosis,* administer cardiac compressions. Place the heel of one hand on the lower half of the sternum just below a line drawn between the nipples or in the same position used for adult CPR. Keep the other hand on the child's forehead (figure 15-15). If the child is larger, two hands can be posi-

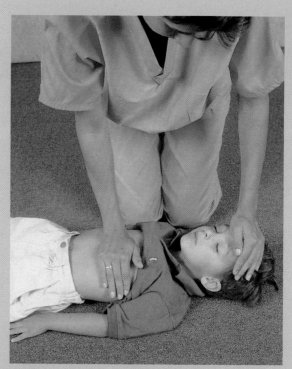

FIGURE 15-15 Use one hand to give chest compressions to a child. Keep the other hand on the child's forehead.

PROCEDURE 15:2D

tioned on the chest for compressions. Give compressions at the rate of 100 per minute. Make sure the child is on a firm surface, or use one hand to support the child's back while administering compressions. Press hard, fast, and deep enough to compress the child's chest ⅓ to ½ the depth of the chest. Give 30 compressions at the rate of 100 per minute. Allow the chest to recoil or re-expand completely between compressions.

10. After every 30 compressions, give 2 breaths until the chest rises visibly.

11. Continue the cycle of 30 compressions followed by 2 ventilations. To establish the correct rate, count, "One, two, three, four, five."

12. If a second rescuer arrives to assist, the second rescuer should activate EMS if this has not been done. Then both rescuers can perform CPR on the child.

   a. The first rescuer should finish a cycle of 30 compressions followed by 2 respirations.

   b. The second rescuer should locate the proper position on the sternum for compressions. As soon as the first rescuer delivers the 2 respirations, the second rescuer should administer 15 compressions.

   c. After 15 compressions, the person giving compressions pauses very briefly so the other rescuer can give 2 ventilations.

   NOTE: The ratio of compressions to ventilations is 15:2 for a two-person rescue on a child.

   d. The rescuers should switch positions after every six to eight cycles (approximately 2 minutes) of CPR.

13. If an AED is available, one rescuer should set up the AED while the other rescuer is giving cycles of CPR. When the AED is ready to analyze the heart rhythm, the rescuer operating the AED must make sure the other rescuer is clear of the vic-

tim. The steps for using the AED are discussed in detail in step 11 of Procedure 15:2A.

▽ CAUTION: Adult electrode pads should be used on any child 8 years or older. Child or pediatric electrodes are used only on children from 1–8 years of age.

14. The rescuers should continue the cycles of CPR until qualified medical help arrives, the child recovers, a doctor or other legally qualified person orders CPR discontinued, or they are presented with a legally valid do not resuscitate (DNR) order.

15. After the practice session, use a gauze pad saturated with 70-percent alcohol or a 10-percent bleach disinfecting solution to clean the manikin. Wipe the face and clean inside the mouth thoroughly. Saturate a clean gauze pad with the solution and lay it on the mouth area for at least 30 seconds. Use another gauze pad to wipe the area dry. Follow manufacturer's instructions for specific cleaning.

NOTE: The 10-percent bleach solution is more effective than alcohol. Some manikins have disposable mouthpieces that are discarded after use. If the mouthpiece is discarded, the remainder of the face should still be disinfected.

16. Replace all equipment used. Wash hands.

Practice
Go to the workbook and use the evaluation sheet for 15:2D, Performing CPR on Children, to practice this procedure. When you believe you have mastered this skill, sign the sheet and give it to your instructor for further action.

 Final Checkpoint Using the criteria listed on the evaluation sheet, your instructor will grade your performance.

PROCEDURE 15:2E

Performing CPR— Obstructed Airway on Conscious Adult or Child

Equipment and Supplies

CPR manikin or choking manikin

Procedure

▽ **CAUTION:** Only a manikin should be used to practice this procedure. Do not practice on another person. Hand placement can be tried on another person, but the actual abdominal thrust should *never* be performed unless the person is choking.

1. Assemble equipment. Position the manikin in an upright position sitting on a chair.

2. Determine whether the victim has an airway obstruction. Ask, "Are you choking?" Check to see whether the victim can cough or speak.

▽ **CAUTION:** If the victim is coughing forcefuly, the airway is not completely obstructed. Encourage the victim to remain calm and cough hard. Coughing is usually very effective for removing an obstruction.

3. If the victim cannot cough, talk, make noise, or breathe, call for help.

4. Perform abdominal thrusts to try to remove the obstruction. Follow these steps:

   a. Stand behind the victim.

   b. Wrap both arms around the victim's waist.

   c. Make a fist of one hand (figure 15-16A). Place the thumb side of the fist in the middle of the victim's abdomen, slightly above the navel (umbili-

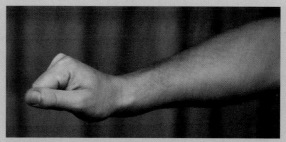

FIGURE 15-16A Make a fist of one hand.

cus) but well below the xiphoid process at the end of the sternum.

   d. Grasp the fist with your other hand (figure 15-16B).

   e. Use quick, upward thrusts to press into the victim's abdomen (figure 15-16C).

NOTE: The thrusts should be delivered hard enough to cause a force of air to push the obstruction out of the airway.

▽ **CAUTION:** Make sure that your forearms do not press against the victim's rib cage while the thrusts are being performed.

   f. If you cannot reach around the victim to give abdominal thrusts (the victim is very obese), or if a victim is in the later stages of pregnancy, give chest thrusts. Stand behind the victim. Wrap your arms under the victim's axilla (armpits) and around to the center of the chest. Make a fist

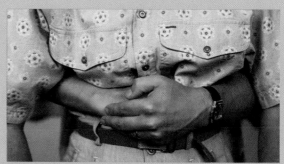

FIGURE 15-16B Place the thumb side of the fist above the umbilicus but well below the xiphoid process at the end of the sternum. Grasp the fist with your other hand.

PROCEDURE 15:2E

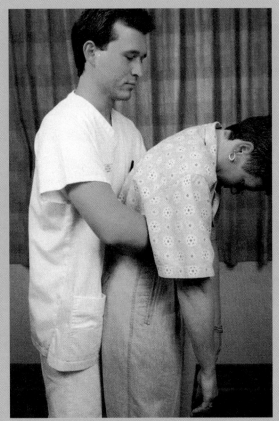

FIGURE 15-16C Use quick, upward thrusts to press into the victim's abdomen.

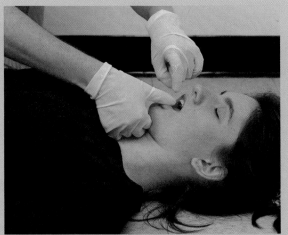

FIGURE 15-17 If an object is visible in the mouth, use a C-shaped, or hooking, motion to remove the object.

with one hand and place the thumb side of the fist against the center of the sternum but well above the xiphoid process. Grab your fist with your other hand and thrust inward.

g. Repeat the thrusts until the object is expelled or until the victim becomes unconscious.

5. If the victim loses consciousness, begin CPR. Activate EMS if this has not already been done. Then start the cycle of CPR by opening the airway and checking breathing. The only difference in CPR for a choking victim is that every time you open the airway you should look in the mouth before giving breaths. If you see an object, use a C-shaped or hooking motion to remove the object (figure 15-17). Perform CPR.

a. Open the airway.

b. Check breathing for at least 5 but not more than 10 seconds.

c. Look in the mouth and remove the object if it is visible.

d. Try giving two breaths.

e. Check the carotid pulse for at least 5 but not more than 10 seconds.

f. If there is a pulse, continue to try to give breaths and check the pulse every 2 minutes.

g. If there is no pulse, give CPR cycles of 30 compressions followed by 2 respirations.

h. Check the mouth for the object every time you are ready to give breaths.

6. Do *not* stop CPR unless the victim recovers, help arrives to take over, a physician or other legally qualified person orders you to discontinue the attempt, you are so physically exhausted you cannot continue, or the scene suddenly becomes unsafe.

7. Make every effort to obtain medical help for the victim as soon as possible.

PROCEDURE 15:2E

8. After the practice session, replace all equipment used. Wash hands.

 Final Checkpoint Using the criteria listed on the evaluation sheet, your instructor will grade your performance.

Practice
Go to the workbook and use the evaluation sheet for 15:2E, Performing CPR—Obstructed Airway on Conscious Adult or Child, to practice this procedure. When you believe you have mastered this skill, sign the sheet and give it to your instructor for further action.

PROCEDURE 15:2F

Performing CPR— Obstructed Airway on Conscious Infant

Equipment and Supplies

CPR infant manikin, alcohol or disinfecting solution, gauze sponges

Procedure

▽ **CAUTION:** Only an infant manikin should be used to practice this procedure. Do *not* practice on a real infant.

1. Assemble equipment. Kneel or sit with the infant in your lap.

   NOTE: An infant is any baby to 1 year of age. Health care providers should use the adult choking sequence for any child older than 1 year.

2. Shake the infant gently. Ask, "Are you OK?"

3. If the infant is conscious and coughing forcefully, allow the infant to cough. The airway is not completely obstructed and the coughing may expel the object.

4. If the infant cannot cry, make any sounds, is making a high-pitched noise while inhaling or no noise at all, is turning cyanotic, and does not appear to be breathing, the airway is completely obstructed. Activate EMS immediately.

5. Quickly bare the infant's chest to expose the sternum (breastbone).

6. Give five back blows. Hold the infant face down, with your arm supporting the infant's body and your hand supporting the infant's head and jaw. Position the head lower than the chest (figure 15-18A). Use the heel of your other hand to give five firm back blows between the infant's shoulder blades.

   ▽ **CAUTION:** When performing back blows on an infant, do not use excessive force.

7. Support the infant's head and neck to turn the infant face up. Hold the infant with your forearm resting on your thigh. Keep the infant's head lower than the chest.

8. Give five chest thrusts. Position two to three fingers on the sternum just below

PROCEDURE 15:2F

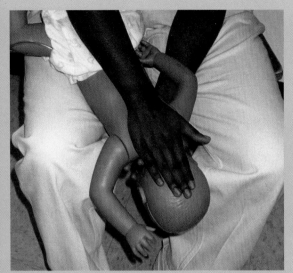

FIGURE 15-18A To give an infant five back blows, position the infant face down, with the head lower than the chest.

an imaginary line drawn between the nipples. Press straight down five times (figure 15-18B), to compress the sternum ⅓ to ½ the depth of the chest.

9. Continue the cycle of five back blows followed by five chest thrusts until EMS arrives or the infant becomes unresponsive.

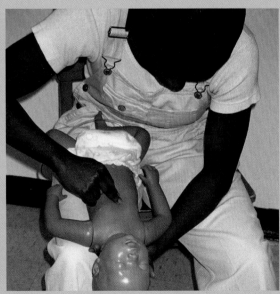

FIGURE 15-18B Give the infant five chest thrusts, keeping the head lower than the chest.

10. If the infant becomes unresponsive, place the infant on a firm surface. Open the airway and look for an object. If an object is visible, use a C-shaped or hooking motion to remove it. Then perform CPR following the normal procedure for an infant, except look in the mouth every time you are ready to give breaths.

    a. Attempt to give two breaths.

    b. Check the brachial pulse for at least 5 but not more than 10 seconds.

    c. If there is a pulse, continue to try to give breaths and check the pulse every 2 minutes.

    d. If there is no pulse, give CPR cycles of 30 compressions followed by 2 respirations.

    e. Check the mouth for the object every time you are ready to give breaths.

11. Do *not* stop CPR unless the infant recovers, help arrives to take over, a physician or other legally qualified person orders you to discontinue the attempt, you are so physically exhausted you cannot continue, or the scene suddenly becomes unsafe.

12. Make every effort to obtain medical help for the infant as soon as possible.

13. After the practice session, use a gauze pad saturated with 70-percent alcohol or a 10-percent bleach disinfecting solution to clean the manikin. Wipe the face and clean inside the mouth thoroughly. Saturate a clean gauze pad with the solution and lay it on the mouth area for at least 30 seconds. Use another gauze pad to wipe the area dry. Follow manufacturer's recommendations for specific cleaning or care.

NOTE: A 10-percent bleach solution is more effective than alcohol. Some manikins have disposable mouthpieces that are discarded after use. If the mouth-

PROCEDURE 15:2F

piece is discarded, the remainder of the face should still be disinfected.

14. Replace all equipment used. Wash hands.

✔ **Final Checkpoint** Using the criteria listed on the evaluation sheet, your instructor will grade your performance.

Practice
Go to the workbook and use the evaluation sheet for 15:2F, Performing CPR—Obstructed Airway on Conscious Infant, to practice this procedure. When you believe you have mastered this skill, sign the sheet and give it to your instructor for further action.

15:3 INFORMATION

Providing First Aid for Bleeding and Wounds

INTRODUCTION

In any health career, as well as in your personal life, you may need to provide first aid to control bleeding or care for wounds. A **wound** involves injury to the soft tissues. Wounds are usually classified as open or closed. With an open wound, there is a break in the skin or mucous membrane. With a closed wound, there is no break in the skin or mucous membrane but injury occurs to the underlying tissues. An example of a closed wound is a bruise or hematoma. Wounds can result in bleeding, infection, and/or tetanus (lockjaw, a serious infection caused by bacteria). First aid care must be directed toward controlling bleeding before the bleeding leads to death, and toward preventing or obtaining treatment for infection.

TYPES OF OPEN WOUNDS

Open wounds are classified into types according to the injuries that occur. Some main types are abrasions, incisions, lacerations, punctures, avulsions, and amputations.

♦ **Abrasion:** With this type of wound the skin is scraped off. Bleeding is usually limited, but infection must be prevented because dirt and contaminants often enter the wound.

♦ **Incision:** This is a cut or injury caused by a sharp object such as a knife, scissors, or razor blade. The edges of the wound are smooth and regular. If the cut is deep, bleeding can be heavy and can lead to excessive blood loss. In addition, damage to muscles, nerves, and other tissues can occur (figure 15-19).

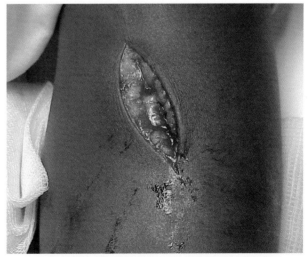

FIGURE 15-19 An incision, caused by a sharp object such as a knife or razor blade, can cause heavy bleeding and/or damage to muscles, nerves, and other tissues. *(Courtesy of Ron Stram, MD, Albany Medical Center, Albany, NY)*

♦ **Laceration:** This type of wound involves tearing of the tissues by way of excessive force. The wound often has jagged, irregular edges. Bleeding may be heavy. If the wound is deep, contamination may lead to infection.

♦ **Puncture:** This type of wound is caused by a sharp object such as a pin, nail, or pointed instrument. Gunshot wounds can also cause puncture wounds that are extremely dangerous because the damage is hidden under the skin and not visible. With all puncture wounds, external bleeding is usually limited, but internal bleeding can occur. In addition, the chance for infection is increased and tetanus may develop if tetanus bacteria enter the wound.

♦ **Avulsion:** This type of wound occurs when tissue is torn or separated from the victim's body. It can result in a piece of torn tissue hanging from the ear, nose, hand, or other body part. Bleeding is heavy and usually extensive. It is important to preserve the body part while caring for this type of wound, because a surgeon may be able to reattach it.

♦ **Amputation:** This type of injury occurs when a body part is cut off and separated from the body. Loss of a finger, toe, hand, or other body part can occur. Bleeding can be heavy and extensive. Care must be taken to preserve the amputated part because a surgeon may be able to reattach it. The part should be wrapped in a cool, moist dressing (use sterile water or normal saline, if possible) and placed in a plastic bag. The plastic bag should be kept cool or placed in ice water and transported with the victim. The body part should never be placed directly on ice because ice can freeze the tissue.

CONTROLLING BLEEDING

Controlling bleeding is the first priority in caring for wounds, because it is possible for a victim to bleed to death in a short period of time. Bleeding can come from arteries, veins, and capillaries. *Arterial blood* usually spurts from a wound, results in heavy blood loss, and is bright red. Arterial bleeding is life-threatening and must be controlled quickly. *Venous blood* is slower, steadier, and dark red or maroon. Venous bleeding is con-

stant and can lead to a large blood loss, but it is easier to control. *Capillary blood* "oozes" from the wound slowly, is less red than arterial blood, and clots easily. The four main methods for controlling bleeding are listed in the order in which they should be used: direct pressure, elevation, pressure bandage, and pressure points.

🔲 **CAUTION:** If possible, use some type of protective barrier, such as gloves or plastic wrap, while controlling bleeding. If this is not possible in an emergency, use thick layers of dressings and try to avoid contact of blood with your skin. Wash your hands thoroughly and as soon as possible after giving first aid to a bleeding victim.

♦ *Direct pressure*: Using your gloved hand over a thick dressing or sterile gauze, apply pressure directly to the wound (figure 15-20A). If no dressing is available, use a clean cloth or linen-type towel. In an emergency when no materials are available, it may even be necessary to use a bare hand. Continue to apply pressure for 5–10 minutes or until the bleeding stops. If blood soaks through the dressing, apply a second dressing over the first and continue to apply direct pressure. Do *not* disturb blood clots once they have formed. Direct pressure will usually stop most bleeding.

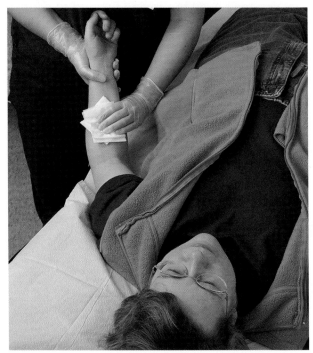

FIGURE 15-20A If possible, use some type of protective barrier, such as gloves or plastic wrap, while applying direct pressure to control bleeding.

♦ *Elevation*: Raise the injured part above the level of the victim's heart to allow gravity to aid in stopping the blood flow from the wound. Continue applying direct pressure while elevating the injured part (figure 15-20B).

▽ **CAUTION:** If fractures (broken bones) are present or suspected, the part should *not* be elevated.

♦ *Pressure bandage*: Apply a pressure bandage to hold the dressings in place. Maintain direct pressure and elevation while applying the pressure bandage. The procedure for applying a pressure bandage is described in step 4 of Procedure 15:3.

♦ *Pressure points*: If direct pressure, elevation, and the pressure bandage do not stop severe bleeding, it may be necessary to apply pressure to pressure points. By applying pressure to a main artery and pressing it against an underlying bone, the main blood supply to the injured area can be cut off. However, because this technique also stops circulation to other parts of the limb, it should *not* be used any longer than is absolutely necessary. Direct pressure and elevation should also be continued while pressure is being applied to the pressure point.

The main pressure point for the arm is the brachial artery. It is located on the inside of the arm, approximately halfway between the armpit and the elbow (figure 15-20C). The main pressure point for the leg is the femoral artery. The pulsation can be felt at the groin (the front middle point of the upper leg, in the crease where the thigh joins the body) (figure 15-20D). When bleeding stops, slowly release pressure on the pressure point. Continue using direct pressure and elevation. If bleeding starts again, be ready to reapply pressure to the correct pressure point.

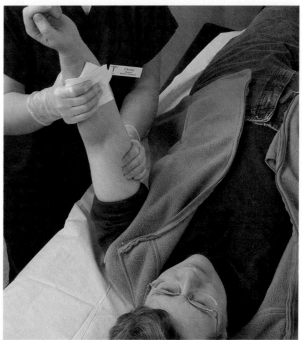

FIGURE 15-20C The main pressure point for the arm is the brachial artery. Pressure is applied to the artery only until the bleeding stops.

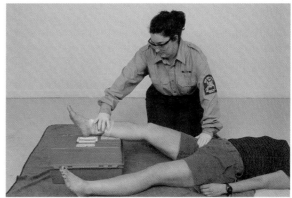

FIGURE 15-20D The main pressure point in the leg is the femoral artery. Pressure is applied while maintaining direct pressure to and elevation of the injured part.

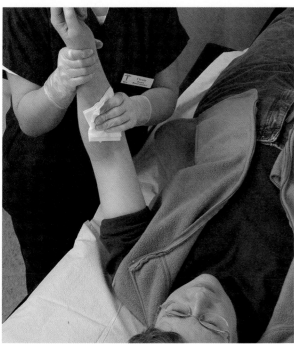

FIGURE 15-20B Continue to apply direct pressure while elevating the injured part above the level of the heart.

After severe bleeding has been controlled, obtain medical help for the victim. Do not disturb any blood clots or remove the dressings that were used to control the bleeding, because this may result in additional bleeding. Make no attempt to clean the wound, because this too is likely to result in additional bleeding.

MINOR WOUNDS

In treating minor wounds that do not involve severe bleeding, prevention of infection is the first priority. Wash your hands thoroughly before treating the wound. Put on gloves to avoid contamination from blood or fluid draining from the wound. Use soap and water and sterile gauze, if possible, to wash the wound. Wipe in an outward direction, away from the wound. Discard the wipe after each use. Rinse the wound thoroughly with cool water. Use sterile gauze to gently blot the wound dry. Apply a sterile dressing or bandage. Watch for any signs of infection. Be sure to tell the victim to obtain medical help if any signs of infection appear.

Infection can develop in any wound. It is important to recognize the signs of infection and to seek medical help if they appear. Some signs and symptoms are swelling, heat, redness, pain, fever, pus, and red streaks leading from the wound. Prompt medical care is needed if any of these symptoms occur.

Tetanus bacteria can enter an open wound and lead to serious illness and death. Tetanus infection is most common in puncture wounds and wounds that involve damage to tissue underneath the skin. When this type of wound occurs, it is important to obtain information from the patient regarding his or her last tetanus shot and to get medical advice regarding protection in the form of a tetanus shot or booster.

With some wounds, objects can remain in the tissues or become embedded in the wound. Examples of such objects include splinters, small pieces of glass, small stones, and other similar objects. If the object is at the surface of the skin, remove it gently with sterile tweezers or tweezers wiped clean with alcohol or a disinfectant. Any objects embedded in the tissues should be left in the skin and removed by a physician.

CLOSED WOUNDS

Closed wounds (those not involving breaks in the skin) can occur anywhere in the body as a result of injury. If the wound is a bruise, cold applications can be applied to reduce swelling. Other closed wounds can be extremely serious and cause internal bleeding that may lead to death. Signs and symptoms may include pain, tenderness, swelling, deformity, cold and clammy skin, rapid and weak pulse, a drop in blood pressure, uncontrolled restlessness, excessive thirst, vomited blood, or blood in the urine or feces. Get medical help for the victim as soon as possible. Check breathing, treat for shock, avoid unnecessary movement, and avoid giving any fluids or food to the victim.

SUMMARY

While caring for any victim with severe bleeding or wounds, always be alert for the signs of shock. Be prepared to treat shock while providing care to control bleeding and prevent infection in the wound.

At all times, remain calm while providing first aid. Reassure the victim. Obtain appropriate assistance or medical care as soon as possible in every case requiring additional care.

STUDENT: *Go to the workbook and complete the assignment sheet for 15:3, Providing First Aid for Bleeding and Wounds. Then return and continue with the procedure.*

PROCEDURE 15:3

Providing First Aid for Bleeding and Wounds

Equipment and Supplies

Sterile dressings and bandages, disposable gloves

Procedure

Severe Wounds

1. Follow the steps of priority care, if indicated.

   a. Check the scene. Move the victim only if absolutely necessary.

   b. Check the victim for consciousness and breathing.

   c. Call emergency medical services (EMS).

   d. Provide care to the victim.

2. To control severe bleeding, proceed as follows:

   a. If possible, put on gloves or wrap your hands in plastic wrap to provide a protective barrier while controlling bleeding. If this is not possible in an emergency, use thick layers of dressings and try to avoid contact of blood with your skin.

   b. Using your hand over a thick dressing or sterile gauze, apply pressure directly to the wound.

   c. Continue to apply pressure to the wound for approximately 5–10 minutes. Do *not* release the pressure to check whether the bleeding has stopped.

   d. If blood soaks through the first dressing, apply a second dressing on top of the first dressing, and continue to apply direct pressure.

   NOTE: If sterile gauze is *not* available, use clean material or a bare hand.

CAUTION: Do *not* disturb blood clots once they have formed. This will cause the bleeding to start again.

3. Elevate the injured part above the level of the victim's heart unless a fracture or broken bone is suspected.

   NOTE: This allows gravity to help stop the blood flow to the area.

   NOTE: Direct pressure and elevation are used together. Do *not* stop direct pressure while elevating the part.

4. To hold the dressings in place, apply a pressure bandage. Maintain direct pressure and elevation while applying the pressure bandage. To apply a pressure bandage, proceed as follows:

   a. Apply additional dressings over the dressings already on the wound.

   b. Use a roller bandage to hold the dressings in place by wrapping the roller bandage around the dressings. Use overlapping turns to cover the dressings and to hold them securely in place.

   c. Tie off the ends of the bandage by placing the tie directly over the dressings (figure 15-21).

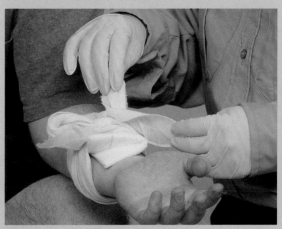

FIGURE 15-21 Tie the ends of the bandage directly over the dressings to secure a pressure bandage.

PROCEDURE 15:3

d. Make sure the pressure bandage is secure. Check a pulse site below the pressure bandage to make sure the bandage is not too tight. A pulse should be present and there should be no discoloration of the skin to indicate impaired circulation. If any signs of impaired circulation are present, loosen and replace the pressure bandage.

5. If the bleeding continues, it may be necessary to apply pressure to the appropriate pressure point. Continue using direct pressure and elevation, and apply pressure to the pressure point as follows:

a. If the wound is on the arm or hand, apply pressure to the brachial artery. Place the flat surface of your fingers (not your fingertips) against the inside of the victim's upper arm, approximately halfway between the elbow and axilla area. Position your thumb on the outside of the arm. Press your fingers toward your thumb to compress the brachial artery and decrease the supply of blood to the arm (refer to figure 15-20C).

b. If the wound is on the leg, place the flat surfaces of your fingers or the heel of one hand directly over the femoral artery where it passes over the pelvic bone. The position is on the front, middle part of the upper thigh (groin) where the leg joins the body. Straighten your arm and apply pressure to compress the femoral artery and to decrease the blood supply to the leg (refer to figure 15-20D).

6. When the bleeding stops, slowly release the pressure on the pressure point while continuing to use direct pressure and elevation. If the bleeding starts again, be ready to reapply pressure to the pressure point.

7. Obtain medical help for the victim as soon as possible. Severe bleeding is a life-threatening emergency.

8. While caring for any victim experiencing severe bleeding, be alert for the signs and symptoms of shock. Treat the victim for shock if any signs or symptoms are noted.

9. During treatment, constantly reassure the victim. Encourage the victim to remain calm by remaining calm yourself.

10. After controlling the bleeding, wash your hands as thoroughly and quickly as possible to avoid possible contamination from the blood. Wear gloves and use a disinfectant solution to wipe up any blood spills. Always wash your hands thoroughly after removing gloves.

Procedure
Minor Wounds

1. Wash hands thoroughly with soap and water. Put on gloves.

2. Use sterile gauze, soap, and water to wash the wound. Start at the center and wash in an outward direction. Discard the gauze after each pass.

3. Rinse the wound thoroughly with cool water to remove all of the soap.

4. Use sterile gauze to dry the wound. Blot it gently.

5. Apply a sterile dressing to the wound.

6. Caution the victim to look for signs of infection. Tell the victim to obtain medical care if any signs of infection appear.

7. If tetanus infection is possible (for example, in cases involving puncture wounds), tell the victim to contact a doctor regarding a tetanus shot.

CAUTION: Do *not* use any antiseptic solutions to clean the wound and do *not*

PROCEDURE 15:3

apply any substances to the wound unless specifically instructed to do so by a physician or your immediate supervisor.

8. Obtain medical help as soon as possible for any victim requiring additional care. Any victim who has particles embedded in a wound, risk for tetanus, severe bleeding, or other complications must be referred for medical care.

9. When care is complete, remove gloves and wash hands thoroughly.

Practice

Go to the workbook and use the evaluation sheet for 15:3, Providing First Aid for Bleeding and Wounds, to practice these procedures. When you believe you have mastered these skills, sign the sheet and give it to your instructor for further action.

✔ **Final Checkpoint** Using the criteria listed on the evaluation sheet, your instructor will grade your performance.

15:4 INFORMATION

Providing First Aid for Shock

INTRODUCTION

Shock is a state that can exist with any injury or illness requiring first aid. It is important that you are able to recognize it and provide treatment.

Shock, also called *hypoperfusion*, can be defined as "a clinical set of signs and symptoms associated with an inadequate supply of blood to body organs, especially the brain and heart." If it is not treated, shock can lead to death, even when a victim's injuries or illness might not themselves be fatal. After just 4–6 minutes of hypoperfusion, brains cells are damaged irreversibly.

CAUSES OF SHOCK

Many different things can cause the victim to experience shock: **hemorrhage** (excessive loss of blood); excessive pain; infection; heart attack; stroke; poisoning by chemicals, drugs, or gases; lack of oxygen; psychological trauma; and dehydration (loss of body fluids) from burns, vomiting, or diarrhea. The eight main types of shock are shown in Table 15-1. All types of shock impair circulation and decrease the supply of oxygen to body cells, tissues, and organs.

SIGNS AND SYMPTOMS

When shock occurs, the body attempts to increase blood flow to the brain, heart, and vital organs by reducing blood flow to other body parts. This can lead to the following signs and symptoms that indicate shock:

♦ Skin is pale or cyanotic (bluish gray) in color. Check the nail beds and the mucous membrane around the mouth.

♦ Skin is cool to the touch.

♦ **Diaphoresis,** or excessive perspiration, may result in a wet, clammy feeling when the skin is touched.

♦ Pulse is rapid, weak, and difficult to feel. Check the pulse at one of the carotid arteries in the neck.

♦ Respirations are rapid, shallow, and may be irregular.

♦ Blood pressure is very low or below normal, and may not be obtainable.

♦ Victim experiences general weakness. As shock progresses, the victim becomes listless

TABLE 15-1 Types of Shock

TYPE OF SHOCK	CAUSE	DESCRIPTION
Anaphylactic	Hypersensitive or allergic reaction to a substance such as food, medications, insect stings or bites, or snake bites	Body releases histamine causing vasodilation (blood vessels get larger) Blood pressure drops and less blood goes to body cells Urticaria (hives) and respiratory distress may occur
Cardiogenic	Damage to heart muscle from heart attack or cardiac arrest	Heart cannot effectively pump blood to body cells
Hemorrhagic	Severe bleeding or loss of blood plasma	Decrease in blood volume causes blood pressure to drop Decreased blood flow to body cells
Metabolic	Loss of body fluid from severe vomiting, diarrhea, or a heat illness Disruption in acid–base balance as occurs in diabetes	Decreased amount of fluid causes dehydration and disruption in normal acid–base balance of body Blood pressure drops and less blood circulates to body cells
Neurogenic	Injury and trauma to brain and/or spinal cord	Nervous system loses ability to control the size of blood vessels Blood vessels dilate and blood pressure drops Decreased blood flow to body cells
Psychogenic	Emotional distress such as anger, fear, or grief	Emotional response causes sudden dilation of blood vessels Blood pools in areas away from the brain Some individuals faint
Respiratory	Trauma to respiratory tract Respiratory distress or arrest (chronic disease, choking)	Interferes with exchange of oxygen and carbon dioxide between lungs and bloodstream Insufficient oxygen supply for body cells
Septic	Acute infection (toxic shock syndrome)	Poisons or toxins in blood cause vasodilation Blood pressure drops Less oxygen to body cells

and confused. Eventually, the victim loses consciousness.

♦ Victim experiences anxiety and extreme restlessness.

♦ Victim may experience excessive thirst, nausea, and/or vomiting.

♦ Victim may complain of blurred vision. As shock progresses, the victim's eyes may appear sunken and have a vacant or confused expression. The pupils may dilate or become large.

TREATMENT FOR SHOCK

It is essential to get medical help for the victim as soon as possible because shock is a life-threatening condition. Treatment for shock is directed toward (1) eliminating the cause of shock; (2) improving circulation, especially to the brain and heart; (3) providing an adequate oxygen supply; and (4) maintaining body temperature. Some of the basic principles for treatment are as follows:

♦ Reduce the effects of or eliminate the cause of shock: control bleeding, provide oxygen if available, ease pain through position change, and/or provide emotional support.

♦ The position for treating shock must be based on the victim's injuries.

 CAUTION: If neck or spine injuries are suspected, the victim should not be moved unless it is necessary to remove him or her from danger.

The best position for treating shock is usually to keep the victim lying flat on the back, because this improves circulation. Raising the feet and legs approximately 12 inches can also provide additional blood for the heart and brain. However, if the victim is vomiting or has bleeding and injuries of the jaw or mouth, the victim should be positioned on the side to prevent him or her from choking on blood and/or vomitus. If a victim is experiencing breathing problems, it may be necessary to raise the victim's head and shoulders to make breathing easier. If the victim has a *head* (not neck) injury and has difficulty breathing, the victim should be positioned lying flat or with the head raised slightly. It is important to position the victim based on the injury or illness involved.

♦ Cover the patient with blankets or additional clothing to prevent chilling or exposure to the cold. Blankets may also be placed between the ground and the victim. However, it is impor-tant to avoid overheating the victim. If the skin is very warm to the touch and perspiration is noted, remove some of the blankets or coverings.

♦ Avoid giving the victim anything to eat or drink. If the victim complains of excessive thirst, a wet cloth can be used to provide some comfort by moistening the lips and mouth.

Remember that it is important to look for signs of shock while providing first aid for any injury or illness. Provide care that will reduce the effect of shock. Obtain medical help for the victim as soon as possible.

STUDENT: *Go to the workbook and complete the assignment sheet for 15:4, Providing First Aid for Shock. Then return and continue with the procedure.*

PROCEDURE 15:4

Providing First Aid for Shock

Equipment and Supplies

Blankets, watch with second hand (optional), disposable gloves

Procedure

1. Follow the steps of priority care, if indicated.

    a. Check the scene. Move the victim only if absolutely necessary.

    b. Check the victim for consciousness and breathing.

    c. Call emergency medical services (EMS).

    d. Provide care to the victim.

    e. Control severe bleeding.

    CAUTION: If possible, wear gloves or use a protective barrier while controlling bleeding.

2. Obtain medical help for the victim as soon as possible. Call or send someone to obtain help.

3. Observe the victim for any signs of shock. Look for a pale or cyanotic (bluish) color to the skin. Touch the skin and note if it is cool, moist, or clammy to the touch. Note diaphoresis, or excessive perspiration. Check the pulse to see if it is rapid, weak, or irregular. If you are unable to feel a radial pulse, check the carotid pulse. Check the respirations to see if they are rapid, weak, irregular, shallow, or labored. If equipment is available, check blood pressure to see if it is low. Observe the victim for signs of weakness, apathy, confusion, or consciousness. Note if the victim is nauseated or vomiting, complaining of excessive thirst, restless or anxious, or complaining of blurred vision. Examine the eyes for a sunken, vacant, or confused appearance, and dilated pupils.

4. Try to reduce the effects or eliminate the cause of shock:

    a. Control bleeding by applying pressure at the site.

    b. Provide oxygen, if possible.

    c. Attempt to ease pain through position changes and comfort measures.

    d. Give emotional support.

PROCEDURE 15:4

5. Position the victim based on the injuries or illness present.

   a. If an injury of the neck or spine is present or suspected, do not move the victim.

   b. If the victim has bleeding and injuries to the jaw or mouth, or is vomiting, position the victim's body on either side. This allows fluids, vomitus, and/or blood to drain and prevents the airway from becoming blocked by these fluids.

   c. If the victim is having difficulty breathing, position the victim on the back, but raise the head and shoulders slightly to aid breathing.

   d. If the victim has a head injury, position the victim lying flat or with the head raised slightly.

   NOTE: Never allow the head to be positioned lower than the rest of the body.

   e. If none of these conditions exist, position the victim lying flat on the back. To improve circulation, raise the feet and legs approximately 12 inches (figure 15-22). If raising the legs causes pain or leads to difficult breathing, however, lower the legs to the flat position.

   CAUTION: Do not raise the legs if the victim has head, neck, or back injuries, or if there are possible fractures of the hips or legs.

   f. If in doubt on how to position a victim according to the injuries involved, keep the victim lying down flat or in the position in which you found him or her. Avoid any unnecessary movement.

6. Place enough blankets or coverings on the victim to prevent chilling. Sometimes, a blanket can be placed between the victim and the ground. Avoid overheating the victim.

7. Do not give the victim anything to eat or drink. If the victim complains of excessive thirst, use a moist cloth to wet the lips, tongue, and inside of the mouth.

8. Constantly reassure the victim. Encourage the victim to remain calm by remaining calm yourself.

9. Observe and provide care to the victim until medical help is obtained.

10. Replace all equipment used. Wash hands.

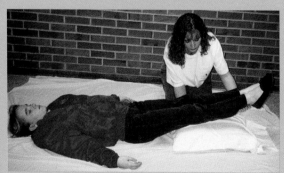

FIGURE 15-22 Position a shock victim flat on the back and elevate the feet and legs approximately 12 inches. Do *not* use this position if the victim has a neck, spinal, head, or jaw injury, or if the victim is having difficulty breathing.

Practice

Go to the workbook and use the evaluation sheet for 15:4, Providing First Aid for Shock, to practice this procedure. When you believe you have mastered this skill, sign the sheet and give it to your instructor for further action.

 Final Checkpoint Using the criteria listed on the evaluation sheet, your instructor will grade your performance.

15:5 INFORMATION

Providing First Aid for Poisoning

INTRODUCTION

Poisoning can occur anywhere, anytime—not only in health care settings, but also in your personal life. **Poisoning** can happen to any individual, regardless of age. It can be caused by ingesting (swallowing) various substances, inhaling poisonous gases, injecting substances, or contacting the skin with poison. Any substance that causes a harmful reaction when applied or ingested can be called a poison. Immediate action is necessary for any poisoning victim. Treatment varies depending on the type of poison, the injury involved, and the method of contact.

If the poisoning victim is unconscious, check for breathing. Provide artificial respiration if the victim is not breathing. Obtain medical help as soon as possible. If the unconscious victim is breathing, position the victim on his or her side so fluids can drain from the mouth. Obtain medical help quickly.

INGESTION POISONING

If a poison has been swallowed, immediate care must be provided before the poison can be absorbed into the body. Basic steps of first aid include:

♦ Call a poison control center (PCC) or a physician immediately. If you cannot contact a PCC, call emergency medical services (EMS). Most areas have poison control centers that provide information on specific antidotes and treatment.

♦ Save the label or container of the substance taken so this information can be given to the PCC or physician.

♦ Calculate or estimate how much was taken and the time at which the poisoning occurred.

♦ If the victim vomits, save a sample of the vomited material.

♦ If the PCC tells you to induce vomiting, get the victim to vomit. To induce vomiting, tickle the back of the victim's throat or give the victim warm saltwater to drink. In some cases, the PCC may recommend giving syrup of ipecac followed by a glass of water. Recent studies have shown that syrup of ipecac can cause dehydration and confusion, so it should only be given if recommended by the PCC or a physician. Follow dosage recommended on bottle. Syrup of ipecac is available in most drug stores and can be kept in a first aid kit for poisoning victims.

▽ **CAUTION:** Vomiting must *not* be induced in unconscious victims, victims who swallowed an acid or alkali, victims who swallowed petroleum products, victims who are convulsing, or victims who have burns on the lips and mouth.

♦ Activated charcoal may be recommended by the PCC to bind to the poison so it is not absorbed into the body. Activated charcoal should only be given to victims who are conscious and able to swallow. It is available in most drug stores. The directions on the bottle should be followed to determine the correct dosage.

INHALATION POISONING

If poisoning is caused by inhalation of dangerous gases, the victim must be removed immediately from the area before being treated. A commonly inhaled poison is carbon monoxide. It is odorless, colorless, and very difficult to detect. Basic steps of first aid include:

♦ Before entering the danger area, take a deep breath of fresh air and do *not* breathe the gas while you are removing the victim from the area.

♦ After rescuing the victim, immediately check for breathing.

♦ Provide artificial respiration if needed.

♦ Obtain medical help immediately; death may occur very quickly with this type of poisoning.

CONTACT POISONING

If poisoning is caused by chemicals or poisons coming in contact with the victim's skin, care for the victim includes:

♦ Use large amounts of water to wash the skin for at least 15–20 minutes to dilute the substance and remove it from the skin.

♦ Remove any clothing and jewelry that contain the substance.

♦ Call a PCC or physician for additional information.

♦ Obtain medical help as soon as possible for burns or injuries that may result from contact with the poison.

Contact with a poisonous plant such as poison ivy, oak, or sumac can cause a serious skin reaction if not treated immediately. Basic steps of first aid include:

♦ Wash the area thoroughly with soap and water

♦ If a rash or weeping sores develop after 2–3 days, lotions such as Calamine or Caladryl, or a paste made from baking soda and water may help relieve the discomfort.

♦ If the condition is severe and affects large areas of the body or face, obtain medical help.

INJECTION POISONING

Injection poisoning occurs when an insect, spider, or snake bites or stings an individual. If an arm or leg is affected, position the affected area below the level of the heart. For an insect sting, first aid treatment includes:

♦ Remove any embedded stinger by scraping the stinger away from the skin with the edge of a rigid card, such as a credit card, or a tongue depressor. Do not use tweezers because tweezers can puncture the venom sac attached to the stinger, injecting more poison into body tissues.

♦ Wash the area well with soap and water.

♦ Apply a sterile dressing and a cold pack to reduce swelling.

If a tick is embedded in the skin, first aid treatment includes:

♦ Use tweezers to slowly pull the tick out of the skin.

♦ Wash the area thoroughly with soap and water.

♦ Apply an antiseptic.

♦ Watch for signs of infection.

♦ Obtain medical help if needed.

Ticks can cause Rocky Mountain spotted fever or Lyme disease, dangerous diseases if untreated.

For a snakebite or spider bite, first aid treatment includes:

♦ Wash the wound.

♦ Immobilize the injured area, positioning it lower than the heart, if possible.

♦ Do *not* cut the wound or apply a tourniquet.

♦ Monitor the breathing of the victim and give artificial respiration if necessary.

♦ Obtain medical help for the victim as soon as possible.

For any type of injection poisoning, watch for allergic reaction in all victims (figure 15-23). Signs and symptoms of allergic reaction include redness and swelling at the site, itching, hives, pain, swelling of the throat, difficult or labored breathing, dizziness, and a change in the level of consciousness. Maintain respirations and obtain medical help as quickly as possible for the victim who experiences an allergic reaction.

SUMMARY

In all poisoning victims, observe for signs of anaphylactic shock. Treat the victim for shock, if necessary. Try to remain calm and confident while providing first aid for poisoning victims. Reassure the victim as needed. Act quickly and in an organized, efficient manner.

STUDENT: *Go to the workbook and complete the assignment sheet for 15:5, Providing First Aid for Poisoning. Then return and continue with the procedure.*

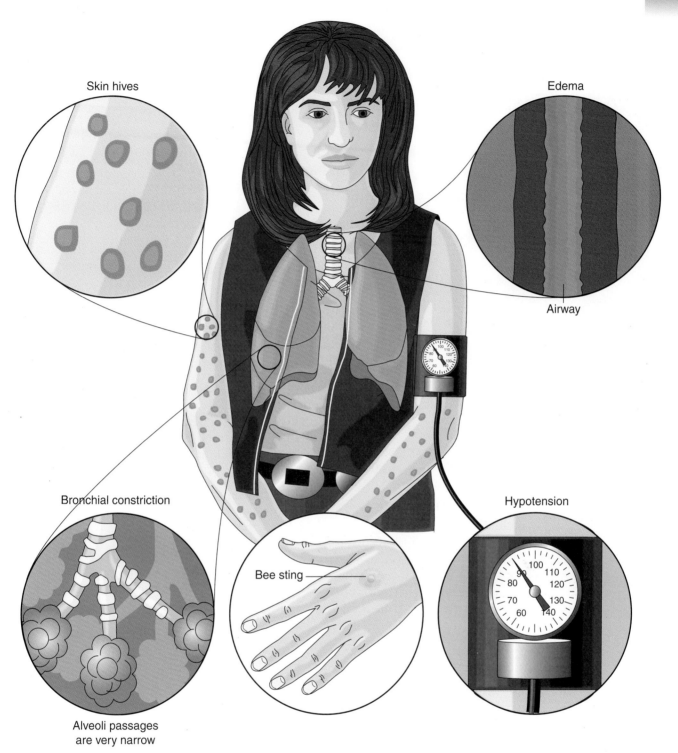

Skin hives

Edema

Airway

Bronchial constriction

Bee sting

Hypotension

Alveoli passages
are very narrow

FIGURE 15-23 Watch for allergic reactions in all poisoning victims.

PROCEDURE 15:5

Providing First Aid for Poisoning

Equipment and Supplies

Telephone, disposable gloves

Procedure

1. Follow the steps of priority care, if indicated:

   a. Check the scene. Move the victim only if absolutely necessary.

   b. Check the victim for consciousness and breathing.

   c. Call emergency medical services (EMS).

   d. Provide care to the victim.

   e. Control severe bleeding.

   CAUTION: If possible, wear gloves or use a protective barrier while controlling bleeding.

2. Check the victim for signs of poisoning. Signs may include burns on the lips or mouth, odor, a container of poison, or presence of the poisonous substance on the victim or in the victim's mouth. Information may also be obtained from the victim or from an observer.

3. If the victim is conscious, not convulsing, and has swallowed a poison:

   a. Try to determine the type of poison, how much was taken, and when the poison was taken. Look for the container near the victim.

   b. Call a poison control center (PCC) or physician immediately for specific information on how to treat the poisoning victim. Provide as much information as possible.

   c. Follow the instructions received from the PCC. Obtain medical help if needed.

   d. If the victim vomits, save a sample of the vomited material.

4. If the PCC tells you to get the victim to vomit, induce vomiting. Give the victim warm salt water or tickle the back of the victim's throat. Syrup of ipecac is also used to induce vomiting, but it should not be given to a victim unless the PCC or a physician tells you to use it.

   CAUTION: Do *not* induce vomiting if the victim is unconscious or convulsing, has burns on the lips or mouth, or has swallowed an acid, alkali, or petroleum product.

5. If the PCC tells you to give the victim activated charcoal, follow the directions on the container. Make sure the victim is conscious and able to swallow before giving the charcoal.

   NOTE: Activated charcoal binds to the poison so it is not absorbed into the body.

6. If the victim is unconscious:

   a. Check for breathing. If the victim is not breathing, give artificial respiration and/or CPR as needed.

   b. If the victim is breathing, position the victim on his or her side to allow fluids to drain from the mouth.

   c. Call a PCC or physician for specific treatment. Obtain medical help immediately.

   d. If possible, save the poison container and a sample of any vomited material. Check with any observers to find out what was taken, how much was taken, and when the poison was taken.

7. If chemicals or poisons have splashed on the victim's skin, wash the area thoroughly with large amounts of water.

PROCEDURE 15:5

Remove any clothing and jewelry containing the substance. If a large area of the body is affected, a shower, tub, or garden hose may be used to rinse the skin. Obtain medical help immediately for burns or injuries caused by the poison.

8. If the victim has come in contact with a poisonous plant such as poison ivy, oak, or sumac, wash the area of contact thoroughly with soap and water. Remove any contaminated clothing. If a rash or weeping sores develop in the next few days after exposure, lotions such as Calamine or Caladryl, or a paste made from baking soda and water, may help relieve the discomfort. If the condition is severe and affects large areas of the body or face, obtain medical help.

9. If the victim has inhaled poisonous gas, do not endanger your life by trying to treat the victim in the area of the gas. Take a deep breath of fresh air before entering the area and hold your breath while you remove the victim from the area. When the victim is in a safe area, check for breathing. Provide artificial respiration and/or CPR as needed. Obtain medical help immediately.

10. If poisoning is caused by injection from an insect bite or sting or a snakebite, proceed as follows:

    a. If an arm or leg is affected, position the affected area below the level of the heart.

    b. For an insect bite, remove any embedded stinger by scraping it off with an object like a credit card. Wash the area well with soap and water. Apply a sterile dressing and a cold pack to reduce swelling.

    c. If a tick is embedded in the skin, use tweezers to gently pull the tick out of the skin. Wash the area thoroughly with soap and water, and apply an antiseptic. Obtain medical help if needed.

    d. For a snakebite, wash the wound. Immobilize the injured area, positioning it lower than the heart if possible. Monitor the breathing of the victim and give artificial respiration if necessary. Obtain medical help for the victim as soon as possible.

    e. Watch for the signs and symptoms of allergic reaction in all victims. Signs and symptoms of allergic reaction include redness and swelling at the site, itching, hives (figure 15-24), pain, swelling of the throat, difficult or labored breathing, dizziness, and a change in the level of consciousness. Maintain respirations and obtain medical help as quickly as possible for the victim experiencing an allergic reaction.

11. Observe for signs of anaphylactic shock while treating any poisoning victim. Treat for shock as necessary.

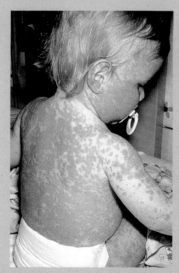

FIGURE 15-24 Hives are a common sign of an allergic reaction. *(Courtesy of Robert A. Silverman, MD, Clinical Associate Professor, Department of Pediatrics, Georgetown University, Georgetown, MD)*

PROCEDURE 15:5

12. Remain calm while treating the victim. Reassure the victim.

13. Always obtain medical help for any poisoning victim. Some poisons may have delayed reactions. Always keep the telephone numbers of a PCC and other sources of medical assistance in a convenient location so you will be prepared to provide first aid for poisoning.

14. Wash hands thoroughly after providing care.

Practice
Go to the workbook and use the evaluation sheet for 15:5, Providing First Aid for Poisoning, to practice this procedure. When you believe you have mastered this skill, sign the sheet and give it to your instructor for further action.

✔ **Final Checkpoint** Using the criteria listed on the evaluation sheet, your instructor will grade your performance.

15:6 INFORMATION

Providing First Aid for Burns

TYPES OF BURNS

A **burn** is an injury that can be caused by fire, heat, chemical agents, radiation, and/or electricity. Burns are classified as either superficial, partial thickness, or full thickness (figure 15-25). Characteristics of each type of burn are as follows:

♦ *Superficial, or first-degree, burn*: This is the least severe type of burn. It involves only the top layer of skin, the epidermis, and usually heals in 5–6 days without permanent scarring. The skin is usually reddened or discolored. There may be some mild swelling, and the victim feels pain. Three common causes are overexposure to the sun (sunburn), brief contact with hot objects or steam, and exposure of the skin to a weak acid or alkali.

♦ *Partial-thickness, or second-degree, burn*: This type of burn involves injury to the top layers of skin, including both the epidermis and dermis. A blister or vesicle forms. The skin is red or has a mottled appearance. Swelling usually occurs, and the surface of the skin frequently appears to be wet. This is a painful burn and

may take 3–4 weeks to heal. Frequent causes include excessive exposure to the sun, a sunlamp, or artificial radiation; contact with hot or boiling liquids; and contact with fire.

♦ *Full-thickness, or third-degree, burn*: This is the most severe type of burn and involves injury to all layers of the skin plus the underlying tissue. The area involved has a white or charred appearance. This type of burn can be either extremely painful or, if nerve endings are destroyed, relatively painless. Third-degree burns can be life-threatening because of fluid loss, infection, and shock. Frequent causes include exposure to fire or flames, prolonged contact with hot objects, contact with electricity, and immersion in hot or boiling liquids.

TREATMENT

First aid treatment for burns is directed toward removing the source of heat, cooling the affected skin area, covering the burn, relieving pain, observing and treating for shock, and preventing infection. Medical treatment is not usually required for superficial and mild partial-thickness burns. However, medical care should be obtained if more than 15 percent of the surface of an adult's body is burned (10 percent in a child).

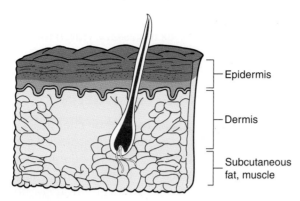

- Epidermis
- Dermis
- Subcutaneous fat, muscle

Skin red, dry

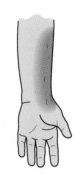

Superficial, first degree

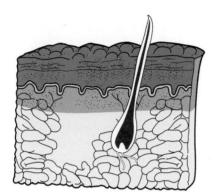

Blistered, skin moist, pink or red

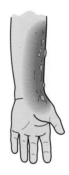

Partial thickness, second degree

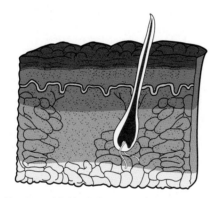

Charring, skin black, brown, red

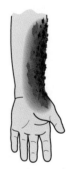

Full thickness, third degree

FIGURE 15-25 Types of burns

The rule of nines is used to calculate the percentage of body surface burned (figure 15-26). Medical care should also be obtained if the burns affect the face or respiratory tract; if the victim has difficulty breathing; if burns cover more than one body part; if the victim has a partial-thickness burn and is under 5 or over 60 years of age; or if the burns resulted from chemicals, explosions, or electricity. All victims with full-thickness burns should receive medical care.

Superficial and Mild Partial-Thickness Burns

The main treatment for superficial and mild partial-thickness burns is to cool the area by flushing it with large amounts of cool water. Do *not* use ice or ice water on burns because doing so causes the body to lose heat. After the pain subsides, use dry, sterile gauze to blot the area dry. Apply a dry, sterile dressing to prevent infec-

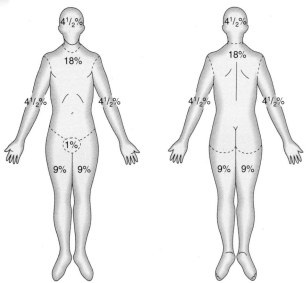

FIGURE 15-26 The *rule of nines* is used to calculate the percentage of body surface burned.

tion. If nonadhesive dressings are available, it is best to use them because they will not stick to the injured area. If possible, elevate the affected part to reduce swelling caused by inflammation. If necessary, obtain medical help.

 CAUTION: Do *not* apply cotton, tissues, ointment, powders, oils, grease, butter, or any other substances to the burned area unless you are instructed to do so by a physician or your immediate supervisor. Do *not* break or open any blisters that form on burns because doing so will just cause an open wound that is prone to infection.

Severe Partial-Thickness and Full-Thickness Burns

Call for medical help immediately if the victim has severe partial-thickness or full-thickness burns. Cover the burned areas with thick, sterile dressings. Elevate the hands or feet if they are burned. If the feet or legs are burned, do *not* allow the victim to walk. If particles of clothing are attached to the burned areas, do *not* attempt to remove these particles. Watch the victim closely for signs of respiratory distress and/or shock.

Provide artificial respiration and treatment for shock, as necessary. Watch the victim closely until medical help arrives.

Chemical Burns

For burns caused by chemicals splashing on the skin, use large amounts of water to flush the affected areas for 15–30 minutes or until medical help arrives. Gently remove any clothing, socks and shoes, or jewelry that contains the chemical to minimize the area injured. Continue flushing the skin with cool water and watch the victim for signs of shock until medical help can be obtained.

If the *eyes* have been burned by chemicals or irritating gases, flush the eyes with large amounts of water for at least 15–30 minutes or until medical help arrives. If only one eye is injured, be sure to tilt the victim's head in the direction of the injury so the injured eye can be properly flushed. Start at the inner corner of the eye and allow the water to run over the surface of the eye and to the outside. Continue flushing the eye with cool water and watch the victim for signs of shock until medical help can be obtained.

 CAUTION: Make sure that the water (or remaining chemical) does not enter the *uninjured* eye.

SUMMARY

Loss of body fluids (dehydration) can occur very quickly with severe burns, so shock is frequently noted in burn victims. Be alert for any signs of shock and treat the burn victim for shock immediately.

Remain calm while treating the burn victim. Reassure the victim. Obtain medical help as quickly as possible for any burn victim requiring medical assistance.

STUDENT: *Go to the workbook and complete the assignment sheet for 15:6, Providing First Aid for Burns. Then return and continue with the procedure.*

PROCEDURE 15:6

Providing First Aid for Burns

Equipment and Supplies

Water, sterile dressings, disposable gloves

Procedure

1. Follow the priorities of care, if indicated:

    a. Check the scene. Move the victim only if absolutely necessary.

    b. Check the victim for consciousness and breathing.

    c. Call emergency medical services (EMS) if necessary.

    d. Provide care to the victim.

    e. Check for bleeding. Control severe bleeding.

    ⊞ **CAUTION:** If possible, wear gloves or use a protective barrier while controlling bleeding.

2. Check the burned area carefully to determine the type of burn. A reddened or discolored area is usually a superficial, or first-degree, burn. If the skin is wet, red, swollen, painful, and blistered, the burn is usually a partial-thickness, or second-degree, burn (figure 15-27A). If the skin is white or charred and there is destruction of tissue, the burn is a full-thickness, or third-degree, burn (figure 15-27B).

    NOTE: Victims can have more than one type of burn at one time. Treat for the most severe type of burn present.

3. For a superficial or mild partial-thickness burn:

    a. Cool the burn by flushing it with large amounts of cool water. If this is not possible, apply clean or sterile cloths that are cold and wet. Continue

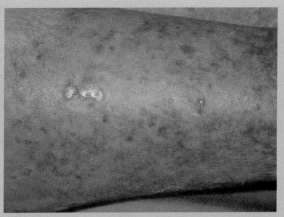

FIGURE 15-27A The skin is wet, red, swollen, painful, and blistered when a partial-thickness burn is present. *(Courtesy of the Phoenix Society of Burn Survivors, Inc.)*

applying cold water until the pain subsides.

    b. Use sterile gauze to gently blot the injured area dry.

    c. Apply dry, sterile dressings to the burned area. If possible, use nonadhesive (nonstick) dressings, because they will not stick to the burn.

    d. If blisters are present, do *not* break or open them.

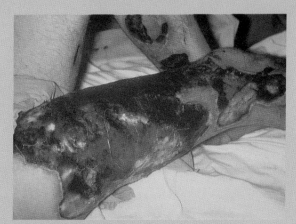

FIGURE 15-27B A full-thickness burn destroys or affects all layers of the skin plus fat, muscle, bone, and nerve tissue. The skin is white or charred in appearance. *(Courtesy of the Phoenix Society of Burn Survivors, Inc.)*

PROCEDURE 15:6

e. If possible, elevate the burned area to reduce swelling caused by inflammation.

f. Obtain medical help for burns to the face, or if burns cover more than 15 percent of the surface of an adult's body or 10 percent of the surface of a child's body. If the victim is having difficulty breathing, or any other distress is noted, obtain medical help.

g. Do *not* apply any cotton, ointment, powders, grease, butter, or similar substances to the burned area.

NOTE: These substances may increase the possibility of infection.

4. For a severe partial-thickness or any full-thickness burn:

a. Call for medical help immediately.

b. Use thick, sterile dressings to cover the injured areas.

c. Do *not* attempt to remove any particles of clothing that have stuck to the burned areas.

d. If the hands and arms or legs and feet are affected, elevate these areas.

e. If the victim has burns on the face or is experiencing difficulty in breathing, elevate the head.

f. Watch the victim closely for signs of shock and provide care if necessary.

5. For a burn caused by a chemical splashing on the skin:

a. Using large amounts of water, immediately flush the area for 15–30 minutes or until medical help arrives.

b. Remove any articles of clothing, socks and shoes, or jewelry contaminated by the substance.

c. Continue flushing the area with large amounts of cool water.

d. Obtain medical help immediately.

6. If the eye has been burned by chemicals or irritating gases:

a. If the victim is wearing contact lenses or glasses, ask him or her to remove them quickly.

b. Tilt the victim's head toward the injured side.

c. Hold the eyelid of the injured eye open. Pour cool water from the inner part of the eye (the part closest to the nose) toward the outer part (figure 15-28).

d. Use cool water to irrigate the eye for 15–30 minutes or until medical help arrives.

▽ **CAUTION:** Take care that the water or chemicals do not enter the uninjured eye.

e. Obtain medical help immediately.

7. Observe for the signs of shock in all burn victims. Treat for shock as necessary.

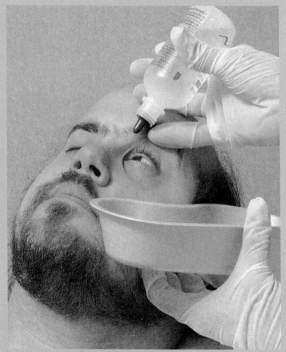

FIGURE 15-28 To irrigate an eye, hold the eyelid open and irrigate from the inner part of the eye toward the outer part.

PROCEDURE 15:6

8. Reassure the victim as you are providing treatment. Remain calm and encourage the victim to remain calm.

9. Obtain medical help immediately for any burn victim with extensive burns, full-thickness burns, burns to the face, signs of shock, respiratory distress, eye burns, and/or chemical burns to the skin.

10. Wash hands thoroughly after providing care.

Practice

Go to the workbook and use the evaluation sheet for 15:6, Providing First Aid for Burns, to practice this procedure. When you believe you have mastered this skill, sign the sheet and give it to your instructor for further action.

 Final Checkpoint Using the criteria listed on the evaluation sheet, your instructor will grade your performance.

15:7 INFORMATION

Providing First Aid for Heat Exposure

Excessive exposure to heat or high external temperatures can lead to a life-threatening emergency (figure 15-29). Overexposure to heat can cause a chemical imbalance in the body that can eventually lead to death. Harmful reactions can occur when water or salt are lost through perspiration or when the body cannot eliminate excess heat.

Heat cramps are caused by exposure to heat. They are muscle pains and spasms that result from the loss of water and salt through perspiration. Firm pressure applied to the cramped muscle will provide relief from the discomfort. The victim should rest and move to a cooler area. In addition, small sips of water or an electrolyte solution, such as sport drinks, can be given to the victim.

Heat exhaustion occurs when a victim is exposed to heat and experiences a loss of fluids through sweating. Signs and symptoms include pale and clammy skin, profuse perspiration (diaphoresis), fatigue or tiredness, weakness, headache, muscle cramps, nausea and/or vomiting, and dizziness and/or fainting. Body temperature is about normal or just slightly elevated. It is important to treat heat exhaustion as quickly as

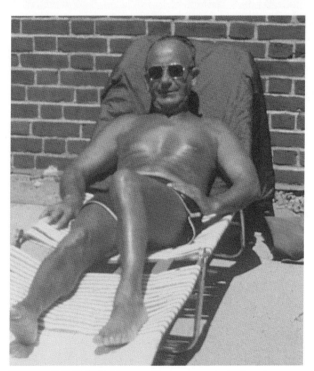

FIGURE 15-29 Excessive exposure to heat or high external temperatures can lead to a life-threatening emergency. *(Courtesy of the Phoenix Society of Burn Survivors, Inc.)*

possible. If it is not treated, it can develop into heat stroke. Treatment methods include moving the victim to a cooler area whenever possible; loosening or removing excessive clothing; applying cool, wet cloths; laying the victim down and elevating the victim's feet 12 inches; and giving the victim small sips of cool water, approximately 4 ounces every 15 minutes if the victim is alert and conscious. If the victim vomits, develops shock, or experiences respiratory distress, medical help should be obtained immediately.

Heat stroke is caused by prolonged exposure to high temperatures. It is a medical emergency. The body is unable to eliminate the excess heat, and internal body temperature rises to 105°F (40.6°C) or higher. Normal body defenses such as the sweating mechanism no longer function. Signs and symptoms in addition to the high body temperature include red, hot, and dry skin. The pulse is usually rapid, but may remain strong. The victim may lose consciousness. Treatment is geared primarily toward ways of cooling the body quickly, because a high body temperature can

cause convulsions and/or death in a very short period of time. The victim can be placed in a tub of cool water, or the skin can be sponged with cool water. Ice or cold packs can be placed on the victim's wrists, ankles, in each axillary (armpit) area, and in the groin. Be alert for signs of shock at all times. Obtain medical help immediately.

After victims have recovered from any condition caused by heat exposure, they must be warned to avoid abnormally warm or hot temperatures for several days. They should also be encouraged to drink sufficient amounts of water and/or electrolyte solutions.

STUDENT: *Go to the workbook and complete the assignment sheet for 15:7, Providing First Aid for Heat Exposure. Then return and continue with the procedure.*

PROCEDURE 15:7

Providing First Aid for Heat Exposure

Equipment and Supplies

Water, wash cloths or small towels

Procedure

1. Follow the priorities of care, if indicated:

   a. Check the scene. Move the victim only if absolutely necessary.

   b. Check the victim for consciousness and breathing.

   c. Call emergency medical services (EMS) if necessary.

   d. Provide care to the victim.

   e. Check for bleeding. Control severe bleeding.

   CAUTION: If possible, wear gloves or use a protective barrier while controlling bleeding.

2. Observe the victim closely for signs and symptoms of heat exposure. Informa-

tion may also be obtained directly from the victim or from observers. If the victim has been exposed to heat or has been exercising strenuously, and is complaining of muscular pain or spasm, he or she is probably experiencing heat cramps. If the victim has close-to-normal body temperature but has pale and clammy skin, is perspiring excessively, and complains of nausea, headache, weakness, dizziness, or fatigue, he or she is probably experiencing heat exhaustion. If body temperature is high (105°F, or 40.6°C, or higher); skin is red, dry, and hot; and the victim is weak or unconscious, he or she is experiencing heat stroke.

3. If the victim has heat cramps:

   a. Use your hand to apply firm pressure to the cramped muscle(s). This helps relieve the spasms.

   b. Encourage relaxation. Allow the victim to lie down in a cool area, if possible.

   c. If the victim is alert and conscious and is not nauseated or vomiting, give him or her small sips of cool

PROCEDURE 15:7

water or an electrolyte solution such as a sport drink. Encourage the victim to drink approximately 4 ounces every 15 minutes.

   d. If the heat cramps continue or get worse, obtain medical help.

4. If the victim has heat exhaustion:

   a. Move the victim to a cool area, if possible. An air-conditioned room is ideal, but a fan can also help circulate air and cool the victim.

   b. Help the victim lie down flat on the back. Elevate the victim's feet and legs 12 inches.

   c. Loosen any tight clothing. Remove excessive clothing such as jackets and sweaters.

   d. Apply cool, wet cloths to the victim's face.

   e. If the victim is conscious and is not nauseated or vomiting, give him or her small sips of cool water or an electrolyte solution such as a sport drink. Encourage the victim to drink approximately 4 ounces every 15 minutes.

   f. If the victim complains of nausea and/or vomits, discontinue the water. Obtain medical help.

5. If the victim has heat stroke:

   a. Immediately move the victim to a cool area, if at all possible.

   b. Remove excessive clothing.

   c. Sponge the bare skin with cool water, or place ice or cold packs on the victim's wrists, ankles, and in the axillary and groin areas. The victim can also be placed in a tub of cool water to lower body temperature.

CAUTION: Watch that the victim's head is not submerged in water. If the victim is unconscious, you may need assistance to place him or her in the tub.

   d. If vomiting occurs, position the victim on his or her side. Watch for signs of difficulty in breathing and provide care as indicated.

   e. Obtain medical help immediately. This is a life-threatening emergency.

6. Shock can develop quickly in all victims of heat exposure. Be alert for the signs of shock and treat as necessary.

CAUTION: Obtain medical help for heat cramps that do not subside, heat exhaustion with signs of shock or vomiting, and *all* heat stroke victims as soon as possible.

7. Reassure the victim as you are providing treatment. Remain calm.

8. Wash hands thoroughly after providing care.

Practice

Go to the workbook and use the evaluation sheet for 15:7, Providing First Aid for Heat Exposure, to practice this procedure. When you believe you have mastered this skill, sign the sheet and give it to your instructor for further action.

 Final Checkpoint Using the criteria listed on the evaluation sheet, your instructor will grade your performance.

15:8 INFORMATION

Providing First Aid for Cold Exposure

Exposure to cold external temperatures can cause body tissues to freeze and body processes to slow. If treatment is not provided immediately, the victim can die. Factors such as wind velocity, amount of humidity, and length of exposure all affect the degree of injury.

Prolonged exposure to the cold can result in **hypothermia,** a condition in which the body temperature is less than 95°F (35°C). Elderly individuals are more susceptible to hypothermia than are younger individuals (figure 15-30). Signs and symptoms include shivering, numbness, weakness or drowsiness, low body temperature, poor coordination, confusion, and loss of consciousness. If prolonged exposure continues, body processes will slow down and death can occur. Treatment consists of getting the victim to a warm area, removing wet clothing, slowly warming the victim by wrapping in blankets or putting on dry clothing, and, if the victim is fully conscious, giving warm nonalcoholic, noncaffeinated liquids by mouth. Avoid warming the victim too quickly, because rapid warming can cause dangerous heart arrhythmias.

Frostbite is actual freezing of tissue fluids accompanied by damage to the skin and underlying tissues (figure 15-31). It is caused by exposure to freezing or below-freezing temperatures.

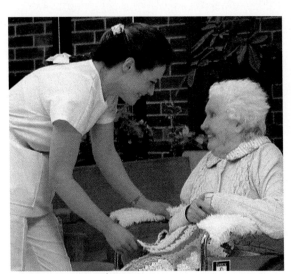

FIGURE 15-30 Elderly individuals are more susceptible to hypothermia than are younger individuals.

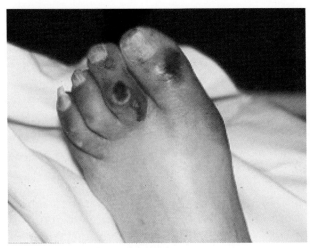

FIGURE 15-31 Frostbite is actual freezing of tissue fluids accompanied by damage to skin and underlying tissues. *(Courtesy of Deborah Funk, MD, Albany Medical Center, Albany, NY)*

Early signs and symptoms include redness and tingling. As frostbite progresses, signs and symptoms include pale, glossy skin, white or grayish yellow in color; blisters; skin that is cold to the touch; numbness; and sometimes, pain that gradually subsides until the victim does not feel any pain. If exposure continues, the victim may become confused, lethargic, and incoherent. Shock may develop followed by unconsciousness and death. First aid for frostbite is directed at maintaining respirations, treating for shock, warming the affected parts, and preventing further injury. Frequently, small areas of the body are affected by frostbite. Common sites include the fingers, toes, ears, nose, and cheeks. Extreme care must be taken to avoid further injury to areas damaged by frostbite. Because the victim usually does not feel pain, the part must be warmed carefully, taking care not to burn the injured tissue. The parts affected may be immersed in warm water at 100–104°F (37.8–40°C).

 CAUTION: Heat lamps, hot water above 104°F (40°C), or heat from a stove or oven should *not* be used. Furthermore, the parts should *not* be rubbed or massaged, because this may cause gangrene (death of the tissue). Avoid opening or breaking any blisters that form because doing so will create an open wound. Do *not* allow the victim to walk or stand if the feet, legs, or toes are affected. Dry, sterile dressings can be placed between toes or fingers to prevent them from rubbing and causing further injury.

Medical help should be obtained as quickly as possible.

Shock is frequently noted in victims exposed to the cold. Be alert for all signs of shock and treat for shock as necessary.

STUDENT: *Go to the workbook and complete the assignment sheet for 15:8, Providing First Aid for Cold Exposure. Then return and continue with the procedure.*

PROCEDURE 15:8

Providing First Aid for Cold Exposure

Equipment and Supplies

Blankets, bath water and thermometer, sterile gauze sponges

Procedure

1. Follow the priorities of care, if indicated:

   a. Check the scene. Move the victim only if absolutely necessary.

   b. Check the victim for consciousness and breathing.

   c. Call emergency medical services (EMS) if necessary.

   d. Provide care to the victim.

   e. Check for bleeding. Control severe bleeding.

   ⊞ **CAUTION:** If possible, wear gloves or use a protective barrier while controlling bleeding.

2. Observe the victim closely for signs and symptoms of cold exposure. Information may also be obtained directly from the victim or observers. Note shivering, numbness, weakness or drowsiness, confusion, low body temperature, and lethargy. Check the skin, particularly on the toes, fingers, ears, nose, and cheeks. Suspect frostbite if any areas are pale, glossy, white or grayish yellow, and cold to the touch, and if the victim complains of any part of the body feeling numb or painless.

3. Move the victim to a warm area as soon as possible.

4. Immediately remove any wet or frozen clothing. Loosen any tight clothing that decreases circulation.

5. Slowly warm the victim by wrapping the victim in blankets or dressing the victim in dry, warm clothing. If a body part is affected by frostbite, immerse the part in warm water measuring 100–104°F (37.8–40°C).

   ▽ **CAUTION:** Warm a victim of hypothermia slowly. Rapid warming can cause heart problems or increase circulation to the surface of the body, which causes additional cooling of vital organs.

   ▽ **CAUTION:** Do *not* use heat lamps, hot water above the stated temperatures, or heat from stoves or ovens. Excessive heat can burn the victim.

6. After the body part affected by frostbite has been thawed and the skin becomes flushed, discontinue warming the area because swelling may develop rapidly. Dry the part by blotting gently with a towel or soft cloth. Gently wrap the part in clean or sterile cloths. Use sterile gauze to separate the fingers and/or toes to prevent them from rubbing together.

   ▽ **CAUTION:** *Never* rub or massage the frostbitten area, because doing so can cause gangrene.

7. Help the victim lie down. Do not allow the victim to walk or stand if the legs, feet, or toes are injured. Elevate any injured areas.

PROCEDURE 15:8

8. Observe the victim for signs of shock. Treat for shock as necessary.

9. If the victim is conscious and is not nauseated or vomiting, give warm liquids to drink.

     CAUTION: Do *not* give beverages containing alcohol or caffeine. Give the victim warm broth, water, or milk.

10. Reassure the victim while providing treatment. Remain calm and encourage the victim to remain calm.

11. Obtain medical help as soon as possible.

12. Wash hands thoroughly after providing care.

15:9 INFORMATION

Providing First Aid for Bone and Joint Injuries

Injuries to bones and joints are common in accidents and falls. A variety of injuries can occur to bones and joints. Such injuries sometimes occur together; other times, these injuries occur by themselves. Examples of injuries to bones and joints are fractures, dislocations, sprains, and strains.

FRACTURES

A **fracture** is a break in a bone. A closed, or simple, fracture is a bone break that is not accompanied by an external or open wound on the skin. A compound, or open, fracture is a bone break that is accompanied by an open wound on the skin. The types of fractures are discussed in Chapter 7:4 and shown in figure 7-22.

Signs and symptoms of fractures can vary. Not all signs and symptoms will be present in every victim. Common signs and symptoms include:

♦ deformity

♦ limited motion or loss of motion

♦ pain and tenderness at the fracture site

♦ swelling and discoloration

♦ the protrusion of bone ends through the skin

♦ the victim heard a bone break or snap or felt a grating sensation (crepitation)

♦ abnormal movements within a part of the body

Basic principles of treatment for fractures include:

♦ maintain respirations

♦ treat for shock

♦ keep the broken bone from moving

♦ prevent further injury.

♦ use devices such as splints and slings to prevent movement of the injured part.

♦ obtain medical help whenever a fracture is evident or suspected

DISLOCATIONS

A **dislocation** is when the end of a bone is either displaced from a joint or moved out of its normal position within a joint. This injury is frequently accompanied by a tearing or stretching of ligaments, muscles, and other soft tissue.

Signs and symptoms that may occur include:

♦ deformity

♦ limited or abnormal movement

♦ swelling

♦ discoloration

♦ pain and tenderness

♦ a shortening or lengthening of the affected arm or leg

First aid for dislocations is basically the same as that for fractures. No attempt should be made to reduce the dislocation (that is, replace the bone in the joint). The affected part must be immobilized in the position in which it was found. Immobilization is accomplished by using splints and/or slings. Movement of the injured part can lead to additional injury to nerves, blood vessels, and other tissue in the area. Obtain medical help immediately.

SPRAINS

A **sprain** is an injury to the tissues surrounding a joint; it usually occurs when the part is forced beyond its normal range of movement. Ligaments, tendons, and other tissues are stretched or torn. Common sites for sprains include the ankles and wrists.

Signs and symptoms of a sprain include swelling, pain, discoloration, and sometimes, impaired motion. Frequently, sprains resemble fractures or dislocations. If in doubt, treat the injury as a fracture.

First aid for a sprain includes:

♦ Apply a cold application to decrease swelling and pain

♦ Elevate the affected part

♦ Encourage the victim to rest the affected part

♦ Apply an elastic bandage to provide support for the affected area but avoid stretching the bandage too tightly

♦ Obtain medical help if swelling is severe or if there is any question of a fracture

STRAINS

A **strain** is the overstretching of a muscle; it is caused by overexertion or lifting. A frequent site for strains is the back. Signs and symptoms of a

strain include sudden pain, swelling, and/or bruising.

Basic principles of first aid treatment for a strain include:

♦ Encourage the victim to rest the affected muscle while providing support

♦ Recommend bedrest with a backboard under the mattress for a strained back

♦ Apply cold applications to reduce the swelling

♦ After the swelling decreases, apply warm, wet applications because warmth relaxes the muscles; different types of cold and heat packs are available (figure 15-32)

♦ Obtain medical help for severe strains and all back injuries

SPLINTS

Splints are devices that can be used to immobilize injured parts when fractures, dislocations, and other similar injuries are present or suspected. Many commercial splints are available, including inflatable, or air, splints, padded boards, and traction splints. Splints can also be made from cardboard, newspapers, blankets, pillows, boards, and other similar materials. Some basic principles regarding the use of splints are:

♦ Splints should be long enough to immobilize the joint above and below the injured area (figure 15-33). By preventing movement in these joints, the injured bone or area is held in position and further injury is prevented.

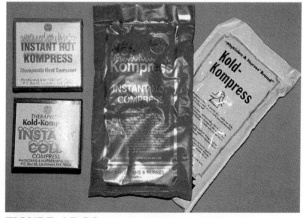

FIGURE 15-32 Disposable heat and cold packs contain chemicals that must be activated before using.

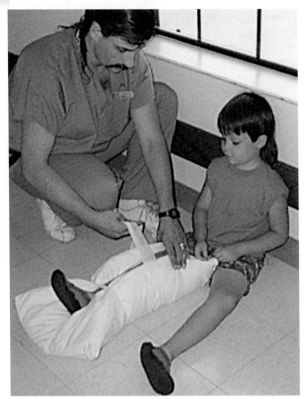

FIGURE 15-33 Splints should be long enough to immobilize the joint above and below the injured area.

♦ Splints should be padded, especially at bony areas and over the site of injury. Cloths, thick dressings, towels, and similar materials can be used as padding.

♦ Strips of cloth, roller gauze, triangular bandages folded into bands or strips, and similar materials can be used to tie splints in place.

♦ Splints must be applied so that they do not put pressure directly over the site of injury.

♦ If an open wound is present, use a sterile dressing to apply pressure and control bleeding.

➕ **CAUTION:** Wear gloves or use a protective barrier while controlling bleeding to avoid contamination from the blood.

▽ **CAUTION:** Leave the dressing in place, and apply the splint in such a way that it does *not* put pressure on the wound.

♦ *Never* make any attempt to replace broken bones or reduce a fracture or dislocation. Do *not* move the victim. Splint wherever you find the victim.

♦ *Pneumatic* splints are available in various sizes and shapes for different parts of the arms and legs. Care must be taken to avoid any unnecessary movement while the splint is being positioned. There are two main types of pneumatic splints: air (inflatable) and vacuum (deflatable).

If an *air splint* is positioned over a fracture site, air pressure is used to inflate the splint (figure 15-34A). Some air splints have nozzles; these splints are inflated by blowing into the nozzles. Other air splints require the use of pressurized material in cans, while still others are inflated with cool air from a refrigerant solution. The coldness reduces swelling. Care must be taken to avoid overinflating air splints. To test whether the splint is properly inflated, use a thumb to apply slight pressure to the splint; an indentation mark should result.

Vacuum pneumatic splints are deflated after being positioned over a fracture site. Air is removed from the splint with a hand pump or suction pump until the splint molds to the fracture site to provide support (figure 15-34B). Care must be taken to avoid overdeflation of the splint. A pulse site below the splint should be checked to make sure the splint is not applying too much pressure and cutting off circulation.

♦ *Traction splints* are special devices that provide a pulling or traction effect on the injured bone. They are frequently used for fractures of the femur, or thigh bone.

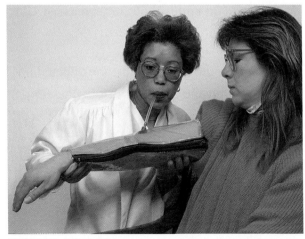

FIGURE 15-34A Some air splints are inflated by blowing into a nozzle. Care must be taken to avoid overinflating this type of splint.

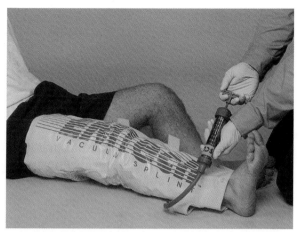

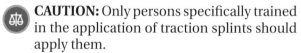

FIGURE 15-34B Vacuum pneumatic splints are deflated until the splint molds to the fracture site to provide support.

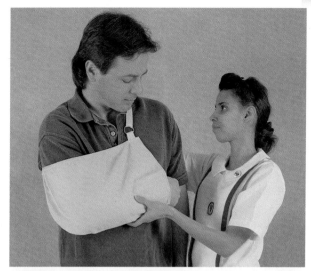

FIGURE 15-35 Commercial slings usually have a series of straps that extend around the neck and/or thoracic region.

CAUTION: Only persons specifically trained in the application of traction splints should apply them.

♦ After a splint is applied, it is essential to note the circulation and the effects on the nerve endings of the skin below the splint to make sure the splint is not too tight. Check skin temperature (it should be warm to the touch), skin color (pale or blue indicates poor circulation), swelling or edema, numbness or tingling, and pulse, if possible.

CAUTION: If any signs of impaired circulation or impaired neurological status are present, immediately loosen the ties holding the splint.

SLINGS

Slings are available in many different forms. Commercial slings usually have a series of straps that extend around the neck and/or thoracic (chest) region (figure 15-35). A common type of sling used for first aid is the triangular bandage. Slings are usually used to support the arm, hand, forearm, and shoulder. They may be used when casts are in place. In addition, they are also used to provide immobility if a fracture of the arm or shoulder is suspected. Basic principles to observe with slings include:

♦ When a sling is applied to an arm, the sling should be positioned in such a way that the hand is higher than the elbow. The purpose of elevating the hand is to promote circulation, prevent swelling (edema), and decrease pain.

♦ Circulation in the limb and nerve supply to the limb must be checked frequently. Specifically, check for skin temperature (should be warm if circulation is good), skin color (blue or very pale indicates poor circulation), swelling (edema), amount of pain, and tingling or numbness. Nail beds can also be used to check circulation. When the nail beds are pressed slightly, they blanch (turn white). If circulation is good, the pink color should return to the nail beds immediately after the pressure is released.

♦ If a sling is being applied because of a suspected fracture to the bone, extreme care must be taken to move the injured limb as little as possible while the sling is being applied. The victim can sometimes help by holding the injured limb in position while the sling is slipped into place.

♦ If a triangular bandage is used, care must be taken so that the knot tied at the neck does not press against a bone. The knot should be tied to either side of the spinal column. Place gauze or padding under the knot of the sling to protect the skin.

♦ When shoulder injuries are suspected, it may be necessary to keep the arm next to the body. After a sling has been applied, another bandage can be placed around the thoracic region to hold the arm against the body.

NECK AND SPINE INJURIES

Injuries to the neck or spine are the most dangerous types of injuries to bones and joints.

 CAUTION: If a victim who has such injuries is moved, permanent damage resulting in paralysis can occur. If at all possible, avoid any movement of a victim with neck or spinal injuries. Wait until a backboard, cervical collar, and adequate help for transfer is available.

SUMMARY

Victims with injuries to bones and/or joints also experience shock. Always be alert for signs of shock and treat as needed.

Injuries to bones and/or joints usually involve a great deal of anxiety, pain, and discomfort, so constantly reassure the victim. Encourage the victim to relax, and position the victim as comfortably as possible. Advise the victim that medical help is on the way. First aid measures are directed toward relieving the pain as much as possible.

Obtain medical help for all victims of bone or joint injuries. The only definite diagnosis of a closed fracture is an X-ray of the area. Whenever a fracture and/or dislocation is suspected, treat the victim as though one of these injuries has occurred.

STUDENT: *Go to the workbook and complete the assignment sheet for 15:9, Providing First Aid for Bone and Joint Injuries. Then return and continue with the procedure.*

PROCEDURE 15:9

Providing First Aid for Bone and Joint Injuries

Equipment and Supplies

Blankets, splints of various sizes, air or inflatable splints, triangular bandages, strips of cloth or roller gauze, disposable gloves

Procedure

1. Follow the priorities of care, if indicated:

   a. Check the scene. Move the victim only if absolutely necessary. If the victim must be moved from a dangerous area, pull in the direction of the long axis of the body (that is, from the head or feet). If at all possible, tie an injured leg to the other leg or secure an injured arm to the body before movement.

   CAUTION: If neck or spinal injuries are suspected, avoid any movement of the victim unless movement is necessary to save the victim's life.

   b. Check the victim for consciousness and breathing.

   c. Call emergency medical services (EMS) if necessary.

   d. Provide care to the victim.

   e. Control severe bleeding. If an open wound accompanies a fracture, take care not to push broken bone ends into the wound.

    CAUTION: If possible, wear gloves or use a protective barrier while controlling bleeding.

2. Observe for signs and symptoms of a fracture, dislocation, or joint injury. Note deformities (such as a shortening or lengthening of an extremity), limited motion or loss of motion, pain, tenderness, swelling, discoloration, and bone

PROCEDURE 15:9

fragments protruding through the skin. Also, the victim may state that he or she heard a bone snap or crack, or may complain of a grating sensation.

3. Immobilize the injured part to prevent movement.

▽ **CAUTION:** Do *not* attempt to straighten a deformity, replace broken bone ends, or reduce a dislocation. Avoid any unnecessary movement of the injured part. If a bone injury is suspected, treat the victim as though a fracture or dislocation has occurred. Use splints or slings to immobilize the injury.

4. *To apply splints:*

a. Obtain commercial splints or improvise splints by using blankets, pillows, newspapers, boards, cardboard, or similar supportive materials.

b. Make sure that the splints are long enough to immobilize the joint both above and below the injury.

c. Position the splints, making sure that they do *not* apply pressure directly at the site of injury. Two splints are usually used. However, if a pillow, blanket, or similar item is used, one such item can be rolled around the area to provide support on all sides.

d. Use thick dressings, cloths, towels, or other similar materials to pad the splints. Make sure bony areas are protected. Avoid direct contact between the splint material and the skin.

NOTE: Many commercial splints are already padded. However, additional padding is often needed to protect the bony areas.

e. Use strips of cloth, triangular bandages folded into strips, roller gauze, or other similar material to tie or anchor the splints in place. The use of elastic bandage is discouraged because the bandage may cut off or interfere with circulation. If splints are long, three to five ties may be required. Tie the strips above and below the upper joint and above and below the lower joint. An additional tie should be placed in the center region of the splint.

f. Avoid any unnecessary movement of the injured area while splints are being applied. If possible, have another individual support the area while you are applying the splints.

5. *To apply air (inflatable) splints:*

a. Obtain the correct splint for the injured part.

NOTE: Most air splints are available for full arm, lower arm, wrist, full leg, lower leg, and ankle/foot.

b. Some air splints have zippers for easier application, but others must be slipped into position on the victim. If the splint has a zipper, position the open splint on the injured area, taking care to avoid any movement of the affected part. Use your hand to support the injured area. Close the zipper. If the splint must be slipped into position, slide the splint onto your arm first. Then hold the injured leg or arm and slide the splint from your arm to the victim's injured extremity. This technique prevents unnecessary movement.

c. Inflate the splint. Many splints are inflated by blowing into the nozzle. Others require the use of a pressure solution in a can. Follow instructions provided by the manufacturer of the splint.

d. Check to make sure that the splint is not overinflated. Use your thumb to press a section of the splint. Your thumb should leave a slight indentation if the splint is inflated correctly.

PROCEDURE 15:9

6. *To apply a sling*, follow the manufacturer's instructions for commercial slings. To use a triangular bandage for a sling (figure 15-36), proceed as follows:

   a. If possible, obtain the help of another individual to support the injured arm while the sling is being applied. Sometimes, the victim can hold the injured arm in place.

   b. Place the long straight edge of the triangular bandage on the uninjured side. Allow one end to extend over the shoulder of the uninjured arm. The other end should hang down in front of the victim's chest. The short edge of the triangle should extend back and under the elbow of the injured arm.

   ▽ **CAUTION:** Avoid excessive movement of the injured limb while positioning the sling.

   c. Bring the long end of the bandage up and over the shoulder of the injured arm.

   d. Use a square knot to tie the two ends together near the neck. Make sure the knot is not over a bone. Tie it to either side of the spinal column. Place gauze or padding between the knot and the skin. Make sure the hand is elevated 5–6 inches above the elbow.

   e. The point of the bandage is now near the elbow. Bring the point forward, fold it, and pin it to the front of the sling. If no pin is available, coil the end and tie it in a knot.

   ▽ **CAUTION:** If you use a pin, put your hand between the pin and the victim's skin while inserting the pin.

   f. Check the position of the sling. The fingers of the injured hand should extend beyond the edge of the triangular bandage. In addition, the hand should be slightly elevated to prevent swelling (edema).

   g. If a shoulder injury is suspected, it may be necessary to secure the arm close to the body. Apply a large bandage around the thoracic region to stabilize the shoulder joint (figure 15-37).

7. After splints and/or slings have been applied, check for signs of impaired circulation. Skin color should be pink. A

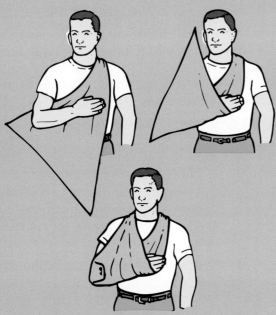

FIGURE 15-36 Steps for applying a triangular bandage as a sling.

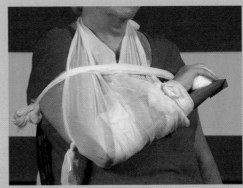

FIGURE 15-37 If a shoulder injury is suspected, use a long bandage to secure the arm against the body to stabilize the shoulder joint.

PROCEDURE 15:9

pale or cyanotic (bluish) color is a sign of poor circulation. The skin should be warm to the touch. Swelling can indicate poor circulation. If the victim complains of pain or pressure from the splints and/or slings, or of numbness or tingling in the area below the splints/sling, circulation may be impaired. Slightly press the nail beds on the foot or hand so they temporarily turn white. If circulation is good, the pink color will return to the nail beds immediately after pressure is released. If you note any signs of impaired circulation, loosen the splints and/or sling immediately.

8. Watch for signs of shock in any victim with a bone and/or joint injury. Remember, inadequate blood flow is the main cause of shock. Watch for signs of impaired circulation, such as a cyanotic (bluish) tinge around the lips or nail beds. Treat for shock, as necessary.

9. If medical help is delayed, cold applications such as cold compresses or an ice bag can be used on the injured area to decrease swelling.

▽ **CAUTION:** To prevent injury to the skin, make sure that the ice bag is covered with a towel or other material.

10. Place the victim in a comfortable position, but avoid any unnecessary movement.

▽ **CAUTION:** Avoid *any* movement if a neck or spinal injury is suspected.

11. Reassure the victim while providing first aid. Try to relieve the pain by carefully positioning the injured part, avoiding unnecessary movement, and applying cold.

12. Obtain medical help as quickly as possible.

13. Wash hands thoroughly after providing care.

Practice

Go to the workbook and use the evaluation sheet for 15:9, Providing First Aid for Bone and Joint Injuries, to practice this procedure. When you believe you have mastered this skill, sign the sheet and give it to your instructor for further action.

✔ **Final Checkpoint** Using the criteria listed on the evaluation sheet, your instructor will grade your performance.

15:10 INFORMATION

Providing First Aid for Specific Injuries

Although treatment for burns, bleeding, wounds, poisoning, and fractures is basically the same for all regions of the body, injuries to specific body parts require special care. Examples of these parts are the eyes, ears, nose, brain, chest, abdomen, and genital organs.

EYE INJURIES

Any eye injury always involves the danger of vision loss, especially if treated incorrectly. In most cases involving serious injury to the eyes, it is best *not* to provide major treatment. Obtaining medical help, preferably from an eye specialist, is a top priority of first aid care.

♦ *Foreign objects* such as dust, dirt, and similar small particles frequently enter the eye. These objects cause irritation and can scratch the eye or become embedded in the eye tissue. Signs and symptoms include redness, a burning sensation, pain, watering or tearing of the eye, and/or the presence of visible objects in the eye. If the foreign body is floating freely, prevent the victim from rubbing the eye, wash your hands thoroughly, and gently draw the upper lid down over the lower lid. This stimulates the formation of tears. The proximity of the lids also creates a wiping action, which may remove the particle. If this does not remove the foreign body, use your thumb and forefinger to grasp the eyelashes and gently raise the upper eyelid. Tell the victim to look down and tilt his or her head toward the injured side. Use water to gently flush the eye or use the corner of a piece of sterile gauze to gently remove the object.

 CAUTION: If this does not remove the object or if the object is embedded, make *no* attempt to remove it.

Apply a dry, sterile dressing and obtain medical help for the victim. Serious injury can occur if any attempt is made to remove an object embedded in the eye tissue.

♦ *Blows to the eye* from a fist, accident, or explosion may cause contusions or black eyes as a result of internal bleeding and torn tissues inside the eye. Because this can lead to loss of vision, the victim should be examined as soon as possible by an eye specialist. Apply sterile dressings or an eye shield, keep the victim lying flat, and obtain medical help. It is sometimes best to cover both eyes to prevent involuntary movement of the injured eye.

♦ *Penetrating injuries* that cut the eye tissue are extremely dangerous.

 CAUTION: If an object is protruding from the eye, make *no* attempt to remove the object. Rather, support it by *loosely* applying dressings. A paper cup with a hole cut in the bottom can also be used to stabilize the object and prevent it from moving (figure 15-38).

Apply dressings to both eyes to prevent involuntary movement of the injured eye. Avoid applying pressure to the eye while applying the dressings. Keep the victim lying flat on his or her back to prevent fluids from draining out of the eye. Obtain medical help immediately.

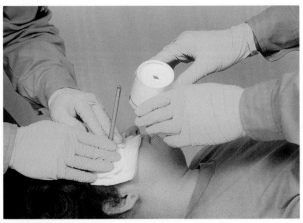

FIGURE 15-38 A cup can be used to stabilize an object impaled in the eye and to prevent it from moving.

EAR INJURIES

Injuries to the ear can result in rupture or perforation of the eardrum. These injuries also require medical care. Treatment for specific types of ear injuries is as follows:

♦ Wounds of the ear frequently result in torn or detached tissue. Apply sterile dressings with light pressure to control bleeding.

 CAUTION: If possible, wear gloves or use a protective barrier while controlling bleeding.

Save any torn tissue and wrap it in gauze moistened with cool sterile water or sterile normal saline solution. Put the gauze wrapped tissue in a plastic bag to keep it cool and moist. Send the torn tissue to the medical facility along with the victim.

NOTE: If sterile water is not available, use cool, clean water.

♦ Keep the victim lying flat, but raise his or her head (if no other conditions prohibit raising the head).

♦ If the eardrum is ruptured or perforated, place sterile gauze loosely in the outer ear canal. Do *not* allow the victim to hit the side of the head in an attempt to restore hearing. Do *not* put any liquids into the ear. Obtain medical help for the victim.

♦ Clear or blood-tinged fluid draining from the ear can be a sign of skull or brain injury. Allow the fluid to flow from the ear. Keep the victim lying down. If possible, turn the victim on his or her injured side and elevate the head and shoulders slightly to allow the fluid to drain. Obtain medical help immediately and report the presence and description of the fluid.

CAUTION: Wear gloves or use a protective barrier to avoid skin contact with fluid draining from the ear.

HEAD OR SKULL INJURIES

Wounds or blows to the head or skull can result in injury to the brain. Again, it is important to obtain medical help as quickly as possible for the victim.

♦ Signs and symptoms of brain injury include clear or blood-tinged cerebrospinal fluid draining from the nose or ears, loss of consciousness, headache, visual disturbances, pupils unequal in size, muscle paralysis, speech disturbances, convulsions, and nausea and vomiting.

♦ Keep the victim lying flat and treat for shock. If there is no evidence of neck or spinal injury, raise the victim's head slightly by supporting the head and shoulders on a small pillow or a rolled blanket or coat.

♦ Watch closely for signs of respiratory distress and provide artificial respiration as needed.

♦ Make *no* attempt to stop the flow of fluid. Loose dressings can be positioned to absorb the flow.

CAUTION: Wear gloves or use a protective barrier to avoid contamination from the cerebrospinal fluid.

♦ Do *not* give the victim any liquids. If the victim complains of excessive thirst, use a clean, cool, wet cloth to moisten the lips, tongue, and inside of the mouth.

♦ If the victim loses consciousness, note how long the victim is unconscious and report this to the emergency rescue personnel.

NOSE INJURIES

Injuries to the nose frequently cause a nosebleed, also called an *epistaxis*. Nosebleeds are usually more frightening than they are serious. Nosebleeds can also be caused by change in altitude, strenuous activity, high blood pressure, and rupture of small blood vessels after a cold. Treatment for a nosebleed includes:

♦ Keep the victim quiet and remain calm.

♦ If possible, place the victim in a sitting position with the head leaning slightly forward.

♦ Apply pressure to control bleeding by pressing the bleeding nostril toward the midline. If both nostrils are bleeding, press both nostrils toward the midline.

> **NOTE:** If both nostrils are blocked, tell the victim to breathe through the mouth.

CAUTION: Wear gloves or use a protective barrier to avoid contamination from blood.

♦ If application of pressure against the midline or septum does not stop the bleeding, insert a small piece of gauze in the nostril and then apply pressure on the outer surface of the nostril. Be sure to leave a portion of the gauze extending out of the nostril so that the packing can be removed later.

CAUTION: Do not use cotton balls because the fibers will shed and stick.

♦ Apply a cold compress to the bridge of the nose. A covered ice pack or a cold, wet cloth can be used.

♦ If the bleeding does not stop or a fracture of the nose is suspected, obtain medical assistance. If a person has repeated nosebleeds, a referral for medical attention should be made. Nosebleeds can indicate an underlying condition that requires medical care and treatment, such as high blood pressure.

CHEST INJURIES

Injuries to the chest are usually medical emergencies because the heart, lungs, and major blood vessels may be involved. Chest injuries include sucking chest wounds, penetrating wounds, and crushing injuries. In all cases, obtain medical help immediately.

♦ *Sucking chest wound*: This is a deep, open chest wound that allows air to flow directly in and out with breathing. The partial vacuum that is usually present in the pleura (sacs surrounding the lungs) is destroyed, causing the lung on the injured side to collapse. Immediate medical help must be obtained. An airtight dressing must be placed over the wound to prevent air flow into the wound. Aluminum foil, plastic wrap, or other nonporous material should be used to cover the wound. Tape or a bandage can be used to hold the nonporous material in place on three sides. The fourth side should be left loose to allow air to escape when the victim exhales. When the victim inhales, the negative pressure of inspirations will draw the dressing against the wound to create an airtight seal. Maintain an open airway (through the nose or mouth) and provide artificial respiration as needed. If possible, position the victim on his or her injured side and elevate the head and chest slightly. This allows the uninjured lung to expand more freely and prevents pressure on the uninjured lung from blood and damaged tissue.

♦ *Penetrating injuries to the chest*: These injuries can result in sucking chest wounds or damage to the heart and blood vessels. If an object (for example, a knife) is protruding from the chest, do *not* attempt to remove the object. If possible, immobilize the object by placing dressings around it and taping the dressings in position (figure 15-39). Place the victim in a

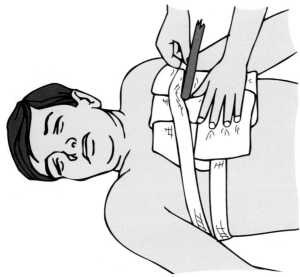

FIGURE 15-39 Immobilize an object protruding from the chest by placing dressings around the object and taping the dressings in place.

comfortable position, maintain respirations, and obtain medical help immediately.

♦ *Crushing chest injuries*: These injuries are caused in vehicular accidents or when heavy objects strike the chest. Fractured ribs and damage to the lungs and/or heart can occur. Place the victim in a comfortable position and, if possible, elevate the head and shoulders to aid breathing. If an injury to the neck or spine is suspected, avoid moving the victim. Obtain medical help immediately.

ABDOMINAL INJURIES

Abdominal injuries can damage internal organs and cause bleeding in major blood vessels. The intestines and other abdominal organs may protrude from an open wound. Medical help must be obtained immediately; bleeding, shock, and organ damage can lead to death in a short period of time.

♦ Signs and symptoms include severe abdominal pain or tenderness, protruding organs, open wounds, nausea and vomiting (particularly of blood), abdominal muscle rigidity, and symptoms of shock.

♦ Position the victim flat on his or her back. Place a pillow or rolled blanket under the knees to bend the knees slightly. This helps relax the abdominal muscles. Elevate the head and shoulders slightly to aid breathing.

♦ Remove clothing from around the wound or protruding organs. Use a large sterile dressing moistened with sterile water or normal saline solution to cover the area. If sterile water or normal saline is not available, use warm tap water to moisten the dressings. Cover the dressings with plastic wrap, if available, to keep the dressings moist. Then cover the dressings with aluminum foil or a folded towel to keep the area warm.

⚠ **CAUTION:** Make no attempt to reposition protruding organs.

♦ Avoid giving the victim any fluids or food. If the victim complains of excessive thirst, use a cool, wet cloth to moisten the lips, tongue, and inside of the mouth.

INJURIES TO GENITAL ORGANS

Injuries to genital organs can result from falls, blows, or explosions. Zippers catching on genitals and other accidents sometimes bruise the genitals. Because injuries to the genitals may cause severe pain, bleeding, and shock, medical help is required. Basic principles of first aid include the following:

♦ Control severe bleeding by using a sterile (or clean) dressing to apply direct pressure to the area.

✚ **CAUTION:** Wear gloves or use a protective barrier to avoid contamination from blood.

♦ Treat the victim for shock.

♦ Do not remove any penetrating or inserted objects.

♦ Save any torn tissue and wrap it in gauze moistened with cool sterile water or sterile normal saline. Put the gauze-wrapped tissue in a plastic bag to keep it cool and moist. Send the torn tissue to the medical facility along with the victim.

♦ Use a covered ice pack or other cold applications to decrease bleeding and relieve pain.

♦ Obtain medical help.

SUMMARY

Shock frequently occurs in victims with specific injuries to the eyes, ears, chest, abdomen, or other vital organs. Be alert for the signs of shock and immediately treat all victims.

Most of the specific injuries discussed in this section result in extreme pain for the victim. It is essential that you reassure the victim constantly and encourage the victim to relax as much as possible. Direct first aid care toward providing as much relief from pain as possible.

STUDENT: *Go to the workbook and complete the assignment sheet for 15:10, Providing First Aid for Specific Injuries. Then return and continue with the procedure.*

PROCEDURE 15:10

Providing First Aid for Specific Injuries

Equipment and Supplies

Blankets, pillows, dressings, bandages, tape, aluminum foil or plastic wrap, eye shields or sterile dressings, sterile water, disposable gloves

Procedure

1. Follow the priorities of care, if indicated:

   a. Check the scene. Move the victim only if absolutely necessary.

   b. Check the victim for consciousness and breathing.

   c. Call emergency medical services (EMS), if necessary.

   d. Provide care to the victim.

   e. Check for bleeding. Control severe bleeding.

   ✚ **CAUTION:** If possible, wear gloves or use a protective barrier while controlling bleeding.

2. Observe the victim closely for signs and symptoms of specific injuries. Do a systematic examination of the victim. Always have a reason for everything you do. Explain what you are doing to the victim and/or observers.

3. If the victim has an eye injury, proceed as follows:

   a. If the victim has a free-floating particle or foreign body in the eye, warn the victim *not* to rub the eye. Wash your hands thoroughly to prevent infection. Gently grasp the upper eyelid and draw it down over the lower

PROCEDURE 15:10

eyelid. If this does not remove the object, use your thumb and forefinger to grasp the eyelashes and gently raise the upper eyelid. Tell the victim to look down and tilt his or her head slightly to the injured side. Use water to gently flush the eye or use the corner of a piece of sterile gauze to gently remove the object. If this does not remove the object or if the object is embedded, proceed to step b.

b. If an object is embedded in the eye, make *no* attempt to remove it. Rather, apply a dry, sterile dressing to loosely cover the eye. Obtain medical help.

c. If an eye injury has caused a contusion, a black eye, internal bleeding, and/or torn tissue in the eye, apply sterile dressings or eye shields to both eyes. Keep the victim lying flat. Obtain medical help.

NOTE: Both eyes are covered to prevent involuntary movement of the injured eye.

d. If an object is protruding from the eye, make *no* attempt to remove the object. If possible, support the object in position by loosely placing dressings around it. A paper cup with the bottom removed can also be used to surround and prevent any movement of the object. Apply dressings to the uninjured eye to prevent movement of the injured eye. Keep the victim lying flat. Obtain medical help immediately.

4. If the victim has an ear injury:

a. Control severe bleeding from an ear wound by using a sterile dressing to apply light pressure.

CAUTION: Wear gloves or use a protective barrier to prevent contamination from the blood.

b. If any tissue has been torn from the ear, preserve the tissue by placing it in gauze moistened with cool, sterile water or normal saline solution. Place the gauze-wrapped tissue in a plastic bag. Send the torn tissue to the medical facility along with the victim.

NOTE: If sterile water is not available, use cool, clean water.

c. If a rupture or perforation of the eardrum is suspected or evident, place sterile gauze loosely in the outer ear canal. Caution the victim against hitting the side of the head to restore hearing. Obtain medical help.

d. If cerebrospinal fluid is draining from the ear, make no attempt to stop the flow of the fluid. If no neck or spinal injury is suspected, turn the victim on his or her injured side and slightly elevate the head and shoulders to allow the fluid to drain. A dressing may be positioned to absorb the flow. Obtain medical help immediately.

CAUTION: Wear gloves or use a protective barrier to prevent contamination from the cerebrospinal fluid.

5. If the victim has a brain injury:

a. Keep the victim lying flat. Treat for shock. If there is no evidence of a neck or spinal injury, place a small pillow or a rolled blanket or coat under the victim's head and shoulders to elevate the head slightly.

CAUTION: Never position the victim's head lower than the rest of the body.

b. Watch closely for signs of respiratory distress. Provide artificial respiration if needed.

NOTE: Remove the pillow if artificial respiration is given.

c. If cerebrospinal fluid is draining from the ears, nose, and/or mouth, make *no* attempt to stop the flow. Position dressings to absorb the flow.

PROCEDURE 15:10

 CAUTION: Wear gloves or use a protective barrier to prevent contamination from the cerebrospinal fluid.

d. Avoid giving the victim any fluids by mouth. If the victim complains of excessive thirst, use a cool, wet cloth to moisten the lips, tongue, and inside of the mouth.

e. If the victim is unconscious, note for how long and report this information to the emergency rescue personnel.

f. Obtain medical help as quickly as possible.

6. If the victim has a nosebleed:

a. Try to keep the victim calm. Remain calm yourself.

b. Position the victim in a sitting position, if possible. Lean the head forward slightly. If the victim cannot sit up, slightly elevate the head.

c. Apply pressure by pressing the nostril(s) toward the midline. Continue applying pressure for at least 5 minutes and longer if necessary to control the bleeding.

NOTE: If both nostrils are bleeding and must be pressed toward the midline, tell the victim to breathe through the mouth.

 CAUTION: Wear gloves or use a protective barrier to prevent contamination from the blood.

d. If application of pressure does not control the bleeding, insert gauze into the bleeding nostril, taking care to allow some of the gauze to hang out. Then apply pressure again by pushing the nostril toward the midline.

e. Apply cold compresses to the bridge of the nose. Use cold, wet cloths or a covered ice bag.

f. If the bleeding does not stop, a fracture is suspected, or if the victim has repeated nosebleeds, obtain medical help.

NOTE: Nosebleeds can indicate a serious underlying condition that requires medical attention, such as high blood pressure.

7. If the victim has a chest injury:

a. If the wound is a sucking chest wound, apply a nonporous dressing. Use plastic wrap or aluminum foil to create an airtight seal. Use tape on three sides to hold the dressing in place. Leave the fourth side loose to allow excess air to escape when the victim exhales (figure 15-40).

b. Maintain an open airway. Constantly be alert for signs of respiratory distress. Provide artificial respiration as needed.

c. If there is no evidence of a neck or spinal injury, position the victim with his or her injured side down. Slightly elevate the head and chest by placing small pillows or blankets under the victim.

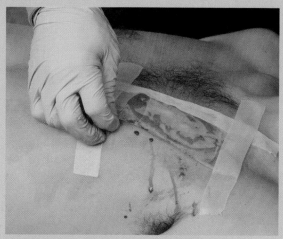

FIGURE 15-40 An airtight dressing is used to cover a sucking chest wound. It is taped on three sides. The fourth side is left open to allow excess air to escape when the victim exhales.

PROCEDURE 15:10

d. If an object is protruding from the chest, make *no* attempt to remove it. If possible, immobilize the object with dressings, and tape around it.

e. Obtain medical help immediately for all chest injuries.

8. If the victim has an abdominal injury:

a. Position the victim flat on the back. Place a small pillow or a rolled blanket or coat under the victim's knees to flex them slightly. Elevate the head and shoulders to aid breathing. If movement of the legs causes pain, leave the victim lying flat.

b. If abdominal organs are protruding from the wound, make *no* attempt to reposition the organs. Remove clothing from around the wound or protruding organs. Use a sterile dressing that has been moistened with sterile water or normal saline solution to cover the area. If sterile water or normal saline is not available, use warm tap water to moisten the dressings.

c. Cover the dressing with plastic wrap, if available, to keep the dressing moist. Then apply a folded towel or aluminum foil to keep the area warm.

d. Avoid giving the victim any fluids or food. If the victim complains of excessive thirst, use a cool, wet cloth to moisten the lips, tongue, and inside of the mouth.

e. Obtain medical help immediately.

9. If the victim has an injury to the genital organs:

a. Control severe bleeding by using a sterile dressing to apply direct pressure.

CAUTION: Wear gloves or use a protective barrier to prevent contamination from the blood.

b. Position the victim flat on the back. Separate the legs to prevent pressure on the genital area.

c. If any tissue is torn from the area, preserve the tissue by wrapping it in gauze moistened with cool, sterile water or normal saline solution. Put the gauze-wrapped tissue in a plastic bag and send it to the medical facility along with the victim.

d. Apply cold compresses such as covered ice bags to the area to relieve pain and reduce swelling.

e. Obtain medical help for the victim.

10. Be alert for the signs of shock in all victims. Treat for shock immediately.

11. Constantly reassure all victims while providing care. Remain calm. Encourage the victim to relax as much as possible.

12. Always obtain medical help as quickly as possible. Shock, pain, and injuries to vital organs can cause death in a very short period of time.

13. Wash hands thoroughly after providing care.

Practice

Go to the workbook and use the evaluation sheet for 15:10, Providing First Aid for Specific Injuries, to practice this procedure. When you believe you have mastered this skill, sign the sheet and give it to your instructor for further action.

 Final Checkpoint Using the criteria listed on the evaluation sheet, your instructor will grade your performance.

15:11 INFORMATION

Providing First Aid for Sudden Illness

The victim of a sudden illness requires first aid until medical help can be obtained. Sudden illness can occur in any individual. At times, it is difficult to determine the exact illness being experienced by the victim. However, by knowing the signs and symptoms of some major disorders, you should be able to provide appropriate first aid care. Information regarding a specific condition or illness may also be obtained from the victim, medical alert bracelets or necklaces, or medical information cards. Be alert to all of these factors while caring for the victim of a sudden illness.

HEART ATTACK

A **heart attack** is also called a *coronary thrombosis, coronary occlusion,* or *myocardial infarction.* It may occur when one of the coronary arteries supplying blood to the heart is blocked. If the attack is severe, the victim may die. If the heart stops beating, cardiopulmonary resuscitation (CPR) must be started. Main facts regarding heart attacks are as follows:

♦ Signs and symptoms of a heart attack may vary depending on the amount of heart damage. Severe, painful pressure under the breastbone (sternum) with pain radiating to the shoulders, arms, neck, and jaw is a common symptom (figure 15-41). The victim usually experiences intense shortness of breath. The skin, especially near the lips and nail beds, becomes pale or cyanotic (bluish). The victim feels very weak but is also anxious and apprehensive. Nausea, vomiting, diaphoresis (excessive perspiration), and loss of consciousness may occur.

♦ First aid for a heart attack is directed toward encouraging the victim to relax, placing the victim in a comfortable position to relieve pain and assist breathing, and obtaining medical help. Shock frequently occurs, so provide treatment for shock. Prevent any unnecessary stress and avoid excessive movement because any activity places additional strain on the heart. Reassure the victim constantly, and

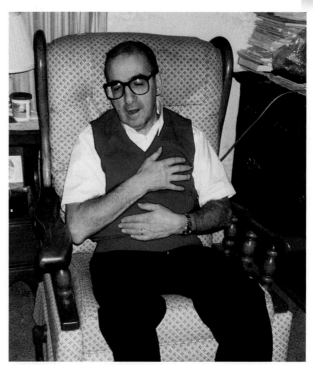

FIGURE 15-41 Severe pressure under the sternum with pain radiating to the shoulders, arms, neck, and jaw is a common symptom of a heart attack.

obtain appropriate medical assistance as soon as possible.

♦ After calling EMS, the American Heart Association recommends that patients who can should take an aspirin. Aspirin keeps platelets in the blood from sticking together to cause a clot. However, there are legal restrictions to which health care providers can administer medications. Only qualified individuals should give the victim aspirin.

CEREBROVASCULAR ACCIDENT OR STROKE

A *stroke* is also called a **cerebrovascular accident** (CVA), *apoplexy,* or *cerebral thrombosis.* It is caused by either the presence of a clot in a cerebral artery that provides blood to the brain or hemorrhage from a blood vessel in the brain.

♦ Signs and symptoms of a stroke vary depending on the part of the brain affected. Some common signs and symptoms are numbness, paralysis, eye pupils unequal in size, mental confusion, slurred speech, nausea, vomiting, difficulty breathing and swallowing, and loss of consciousness.

♦ First aid for a stroke victim is directed toward maintaining respirations, laying the victim flat on the back with the head slightly elevated or on the side to allow secretions to drain from the mouth, and avoiding any fluids by mouth. Reassure the victim, prevent any unnecessary stress, and avoid any unnecessary movement.

🔘 NOTE: Always remember that although the victim may be unable to speak or may appear to be unconscious, he or she may be able to hear and understand what is going on.

♦ Obtain medical help as quickly as possible. Immediate care during the first 3 hours can help prevent brain damage. If the CVA is caused by a blood clot, treatment with thrombolytic or "clot busting" drugs such as TPA (tissue plasminogen activator) or angioplasty of the cerebral arteries can dissolve a blood clot and restore blood flow to the brain.

FAINTING

Fainting occurs when there is a temporary reduction in the supply of blood to the brain. It may result in partial or complete loss of consciousness. The victim usually regains consciousness after being in a supine position (that is, lying flat on the back).

♦ Early signs of fainting include dizziness, extreme pallor, diaphoresis, coldness of the skin, nausea, and a numbness and tingling of the hands and feet.

♦ If early symptoms are noted, help the victim to lie down or to sit in a chair and position his or her head at the level of the knees.

♦ If the victim loses consciousness, try to prevent injury. Provide first aid by keeping the victim in a supine position. If no neck or spine injuries are suspected, use a pillow or blankets to elevate the victim's legs and feet 12 inches. Loosen any tight clothing and maintain an open airway. Use cool water to gently bathe the victim's face. Check for any injuries that may have been caused by the fall. Permit the victim to remain flat and quiet until color improves and the victim has recovered. Then allow the victim to get up gradually. If recovery is not prompt, if other injuries occur or are suspected, or if fainting occurs again, obtain medical help. Fainting can be a sign of a serious illness or condition that requires medical attention.

CONVULSION

A **convulsion,** which is a type of *seizure*, is a strong, involuntary contraction of muscles. Convulsions may occur in conjunction with high body temperatures, head injuries, brain disease, and brain disorders such as epilepsy.

♦ Convulsions cause a rigidity of body muscles followed by jerking movements. During a convulsion, a person may stop breathing, bite the tongue, lose bladder and bowel control, and injure body parts. The face and lips may develop a cyanotic (bluish) color. The victim may lose consciousness. After regaining consciousness at the end of the convulsion, the victim may be confused and disoriented, and complain of a headache.

♦ First aid is directed toward preventing self-injury. Removing dangerous objects from the area, providing a pillow or cushion under the victim's head, and providing artificial respiration, as necessary, are all ways to assist the victim.

♦ Do *not* try to place anything between the victim's teeth. This can cause severe injury to your fingers, and/or damage to the victim's teeth or gums.

♦ Do *not* use force to restrain or stop the muscle movements; this only causes the contractions to become more severe.

♦ When the convulsion is over, watch the victim closely. If fluid, such as saliva or vomit, is in the victim's mouth, position the victim on his or her side to allow the fluid to drain from the mouth. Allow the victim to sleep or rest.

♦ Obtain medical help if the seizure lasts more than a few minutes, if the victim has repeated seizures, if other severe injuries are apparent, if the victim does not have a history of seizures, or if the victim does not regain consciousness.

DIABETIC REACTIONS

Diabetes mellitus is a metabolic disorder caused by a lack or insufficient production of insulin (a hormone produced by the pancreas). Insulin helps the body transport glucose, a form of sugar, from the bloodstream into body cells where the glucose is used to produce energy. When there is a lack of insulin, sugar builds up in the bloodstream. Insulin injections can reduce and control the level of sugar in the blood. Individuals with diabetes are in danger of developing two condi-

tions that require first aid: diabetic coma and insulin shock (figure 15-42).

♦ **Diabetic coma** or *hyperglycemia* is caused by an increase in the level of glucose in the bloodstream. The condition may result from an excess intake of sugar, failure to take insulin, or insufficient production of insulin. Signs and symptoms include confusion; weakness or dizziness; nausea and/or vomiting; rapid, deep respirations; dry, flushed skin; and a sweet or fruity odor to the breath. The victim will eventually lose consciousness and die unless the

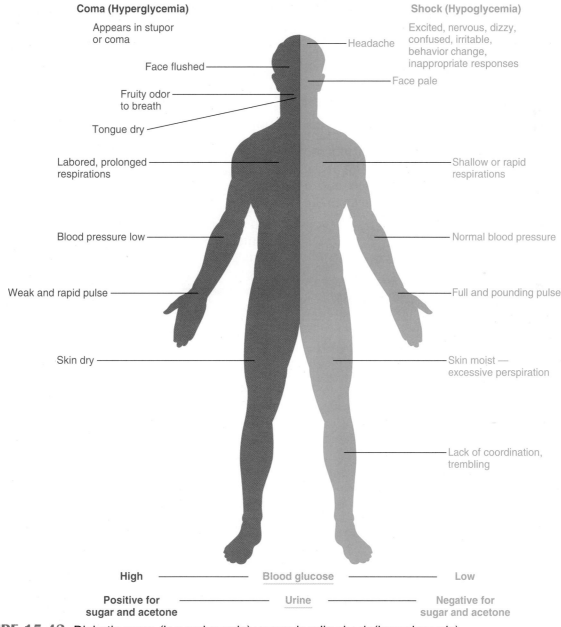

FIGURE 15-42 Diabetic coma (hyperglycemia) versus insulin shock (hypoglycemia).

condition is treated. Medical assistance must be obtained as quickly as possible.

♦ **Insulin shock** or *hypoglycemia* is caused by an excess amount of insulin (and a low level of glucose) in the bloodstream. It may result from failure to eat the recommended amounts, vomiting after taking insulin, or taking excessive amounts of insulin. Signs and symptoms include muscle weakness; mental confusion; restlessness or anxiety; diaphoresis; pale, moist skin; hunger pangs; and/or palpitations (rapid, irregular heartbeats). The victim may lapse into a coma and develop convulsions. The onset of insulin shock is sudden, and the victim's condition can deteriorate quickly; therefore, immediate first aid care is required. If the victim is conscious, give him or her a drink containing sugar, such as sweetened orange juice. A cube or teaspoon of granulated sugar can also be placed in the victim's mouth. If the victim is confused, avoid giving hard candy. Unconsciousness could occur, and the victim could choke on the hard candy. Many individuals with diabetes use tubes of glucose that they carry with them (figure 15-43). If the victim is conscious and can swallow and a glucose tube is available, it can be given to the victim.

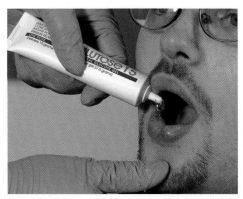

FIGURE 15-43 A victim experiencing insulin shock needs glucose or some form of sugar as quickly as possible.

The intake of sugar should quickly control the reaction. If the victim loses consciousness or convulsions start, provide care for the convulsions and obtain medical assistance immediately.

By observing symptoms carefully and obtaining as much information as possible from the victim, you can usually determine whether the condition is diabetic coma or insulin shock. Ask the victim, "Have you eaten today?" and "Have you taken your insulin?" If the victim has taken insulin but has not eaten, insulin shock is developing because there is too much insulin in the body. If the victim has eaten but has not taken insulin, diabetic coma is developing. In cases when you know that the victim is diabetic but the victim is unconscious and there are no definite symptoms of either condition, you may not be able to determine whether the condition is diabetic coma or insulin shock. In such cases, the recommendation is to put granulated sugar under the victim's tongue and activate emergency medical services (EMS). This is the lesser of two evils. If the patient is in diabetic coma, the blood-sugar level can be lowered as needed when the victim is transported for medical care. If the victim is in insulin shock, however, brain damage can occur if the blood-sugar level is not raised immediately. Medical care cannot correct brain damage.

SUMMARY

In all cases of sudden illness, constantly reassure the victim and make every attempt to encourage the victim to relax and avoid further stress. Be alert for the signs of shock and provide treatment for shock to all victims. The pain, anxiety, and fear associated with sudden illness can contribute to shock.

STUDENT: *Go to the workbook and complete the assignment sheet for 15:11, Providing First Aid for Sudden Illness. Then return and continue with the procedure.*

PROCEDURE 15:11

Providing First Aid for Sudden Illness

Equipment and Supplies

Blankets, pillows, sugar, clean cloth, cool water, disposable gloves

Procedure

1. Follow the priorities of care, if indicated.

   a. Check the scene. Move the victim only if absolutely necessary.

   b. Check the victim for consciousness and breathing.

   c. Call emergency medical services (EMS), if necessary.

   d. Provide care to the victim.

   e. Check for bleeding. Control severe bleeding.

   CAUTION: If possible, wear gloves or use a protective barrier while controlling bleeding.

2. Closely observe the victim for specific signs and symptoms. If the victim is conscious, obtain information about the history of the illness, type and amount of pain, and other pertinent details. If the victim is unconscious, check for a medical bracelet or necklace or a medical information card. Always have a reason for everything you do. Explain your actions to any observers, especially if it is necessary to check the victim's wallet for a medical card.

3. If you suspect the victim is having a *heart attack*, provide first aid as follows:

   a. Place the victim in the most comfortable position possible, but avoid unnecessary movement. Some victims will want to lie flat, but others will want to be in a partial or complete sitting position. If the victim is having difficulty breathing, use pillows or rolled blankets to elevate the head and shoulders.

   b. Obtain medical help for the victim immediately. Advise EMS that oxygen may be necessary.

   c. Encourage the victim to relax. Reassure the victim. Remain calm and encourage others to remain calm.

   d. Watch for signs of shock and treat for shock as necessary. Avoid overheating the victim.

   e. If the victim complains of excessive thirst, use a wet cloth to moisten the lips, tongue, and inside of the mouth. Small sips of water can also be given to the victim, but avoid giving large amounts of fluid.

   CAUTION: Do *not* give the victim ice water or very cold water because the cold can intensify shock.

4. If you suspect that the victim has had a *stroke*:

   a. Place the victim in a comfortable position. Keep the victim lying flat or slightly elevate the victim's head and shoulders to aid breathing. If the victim has difficulty swallowing, turn the victim on his or her side to allow secretions to drain from the mouth and prevent choking on the secretions.

   b. Reassure the victim. Encourage the victim to relax.

   c. Avoid giving the victim any fluids or food by mouth. If the victim complains of excessive thirst, use a cool, wet cloth to moisten the lips, tongue, and inside of the mouth.

   d. Obtain medical help for the victim as quickly as possible.

PROCEDURE 15:11

5. If the victim has *fainted*:

   a. Keep the victim in a supine position (that is, lying flat on the back). Raise the legs and feet 12 inches.

   b. Check for breathing. Provide artificial respiration, if necessary.

   c. Loosen any tight clothing.

   d. Use cool water to gently bathe the face.

   e. Check for any other injuries.

   f. Encourage the victim to continue lying down until his or her skin color improves.

   g. If no other injuries are suspected, allow the victim to get up slowly. First, elevate the head and shoulders. Then place the victim in a sitting position. Allow the victim to stand slowly. If any signs of dizziness, weakness, or pallor are noted, return the victim to the supine position.

   h. If the victim does not recover quickly, or if any other injuries occur, obtain medical care. If fainting has occurred frequently, refer the victim for medical care.

   NOTE: Fainting can be a sign of a serious illness or condition.

6. If the victim is having a *convulsion*:

   a. Remove any dangerous objects from the area. If the victim is near heavy furniture or machinery that cannot be moved, move the victim to a safe area.

   b. Place soft material such as a blanket, small pillow, rolled jacket, or other similar material under the victim's head to prevent injury.

   c. Closely observe respirations at all times. During the convulsion, there will be short periods of apnea (cessation of breathing).

NOTE: If breathing does not resume quickly, artificial respiration may be necessary.

   d. Do *not* try to place anything between the victim's teeth. This can cause injury to the teeth and/or gums.

   e. Do *not* attempt to restrain the muscle contractions. This only makes the contractions more severe.

   f. Note how long the convulsion lasts and what parts of the body are involved. Be sure to report this information to the EMS personnel.

   g. After the convulsion ends, closely watch the victim. Encourage the victim to rest.

   h. Obtain medical assistance if the convulsion lasts more than a few minutes, if the victim has repeated convulsions, if other severe injuries are apparent, if the victim does not have a history of convulsions, or if the victim does not regain consciousness.

7. If the victim is in *diabetic coma*:

   a. Place the victim in a comfortable position. If the victim is unconscious, position him or her on either side to allow secretions to drain from the mouth.

   b. Frequently check respirations. Provide artificial respiration as needed.

   c. Obtain medical help immediately so the victim can be transported to a medical facility.

8. If the victim is in *insulin shock*:

   a. If the victim is conscious and can swallow, offer a drink containing sugar or oral glucose if a tube is available.

   b. If the victim is unconscious, place a small amount of granulated sugar under the victim's tongue.

PROCEDURE 15:11

c. Place the victim in a comfortable position. Position an unconscious victim on either side to allow secretions to drain from the mouth.

d. If recovery is not prompt, obtain medical help immediately.

9. Observe all victims of sudden illness for signs of shock. Treat for shock as necessary.

10. Constantly reassure any victim of sudden illness. Encourage relaxation to decrease stress.

11. Wash hands thoroughly after providing care.

Practice

Go to the workbook and use the evaluation sheet for 15:11, Providing First Aid for Sudden Illness, to practice this procedure. When you believe you have mastered this skill, sign the sheet and give it to your instructor for further action.

✔ **Final Checkpoint** Using the criteria listed on the evaluation sheet, your instructor will grade your performance.

15:12 INFORMATION

Applying Dressings and Bandages

In many cases requiring first aid, it will be necessary for you to apply dressings and bandages. This section provides basic information on types of bandages and dressings and on application methods.

A **dressing** is a sterile covering placed over a wound or an injured part. It is used to control bleeding, absorb blood and secretions, prevent infection, and ease pain. Materials that may be used as dressings include gauze pads in a variety of sizes and compresses of thick, absorbent material (figure 15-44). Fluff cotton should *not* be used as a dressing because the loose cotton fibers may contaminate the wound. In an emergency when no dressings are available, a clean handkerchief or pillowcase may be used. The dressing is held in place with tape or a bandage.

Bandages are materials used to hold dressings in place, to secure splints, and to support and protect body parts. Bandages should be applied snugly enough to control bleeding and prevent movement of the dressing, but not so tightly that they interfere with circulation. Types of bandages include roller gauze bandages, triangular bandages, and elastic bandages (figure 15-45).

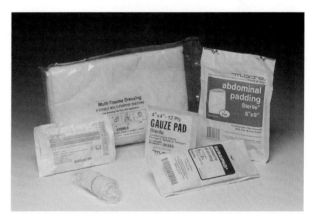

FIGURE 15-44 Dressings to cover a wound are available in many different sizes.

♦ *Roller gauze bandages* come in a variety of widths, most commonly 1-, 2-, and 3-inch widths. They can be used to hold dressings in place on almost any part of the body.

♦ *Triangular bandages* can be used to secure dressings on the head/scalp or as slings. A triangular bandage is sometimes used as a covering for a large body part such as a hand, foot, or shoulder. By folding the triangular bandage into a band of cloth called a *cravat* (figure 15-46), the bandage can be used to secure splints or dressings on body parts.

♦ *Elastic bandages* are easy to apply because they readily conform, or mold, to the injured

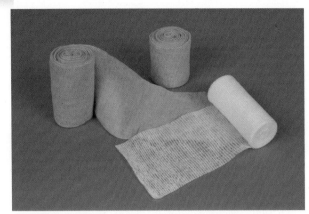

FIGURE 15-45 Roller gauze and elastic bandages can be used to hold dressings in place.

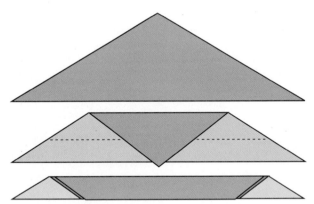

FIGURE 15-46 Folding a cravat bandage from a triangular bandage.

part. However, they can be quite hazardous; if they are applied too tightly or are stretched during application, they can cut off or constrict circulation. Elastic bandages are sometimes used to provide support and stimulate circulation.

Several methods are used to wrap bandages. The method used depends on the body part involved. Some common wraps include the spiral wrap, the figure-eight wrap for joints, and the finger, or recurrent, wrap. The wraps are described in Procedure 15:12, immediately following this information section.

After any bandage has been applied, it is important to check the body part below the bandage to make sure the bandage is not so tight as to interfere with blood circulation. Signs that indicate poor circulation include swelling, a pale or blue (cyanotic) color to the skin, coldness to the touch, and numbness or tingling. If the bandage has been applied to the hand, arm, leg, or foot, press lightly on the nail beds to blanch them (that is, make them turn white). The pink color should return to the nail beds immediately after pressure is released. If the pink color does not return or returns slowly, this is an indication of poor or impaired circulation. If any signs of impaired circulation are noted, loosen the bandages immediately.

STUDENT: *Go to the workbook and complete the assignment sheet for 15:12, Applying Dressings and Bandages. Then return and continue with the procedure.*

PROCEDURE 15:12

Applying Dressings and Bandages

Equipment and Supplies

Sterile gauze pads, triangular bandage, roller gauze bandage, elastic bandage, tape, disposable gloves

Procedure

1. Assemble equipment.

2. Wash hands. Put on gloves if there is any chance of contact with blood or body fluids.

3. Apply a dressing to a wound as follows:

   a. Obtain the correct size dressing. The dressing should be large enough to extend at least 1 inch beyond the edges of the wound.

   b. Open the sterile dressing package, taking care not to touch or handle the sterile dressing with your fingers.

PROCEDURE 15:12

c. Use a pinching action to pick up the sterile dressing so you handle only one part of the outside of the dressing. The ideal situation would involve the use of sterile transfer forceps or sterile gloves to handle the dressing. However, these items are usually not available in emergency situations.

d. Place the dressing on the wound. The untouched (sterile) side of the dressing should be placed on the wound. Do *not* slide the dressing into position. Instead, hold the dressing directly over the wound and then lower the dressing onto the wound.

e. Secure the dressing in place with tape or with one of the bandage wraps.

▽ **CAUTION:** If tape is used, do not wrap it completely around the part. This can lead to impaired circulation.

4. Apply a triangular bandage to the head or scalp (figure 15-47):

a. Fold a 2-inch hem on the base (longest side) of the triangular bandage.

b. Position and secure a sterile dressing in place over the wound.

c. Keeping the hem on the outside, position the middle of the base of the bandage on the forehead, just above the eyebrows.

d. Bring the point of the bandage down over the back of the head.

e. Bring the two ends of the base of the bandage around the head and above the ears. Cross the ends when they meet at the back of the head. Bring them around to the forehead.

f. Use a square knot to tie the ends in the center of the forehead.

g. Use one hand to support the head. Use the other hand to gently but firmly pull down on the point of the bandage at the back of the head until

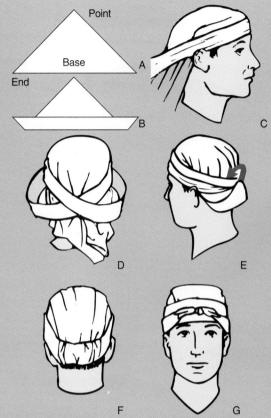

FIGURE 15-47 Steps for applying a triangular bandage to the head or scalp.

the bandage is snug against the head.

h. Bring the point up and tuck it into the bandage where the bandage crosses at the back of the head.

5. Make a cravat bandage from a triangular bandage (review figure 15-46):

a. Bring the point of the triangular bandage down to the middle of the base (the long end of the bandage).

b. Continue folding the bandage lengthwise until the desired width is obtained.

6. Apply a circular bandage with the cravat bandage (figure 15-48):

a. Place a sterile dressing on the wound.

PROCEDURE 15:12

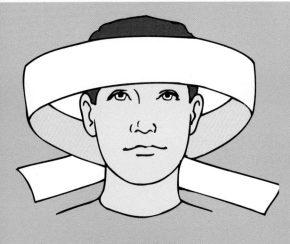

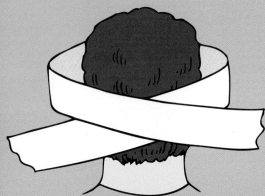

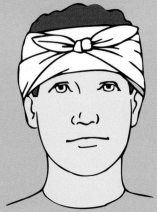

FIGURE 15-48 Steps for applying a circular bandage with a cravat bandage.

b. Place the center of the cravat bandage over the sterile dressing.

c. Bring the ends of the cravat around the body part and cross them when they meet.

d. Bring the ends back to the starting point.

e. Use a square knot to tie the ends of the cravat over the dressing.

▽ **CAUTION:** Avoid tying or wrapping the bandage too tightly. This could impair circulation.

NOTE: Roller gauze bandage can also be used.

▽ **CAUTION:** This type of wrap is *never* used around the neck because it could strangle the victim.

7. Apply a spiral wrap using roller gauze bandage or elastic bandage:

a. Place a sterile dressing over the wound.

b. Hold the roller gauze or elastic bandage so that the loose end is hanging off the bottom of the roll.

c. Start at the farthest end (the bottom of the limb) and move in an upward direction.

d. Anchor the bandage by placing it on an angle at the starting point. To do this, encircle the limb once, leaving a corner of the bandage uncovered. Turn down this free corner and then encircle the part again with the bandage (figure 15-49A).

e. Continue encircling the limb. Use a spiral type motion to move up the limb. Overlap each new turn approximately half the width of the bandage.

f. Use one or two circular turns to finish the wrap at the end point.

PROCEDURE 15:12

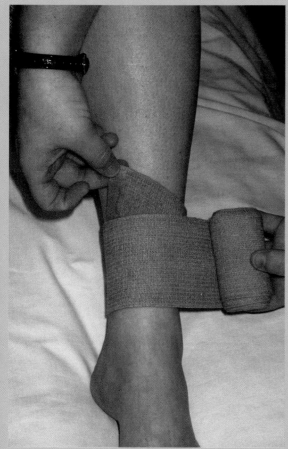

FIGURE 15-49A Anchor the bandage by leaving a corner exposed. This corner is then folded down and covered when the bandage is circled around the limb.

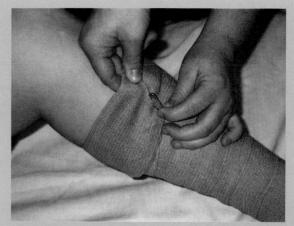

FIGURE 15-49B Place your hand between the bandage and the victim's skin while inserting a pin.

c. Make one or two circular turns around the instep and foot (figure 15-50A).

d. Bring the bandage up over the foot in a diagonal direction. Bring it around the back of the ankle and then down over the top of the foot. Circle it under the instep. This creates the figure-eight pattern.

e. Repeat the figure-eight pattern. With each successive turn, move downward and backward toward the heel

g. Secure the end by taping, pinning, or tying. To avoid injury when pins are used, place your hand under the double layer of bandage and between the pin and the skin before inserting the pin (figure 15-49B). The end of the bandage can also be cut in half and the two halves brought around opposite sides and tied into place.

8. Use roller gauze bandage or elastic bandage to apply a figure-eight ankle wrap:

a. Position a dressing over the wound.

b. Anchor the bandage at the instep of the foot.

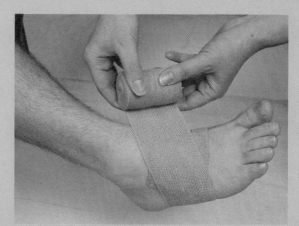

FIGURE 15-50A Bring the bandage over the foot in a diagonal direction for the start of the figure-eight pattern.

PROCEDURE 15:12

(figure 15-50B). Overlap the previous turn by one-half to two-thirds the width of the bandage.

NOTE: Hold the bandage firmly but do not pull it too tightly. If you are using elastic bandage, avoid stretching the material during the application.

f. Near completion, use one or two final circular wraps to circle the ankle.

g. Secure the bandage in place by taping, pinning, or tying the ends, as described in step 7g.

▽ **CAUTION:** To avoid injury to the victim when pins are used, place your hand between the bandage and the victim's skin.

9. Use roller gauze bandage to apply a recurrent wrap to the fingers (figure 15-51).

a. Place a sterile dressing over the wound.

b. Hold the roller gauze bandage so that the loose end is hanging off the bottom of the roll.

c. Place the end of the bandage on the bottom of the finger. Then bring the bandage up to the tip of the finger and down to the bottom of the oppo-

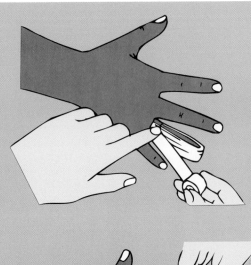

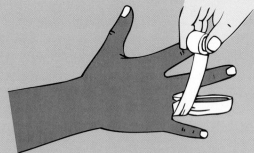

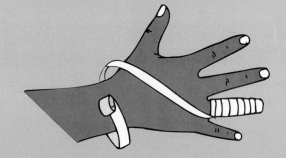

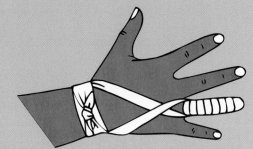

FIGURE 15-51 Recurrent wrap for the finger

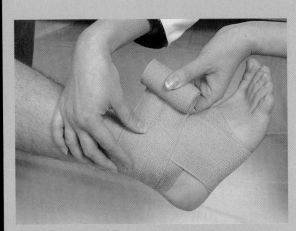

FIGURE 15-50B Keep repeating the figure-eight pattern by moving downward and backward toward the heel with each turn.

PROCEDURE 15:12

site side of the finger. With overlapping wraps, fold the bandage backward and forward over the finger three or four times.

d. Start at the bottom of the finger and use a spiral wrap up and down the finger to hold the recurrent wraps in position.

e. Complete the bandage by using a figure-eight wrap around the wrist. Bring the bandage in a diagonal direction across the back of the hand. Circle the wrist at least two times. Bring the bandage back over the top of the hand and circle the bandaged finger. Repeat this figure-eight motion at least twice.

f. Secure the bandage by circling the wrist once or twice. Tie the bandage at the wrist.

10. After any bandage has been applied, check the circulation below the bandage at frequent intervals. If possible, check for a pulse at a site below the bandage. Note any signs of impaired circulation, including swelling, coldness, numbness or tingling, pallor or cyanosis, and poor return of pink color after nail beds are blanched by lightly pressing on them. If any signs of poor circulation are noted, loosen the bandages immediately.

11. Obtain medical help for any victim who may need additional care.

12. Remove gloves and wash hands.

Practice

Go to the workbook and use the evaluation sheet for 15:12, Applying Dressings and Bandages, to practice this procedure. When you believe you have mastered this skill, sign the sheet and give it to your instructor for further action.

 Final Checkpoint Using the criteria listed on the evaluation sheet, your instructor will grade your performance.

CHAPTER 15 SUMMARY

First aid is defined as "the immediate care given to the victim of an injury or illness to minimize the effect of the injury or illness until experts can take over." Nearly everyone at some time experiences situations for which a proper knowledge of first aid is essential. It is important to follow correct techniques while administering first aid and to provide only the treatment you are qualified to provide.

The basic principles of first aid were presented in this unit. Methods of cardiopulmonary resuscitation (CPR) for infants, children, adults, and choking victims were described. Proper first aid for bleeding, shock, poisoning, burns, heat and cold exposure, bone and joint injuries, specific injuries, and sudden illness were covered. Instructions were given for the application of common dressings and bandages. By learning and following the suggested methods, the health care worker can provide correct first aid treatment in emergency situations until the help of experts can be obtained.

TODAY'S RESEARCH: TOMORROW'S HEALTH CARE

A microchip to cure diabetes?

Diabetes mellitus is a chronic disease caused by a decreased secretion of insulin, a hormone that is needed by body cells to absorb glucose (sugar) from the blood. In the United States, approximately 18.2 million people, or 6.3 percent of the population, have diabetes. Many of these individuals have insulin-dependent diabetes, which means they must inject daily doses of insulin to maintain blood glucose levels. For years, researchers have been looking for a technology that will end the need for individuals with diabetes to use needles to inject insulin and to constantly prick the skin to draw blood for glucose monitoring.

One researcher, Tejal Desai, has been successful in curing rats with diabetes by using a biological microelectromechanical system (MEMS), commonly called bioMEMS. BioMEMS are tiny devices that use microchips. Desai built a small implantable capsule with tiny pores, smaller than 1/100 of a human hair, on the surface. She placed live insulin-secreting pancreatic cells inside the capsule. The tiny pores on the capsule allow nutrients, waste products, and insulin to pass through, but are so small they prohibit harmful antibodies from entering the capsule. Because the body does not like foreign objects in the bloodstream, it produces antibodies to kill the objects. By blocking the antibodies, Desai appears to have eliminated the problem of rejection, allowing the implanted device to remain in the body where it can monitor the blood glucose level and secrete insulin as needed.

It will be several more years before Desai's research will be used on humans, but many scientists are currently using her ideas to create bioMEMS that can be used to cure disease. Some researchers are evaluating capsules that secrete blood-clotting factors for individuals with hemophilia. Others are trying to develop capsules that will carry dopamine to treat Parkinson's disease. Think of a future in which tiny capsules floating in the bloodstream or implanted in the body cure chronic diseases and allow individuals to live long and healthy lives.

INTERNET SEARCHES

Use the suggested search engines in Chapter 17:4 of this textbook to search the Internet for additional information on the following topics:

1. *Organizations*: find Web sites for the American Red Cross, the American Heart Association, Emergency Medical Services, and Poison Control Centers to learn services offered

2. *CPR*: look for sites that discuss the principles of cardiopulmonary resuscitation, abdominal thrusts, and cardiac emergencies

3. *Automated external defibrillators*: search for manufacturers of AEDs and compare different models

4. *First aid treatments*: find information on recommended treatment for bleeding, wounds, shock, poisoning, snakebites, insect stings, ticks, burns, heat exposure, heat stroke, hypothermia, frostbite, fractures, dislocations, sprains, strains, eye injuries, nose injuries, head and skull injuries, spine injuries, chest injuries, abdominal injuries, myocardial infarction, cerebrovascular accident, fainting, convulsions or seizures, diabetic coma, and insulin shock

REVIEW QUESTIONS

Review the following case histories. List the correct first aid care, in proper order of use, that should be used to treat each victim.

1. You are slicing carrots and cut off the end of your finger.

2. You find your 2-year-old brother in the bathroom. An empty bottle of aspirin tablets is on the floor. His mouth is covered with a white powdery residue.

3. You are watching television with your parents. Suddenly your father complains of severe pain in his chest and left arm. He is very short of breath and his lips appear cyanotic.

4. You are working in chemistry lab. Suddenly an experiment boils over and concentrated hydrochloric acid splashes into your lab partner's face and eyes. She starts screaming with pain.

5. You are driving and the car ahead of you loses control, goes off the road, and hits a tree. When you get to the car, the driver is slumped over the wheel. His arm is twisted at an odd angle. You notice a small fire at the rear of the car. A small child is crying in a car seat in the back seat.

6. You are playing tennis on a hot summer day with a friend. Suddenly your friend collapses on the tennis court. When you get to her, her skin is hot, red, and dry. She is breathing but she is unconscious.

For additional information on first aid and emergency care, write to:

♦ American Red Cross—contact your local chapter for First Aid and CPR courses and certification, or check the Web site at: *www.redcross. org*

♦ American Heart Association—contact your local chapter for CPR courses and certification or check the Web site at: *www.americanheart. org*

♦ Contact the National Highway Traffic Safety Administration (NHTSA), U.S. Department of Transportation, Emergency Medical Services Branch N-42-13, Washington, D.C. 20540 or check the Web at: *www.nhtsa.dot.gov* (click link to traffic safety and then emergency medical services)

PART 5

Working in Health Care

CHAPTER 16

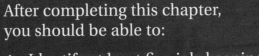

Preparing for the World of Work

Observe Standard Precautions

Instructor's Check—Call Instructor at This Point

Safety—Proceed with Caution

OBRA Requirement—Based on Federal Law

Math Skill

Legal Responsibility

Science Skill

Career Information

Communications Skill

Technology

Chapter Objectives

After completing this chapter, you should be able to:

◆ Identify at least five job-keeping skills and explain why employers consider them to be essential skills

◆ Write a cover letter containing all required information and using correct form for letters

◆ Prepare a résumé containing all necessary information and meeting standards for neatness and correctness

◆ Complete a job application form that meets standards of neatness and accuracy

◆ Demonstrate how to participate in a job interview, including wearing correct dress and meeting standards established in this chapter

◆ Determine gross and net income

◆ Calculate an accurate budget for a one-month period, accounting for fixed expenses and variable expenses without exceeding net monthly income

◆ Define, pronounce, and spell all key terms

KEY TERMS

application forms	fixed expenses	letter of application
budget	gross income	net income
cover letter	income	résumé *(rez'-ah-may)*
deductions	job interview	variable expenses

16:1 INFORMATION

Developing Job-Keeping Skills

To obtain and keep a job you must develop certain characteristics to be a good employee. A recent survey of employers asked for information on the deficiencies of high school graduates. The most frequent complaints included poor written grammar, spelling, speech, and math skills. Other complaints included lack of respect for work, lack of self-initiative, poor personal appearance, not accepting responsibility, excessive tardiness, poor attendance, and inability to accept criticism. Any of these defects would be detrimental in a health care worker.

It is essential that you develop good job-keeping skills to be successful in a health care career. Being aware of and striving to achieve the qualities needed for employment are as important as acquiring the knowledge and skills required in your chosen health care profession.

Job-keeping skills include:

♦ *Use correct grammar at all times.* This includes both the written and spoken word. Patients often judge ability on how well a person speaks or writes information. Use of words like *ain't* indicates a lack of education and does not create a favorable or professional impression. You must constantly strive to use correct grammar. Listen to how other health care professionals speak and review basic concepts of correct grammar. It may even be necessary to take a communications course to learn to speak correctly. Because you will be completing legal written records for health care, the use of correct spelling, punctuation, and sentence structure is also essential. Use a dictionary to check spelling, or use the spell check on a computer system. Refer to standard English books or secretarial manuals for information on sentence structure and punctuation. Constantly strive to improve both oral and written communication skills.

♦ *Report to work on time and when scheduled.* Because many health care facilities provide care 7 days a week, 365 days per year, and often 24 hours per day, an employee who is frequently late or absent can cause a major disruption in schedule and contribute to an insufficiency of personnel to provide patient care. Most health care facilities have strict rules regarding absenteeism, and a series of absences can result in job loss.

♦ *Be prepared to work when you arrive at work.* An employer does not pay workers to socialize, make personal telephone calls, consult others about personal or family problems, bring their children to work, shop on the Internet, play games on a computer, or work in a sloppy and inefficient manner. Develop a good work ethic. Observe all legal and ethical responsibilities. Follow the policies and procedures of your health care facility. Recognize your limitations and seek help when you need it. Be willing to learn new procedures and techniques. Watch efficient and knowledgeable staff members and learn by their examples. Constantly strive to do the best job possible. A worker who has self-initiative, who sees a job that needs to be done and does it, is a valuable employee who is likely to be recognized and rewarded.

♦ *Practice teamwork.* Because health care typically involves a team of different professionals working together to provide patient care, it is important to be willing to work with others. If you are willing to help others when they need help, they will likely be willing to help you. Two or three people working together can lift a heavy patient much more readily than can one.

♦ *Promote a positive attitude.* By being positive, you create a good impression and encourage the same attitude in others. Too often, employees concentrate only on the negative aspects of their jobs. Every job has some bad points; and it is easy to criticize these points. It is also easy to criticize the bad points in others with whom you work. However, this leads to a negative attitude and helps create poor morale in everyone. By concentrating on the good aspects of a job and the rewards it can provide, work will seem much more pleasant, and employees will obtain more satisfaction from their efforts.

♦ *Accept responsibility for your actions.* Most individuals are more than willing to take credit for the good things they have done. In the same manner, it is essential to take responsibility for mistakes. If you make a mistake, report it to your supervisor and make every effort to correct the error. Every human being will do something wrong at some time. Recognizing an error, taking responsibility for it, and making every effort to correct it or prevent it from happening again is a sign of a competent worker. Honesty is essential in health care. Not accepting responsibility for your actions is dishonest. It is often a reason for dismissal and can prevent you from obtaining another position.

♦ *Be willing to learn.* Health care changes constantly because of advances in technology and research. Every health care worker must be willing to learn new things and adapt to change. Participating in staff development programs (figure 16-1), taking courses at technical schools or colleges, attending special seminars or meetings, reading professional journals, and asking questions of other qualified individuals are all ways to improve your knowledge and skills. Employers recognize these efforts. Ambition is often rewarded with a higher salary and/or job advancement.

Without good job-keeping skills, no amount of knowledge will help you keep a job. Therefore, it is essential for you to strive to develop the qualities that employers need in workers. Be courteous, responsible, enthusiastic, cooperative, reliable, punctual, and efficient. Strive hard

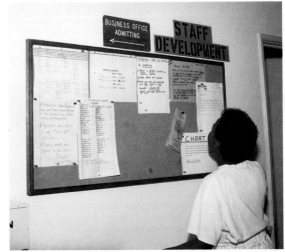

FIGURE 16-1 Participating in staff development programs is one way to improve your own knowledge and skills.

to be the best you can be. If you do this, you will not only be likely to retain your job, but you will probably be rewarded with job advancement, increased salary, and personal satisfaction.

STUDENT: *Go to the workbook and complete the assignment sheet for 16:1, Developing Job-Keeping Skills.*

16:2 INFORMATION

Writing a Cover Letter and Preparing a Résumé

INTRODUCTION

Before you look for a job, evaluate your interests and abilities. Decide what type job you would like. Make sure you obtain the education needed to perform the job. Then look at different job sources to try to find a position you will like. There are many different sources for finding job openings. Some of them include:

♦ Advertisements in newspapers

♦ Job fairs sponsored by schools or employment agencies

♦ Recommendations from friends and relatives

♦ School counselors or bulletin boards

♦ Employment agencies

- Internet job search sites
- Professional organizations: check their Internet site or contact the local organization
- Job listings posted at health care facilities or listed on their Internet site

Once you have identified possible places of employment, prepare to apply for the position. In most cases, this involves writing a cover letter, or letter of application, and a résumé.

COVER LETTER

The purpose of a **cover letter** or **letter of application** is to obtain an interview. You must create a good impression in the letter so that the employer will be interested in hiring you. In many cases, you will be responding to a job advertised either in the newspaper, on the Internet, or through other sources. However a résumé may be sent to potential employers even though they have not advertised a job opportunity. A cover letter should accompany all résumés.

The letter should be computer printed or typewritten on good quality paper. It must be neat, complete, and done according to correct form for letters. The correct form for composing business letters can be found in many English and business books. Care must be taken to ensure that spelling and punctuation are correct. Remember, this letter is the employer's first impression of you.

If possible, the letter should be addressed to the correct individual. If you know the name of the agency or company, call to obtain this information. Be sure you obtain the correct spelling of the person's name as well as the person's correct title. If you are responding to a box number, follow the instructions in the advertisement. Another possibility is to address the letter to the director of human resources or the head of a particular department.

The letter usually contains three to four paragraphs. The contents of each paragraph are described as follows:

- *Paragraph one*: state your purpose for writing and express interest in the position for which you are applying. If you are responding to an advertisement, state the name and date of the publication. If you were referred by another individual, give this person's name and title.

- *Paragraph two*: state why you believe you are qualified for the position. It may also state why you want to work for this particular employer. Information should be brief because most of the information will be included on your résumé.

- *Paragraph three*: state that a résumé is included. You may also want to draw the employer's attention to one or two important features on your résumé. If you are not including a résumé, state that one is available on request. Whenever possible, it is best to enclose a résumé.

- *Paragraph four*: closes the letter with a request for an interview. Be sure you clearly state how the employer can contact you for additional information. Include a telephone number and the times you will be available to respond to a telephone call. Finally, include a thank you to the potential employer for considering your application.

Figure 16-2 is a sample cover letter to serve as a guide to writing a good letter. However, remember this is only one guide. Letters must be varied to suit each circumstance.

RÉSUMÉ

A **résumé** is a record of information about an individual. It is a thorough yet concise summary of an individual's education, skills, accomplishments, and work experience. It is used to provide an employer with basic information that makes you appear qualified as an employee. At the same time, a good résumé will help you clarify your job objective and be better prepared for a job interview.

A résumé should be computer printed or typed and attractive in appearance. Like a cover letter, a résumé creates an impression on the employer. Information should be presented in an organized fashion. At the same time, the résumé should be concise and pertinent. Good-quality paper; correct spelling and punctuation; straight, even margins; and an attractive style are essential. If an individual is sending out a series of résumés, professional copies are permitted. However, the copies must be clear, on good-quality paper, and appealing in appearance.

Résumé format can vary. Review sample sources and find a style that you feel best pre-

18 Hireme Lane
Job City, Ohio 44444
June 3, 20--

Mr. Prospective Employer
Director of Human Resources
Health Care Facility
12 Nursing Lane
Dental City, Ohio 44833

Dear Mr. Employer:

In response to your advertisement in the _____
on _____ , 20 _____ , I would like to apply for
the position of _____ .

I recently graduated from _____ . I majored in
_____ and feel I am well qualified for this
position. I enjoy working with people and have a sincere
interest in additional training in _____ .

My resume is enclosed. I have also enclosed a specific list of
skills that I mastered during my school experience. I feel
that previous positions noted on the resume have provided me
with a good basis for meeting your job requirements.

Thank you for considering my application. I would appreciate
a personal interview at your earliest convenience to discuss
my qualifications. Please contact me at the above address or
by telephone at 589-1111 after 2:00 PM any day.

Sincerely,

Iamjob Hunting

FIGURE 16-2 A sample cover letter.

sents your information. A one-page résumé is usually sufficient.

Parts of a résumé can also vary. Some of the most important parts that should be included are shown in figures 16-3A and 16-3B and are described as follows:

♦ *Personal identification*: This includes your name, address, and telephone number. Be sure to include the area code.

♦ *Employment objective, job desired, or career goal*: Briefly state the title of the position for which you are applying.

Florence Nurse
22 South Main Street
Nursing, Ohio 33303
(400)589-1111

Employment Objective: Nursing Assistant Position

Skills

Recording Vital Signs   Making Beds
Moving and Transferring Patients   Observing Infection Control
Administrering CPR and First Aid   Providing Personal Hygience
Understanding Medical Terminology   Collecting Specimens
Applying Heat or Cold Applications   Ambulating Patients

Education

Career High School   Graduation: June 5, 2008
5 Diamond Street   Major: Health Occupations
Nursing, Ohio 33303   Grade Average: A's and B's

Certification: State Approved Nurse Assistant

Work Experience

Summer 2007 to Present   Country King Fried Chicken
                            5 Southern Lane
                            Mansfield, Ohio 33302

Fast Food Worker   Operate register
                            Record orders
                            Promote customer relations

Summer of 2005 and 2008   Madison Ram Hospital
                            602 Esley Lane
                            Mansfield, Ohio 33301

Volunteer Worker   Deliver mail and flowers
                            Assist nurses with patients

Extracurricular Activities

School Marching Band   Member for 3 years
SkillsUSA   Class treasurer for 2 years
Red Cross Club   Member for 3 years
Red Cross Blood Mobile   Volunteer worker for 3 years
March of Dimes Walkathon   Walker for 5 years
Church Youth Group   Member for 7 years

FIGURE 16-3A A sample résumé with information centered.

THOMAS J. TOOTH

340 DENTAL LANE   FLOSS, OHIO 44598   (524) 333-2435

CAREER GOAL: POSITION AS A DENTAL ASSISTANT IN GENERAL PRACTICE WITH A
                GOAL OF BECOMING A CERTIFIED DENTAL ASSISTANT

EDUCATION: OHIO JOINT VOCATIONAL SCHOOL, OPPORTUNITY, OHIO 44597
                GRADUATED IN JUNE 2007
                MAJORED IN DENTAL ASSISTANT PROGRAM FOR TWO YEARS

SKILLS: IDENTIFICATION OF TEETH, CHARTING CONDITIONS OF THE
                TEETH, MIXING DENTAL CEMENTS AND BASES, POURING MODELS
                AND CUSTOM TRAYS, PREPARING ANESTHETIC SYRINGE, SETTING
                UP BASIC DENTAL TRAYS, STERILIZING OF INSTRUMENTS,
                DEVELOPING AND MOUNTING RADIOGRAPHS, TYPING BUSINESS LETTERS,
                COMPLETING INSURANCE FORMS

WORK   DENTAL LAB PRODUCTS, 55 MODEL STREET, FLOSS, OHIO 44598
EXPERIENCE: EMPLOYED SEPTEMBER 2006 TO PRESENT AS DENTAL LAB ASSISTANT
                PROFICIENT IN MODELS, CUSTOM TRAYS, PROSTHETIC DEVICES

                DRUGGIST STORES, 890 PHARMACY LANE, OPPORTUNITY, OHIO 44597
                EMPLOYED JUNE 2004 TO AUGUST 2006 AS SALESPERSON
                EXPERIENCE IN CUSTOMER RELATIONS, INVENTORY, REGISTER, AND
                SALES PROMOTION

ACTIVITIES: HEALTH OCCUPATIONS STUDENTS OF AMERICA (HOSA) TREASURER
                FIRST PLACE STATE AWARD IN HOSA DENTAL ASSISTANT CONTEST
                VOLUNTEER WORKER DURING DENTAL HEALTH WEEK
                MEMBER OF SCHOOL PEP CLUB
                HOBBIES INCLUDE FOOTBALL, SWIMMING, BASKETBALL, READING
                VOLUNTEER FOR MEALS-ON-WHEELS

PERSONAL   DEPENDABLE, CONSIDERATE OF OTHERS, WILLING TO LEARN,
TRAITS: ADAPTABLE TO NEW SITUATIONS, RESPECTFUL AND HONEST,
                ADEPT AT DENTAL TERMINOLOGY, ABLE TO PERFORM A VARIETY
                OF DENTAL SKILLS

FIGURE 16-3B A sample résumé with left margin highlights.

♦ *Educational background*: List the name and address of your high school. Be sure to include special courses or majors if they relate to the job position. If you have taken additional courses or special training, list them also. If you have completed college or technical school, this information should be placed first.

♦ *Work or employment experience*: This includes previous positions of employment. Always start with the most recent position and work backward. Each entry should include the name and address of the employer, dates employed, your job title, and a brief description of duties. Avoid use of the word *I*. For example, instead of stating, "I sterilized supplies," state, "sterilized supplies," using action verbs to describe duties.

♦ *Skills*: List special knowledge, computer, and work skills you have that can be used in the job you are seeking. The list of skills should be specific and indicate your qualifications and ability to perform the job duties. When work experience is limited, a list of skills is important to show an employer that you are qualified for the position.

♦ *Other activities*: These can include organizations of which you are a member, offices held, community activities, special awards received, volunteer work, hobbies, special interests, and other similar facts. Keep this information brief, but do not hesitate to include facts that indicate school, church, and community involvement. This section can show an employer that you are a well-rounded person who participates in activities, assumes leadership roles, strives to achieve, and practices good citizenship. Write out the full names of organizations rather than the identifying letters.

♦ *References*: Most sources recommend not including references on a resume. Even the statement "references will be furnished on request" is now usually omitted. However, at least three references should be placed on a separate sheet of paper. The paper should be the same paper used for the résumé and include the same heading showing your name, address, and telephone number. The reference sheet can be given to an employer during the job interview. For a high school student with limited experience, references can provide valuable additional information. Always be sure you have an individual's permission before using that person as a reference. List the full name, title, address, and telephone number of the reference. It is best not to use relatives or high school friends as references. Select professionals in your field, clergy, teachers, or other individuals with responsible positions.

Honesty is always the best policy, and this is particularly true regarding résumés. Never give information that you think will look good but is exaggerated or only partly true. Inaccurate or false information can cost you a job. If you have an A to B average in school, include this information. If your average is lower than an A to B, do *not* include this information.

Before preparing your résumé, it is important to list all of the information you wish to include. Then select the format that best presents this information. The two sample résumés shown in figures 16-3A and 16-3B are meant to serve as guidelines only. Do not hesitate to evaluate other formats and present your information in the best possible way.

The envelope should be the correct size for your letter of application and résumé. Do *not* fold the letter into small sections and put it in an undersized envelope. This creates a sloppy impression. When possible, it is best to buy standard business envelopes that match your paper. A 9 × 12 envelope eliminates the need to fold the cover letter and résumé, and helps create a more professional appearance. Be sure the envelope is addressed correctly and neatly. It should also be computer printed or typewritten.

CAREER PASSPORT OR PORTFOLIO

A *career passport* or *portfolio* is a professional way to highlight your knowledge, abilities, and skills as you prepare for employment or extended education. It allows you to present yourself in an organized and efficient manner when you interview for schools or employment. Most career passports or portfolios contain the following types of information:

♦ *Introductory letter*: provides a brief synopsis of yourself including your background, education, and future goals

♦ *Résumé*: provides an organized record of information on education, employment experience, special skills, and activities

♦ *Skill list and competency level*: provides a list of skills you have mastered and the level of competency for each skill; some health occupation programs provide summaries of competency evaluations that can be used; if your program does not provide this, a list of skills and final competency grades can be compiled by using the evaluation sheets in the *Health Science Technology Workbook*

♦ *Letter(s) of recommendation*: include letters of recommendation from your instructors, guidance counselors, supervisors at clinical areas or agencies where you perform volunteer work, respected members of the community, advisors of activities in which you participate, and presidents of organizations of which you are a member

♦ *Copies of work evaluations*: include copies of evaluations you receive at job-training sites, volunteer activities, and/or paid work experiences

♦ *Documentation of mastering job-keeping skills*: the federal government has created SCANS, or the Secretaries Commission on Acquiring Necessary Skills, to designate skills employers desire in employees. SCANS lists three foundation skills that employers desire: *basic skills* (able to read, write, solve math problems, speak, and listen), *thinking skills* (able to learn, reason, think creatively, make decisions, and solve problems), and *personal qualities* (display responsibility, self-initiative, sociability, honesty, and integrity). In addition, SCANS lists five workplace competencies: *manage resources* (demonstrate ability to allocate time, money, materials, and space), *display interpersonal skills* (demonstrate ability to work in a team, lead, negotiate, compromise, teach others, and work with individuals

from diverse backgrounds), *utilize information* (acquire and evaluate data, file information, interpret information, and communicate with others), *comprehend systems* (understand social, organizational, and technical systems), and *use technologies* (use computers, apply technology to specific tasks, and maintain equipment). Write brief paragraphs to document how you have mastered skills such as teamwork, self-motivation, leadership, a willingness to learn, responsibility, organization, and other SCANS qualities

♦ *Leadership and organization abilities*: include information that demonstrates leadership and organization abilities you have mastered; participation in HOSA or Skills USA should be included

Organize the above information in a neat binder or portfolio. Use tab dividers to separate it into organized sections. Make sure that you use correct grammar and punctuation on all written information. The effort you put into creating a professional portfolio or passport will be beneficial when you have this document ready to present during a school or job interview.

STUDENT: *Go to the workbook and complete the assignment sheet for 16:2, Writing a Cover Letter and Résumé. Then return and continue with the procedure.*

PROCEDURE 16:2

Writing a Cover Letter and Preparing a Résumé

Equipment and Supplies

Good-quality paper, inventory sheet for résumés (see workbook), computer with word processing software and a printer, or typewriter

Procedure

1. Assemble equipment.

2. Re-read the preceding information section on a cover letter and résumés.

3. Review the sample letters of application and résumés.

4. Go to the workbook and complete the inventory sheet for résumés. Check dates for accuracy. Be sure that names are spelled correctly. Use the telephone book or other sources to check addresses and zip codes.

5. Carefully evaluate all your information. Determine the best method of presenting your information. Try different ways of writing your material. Do not hesitate

PROCEDURE 16:2

to show several different versions to your instructor or others and get their opinions on which way seems most effective.

6. Type a rough draft of a cover letter. Follow the correct form for letters. Use correct spacing and margins. Check for correct spelling and punctuation.

7. Type a final cover letter. Be sure it contains the required information. Proofread the letter for spelling errors and other mistakes. If possible, ask someone else to proofread your letter and evaluate it.

8. Type a rough draft of your résumé. Position the information in an attractive manner. Be sure that spacing is standard throughout the résumé and margins are even on all sides.

9. Review your sample résumé. Reword any information, if necessary. Be sure all information is pertinent and concise. Ask your instructor or others for opinions regarding suggested changes.

10. Type your final résumé. Take care to avoid errors. If you are not a good typist, it might be wise to have someone else complete the final draft. Proofread the final copy, checking carefully for errors.

If possible, ask someone else to proofread your résumé and evaluate it.

NOTE: Résumés can be copies of the original; but be sure the copies are of good quality. Cover letters must be originals; they are individually tailored for each potential job, and, therefore, are not copied.

11. Replace all equipment.

Practice

Go to the workbook and use the evaluation sheet for 16:2, Writing a Cover Letter and Résumé, to practice this procedure. When you believe you have mastered this skill, sign the sheet and give it to your instructor for further action. Also give your instructor your cover letter and résumé along with the evaluation sheet.

✔ **Final Checkpoint** Using the criteria listed on the evaluation sheet, your instructor will grade your cover letter and résumé.

16:3 INFORMATION

Completing Job Application Forms

Even though you provide each potential employer with a résumé, most employers still require you to complete an application form. **Application forms** are used by employers to collect specific information. Forms vary from employer to employer, but most request similar information.

Before completing any application form, it is essential that you first read the entire form. Note areas where certain information is to be placed. Read instructions that state how the form is to be completed. Some forms request that the applicant type or print all answers. Others request that the form be completed in the person's handwriting. If a scanner is available, an application form can be scanned into a computer so information can be keyed onto the application. The application can then be printed. Some health care facilities are using online applications. A computer is used to key information into the appropriate spaces. The application form is then printed and mailed or sent electronically by e-mail to the employer.

Be sure you have all the required information with you when you go for a job interview. Many employers will ask you to complete the application form at that time. Others will allow you to take the form home. Still others will even send the form to you prior to the interview. The latter two options allow you more time to obtain complete information and print or type the form (unless otherwise requested).

Basic rules for completing a job application form include:

♦ Fill out each item neatly and completely.

♦ Do *not* leave any areas blank. Put "none" or "NA" (meaning "not applicable") when the item requested does not apply to you.

♦ Be sure addresses include zip codes and all other required information.

♦ Watch spelling and punctuation. Errors will not impress the potential employer.

♦ Type or print neatly if the application does not state otherwise.

♦ Use a black pen if printing.

♦ If possible, scan the application into a computer word program, key in all information, check for accuracy, and then print the completed application form. Use spell-check if it is available. This method allows for easy correction of errors.

♦ Make sure all information is legible.

♦ Do *not* write in spaces that state "office use only" or "do not write below this line." Employers often judge how well you follow directions by your reaction to these sections.

♦ Be sure all information is correct and truthful. Remember, material can be checked and verified. A simple half-truth can cost you a job.

♦ Proofread your completed application. Check for completeness, spelling, proper answers to questions, and any errors.

♦ If references are requested, be sure to include all information such as title, address, and telephone number. Before using anyone's name as a reference, it is best to obtain that person's permission. Be prepared to provide reference information when you go for a job interview. Most sources suggest listing at least three references on a separate sheet of the same type of paper used for the résumé.

Even though questions vary on different forms, some basic information is usually requested on all of them. In order to be sure you have this information, it is useful to take a "wallet card" with you. A sample card is included in the workbook (as Assignment 2). Employers will not be impressed if you have to ask for a telephone book to find requested information; you may appear to be unprepared. Of course, if you are allowed to take the application home or if it is mailed or sent electronically (e-mail) to you, looking for information would not be a problem.

Remember that employers use application forms as a screening method. To avoid being eliminated from consideration for a position of employment, be sure your application creates a favorable impression.

STUDENT: *Go to the workbook and complete the assignment sheets for 16:3, Completing Job Application Forms and Wallet Card. Then return and continue with the procedure.*

PROCEDURE 16:3

Completing Job Application Forms

Equipment and Supplies

Typewriter or computer and scanner or pen, wallet card (sample in workbook), sample application forms (sample in workbook)

Procedure

1. Assemble equipment. If a typewriter is used, be sure the ribbon is of good quality. If a scanner is available, scan the application form into the word processing program of a computer. The application form can then be completed with the computer and printed on a printer.

PROCEDURE 16:3

2. Complete all information on the wallet card. A sample is included in the workbook (as Assignment 2). Check dates and be sure information is accurate. List full addresses, zip codes, and names.

3. Review the preceding information section on completing job application forms. Read additional references, as needed.

4. Read the entire sample application form (Assignment 3) in the workbook. Be sure you understand the information requested for each part. Read all directions completely.

5. Unless otherwise directed, type all information requested. If a typewriter is not available, use a black ink pen to print all information. If a scanner and computer are available, scan the application form into a word program. After keying in all information, the completed application can be printed.

6. Complete all areas of the form. Use "none" or "NA" as a reply to items that do not apply to you.

7. Take care not to write in spaces labeled "office use only" or "do not write below this line." Leave these areas blank.

8. In the space labeled "signature," sign your name. Note any statement that may be printed by the signature line. Be sure you are aware of what you are signing and the permission you may be giving. Most employers request permission to contact previous employers and/or references, and a verification that information is accurate.

9. Recheck the entire application. Be sure information is correct and complete. Note and correct any spelling errors. Be sure you have answered all of the questions.

10. Replace all equipment.

Practice

Go to the workbook and use the evaluation sheet for 16:3, Completing Job Application Forms, to practice this procedure. Obtain sample job application forms from your instructor or other sources. When you believe you have mastered this skill, sign the sheet and give it to your instructor for further action.

 Final Checkpoint Using the criteria listed on the evaluation sheet, your instructor will grade your job application form.

16:4 INFORMATION

Participating in a Job Interview

A job interview is what you are seeking when you send a letter of application and a résumé. You must prepare for an interview just as hard as you did when composing your résumé. A poor interview can mean a lost job.

A **job interview** is usually the last step before getting or being denied a particular position of employment. Usually, you have been screened by the potential employer and have been selected for an interview as a result of your résumé and application form. To the employer, the interview serves at least two main purposes:

♦ Provides the opportunity to evaluate you in person, obtain additional information, and ascertain whether you meet the job qualifications

♦ Allows the employer to tell you about the position in more detail

Careful preparation is needed before going to an interview. Be sure you have all required information. Your "wallet card," résumé, and completed application form (if you have done one) must be ready. If you have completed a career passport or portfolio, be sure to take it to the interview. If possible, find out about the position and the agency offering the job. In this way, you will be more aware of the agency's needs.

Be sure of the scheduled date and time of the interview. Know the name of the individual you must contact and the exact place of the interview. Write this information down and take it with you.

Dress carefully. It is best to dress conservatively. Coats and ties are still best for men. Although pantsuits are sometimes acceptable for women, employers still generally prefer dresses or skirts. Even though it shouldn't be the case, first impressions can affect the employer. All clothes should fit well and be clean and pressed, if needed. Avoid bright, flashy colors and very faddish styles.

Check your entire appearance. Hair should be neat, clean, and styled attractively. Nails should be clean. Women should avoid wearing bright nail polish, too much makeup, and perfume. Men should be clean shaven. Be sure that your teeth are clean and your breath is fresh. Jewelry should not be excessive. And last but not least, use a good antiperspirant. When you are nervous, you perspire.

It is best to arrive 5–10 minutes early for your interview. Late arrival could mean a lost job. Allow for traffic, trains blocking the road, and other complications that might interfere with your arriving on time.

During the interview, observe all of the following points:

♦ Greet the interviewer by name when you are introduced. Introduce yourself. Shake hands firmly and smile (figure 16-4A).

♦ Remain standing until the interviewer asks you to sit. Be aware of your posture and sit straight. Keep both feet flat on the floor or cross your legs at the ankles only.

♦ Use correct grammar. Avoid using slang words.

♦ Speak slowly and clearly. Don't mumble.

♦ Be polite. Practice good manners.

♦ ⭕ Maintain eye contact (figure 16-4B). Avoid looking at the floor, ceiling, or away from the interviewer. Looking at the middle of the interviewer's forehead or at the tip of the interviewer's nose can sometimes help when you are nervous and experiencing difficulty with direct eye contact.

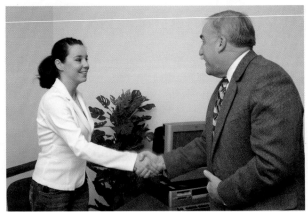

FIGURE 16-4A Shake hands firmly and smile when you greet an interviewer.

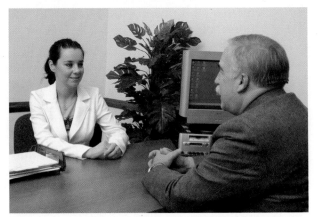

FIGURE 16-4B Sit straight and maintain eye contact during the interview.

♦ Listen closely to the interviewer. Do not interrupt in the middle of a sentence. Allow the interviewer to take the lead.

♦ Answer all questions thoroughly, but don't go into long, drawn-out explanations. Make sure your answers show how you are qualified for the job.

♦ Do *not* smoke, chew gum, or eat candy during the interview.

♦ Smile but avoid excessive laughter or giggling.

♦ Be yourself. Do not try to assume a different personality or different mannerisms; doing so will only increase your nervousness.

♦ Be enthusiastic. Display your positive attitude.

♦ Avoid awkward habits such as swinging your legs, jingling change in your pocket, waving your hands or arms, or patting at your hair.

◆ Never discuss personal problems, finances, or other situations in an effort to get the job. This usually has a negative effect on the interviewer.

◆ Do not criticize former employers or degrade them in any way.

◆ Answer all questions truthfully to the best of your ability.

◆ Think before you respond. Try to organize the information you present.

◆ Be proud of yourself, to a degree. You have skills and are trained. Make sure the interviewer is aware of this. However, be sure to show a willingness to learn and to gain additional knowledge.

◆ Do not immediately question the employer about salary, fringe benefits, insurance, and other similar items. This information is usually mentioned before the end of the interview. If the employer asks whether you have any questions, ask about the job description or responsibilities, type of uniform required, potential for career growth, continuing education or in-service programs, and job orientation. These types of questions indicate a sincere interest in the job rather than a "What's in it for me?" attitude.

◆ Do not expect a definite answer at the end of the interview. The interviewer will usually tell you that he or she will contact you.

◆ Thank the interviewer for the interview as you leave. If the interviewer extends a hand, shake hands firmly. Smile, be polite, and exit with confidence.

◆ Never try to extend the interview if the interviewer indicates that he or she is ready to end it.

After the interview, it is best to send a follow-up note, letter, or electronic message (e-mail) to thank the employer for the interview (figure 16-5). You may indicate that you are still interested in the position. You may also state that you are available for further questioning. When an employer is evaluating several applicants, a thank-you note is sometimes the deciding factor in who gets the job.

Because you may be asked many different questions during an interview, it is impossible to prepare all answers ahead of time. However, it is wise to think about some potential

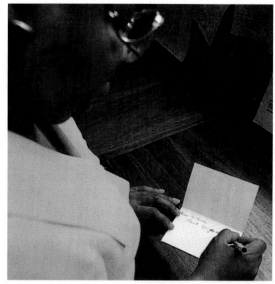

FIGURE 16-5 After a job interview, send a thank-you note, letter, or e-mail to the employer.

questions and your responses to them. The following is a suggested list of questions to review. Additional questions may be found in any book on job interviews.

◆ *Tell me a little about yourself.* (Note: Stick to job-related information.)

◆ *What are your strong points/weak points?* (Note: Be sure to turn a weakness into a positive point. For example, say, "One of my weaknesses is poor spelling, but I use a dictionary to check spelling and try to learn to spell ten new words each week.")

◆ *Why do you feel you are qualified for this position?*

◆ *What jobs have you held in the past? Why did you leave these jobs?* (Note: Avoid criticizing former employers.)

◆ *What school activities are you involved in?*

◆ *What kind of work interests you?*

◆ *Why do you want to work here?*

◆ *What skills do you have that would be of value?*

◆ *What is your attitude toward work?*

◆ *What do you want to know about this job opening?*

◆ *What were your favorite subjects in school and why?*

◆ *What does success mean to you?*

♦ *How do you manage your time?*

♦ *What is your image of the ideal job?*

♦ *How skilled are you with computers?*

♦ *What are the three most important things to you in a job?*

♦ *Do you prefer to work alone or with others? Why?*

♦ *How many days of school did you miss last year?*

♦ *What do you do in your spare time?*

♦ *Do you have any plans for further education?*

⚖ Any questions that may reflect discrimination or bias do *not* have to be answered during a job interview. Federal law prohibits discrimination with regard to age, cultural or ethnic background, marital status, parenthood, disability, religion, race, and sex. Employers are aware that it is illegal to ask questions of this nature, and the large majority will not ask such questions. If an employer does ask a question of this nature, however, you have the right to refuse to answer. An example of this type of question might be, "I see you married recently. Do you plan to start having children in the next year or two?" Be polite but firm in your refusal. A statement such as "I prefer not to answer that question" or "Can I ask you how this would affect the job we are discussing?" is usually sufficient.

⚖ At the end of the interview, you may be asked to provide proof of your eligibility to work. Under the Bureau of Immigration Reform Act of 1986, employers are now required by federal law to ask you to complete an Employment Eligibility Verification Form I-9. This form helps the employer verify that you are legally entitled to work in the United States. To complete this form, you must provide documents that indicate your identity. A birth certificate, passport, and/or immigration card can be used for this purpose. You must also have a photo identification, such as a driver's license, and a social security card. The employer must make copies of these documents and include them in your file. Having these forms readily available shows that you are prepared for a job.

STUDENT: *Go to the workbook and complete the assignment sheet for 16:4, Participating in a Job Interview. Then return and continue with the procedure.*

PROCEDURE 16:4

Participating in a Job Interview

Equipment and Supplies

Desk, two chairs, evaluation sheets, lists of questions

Procedure

1. Assemble equipment. Role-play a mock interview with four persons. Arrange for two people to evaluate the interview, one person to be the interviewer, and you to be the interviewee.

2. Position the two evaluators in such a way that they can observe both the interviewer and you, the person being interviewed. Make sure they will not interfere with the interview.

3. The interviewer should be seated at the desk and have a list of possible questions to ask during the interview.

4. Play the role of the person being interviewed. Prepare for this role by doing the following:

   a. Be sure you have all necessary information. Prepare your wallet card, résumé, job application form, and/or career passport or portfolio.

   b. Dress appropriately for the interview (as outlined in the preceding information section).

   c. Arrive at least 5–10 minutes early for the interview.

PROCEDURE 16:4

5. When you are called for the interview, introduce yourself. Be sure to refer to the interviewer by name.

6. Sit in the chair indicated. Be aware of your posture, making sure to sit straight. Keep your feet flat on the floor or cross your legs at the ankles only.

7. Listen closely to the employer. Answer all questions thoroughly and completely. Think before you speak. Organize your information.

8. Maintain eye contact. Avoid distracting mannerisms.

9. Use correct grammar. Avoid slang expressions. Speak in complete sentences. Practice good manners.

10. When you are asked whether you have any questions, ask questions pertaining to the job responsibilities. Avoid a series of questions on salary, fringe benefits, vacations, time off, and so forth.

11. At the end of the interview, thank the interviewer for his or her time. Shake hands as you leave.

12. Check your performance by looking at the evaluation sheets completed by the two observers. Study suggested changes.

13. Replace all equipment.

Practice

Go to the workbook and use the evaluation sheet for 16:4, Participating in a Job Interview, to practice this procedure. When you believe you have mastered this skill, sign the sheet and give it to your instructor for further action.

✔ **Final Checkpoint** Using the criteria listed on the evaluation sheet, your instructor will grade your performance.

16:5 INFORMATION

Determining Net Income

 Obtaining a job means, in part, that you will be earning your own money. This often means that you will be responsible for your own living expenses. To avoid debt and financial crisis, it is important that you learn about managing your money effectively, including understanding how to determine net income.

The term **income** usually means money that you earn or that is available to you. However, the amount you actually earn and the amount you receive to spend may vary. The following two terms explain the difference.

◆ **Gross income:** This is the total amount of money you earn for hours worked. It is the amount determined before any deductions have been taken out of your pay.

◆ **Net income:** This is commonly referred to as "take-home pay." It is the amount of money available to you after all payroll **deductions** have been taken out of your salary. Some common deductions are Social Security tax, federal and state taxes, and city taxes. Other deductions may include payroll deductions such as those for United Appeal, medical or life insurance, union dues, and other similar items.

To determine gross income, simply multiply your wage per hour times the number of hours worked. For example, if you earn $9.00 per hour and work a 40-hour week, $9 \times 40 = \$360.00$. In this example, then, $360.00 would be your gross income.

To determine net income, you must first determine the amounts of the various deductions that will be taken out of your gross pay. Deduction percentages usually vary depending on your income level. You can usually determine approximate deduction percentages and, therefore, your approximate net income by referring to tax charts. Tax charts for federal taxes are available on the Internet at *www.irs.gov*. Tax charts for cities and states can usually be found on the treasurer's Internet site for the particular city or state. Never hesitate to ask your employer about deduction percentages. It is your responsibility to check your own paycheck for accuracy. Starting with the example of gross pay of $360.00, the following shows how net pay may be determined.

Gross Pay $360.00

◆ Deduction for federal tax in this income range is usually approximately 15 percent. Check tax tables for accuracy.

15%, or 0.15, × 360 = $54.00   −54.00
                                       306.00

◆ Deduction for state tax is approximately 2 percent.

2%, or 0.02, × 360 = $7.20   −7.20
                                       298.80

◆ Deduction for city tax is approximately 1 percent.

1%, or 0.01, × 360 = 3.60   −3.60
                                       295.20

◆ Deduction for F.I.C.A., or Social Security tax, includes 6.2 percent of the first $102,000 in income and a Medicare deduction of 1.45 percent of the total in income, for a total deduction of 7.65 percent.

7.65%, or 0.0765, × 360 = 27.54   −27.54
                                       267.66

◆ Net income after taxes, then, would be $267.66. Therefore, before you even receive your paycheck, $92.34 will be deducted from it. Additional deductions for insurance, union dues, contributions to charity, and other items may also be taken out of your gross pay.

In order to manage your money effectively, it is essential that you be able to calculate your net income. Because this is the amount of money you will have to spend, it will to some extent determine your lifestyle.

STUDENT: *Read and complete Procedure 16:5, Determining Net Income.*

PROCEDURE 16:5

Determining Net Income

Equipment and Supplies

Assignment sheet for 16:5, Determining Net Income; pen or pencil

Procedure

1. Assemble equipment. If a calculator is available, you may use it to complete this assignment.

2. Read the instructions on the assignment sheet in the workbook for 16:5, Determining Net Income. Use the assignment sheet with this procedure.

3. Determine your wage per hour by using your salary in a current job or an amount assigned by your instructor. Multiply this amount by the number of hours you work per week. This is your gross weekly pay.

4. If your instructor has federal tax tables, read the tax tables to determine the percentage, or amount of money, that will be withheld for federal tax. If tax tables are not available, look on the Internet at *www.irs.gov* or check with your employer to obtain this information.

   NOTE: The average withholding tax for an initial income bracket is usually approximately 15 percent. If you cannot find the exact amount or percentage, use this amount (0.15) for an approximate determination.

5. Multiply the percentage for federal tax times your gross weekly pay to deter-

PROCEDURE 16:5

mine the amount deducted for federal tax.

6. Determine the deduction for state tax by reading your state tax tables, checking the state treasurer's site on the Internet, or by consulting your employer.

   NOTE: An average state tax is 2 percent. If you cannot find the exact amount or percentage, use this amount (0.02) for an approximate determination.

7. Multiply the percentage for state tax by your gross weekly pay to determine the amount deducted for state tax.

8. Determine the deduction for any city or corporation tax by reading the city/corporation tax tables, checking the city/corporation treasurer's site on the Internet, or consulting your employer.

   NOTE: An average city/corporation tax is 1 percent. If you cannot find the exact amount or percentage, use this amount (0.01) for an approximate determination.

9. Multiply the percentage for city/corporation tax by your gross weekly pay to determine the amount deducted for city/corporation tax.

10. Check the current deduction for F.I.C.A., or Social Security and Medicare, by checking the Social Security Internet site or asking your employer for this information. Determine the deduction for F.I.C.A. by multiplying your gross weekly pay by this percentage.

    NOTE: In 2008, the F.I.C.A. rate was 6.2 percent of the first $102,000 in income

and 1.45 percent of total income for Medicare. Use this total of 7.65 percent, or 0.0765, if you cannot obtain another percentage.

11. List the amounts for any other deductions. Examples include insurance, charitable donations, union dues, and similar items.

12. Add the amounts determined for federal tax, state tax, city/corporation tax, social security, and other deductions together.

13. Subtract the total amount for deductions from your gross weekly pay. The amount left is your net, or take-home, pay.

14. Recheck any figures, as needed.

15. Replace all equipment.

Practice

Go to the workbook and use the evaluation sheet for 16:5, Determining Net Income. Practice determining net income according to the criteria listed on the evaluation sheet. When you believe you have mastered this skill, sign the sheet and give it to your instructor for further action.

 Final Checkpoint Using the criteria listed on the evaluation sheet, your instructor will grade your performance.

16:6 INFORMATION

Calculating a Budget

In order to use your net income wisely, it is best to prepare a budget. A **budget** is an itemized list of living expenses. It must be realistic to be effective.

A budget usually consists of two main types of expenses: fixed expenses and variable expenses. **Fixed expenses** include items such as rent or house payments, utilities, food, car payments, and insurance payments. **Variable expenses** include items such as entertainment, clothing purchases, and donations.

The easiest way to prepare a budget is to simply list all anticipated expenses for a one-month period. Then determine your net monthly pay. Allow a fair percentage of the net monthly pay for each of the budget items listed.

Savings should be incorporated into every budget. If saving money is regarded as an obligation, it is easier to set aside money for this purpose. When an emergency occurs, money is then available to cover the unexpected expenditure.

Some payments are due once or twice a year. An example is insurance payments. To be realistic, a monthly amount should be budgeted for this purpose. To determine a monthly amount, divide the total yearly cost for the insurance by 12. Then budget this amount each month. In this way, when insurance payments are due, the money is available for payment, and one month's budget will not have to bear the full amount of the insurance payment.

Money Management International (MMI), a nonprofit consumer counseling organization, recommends that the following percentage ranges of total net income be used while preparing a realistic budget:

♦ *Housing*: 20–35 percent
♦ *Food*: 15–30 percent
♦ *Utilities*: 4–7 percent
♦ *Transportation* (including car loan, insurance, gas, and maintenance): 6–20 percent
♦ *Insurance* (including health, life, and/or disability): 4–6 percent
♦ *Health* (including prescriptions, eye care, dental care): 2–8 percent

♦ *Clothing*: 3–10 percent
♦ *Personal care* (including soap, toothpaste, laundry detergents, cosmetics, etc.): 2–4 percent
♦ *Miscellaneous* (including travel, child care, entertainment, gifts, etc.): 1–4 percent
♦ *Savings*: 5–9 percent

It is important to remember that these percentages and line items are just suggested guidelines. Each individual must determine his or her own needs and allocate monies accordingly. However, MMI does state that personal debt should not exceed 10–20 percent of net income. Financial difficulties usually occur when debt exceeds this limit.

It is important that budgeted expenses do *not* exceed net monthly income. It may sometimes be necessary to limit expenses that are not fixed. Entertainment, clothing purchases, and similar items are examples of expenses that can be limited.

The final step is to live by your budget and avoid any spending over the allotted amounts. This is one way to prevent financial problems and excessive debt. If your fixed expenses or net income increases, you will have to revise your budget. Remember, creating a budget leads to careful management of hard-earned money.

STUDENT: *Read Procedure 16:6, Calculating a Budget. Then go to the workbook and complete the corresponding assignment sheet.*

PROCEDURE 16:6

Calculating a Budget

Equipment and Supplies

Assignment sheet for 16:6, Calculating a Budget; pen or pencil

Procedure

1. Assemble equipment. If a calculator is available, you may use it to complete this procedure.

2. Go to the workbook and read the instructions on the assignment sheet for 16:6, Calculating a Budget.

3. Determine your fixed expenses for a one-month period. This includes amounts you must pay for rent, utilities, loans, charge accounts, insurance, and similar items. List these expenses.

4. Determine your variable expenses for a one-month period. This includes amounts for clothing purchases, per-

PROCEDURE 16:6

sonal items, donations, entertainment, and similar items. List these expenses.

5. List any other items that must be included in your monthly budget. Be sure to list a reasonable amount for each item.

6. Determine a reasonable amount for savings. Many people prefer to set aside a certain percentage of their net monthly pay as savings.

7. Determine your net monthly pay. Double-check all figures for accuracy.

8. Add all of your monthly budget expenses together. The sum represents your total expenditures per month.

9. Compare your expense total to your net monthly income. If your expense total is higher than your net income, you will have to revise your budget and reduce any expenses that are not fixed. If your expense total is lower than your net income, you may increase the dollar amounts of your budget items. If the other figures in your budget are realistic, it may be wise to increase the dollar amount of savings.

10. When the expense total in your budget equals your monthly net income, you have a balanced budget. Live by this budget and avoid any expenditures not listed on the budget.

11. Replace all equipment.

Practice

Go to the workbook and use the evaluation sheet for 16:6, Calculating a Budget, to practice this procedure. When you believe you have mastered this skill, sign the sheet and give it to your instructor for further action. Give your instructor a completed budget along with the evaluation sheet.

 Final Checkpoint Using the criteria listed on the evaluation sheet, your instructor will grade your budget.

CHAPTER 16 SUMMARY

Even if an individual is proficient in many skills, it does not necessarily follow that the individual will obtain the "ideal" job. Just as it is important to learn the skills needed in your chosen health care career, it is important to learn the skills necessary to obtain a job.

Job-keeping skills important to an employer include using correct grammar in both oral and written communications, reporting to work on time and when scheduled, being prepared to work, following correct policies and procedures, having a positive attitude, working well with others, taking responsibility for your actions, and being willing to learn. Without good job-keeping skills, no amount of knowledge will help you keep a job.

One of the first steps in obtaining a job involves preparing a cover letter and a résumé. These are the "press releases" that tell a potential employer about your skills and abilities. A properly prepared résumé will help you obtain an interview.

It is important to prepare for an interview. Careful consideration should be given to dress and appearance. Answers should be prepared

TODAY'S RESEARCH: TOMORROW'S HEALTH CARE

A bravery gene?

Anxiety and fear have been felt by every human being. However, some individuals are so anxious or fearful they are not able to function within society. For example, individuals with agoraphobia have an abnormal fear of being helpless in a situation from which they cannot escape, so they stay in an environment in which they feel secure. Many agoraphobic people never leave their homes; they avoid all public or open places. Scientists are not really certain how fear works in the brain, so conditions such as these are difficult to treat.

Recently, scientists working with mice found that by removing a single gene, they could turn normally cautious animals into brave animals that were more willing to explore an unknown territory and were less intimidated by dangers. By analyzing brain tissue, scientists located a gene in a tiny prune-shaped region of the brain called the *amygdala*, an area of the brain that is extremely active when animals or humans are afraid or anxious. This gene produces a protein called *stathmin*, which is highly concentrated in the amygdala but very hard to detect in other areas of the brain. Scientists removed this stathmin gene and bred a line of mice that were all missing this gene. Tests showed that this breed of mice was twice as willing to explore unknown territories as unaltered mice. In addition, if the mice were trained to expect a small electrical shock after being presented with a stimulus such as a sound or sight, this group of mice did not seem as fearful when the sound or sight was given. Researchers are theorizing that stathmin helps form fearful memories in the amygdala of the brain, the area where unconscious fears seemed to be stored. If the production of stathmin could be halted or inhibited by medication, it is possible that fears would not be stored as unconscious memories. This would greatly decrease an individual's anxieties because unconscious fears are a major cause of anxiety. Think of all of the people whose lives are affected by anxiety and fear. If their anxieties and fears could be decreased or eliminated, they could lead normal healthy lives.

for common interview questions. The applicant should also try to learn as much as possible about the potential employer; this way, the applicant will be able to match his or her skills and abilities to the needs of the employer. Finally, practice completing job application forms. A neat, correct, and thorough application form will also help you get a job.

Certain other skills become essential when a person has a job. Everyone should be able to calculate gross and net income. In addition, everyone should be able to develop a budget based on needs and income. Having and following a budget makes it more likely that money earned will be spent wisely and minimizes the chance of debt. Learn the job-seeking and job-keeping skills well. They will benefit you throughout your life as you seek new positions of employment and advance in your chosen health career.

INTERNET SEARCHES

Use the suggested search engines in Chapter 17:4 of this textbook to search the Internet for additional information on the following topics:

1. *Components of a job search*: find information on letters of application or cover letters, résumés, job interviews, and job application forms

3. *Requirements of employers*: locate information on skills and qualities that employers desire

4. *Job search*: look for sites that provide information on employment opportunities. For specific health care careers, look for opportunities under organizations for the specific career. Also check general sites such as *monster.com, job-listing.com, jobsleuth.com, hotjobs.yahoo. com, careerbuilder.com,* and *joblocator.com.*

4. *Salary and wages*: check sites such as the Internal Revenue Service (IRS), state and local tax departments, and Social Security Administration for information on taxes and tax rates; also locate sites on money management, budgeting, and fiscal or financial management for information on how to manage money

REVIEW QUESTIONS

1. Choose four (4) job-keeping skills that you believe you have mastered. Write a paragraph describing why you believe you have mastered these skills.

2. What is the main purpose of a letter of application or cover letter? When is it used?

3. List the main sections of a résumé and briefly describe the information that should be included in each section.

4. State six (6) basic principles that must be followed while completing a job application form.

5. Create answers for the following interview questions.
   a. Why do you believe you are qualified for this job?
   b. Why do you want to leave your current job?
   c. Tell me about two or three of your major accomplishments and why you feel they are important.

6. You have obtained a job and will receive a salary of $8.20 per hour. Calculate the following:
   a. Gross pay for a 40-hour week
   b. Federal tax deduction of 15%
   c. State tax deduction of 3%
   d. City tax deduction of 0.5%
   e. FICA or social security deduction of 7.65%
   f. Net pay after above deductibles

CHAPTER 17

Computer Technology in Health Care

Observe Standard
Precautions

Instructor's Check—Call
Instructor at This Point

Safety—Proceed with
Caution

OBRA Requirement—Based
on Federal Law

Math Skill

Legal Responsibility

Science Skill

Career Information

Communications Skill

Technology

Chapter Objectives

After completing this chapter,
you should be able to:

◆ Identify the three major components of a
computer system

◆ Compare computer capabilities and
limitations

◆ Describe computer applications currently
being used in today's health care computer
systems

◆ Search the Internet for information on a
specific topic

◆ Identify precautions that must be taken to
maintain the confidentiality of patient
information

◆ Differentiate between antivirus and firewall
software, and explain how each helps to
provide computer security

◆ Define, pronounce, and spell all key terms

KEY TERMS

browser

central processing unit (CPU)

computer literacy *(come-pew'-tur lit'-er-ass-see)*

computer-assisted instruction (CAI)

computerized tomography (CT) *(com-pew'-tur-eyesd toe-mawg'-rah-fee)*

database

echocardiograph

electronic mail

file

fields

hardware

input

interactive video (computer-assisted video)

Internet

magnetic resonance imaging (MRI) *(mag-net'-ik rez'-oh-nance im'-adj-ing)*

mainframe computer

microcomputer

modem

networks

output

personal computer

positron emission tomography (PET) *(pos-ee'-tron ee-miss'-shun toe-mawg'-rah-fee)*

random access memory (RAM)

read only memory (ROM)

record

software

spreadsheet

stress test

telemedicine

telepharmacies

ultrasonography *(ul-trah-sawn-ahg'-rah-fee)*

virtual communities

17:1 INFORMATION

Introduction

Computer technology has been called the greatest advance in information processing since Gutenberg invented the printing press. Rapid advances in health care and the explosion of information needed for health care workers to provide quality patient care have made computer use a necessity. Today, it is as common to see a computer terminal in the admissions office of your local hospital or clinic as it is to see a bar code reader being used to add up a grocery bill in your neighborhood supermarket. In fact, many hospitals use this same bar coding method to control inventories and patient costs for hospital supplies.

The computer has become essential in almost every aspect of health care. Computers are used in four general areas:

♦ *Hospital information systems (HIS) or medical information systems (MIS)*: managing budgets, equipment inventories, patient information, laboratory reports, operating room and personnel scheduling, and general records

♦ *Diagnostic testing*: analyzing blood and scanning or viewing body parts by computerized tomography (CT scan), magnetic resonance imaging (MRI), positron emission tomography (PET), and ultrasonography

♦ *Educational tools*: computer-assisted instruction (CAI) and computer-assisted video instruction (interactive video) for professional nurses, physicians, and other allied health personnel

♦ *Research*: statistical analysis of data

It is estimated that the health care industry will spend approximately one billion dollars on computer technology within the next few years. Whether you want to be a physician, registered nurse, lab technician, nurse's aide, radiology technician, dietitian, pharmacist, occupational therapist, physical therapist, or any other type of allied health professional, a working knowledge of the computer is essential. This working knowledge is sometimes called *computer literacy*. **Computer literacy** means a basic understanding of how the computer works and a basic understanding of the applications used in your field or profession. Computer literacy also means feeling comfortable using a computer for your job needs. Practice and experience in using a computer are essential in order to develop computer literacy.

HISTORY OF THE COMPUTER

The first computers were installed in hospitals in the late 1950s and early 1960s. Some of these hospitals had some form of assistance from the International Business Machines (IBM) Corporation.

Today's computers have come a long way from the Electronic Numerical Integrator and Computer (ENIAC) built in 1946 by J.P. Eckert and J. W. Mauchly at the University of Pennsylvania. This huge computer had to be housed in a room that measured 20 by 40 feet. The ENIAC contained approximately 18,000 vacuum tubes. With the invention of the silicon chip in the 1970s, hundreds of thousands of electronic components were able to fit on a single chip smaller than a fingernail. These microchips paved the way for the introduction of the microcomputer.

Computer chips are found in many commonly used items such as watches, cameras, telephones, thermometers, blood pressure gauges, cars, satellite navigation equipment, stoves, burglar alarm systems, and personal desktop computers.

Computers vary in size. Computer size can range anywhere from a **microcomputer** such as a handheld calculator or personal digital assistant (PDA), which can be held in one hand, to a laptop in a compact case (figure 17-1), to a **personal computer,** which can sit on a desktop, to a very large **mainframe computer,** which can control the launching of a rocket to outer space.

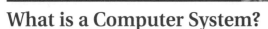

17:2 INFORMATION

What is a Computer System?

A computer system is an electronic device that can be thought of as a complete information-processing center. It can calculate, store, sort, update, manipulate, sequence, organize, and

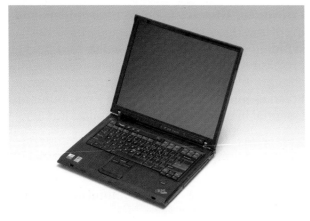

FIGURE 17-1 Today's microcomputers fit easily on a lap or desktop.

process data. It also controls logic operations and can rapidly communicate in graphics, numbers, words, and sound.

COMPONENTS OF A COMPUTER SYSTEM

All computer systems contain essentially the same parts, the hardware and software. The **hardware** consists of the machine components, including the keyboard, central processing unit (CPU), disk drive, and monitor with display screen. The **software** consists of the programs, or instructions, that run the hardware and allow the computer to perform specific tasks.

There are three major components to a computer system (figure 17-2):

♦ **Input:** information that is entered into the computer by means of an input device

♦ **Central processing unit (CPU):** processes the input and performs the operations of the computer by following the instructions in the software

♦ **Output:** the processed information, or final product; it can be displayed on a screen, printed as hard copy, stored on magnetic tape or disks, or transmitted to another user or users

Input Devices

For the computer to work, instructions and data, or input, must be entered into it using some form of input device. One of the most popular input devices is the computer keyboard. This device is similar to the familiar typewriter keyboard. Other input devices include:

♦ *Magnetic tape*: usually used to enter data on large, mainframe computers

♦ *Touch screen monitor*: a monitor with touch-sensitive areas built into the screen; examples are the touch screens found in many fast-food outlets and on many microwave ovens

♦ *Optical scanner*: a machine that can scan a document and read the printed text; an example is the bar code readers found in many supermarkets and used to record and total grocery items

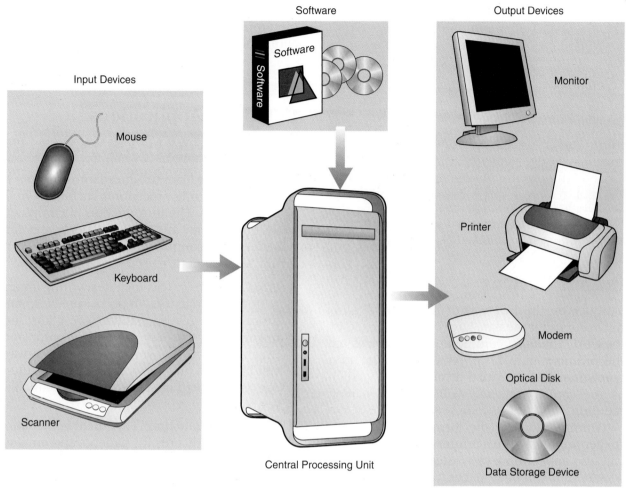

FIGURE 17-2 Components of a computer system.

◆ *Mouse*: a small device that sits on a desktop or is built into the keyboard of a laptop computer; it controls the cursor and performs other functions such as creating graphics

◆ *Light pen*: a device that looks like a pen and is used to perform functions such as selecting menus and drawing graphics on a cathode ray tube, or CRT, which is similar to a television screen (figure 17-3)

Central Processing Unit (CPU)

The CPU processes all information or data entering the computer. It acts as the "brain" of the computer. The CPU is divided into three main units: the internal memory unit, the arithmetic and logic unit, and the control unit (figure 17-4).

◆ *Internal memory unit*: This unit is controlled by two types of memory. A permanent program already built and stored in the computer system by the manufacturer of the computer is called **read only memory (ROM).** A program that is *NOT* permanent because data can be stored, changed, and/or retrieved is called **random access memory (RAM),** or read/write memory.

◆ *Arithmetic and logic unit (ALU)*: This performs all of the calculations, such as addition, subtraction, multiplication, and division. It also provides for a logical, step-by-step handling of data or information as the data or information enters or leaves the computer.

◆ *Control unit*: This unit communicates with the input and output units of the computer system. It initiates, interprets, directs, and controls the processing of information.

FIGURE 17-3 The light pen is a common input device. *(Courtesy of USDA/ARS (K-2656-2)*

Output Devices

Output is the finished work of the computer. Output occurs after the data have been processed by the CPU. The most common output devices are the printer (figure 17-5), which is similar to a typewriter, and the video display monitor, such as the *cathode-ray tube* (CRT) or flat screen monitor.

Output can take the form of a hard copy (paper printout) from a printer or plotter. Output can also appear on a computer monitor display screen. Data can be stored or transferred to magnetic tapes, disks, CDs, DVDs, or flash (travel) drives. Data can also be displayed on a video monitor or heard as music or sound through an audio speaker.

17:3 INFORMATION

Computer Applications

INFORMATION SYSTEMS

Computers were first introduced into hospitals to simplify accounting procedures such as payrolls and inventories. The introduction of computers saved both money and time. Today's health care providers use computers in every health care facility. Computers are used for:

♦ *Word processing*: This includes writing letters, memos, newsletters, reports, policies, and procedures; creating patient care plans; and documenting care on a patient's record. Documents created by word processing software can be edited and corrected, stored for future use, and printed or sent by electronic mail or fax.

♦ *Compiling databases*: This includes creating information records for patients and employees. A **database** is an organized collection of information. Information is entered into areas called **fields.** For example, the database may

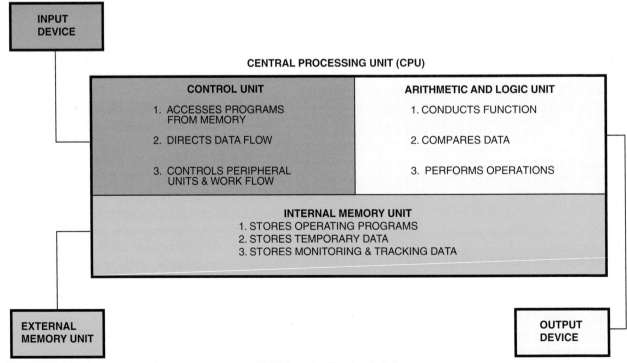

FIGURE 17-4 The central processing unit (CPU) is the "brains" of the computer.

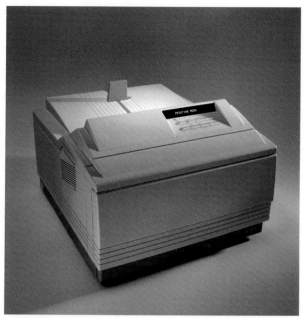

FIGURE 17-5 The printer is a common output device that produces a paper printout called *hard copy*. (*Courtesy of Photodisc*)

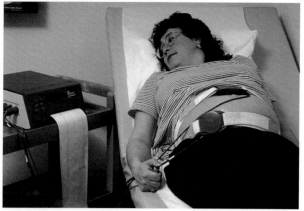

FIGURE 17-6 Computers are used to monitor fetal movements.

contain separate fields for information such as name, address, telephone, insurance information, social security number, place of employment, and medical history. When all of the fields for a particular patient are combined, the information on the patient is a **record.** Most databases that contain patient records are access limited or password protected to maintain patient confidentiality.

♦ *Scheduling*: Scheduling is recording appointments for patients and creating work schedules for employees.

♦ *Maintaining financial records*: This includes processing charges, billing patients, recording payments, completing insurance forms, maintaining accounts, and calculating payrolls for employees.

♦ *Monitoring patients*: This includes recording heart rhythms, pulse, blood pressure, blood oxygen levels, and fetal movements (figure 17-6).

♦ *Performing diagnostic tests*: Diagnostic tests include performing radiological imaging (CT, PET, MRI), blood tests, urine tests, and cardiac and respiratory functions.

♦ *Maintaining inventories*: Inventory maintenance includes ordering and tracking supplies and equipment; coding supplies with bar codes for billing purposes.

♦ *Developing spreadsheets*: A **spreadsheet** uses special software to access a computer's ability to perform high-speed math calculations. The user enters formulas to tell the computer to perform specific math functions (addition, subtraction, multiplication, division, percentage) with numerical data. This allows the user to process bills, maintain accounts, create budgets, develop statistical reports, analyze finances, tabulate nutritional value of foods, evaluate treatments, and project future needs. In addition, once a spreadsheet has been created, the numerical data and statistics can be displayed as a graph or chart.

♦ *Communicating*: Communicating involves using modems or high-speed data transmission networks to communicate with other departments or different facilities, send or receive information by e-mail, order supplies or equipment, and operate security systems.

When a patient is admitted to a hospital, many different health care providers use computers to record the patient's information. Some examples include:

♦ *Health information technician (admissions technician)*: obtains the patient's name, age, and all other vital information to enter, process, and store in the computer's memory; establishes an electronic database so that the information about the patient can be retrieved whenever it is needed

♦ *Physician*: uses word processing to enter all of the findings of the initial admitting physical examination; order all of the patient's medications from the pharmacy; order laboratory tests, including blood and urine studies; and/or order an electrocardiogram, radiographs, dietary restrictions, and specific nursing care

♦ *Pharmacist*: checks the computer regularly for new orders; supplies the nursing departments with ordered medications; warns physicians of drug interactions; monitors pharmacy inventory (figure 17-7)

♦ *Dietitian*: checks the dietary restrictions and creates a spreadsheet to show a nutritional analysis of the prescribed diet

♦ *Laboratory technician*: checks the computers for their new or revised orders; when any test or procedure is completed, records the results in the patient's computerized record

♦ *Environmental service worker (central supply/ central processing worker)*: maintains an inventory of all supplies in the facility, orders required supplies, and provides information for billing supplies. Many facilities use bar codes on each supply item. When the item is

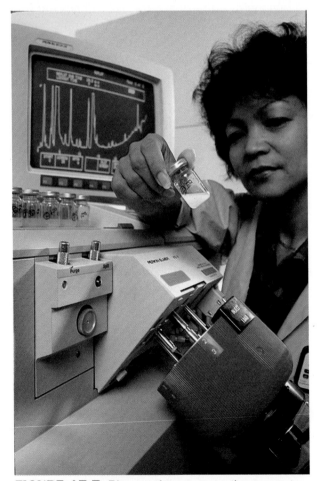

FIGURE 17-7 Pharmacists can use the computer to monitor medications and maintain inventories. *(Courtesy of USDA/ARS #K-3512-3)*

used for a particular patient, the bar code is scanned into the patient's record for automatic billing to the patient.

After each health care worker inputs information into the patient's record, the information is then immediately accessible to the medical, nursing, and allied health teams. These teams no longer have to wait for the results of tests to be typed on a typewriter and hand delivered to the patient care area. Nurses no longer have to manually transcribe physicians' orders or nurses' notes. Because patient care plans are computerized, they can be easily updated. This use of the computer decreases the time health care workers spend on paperwork and away from patient care.

Many health care facilities are using bar codes on patient identification bands. Small scanners are used to scan the band and verify that a treatment or medication is being given to the correct patient. The bar codes are extremely useful for disoriented or unconscious patients.

Handheld portable computers are used in many hospitals. The terminal device contains a miniature keyboard and is linked remotely to the nurse's station. With this small terminal, the health care worker is able to record data at a patient's bedside. Patient information, such as temperature, heart rate, and respirations, is recorded and immediately available to other health care providers. Updated data are also received from other parts of the hospital. Other health care workers can then retrieve this information from the computer.

Eventually this may lead to a "paperless" patient record. All information would be stored in a computer database and sent electronically to insurance companies, pharmacies, and other health care facilities that would require the information. Massive filing systems with tons of paper charts would no longer be required. Safeguards would have to be installed in the computer, however, to meet Health Insurance Portability and Accountability Act (HIPAA) requirements (discussed in Chapters 5:1 and 17:5) and protect the privacy of patient information.

⚖ Confidentiality of patient information must be strictly enforced. This is usually done by means of access codes or special passwords. Computer users must enter the special access code or password to enter or retrieve information. Only authorized workers are given access to the system. Health care workers must keep their code or password confidential to protect themselves and the patient.

A contingency backup plan is always essential when computers are used. At times, a computer must be shut down for reprogramming or adding additional or new software. At other times, power or computer failure will shut down the computer system. When the computer is not functioning, manual recording of all information is required and an alternative plan must be used to avoid losing essential information. Most facilities make frequent backup tapes or disks to prevent a loss of information when computer failure occurs.

INFORMATION MANAGEMENT

Database

Keeping track of huge amounts of data is a challenge in the health care world. Having quick access to information is necessary for tasks such as selecting appropriate courses of treatment,

preparing reports for regulatory agencies, and justifying insurance bills. A major role of the computer is storing and making this information easily accessible in useful formats.

A **database** is a collection of information organized in a structured way. Databases can be set up by the user with application software that can be purchased at a relatively low cost. For example, a small medical office might use a software program to develop a database of all active patients served by a specific insurance company. Complex databases for large facilities are created by computer programmers to meet the specific needs of the facility.

The basic structure of a database is the key to its usefulness. Each collection of related data is called a **record.** For example, the data about each individual are grouped together in a separate record. These data are entered into **fields.** Suppose that a computerized patient record contains five pieces of demographic information, such as name, address, telephone number, occupation, and insurance company name. Each of these items has its own field. A group of related records is called a **file.** See figure 17-8 to see the relation among fields, records, and files.

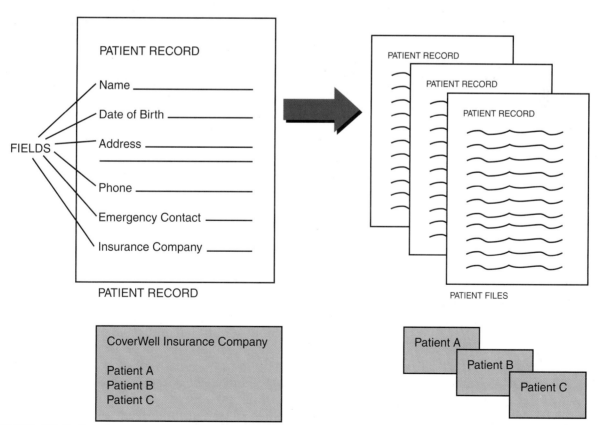

FIGURE 17-8 Databases are structured to provide easy access to needed information.

Computerized databases have many advantages over paper filing systems. The following features make them especially useful in health care information management:

♦ Records can be retrieved quickly and easily.

♦ Records can be sorted, accessed, and reported in many ways. For example, patient records can be organized alphabetically by last name, grouped by ZIP code, grouped by insurance company, or listed chronologically by date of last visit.

♦ Information can be accessed by more than one person at the same time.

♦ Additions and changes can be entered easily.

♦ Reports can be generated as needed.

♦ Quality improvement studies can be conducted.

Many health care workers are responsible for entering data on forms that are displayed on the monitor. Some forms use abbreviations or numerical codes to identify the various fields. The data are converted into a readable form such as the computerized medical history and physical examination in figure 17-9.

Accuracy is critical when entering data. Patient diagnoses, treatment plans, and billing are negatively affected by incorrect data. All input must be carefully reviewed and verified. When an error is made while inputting data, only the incorrect sections should be erased. Reconstructing records can be difficult and time-consuming, as well as being the cause of inconsistent patient care and legal problems.

Health care workers who function as information managers may be required to design and create databases. In these cases, it is important that they carefully study the information needs of the facility. A computerized database is valuable only if it serves the needs of the users.

CREATION OF DOCUMENTS

Computers are excellent tools to help create high-quality written material. Word processing software converts the computer into a "super-typewriter" that gives the user the capability to create customized documents that are error free. Written materials of all types can be produced with word processing software. There are many software programs available that enable the user to perform the following functions:

♦ Design the appearance of text and documents

♦ Edit, correct errors, and check spelling and grammar

♦ Store documents for later use

♦ Print and/or send documents by e-mail, fax, or direct connection to other computers

SPREADSHEETS

Electronic spreadsheet software permits the user to apply the computer's ability to perform high-speed calculations of numerical data. **Spreadsheet** software provides a worksheet that consists of intersecting rows and columns that form squares called *cells.* Numbers and formulas (instructions for performing calculations) are entered into the cells. For example, to create a simple budget using spreadsheet software, the user enters the amounts of income and expenses and the formulas for the desired calculations. A formula may have several steps. The budgeting example would allow the user to calculate monthly income by adding all income and subtracting all expenses.

Electronic spreadsheets provide the basis for billing and accounting programs. In addition to speed and accuracy, these programs allow changes to be reflected throughout the spreadsheet. For example, if the cost of a clinic's rent increases, the effect on income can easily be calculated. All totals affected by the change in rent will automatically be adjusted. Changes or corrections that would take a person many hours to recalculate can be accomplished in seconds.

The methods used for patient billing have been significantly affected by computers. Amounts to be billed are not only calculated electronically, but they are now also sent electronically to payers instead of being mailed. Starting in the year 2000, all Medicare and Medicaid claims had to be submitted electronically. Standardized codes have been developed that correspond to various diagnoses and treatment procedures. The computer matches the codes for various procedures to a fee schedule and prepares bills. Computerized billing is easier and more accurate. Additional numerical codes that

Patient: Leo McKay
Date of Birth: 01/22/44
Visit Date: 04/01/__

Chief Complaint: Abdominal pain
History: Has been ill over the last 2 weeks with progressively worsening abdominal pain.
Review of Symptoms: Patient denies the following:
- Chest pain, Chest pressure, Chest heaviness, Circulation problems, Palpitations, Rapid heartbeat, Irregular heartbeat, Ankle swelling
- Cough, Phlegm, Coughing up blood, Shortness of breath, Wheeze, Change in exercise tolerance
- Burning or pain on urination, Difficulty starting or stopping urination, Dribbling after urination, Incontinence of urine, Blood in urine, Cloudiness of urine
- Change in appetite, Unexpected weight loss, Nausea, Vomiting, Difficulty Swallowing, Belly pains, Gas pains, Change in bowel habit: change in frequency, shape, color, consistency, size of stool; Blood, Mucus, or Slime, Rectal pain or discomfort, Hemorrhoids
- Skin rash, New or changing moles, Excess bruising or bleeding
- Mouth sores, Denture problems, Sinus drainage or stuffiness, Facial pain
- Panic attacks, Anxiety, Depression, Sadness, Seizures, Problems with concentration or memory, Disturbance of sleep, Insomnia, Early wakefulness
- Dizziness, Fainting, Lightheadedness on standing, Headaches, Vision problems, Hearing problems, Numbness or tingling in arms or legs, Weakness in arms or legs

Medications:

Drug	Dose	Freq.	Started
none			

Medical Problem List

Problem	When Dx d	A ctive?
Peptic Ulcer	1985	no

List of Surgeries.

Surgical Procedure	When
none	

Family History: Parents deceased, father died of heart attack, mother of breast cancer.
Social History: Divorced, no children
Habits: Smokes 2 ppd, Several beers daily
Allergies: Penicillin _____

Physical Examination

GENERAL: Well developed and well nourished gentleman in no distress. No jaundice, cyanosis, clubbing, or edema.
VITALS: Weight = 192, Temp = 97.6, Pulse = 78, BP = 152/88
HEENT: Normocephalic and without evidence of trauma, tympanic membranes and external auditory canals are normal. Pharynx and mouth are normal.
NECK: supple, no masses or thyromegaly.
NODES: No cervical nodes palpable. No axillary or inguinal adenopathy.
CARDIOVASCULAR SYSTEM: Heart sounds: no murmurs, rubs or gallops, carotids with good upstrokes, no bruits heard. Peripheral pulses including radials, brachials, and femorals intact. Posterior tibial, and dorsalis pedis pulses intact.
RESPIRATORY SYSTEM: resps 16/min, trachea central, expansion, fremitus, resonance, and breath sounds normal.
ABDOMEN: soft, no masses, organomegaly, or tenderness. No loin or costo-vertebral angle tenderness. Inguinal canals are intact without herniae. Bowel sounds active.
GENITOURINARY: Penis without lesions or discharge, scrotum, testicles, epididymis and cords all normal
RECTAL: no masses, tenderness, or hemorrhoids. Soft brown stool in vault. Prostate normal in size, and shape without nodules or tenderness.
MUSCULOSKELETAL SYSTEM: Joints with full ROM, no joint tenderness or swelling. Muscle bulk symmetric and normal.
SKIN: without masses, skin tags, rash, blisters or ulcerations. Nails are normal without splinter hemorrhages.
NEUROLOGICAL SYSTEM: Alert and oriented to place, person, and time. Communicates with good word recognition and appropriate word usage. Cranial nerves and spinal nerves grossly intact.

Assessment and Plan

Problem	Plan/Status
Abdominal pain	Reports about two weeks of epigastric and retrosternal chest pain radiating up and to the left. Episodes of pain occur usually during the day and last for 3-4 hours. No associated dyspnea, palpitations, sweats, dizziness. No nausea, vomiting or diarrhea. No blood in the stool. To get barium swallow, CBC, Chem 7 and UA.

follow-up appointment: 3 days
Mark Woo MD

FIGURE 17-9 Sample of computer-generated medical history and physical examination.

identify specific insurance companies can be entered that result in automatic preparation of the proper bill format.

The high speed of computer calculations also enables the user to employ "if . . . then" scenarios to explore a variety of options. Questions such as the following can be posed:

♦ "If the number of patients visiting the clinic continues to grow at the current rate, how many full-time medical assistants will be needed next December?"

♦ "If we finance the purchase of new medical equipment at 6.5%, how much will the total cost be if the repayment period is three years? Five years?"

This type of information assists in the delivery of quality patient care and the making of sound business decisions. Electronic spreadsheet programs are also able to create graphs and charts that illustrate numerical concepts and statistics (figure 17-10).

As with databases, it is critical that data entered into the spreadsheet be accurate. One incorrect entry can affect hundreds of numbers. All electronic spreadsheet entries must be carefully checked.

INTEGRATION OF OPERATIONS

The capacity to integrate various types of operations contributes to the power and value of computers. There are a growing number of commercially prepared integrated systems designed for the health care facility. Medical Manager and Medisoft are only two examples of the many that have been developed for medical offices. They include patient record maintenance, appointment scheduling, insurance coding, billing, and report creation. Using an integrated program helps coordinate administrative tasks and eliminates the need to enter data more than once. For example, a patient recordkeeping database that is tied to billing software allows information entered in one place to appear in the medical record and on a bill to be sent to the insurance company.

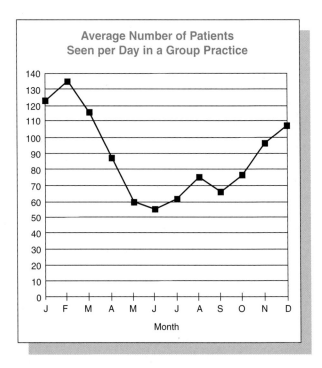

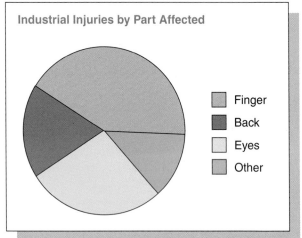

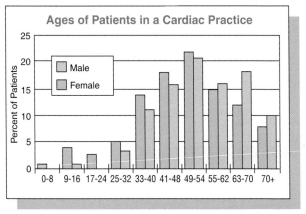

FIGURE 17-10 Graphs and charts can be easily created using computer software. *(Courtesy of GE Medical Systems)*

DIAGNOSTICS

The major goal of health care and medicine is determining exactly what is wrong with the patient. The first step in the process is taking a medical history and doing a physical examination. Based on these findings, several tests may be ordered to diagnose or rule out disease.

Several computer-related diagnostic tests have had a real impact on patient care. These diagnostic aids or specialized technological tools are quite varied. They may be invasive, such as a blood test where a syringe is inserted into a vein and blood is removed, or noninvasive, such as an imaging procedure where no opening into the body is required.

Some computerized instruments automate the step-by-step manual procedure of analyzing blood, urine, serum, and other body-fluid samples. Most laboratories rely heavily on computers for both blood and urine analysis. Smaller units are now used in many medical offices and other health care facilities. The computerized instruments can analyze a drop of serum, blood, urine, or body fluid placed on a slide at rates of over 500 specimens an hour. Such systems have proved to be reliable for clinical chemistry evaluations.

An electrocardiogram (ECG) computerized interpretation system produces visual pictures on a computer monitor and a printout of the electrical activity of a patient's heart. The ECG gives important information concerning the spread of electrical impulses to the heart chambers. It is very important in diagnosing heart disease. An ECG run while the patient is exercising is known as a **stress test** (figure 17-11). This allows the physician to evaluate the function of the patient's heart during activity. An **echocardiograph** utilizes a computer to direct ultrahigh-frequency sound waves through the chest wall and into the heart (figure 17-12). The computer then converts the reflection of the waves into an image of the heart. This test can be used to evaluate cardiac function, reveal valve irregularities, show defects in the heart walls, and visualize the presence of fluid between the layers of the pericardium (membrane that surrounds the outside of the heart). Computers are also used to monitor a patient's pulse and to determine the oxygen level in the blood (figure 17-13).

One advance in medical imaging is the **computerized tomography (CT)** scanner, intro-

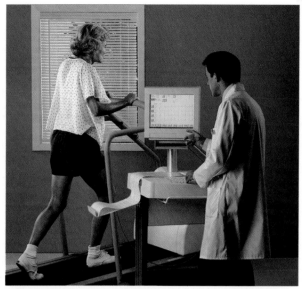

FIGURE 17-11 Computers are used to perform stress tests to evaluate the function of a patient's heart during exercise. *(Courtesy of Spacelabs Medical, Inc.)*

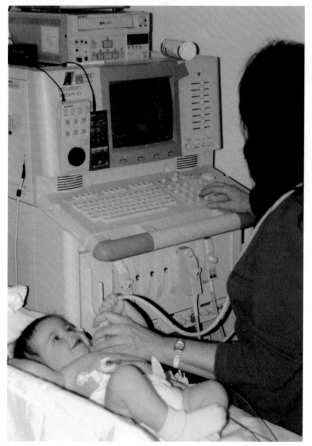

FIGURE 17-12 An echocardiograph utilizes a computer to evaluate cardiac function, reveal heart valve irregularity, and show defects or diseases of the heart.

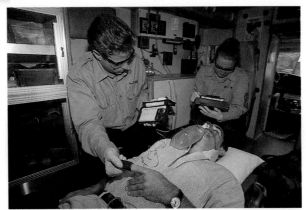

FIGURE 17-13 Pulse oximeters use computer technology to monitor a patient's pulse and determine the oxygen level in the blood.

duced in 1972. The CT scanner was the first computer-based body and brain scanner. This noninvasive, computerized X-ray permits physicians to see clear, cross-sectional views of both bone and body tissues and to find abnormalities such as tumors (figure 17-14). The CT scanner shoots a pencil-thin beam of X-rays through any part of the body and from many different angles. The computer then creates a cross-sectional image of the body part on a screen. A CT scan provides a clear image of the soft tissues inside the body and exposes the patient to less radiation than a conventional radiograph. In addition, a regular radiograph shows little depth, and the soft tissue does not appear clearly.

Another powerful advance in medical imaging is **magnetic resonance imaging (MRI).** This computerized, body-scanning method uses

nuclear magnetic resonance instead of X-ray radiation. Magnetic resonance imaging is the alteration of the magnetic position of hydrogen atoms to produce an image. The patient is placed in a large circular magnet, which uses the magnetic field to measure activity of hydrogen atoms within the body (figure 17-15). A computer translates that activity into cross-sectional images of the body (figure 17-16). For example, a lung tumor

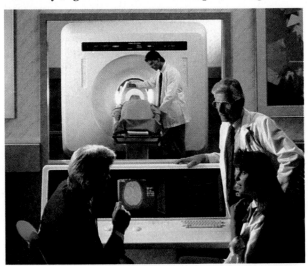

FIGURE 17-15 For magnetic resonance imaging (MRI), the patient is placed in the center of a large magnet that measures the activity of hydrogen ions inside the body and creates an image of the body. *(Courtesy of GE Medical Systems)*

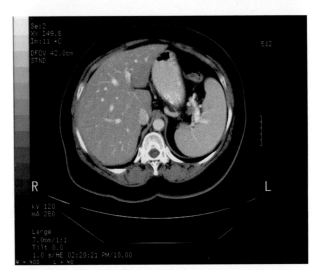

FIGURE 17-14 This computerized tomography (CT) scan highlights the blood vessels of the liver, heart, and spleen.

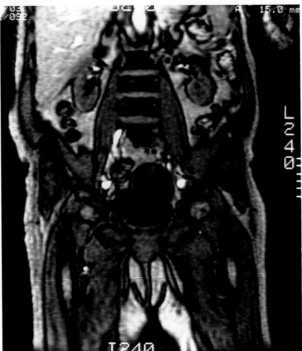

FIGURE 17-16 This magnetic resonance imaging (MRI) scan shows a coronal image of the abdomen.

can be more easily detected by scanning with MRI than by scanning with X-rays or CT. Magnetic resonance imaging allows physicians to see blood moving through veins and arteries, to see a swollen joint shrink in response to medication, and to see the reaction of cancerous tumors to treatment.

Positron emission tomography (PET) is another scanning procedure. A slightly radioactive substance is injected into the patient and detected by the PET scanner. The device's computer then composes a three-dimensional image from the radiation detected. The image allows the doctor to see an organ or bone from all sides. In this way, a PET image is similar to a model that can be picked up and examined.

Ultrasonography (figure 17-17) is another noninvasive scanning method. It uses high-frequency sound waves that bounce back as an echo when they hit different tissues and organs inside the body. A computer then uses the sound wave signals to create a picture of the body part, which can be viewed on a computer screen or processed on a photographic film that resembles a radiograph. Ultrasonography can be used to detect tumors, locate aneurysms and blood vessel abnormalities, and examine the shape and size of internal organs. During pregnancy, when radiation can harm the fetus, ultrasonography is used to detect multiple pregnancies and to determine the size, position, sex, and even abnormalities of the fetus (figure 17-18). A more recent development in sonography is the three-dimensional (3-D) sonogram. This type of ultrasound uses a specialized machine that allows techni-

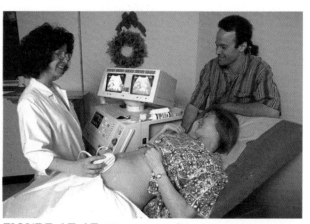

FIGURE 17-17 Ultrasonography is used during pregnancy to determine the size, position, sex, and even abnormalities of the fetus. *(Courtesy of Sandy Clark)*

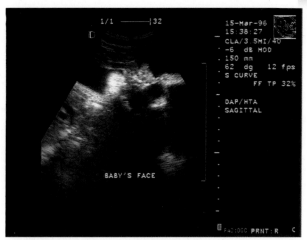

FIGURE 17-18 This ultrasound shows the fetus inside the uterus. *(Courtesy of Sandy Clark)*

cians to store 5 seconds' worth of images in a computer. The technician can then create a 3-D colored picture similar to a portrait of the infant in the uterus. Physicians use the 3-D ultrasound to detect birth defects that are not always visible on a standard sonogram and to determine the severity of a birth defect.

Computers play a major role in oncology (malignancy or cancer) radiology departments. Computers are used to convert information from various scanners to exact data on the location of a tumor. The computer then directs the power of therapeutic radiation precisely to the tumor being irradiated.

EDUCATION

Computers have become commonplace as educational tools. They can be found in elementary, middle, junior high, and high schools, in addition to post-secondary education institutions such as colleges and universities. Research has shown that computer-based learning decreases time on the task and increases achievement and retention of knowledge. Therefore, it comes as no surprise to find computer-based learning in most schools of medicine, nursing, and allied health.

Computer-assisted instruction (CAI) is educational computer programming designed for individualized use. It is user paced, user friendly, and proceeds in an orderly, organized fashion from topic to topic. It may use animated graphics, color, and sound. It may be a drill-and-practice program for learning to calculate medication doses, or may take the form of a tutorial for learning concepts about the heart. In addition, it can be a simulation that allows the learner to do a clinical procedure, such as taking a patient's blood pressure or drawing blood from a vein (venipuncture), while sitting in front of the computer. Computer programs have even been developed to allow a user to perform a simulated operation on a patient.

Patient-education software is available for the patient with osteoarthritis (inflammation of the joints), obesity (overweight), and many other diseases. Software is even available to teach people how to manage stress.

Another advance in computer learning technology is **interactive video,** or **computer-assisted video.** Interactive video is the integration of computer and video technology. It combines the advantages of video (color, sound, and motion) with the advantages of computer-assisted instruction to provide a dynamic new learning medium. Research has shown that this technology greatly enhances learning and retention. Programs available include those that teach medical terminology to health care workers, clinical skills to nurses, physical examination techniques to physicians, and anatomy and physiology to students. Programs are stored on compact disks or CD-ROMs that are inserted into a videodisc player.

The Internet offers a new approach to education called *distance learning.* Students can access a wide variety of courses over the Internet. This allows them to complete the courses in their own homes at times convenient to them. Many health care workers use the Internet to obtain continuing education units (CEUs) or to complete college courses to advance in their professions. Refresher courses to prepare for licensure are also available for many health care careers. Finally, many tests for licensure are now taken on a computer. This allows for immediate grading of the licensure examination. Examples include the licensure tests for registered nurses and physicians.

RESEARCH

Today, health care research without the use of computers is almost nonexistent. A major source used to help health care professionals analyze statistics and obtain information is the National Library of Medicine database, which is the largest research library in the scientific community. It serves as a national resource for all U.S. health science libraries. It is located at the National Institutes of Health in Bethesda, Maryland.

The library's computer-based Medical Literature Analysis and Retrieval System (MEDLARS) is the major source of bibliographic biomedical information database. It can be easily accessed by computer through the Regional Medical Library Network. The MEDLARS includes more than 40 databases, including Index Medicus, a monthly subject/author guide to more than 3,500 journal articles, and Medline, which currently contains more than 10 million references, as well as information about audiovisual materials.

Statistical Package for the Social Sciences (SPSS) is a program used in many universities to prepare and analyze research data. Other programs score and analyze student test scores. Some programs can draw graphs and charts, and others help the user learn how to use the program in a step-by-step fashion.

Research using computer technology is being conducted for almost every disease, infection, or abnormal health condition that exists. Examples include genetic diseases, heart conditions, diabetes, arthritis, patient management systems, and speech recognition patterns. Information acquired during research is frequently organized into large databases and shared with other researchers throughout the world. This process, known as *bioinformatics,* allows for rapid scientific progress through the sharing of information.

In addition, clinical researchers are now using microcomputers for people who have had severe spinal cord injuries. The microcomputers are used to initiate the electrical impulses that stimulate skeletal muscles. This exciting application of computing was used to develop a computer-controlled walking system. This system enables paraplegics and quadriplegics to stand, sit, and walk. Electrodes are applied above the hamstring, quadriceps, and gluteus maximus muscles. These electrodes allow control of flexion and extension of the knees and hips. Sensors applied to the knee provide information to coordinate movement of the knee when the patient is standing or walking. Electrical impulses (controlled by the microcomputer) are delivered through these electrodes to stimulate the muscles through a preprogrammed series of exercises. The computer is programmed to automatically stop the exercise program when the sensors detect that the muscles have become fatigued.

COMMUNICATION

Computers have enhanced communication for health care workers in multiple ways. Through the use of systems called **networks,** computers can be linked together through cables and/or telephone lines. A network can consist of 3 or 4 computers linked together in a medical or dental office, 100 computers linked together in a large health care facility such as a hospital, or the ultimate networked system, the **Internet,** which links millions of computers located throughout the world. Networks allow multiple users to share the same data or information at the same time. They also allow rapid communication between individuals. Examples of using networks for communication include e-mail, telemedicine, telepharmacies, and listservs.

Electronic mail, or e-mail, is the process of creating and sending messages from one computer to another. It allows health care workers to quickly send messages, memos, announcements, reports, and other data to one or more persons. Attachments, such as files created in word-processing programs, insurance forms completed with insurance software, financial data compiled on spreadsheets, X-rays or radiographic images, and/or photographs, can be sent electronically. For example, all claims for Medicare and Medicaid must be submitted electronically. The claim is usually completed on specialized insurance software, attached to an e-mail, and filed electronically as a claim. Most insurance companies also use electronic filing for claims. Electronic messages should be created following the same professional standards for any written document. The message should be clear and concise, correct grammar and spelling must be used, and slang or codes should be avoided. It is also important for all health care personnel to understand that all e-mail messages belong to the employer or owner of the computer. The messages may be stored in backup files and employers have the legal right to read and monitor any messages. Health care personnel should never send or receive personal e-mail correspondence at their place of employment.

Telemedicine, discussed in detail in Chapter 1:2, involves the use of video, audio, and computer systems to provide medical and/or health care services. For example, X-rays or electrocardiograms can be transmitted electronically from one physician to another for consultation. A surgeon can direct the work of another surgeon, or even a robotic arm, by watching the procedure on video. Telemedicine also allows patients to communicate with physicians or health care specialists at a distance, transmit medical information to a physician, or be monitored by health care professionals. A recent advance in telemedicine is a computerized device that has sensors that remind a patient to take medications at specific times and a touchscreen medicine cabinet that recognizes faces and can determine that the patient is taking the correct medication.

E-medicine is another growing practice that allows patients to communicate with a physician by e-mail to ask routine medical questions, ask for renewals of prescriptions, obtain the results of laboratory tests, or obtain financial information about their account. In most cases, the physician and patient form a contract to use e-medicine. Most physicians do not charge for prescription renewals or information on billing or laboratory results. However, physicians may charge for assisting with routine medical problems or evaluating health information sent by patient monitors. The term *Web visit* has been used to describe this interaction between patient and physician. It allows physicians to handle routine medical problems in a quick and efficient manner. If the patient's problems seem more complex, physicians can recommend an office visit.

Telepharmacies allow for rapid dispensing of medications. Prescriptions are sent electronically to a computerized dispensing unit. The unit prepares and dispenses the ordered prescription, which is then mailed or sent by a carrier service to the patient or health care facility.

Health care workers may also receive health information through *Listserv* mailing lists. These are automated systems that send e-mail messages on specific topics, similar to receiving a newsletter or magazine. Some health care Listservs are free, while others charge monthly or annual fees.

Virtual communities consist of individuals who use the Internet to communicate and share information. Discussion groups and methods for exchanging information have valuable health care applications. Both health care workers and patients can share information and experiences about specific health conditions. Patients who are chronically ill, bedridden, or disabled have used the communication capabilities of the computer to break from the isolation that often results from these conditions. There are at least three ways that this can be accomplished:

♦ *Chat rooms*: allow participants to correspond in real time, using typed messages; many groups are organized to create communities of individuals who share similar interests

♦ *Listserv mailing lists*: automated systems that distribute e-mail on specific topics; similar to receiving a newsletter or magazine; mailing lists exist for thousands of topics

♦ *Newsgroups*: provide opportunities for participants to contribute information and comment on items submitted by others; organized by subject, and range from general topics to specific local issues; newsgroups can be accessed using Netscape Navigator or Microsoft Internet Explorer

SUMMARY

Today, computers are used as cost-effective and efficient tools to enhance quality patient care. They are used to analyze blood; regulate electrical impulses to muscles; take pictures of the body; collect patient data; analyze electrocardiograms; schedule hospital personnel; keep hospital and clinic records, inventories, and budgets; and provide information on wellness to the general public. Computer technology has truly invaded the health care field.

17:4 INFORMATION

Using the Internet

The sharing of data over cables and the telephone or wireless devices enables computers to be linked into systems, called **networks,** that allow all types of communication. A simple networked system may consist of four or five personal computers in a small medical office. Patient records are shared, and all staff use the same printer. A large facility may have hundreds of computers linked together that carry out many of the functions described in this chapter. The Internet is the ultimate networked system, consisting of millions of computers located all over the world.

Many types of services and sources of information are offered on the Internet. Through the Internet, health care professionals can readily contact others for medical updates, information on new procedures, aid in making diagnoses, and many other kinds of information.

The Internet began as a method for government authorities to communicate in case of nuclear attack. It has rapidly grown to become a principal means of communicating, conducting business, shopping, learning, and securing needed information. Only four things are needed to access the Internet:

♦ *Computer*

♦ **Modem:** an electronic device that sends or receives computer data over telephone or cable lines

♦ *Service provider*: access to a service that provides a link to the Internet; examples include dial-up, DSL, cable, and wireless services

♦ **Browser:** special software that allows the user to view Web pages and access information on the Internet

One major use of the Internet in health care relates to organ transplants. When an individual needs a transplant, vital information regarding the individual is recorded on the transplant network. The computer monitors all organs as they become available, and can immediately notify the online facility when an organ is suitable for a particular patient. This allows the most expedient use of donor organs and ensures that organs are given to the most compatible recipient. It is another example of modern technology providing a service that saves lives.

Since the Internet contains a wealth of information, every health care provider should be familiar with how to use the Internet as a research tool. In order to do this, the health care provider must first become familiar with search engines. A search engine, or search service, can be defined as a database of Internet files. It usually consists of three parts:

♦ *Search program*: commonly called a spider, wanderer, crawler, robot, or worm, the search program explores different sites and identifies and reads pages

♦ *Index*: the search program creates a main database that contains copies of all the information obtained

♦ *Retrieval program*: a program that searches the database for specific information, lists all sources of the information, and in most cases, ranks the sources with the most relevant first

There are three main types of search engines:

♦ *Crawler based*: creates an index by exploring different sites on the Web and indexing the sites

♦ *Human powered*: creates an index when a description of the information and key words are entered into the index by an individual

♦ *Mixed*: combines results of both crawler-based and human-powered indexes

There are many different search engines available to an Internet user. Many of them use a variety of indexes or directories to provide sources of information. In addition, different search engines partner together to share index listings. Some of the more popular search engines that provide dependable results, are constantly upgraded with new information, and are available to all Internet users include:

♦ *All The Web (FAST search) (www.alltheweb. com)*: one of the largest indexes of the web

♦ *Alta Vista (www.altavista.com)*: one of the oldest and largest crawler-based directories; also offers news search, shopping search, multimedia search, and human-powered directory results from other search engines

♦ *America On Line (AOL) (http:search.aol.com)*: provides web search services to AOL subscribers by using both crawler-based and human-powered directories of other search engines

♦ *Ask (www.ask.com)*: human-powered search that attempts to provide an exact page of information in response to a question

♦ *Google (www.google.com)*: has the largest collection of Web pages for a crawler-based search engine, provides links to other sites, provides Web page search results to other search engines

♦ *Look Smart (www.looksmart.com)*: human-powered directory of Web sites, provides search results to many other search engines

♦ *Lycos (www.lycos.com)*: began as crawler-based but switched to human-powered directory, obtains search results from other search engines

♦ *MSN (http:search.msn.com)*: Microsoft's search service that uses results from many other search engines

♦ *Yahoo (www.yahoo.com)*: most popular search service, largest human-powered directory on the Web with over 1 million sites listed, also uses results from other search engines

To find relevant material on the Internet, it is important to develop a strategy to locate information on a specific topic in an efficient and effective way. Searching for information on a topic such as "Does smoking or drinking alcohol during pregnancy increase the chance of a premature birth?" can result in hundreds or even thousands of listings. Some of the listings may be relevant; others will not be. Various techniques can be used to limit the search and produce only information that is specific to the topic. Basic steps that should be followed include:

♦ *Identify key words*: Always try to determine the main words that pertain to the information you desire. In the example above, the key words are *smoking, alcohol, pregnancy*, and *premature birth*. Other words that are alternative ways of expressing the key words might include *cigarettes, premature infants*, and *alcoholism*.

♦ *Combine key words*: If any of the above key words are entered as separate searches, a large amount of information generated would not be pertinent. More specific information can be obtained by telling the search engine to limit the search. This can be accomplished in several ways. One of the easiest methods, recognized by most major search engines, is to use math symbols:

a. *Plus (+) symbol*: tells an engine that you want all words entered; for example, *+pregnancy +alcohol +premature birth* will produce only listings that contain all three words

b. *Minus (−) symbol*: tells the search engine that you want to find information with one word but not another word; for example, *search +engines −car −automobile* will eliminate information on car or automobile engines

c. *Quotation marks (")*: placed around a phrase or group of words tell a search engine to locate pages that contain the exact same phrase in the order specified; for example, *"hearing aids"* will provide information only on hearing aids, not the disease AIDS.

◆ Boolean operators/connectors are also used to tell a search engine how to limit a search. Common connectors include *AND* (used like the plus sign), *NOT* used like the minus sign, *OR* used to present an alternative word such as *cigarettes OR smoking*, and *NEAR* to indicate words that should be used close to one another. Most search engines that recognize Boolean operators require that the word be keyed in capital letters.

◆ *Vary your search*: To obtain as much information as possible on a specific topic, it is wise to use a variety of key word combinations. For example, to obtain information on the relationship of smoking and alcohol during pregnancy on premature births, one search could be + *smoking OR cigarettes + alcohol OR alcoholism + pregnancy + premature births*. This search would bring up all information that contains all of the terms. A second search such as + *alcohol OR alcoholism + pregnancy + premature birth*, or even + *alcohol OR alcoholism + pregnancy* would provide additional information on just the effects of alcohol. Many articles might discuss the effects of alcohol on pregnancy and not discuss smoking. Similarly, other articles might discuss the effects of smoking, but not alcohol. By changing key words, additional pertinent information can be located.

◆ *Use different search engines*: If one search engine does not locate pertinent information, try different search engines. No search engine has access to all the information on the Internet.

◆ *Evaluate the source of all information*: The Internet can provide a wealth of information to health care providers, but individuals using it must also evaluate the information.

At this time, material placed on the Internet is not regulated. Anyone can say anything and make any claims. Not all information is accurate or current. Much of it consists of personal opinions or is motivated by the desire to sell products. Health care workers must take care to determine the reliability of any information taken from the Internet. The following guidelines, suggested by Leshin (1998), are designed to help evaluate sites:

◆ *Identify the source*: Universities and government agencies tend to be reliable sources of information. Research and professional organizations, if not organized for the purpose of selling specific products, may also be reliable. Examples include the American Heart Association and the American Association of Medical Assistants.

◆ *Determine the author*: Is the person an expert in the field? Does he or she have appropriate education and credentials? Is the purpose of the material to share information and/or report research findings? Or to persuade readers and sell ideas or products?

◆ *Check for accuracy*: Is a reference given for the information? Is the reference from a reliable source?

◆ *Verify important data*: Cross-check statistics and other numerical data.

◆ *Look for signs of quality*: Are the ideas well-supported? Is the spelling accurate and vocabulary used correctly?

◆ *Check for currency*: Is the information recent and up to date?

Health care providers can research many topics on the Internet. They can obtain current health care information; learn about new diagnostic tests; research diseases, medications, therapies, and other health concerns; and communicate with other health care providers. The Internet is an excellent learning tool and another example of how technology has enhanced health care.

Some reliable sources for medical information on the Internet include:

◆ *www.aap.org*: the American Academy of Pediatrics

◆ *www.ama-assn.org*: the American Medical Association

◆ *www.amhrt.org*: heart and stroke guide from the American Heart Association

◆ *www.cancer.gov*: the National Cancer Institute

◆ *www.cdc.gov*: the Centers for Disease Control and Prevention

◆ *www.familydoctor.org*: health information from the American Academy of Family Physicians

◆ *www.healthtouch.com*: provides links to specific health organizations

◆ *www.healthypeople.gov/healthfinder*: a health information site provided by the U. S. government

♦ *www.medicinenet.com*: medical information site that includes an "ask the experts" feature

♦ *www.medscape.com*: a news service that has full-text medical articles

♦ *www.nih.gov*: the National Institutes of Health

♦ *www.webmd.com*: provides health and medical news provided by physicians

17:5 INFORMATION

Computer Protection and Security

The widespread use of computerized records in health care has created the need for protecting and securing the information. Electrical surges, power outages, viruses, and hackers (individuals who use the Internet or networks to obtain unauthorized access to the computer) can all result in a loss of information and/or damage to the software and hardware of the computer.

To protect the computer from electrical surges and power outages, an *Uninterrupted Power Supply (UPS)* device should be used. The computer plugs into the UPS, which has a surge protector and a battery backup. If an electrical failure occurs, the computer operates on the battery backup in the UPS. Even when a UPS is in use, it is still important to backup data on the computer frequently. A computer "crash" can cause a loss of all data and programs. Most health care facilities perform daily backups onto disks or tapes. To protect against loss by fire, natural disasters, or theft, the backups should be stored in a safe and secure location outside the health care facility. Many health care facilities have contracts with computer security companies to have backups performed and stored in an off-site facility.

Viruses are programs that contain instructions to alter the operation of the computer programs, erase or scramble data on the computer, and/or allow access to information on the computer. Viruses can enter a computer by downloading information from the Internet, opening e-mails, or using disks or tapes that contain viruses. Antivirus software must be installed on every computer to protect against these invasive programs. The software should be updated on a daily basis. When the software issues a virus alert, the computer user should follow the recommendations of the software.

Firewalls are protective programs that limit the ability of other computers to access a computer. A firewall alert will usually inform the user that an outside program is trying to access the computer. A strong firewall will prevent some programs and hackers from entering the database, but no firewall is foolproof. The best way to prevent access to the database is to use only a dedicated computer to communicate with an outside network or the Internet. Computers that contain the databases should be networked only within the health care facility. When information must be transferred to an outside source, the information can be copied, placed on the dedicated computer, and then sent to the correct recipient.

Security to protect confidential patient information is essential for any health care facility. Guidelines to protect patient privacy have been established by many health care organizations including the American Medical Association and the American Health Information Management Association. In addition, specific standards have been established through the Privacy Rule of the Health Insurance Portability and Accountability Act (HIPAA). (HIPAA is discussed in detail in Chapter 5:1.) The main requirements established by HIPAA to protect the confidentiality of health care information include:

♦ Develop and implement a security plan to ensure compliance with HIPAA policies and procedures

♦ Prepare documents that patients sign to stipulate consent for the use and dissemination of health information

♦ Establish a certification process and educational program to ascertain that all employees understand the security plan

♦ Require individuals to sign a contract verifying that they will follow the security and privacy regulations

♦ Determine the level of security necessary for each job classification

♦ Establish access levels that provide authorization to confidential information on a need-to-know basis

♦ Create a system that identifies date, time, and name of the individual who enters information into any database

♦ Incorporate periodic password expirations

TODAY'S RESEARCH: TOMORROW'S HEALTH CARE

A computer that reads and interprets X-rays?

A major tool used to diagnose tumors and cancer is imaging. Physicians use X-rays, ultrasound, magnetic resonance imaging (MRI), computerized tomography (CT), and mammography to find cancer in its early stages. However, every type of image must be read by a radiologist, a physician specializing in the study of radiographic images and radiation. Radiologists are human. At times, they miss the early signs of a cancerous tumor on the image. For example, studies have shown that radiologists reading mammograms (diagnostic images used to detect breast cancer) miss more than 25 percent, or 1 of every 4, early tumors.

Now, computer-aided detection (CAD) systems have been developed to help the radiologist pinpoint suspicious areas. These systems use computing equipment and a special image scanner to change images into numeric patterns that can be understood by the computer. The CAD system then uses these patterns to locate suspicious areas and pinpoint them for the radiologist. In short, the computer becomes a second pair of "eyes."

Currently, the U. S. Food and Drug Administration (FDA) is evaluating a MammoReader developed to aid radiologists in interpreting mammograms. Other CAD systems are being developed for other types of diagnostic images. The systems may produce some "false" positives, or areas that appear suspicious but are in fact harmless. This may lead to the need for additional tests and increased health care expense. However, if the CAD system locates the 25 percent of tumors that are missed by the human eye, it will save thousands of lives.

♦ Secure workstations, record storage areas, and computer hardware

♦ Use encryption technology when health care information is transmitted electronically

♦ Create a system for destruction of duplicate or obsolete records (electronic and hard copy)

Health care workers must make every effort to protect and secure computerized records. Passwords should be kept confidential and never given to any other individual. When a password is keyed into a computer, no other individual should be able to see the keyboard. Other individuals should not be able to read the computer screen when confidential patient information is on the screen. Monitor screens that contain confidential data should be cleared before leaving the work area. E-mails or files from unknown parties must never be opened or downloaded onto the computer. If a virus or firewall alert occurs, instructions provided by the program should be followed. Discarded hard copies or printouts should be shredded. If every worker in a health care facility follows the established security and privacy policy, the confidentiality of patient information will be protected.

STUDENT: *Go to the workbook and complete the assignment sheet for Chapter 17, Computer Technology in Health Care.*

CHAPTER 17 SUMMARY

The use of computers in health care has almost become a necessity. All health care workers should have basic computer literacy, meaning an understanding of how the computer works and an understanding of the applications used in their particular health careers.

A computer system is a complete information-processing center. All computer systems contain essentially the same parts: hardware and software. The hardware consists of the machine components. The software consists of the programs, or instructions, that run the hardware and allow the computer to perform specific tasks. Each computer system also requires input, or the information entered into the computer, and a central processing unit (CPU), which performs the operations of the computer by following the directions in the software. This results in output (the processed information, or final product), which can be displayed on a screen, printed, stored, or transmitted to another user.

Computers are used in many aspects of health care. They serve as information centers to provide patient information, schedule personnel, and maintain records and inventory. Computers are also used as diagnostic tools by performing blood tests or viewing body parts. They are major educational tools, and many computer-assisted instructional programs exist to teach both health care workers and patients. Computers are critical components in health care research. They are also a major way of communicating for health care professionals and patients. The use of computers in health care has proved they are efficient tools that enhance the quality of patient care.

The Internet is used by almost every health care worker. By using search engines and specific techniques to obtain correct information, a health care worker can find a wealth of information. It is important to ensure that any information obtained is from reliable sources.

The widespread use of computers in health care makes it essential to protect and secure the data to maintain patient confidentiality. Uninterrupted Power Supply devices, antivirus programs, firewalls, and strict control of access to computers can help protect both the computer and the information it contains.

INTERNET SEARCHES

Use the suggested search engines in the Using the Internet section in this chapter to search the Internet for additional information on the following topics:

1. *Computer hardware*: obtain information about different computer systems and compare and contrast the systems by searching the sites of computer manufacturers such as Gateway, Dell, Compaq, and IBM

2. *Computer software*: search for different types of software for health care providers

3. *Diagnostic devices*: search for additional information on blood analyzers, echocardiographs, computerized tomography, magnetic resonance imaging, positron emission tomography, and ultrasonography

4. *Organizations*: search for additional information and Internet links to the National Library of Medicine, National Institute of Health, Medical Literature Analysis and Retrieval System (MEDLARS), and the Statistical Package for Social Sciences (SPSS)

5. *Search engines*: search for information on the main search engines, advantages and disadvantages of the engines, and ways to use the engines most effectively

6. *Computer security*: search for information on antivirus and firewall programs, the effectiveness of these programs, ways to protect a computer from hackers, and encryption coding

REVIEW QUESTIONS

1. Define *computer literacy*.

2. Differentiate between hardware and software.

3. List five (5) examples of input devices and two (2) examples of output devices.

4. Identify ways confidentiality of patient information can be maintained while using computers.

5. Why is a contingency backup plan essential when computers are used to record information?

6. Briefly describe the main uses of the following imaging techniques:
   a. computerized tomography (CT)
   b. magnetic resonance imaging (MRI)
   c. positron emission tomography (PET)
   d. ultrasonography

7. You are conducting an Internet search for information on the following research question: "Does hypertension affect some cultures and/or races more readily than others?"
   a. Identify the key words in the question.
   b. List at least three (3) possible search phrases using math symbols and/or Boolean connectors.
   c. Which search engine will you use? Why?

8. Differentiate between an antivirus program and a firewall program.

9. List five (5) ways a health care worker can help meet HIPAA standards for maintaining confidentiality of health care information while using computer technology.

Source: Mitchell, Joyce & Haroun, Lee. *Introduction to Health Care, 2/E, Cengage Learning, 2007.*

CHAPTER 18 Medical Math

Chapter Objectives

After completing this chapter,
you should be able to:

◆ Perform basic math calculations on whole numbers, decimals, fractions, percentages, and ratios

◆ Convert between the following numerical forms: decimals, fractions, percentages, and ratios

◆ Round off numbers correctly

◆ Solve mathematical problems with proportions

◆ Express numbers using Roman numerals

◆ Estimate angles from a reference plane

◆ Use household, metric, and apothecary units to express length, volume, and weight

◆ Convert between the Fahrenheit and Celsius temperature scales

◆ Express time using the 24-hour clock (military time)

◆ Define, pronounce, and spell all key terms

 Observe Standard Precautions

 Instructor's Check—Call Instructor at This Point

 Safety—Proceed with Caution

 OBRA Requirement—Based on Federal Law

 Math Skill

 Legal Responsibility

 Science Skill

 Career Information

 Communications Skill

 Technology

KEY TERMS

angles
apothecary system
  (ah-pa'-the-ker-E)
Celsius
centigrade
decimals
degrees
estimating

Fahrenheit
fractions
household system
improper fractions
metric system
military time
nomenclature
  (no'-men-kla-shure)

percentages
proportion
ratios
reciprocal *(ree-si'-pre-kal)*
reference plane
Roman numerals
rounding numbers
whole numbers

INTRODUCTION

Working in health care requires the use of math skills to measure and perform various types of calculations. There are applications in all types of occupations:

♦ Calculating medication dosages

♦ Taking height and weight readings

♦ Measuring the amount of intake (fluids consumed or infused) and output (fluids expelled, e.g., urine, vomit)

♦ Billing and bookkeeping tasks

♦ Performing lab tests

♦ Mixing cleaning solutions

Errors in math can have negative effects on patients. For example, administering the wrong dosage of medication is a serious mistake and can harm the patient. Health care workers must strive for 100% accuracy. *If there is any doubt, it is essential to ask your supervisor or a qualified coworker to double-check calculations.*

18:1 INFORMATION

Basic Calculations

To work safely in health care, it is essential to be able to add, subtract, multiply, and divide whole numbers, decimals, fractions, and percentages. Health care workers also need to understand equivalents when using decimals, fractions, and percentages (figure 18-1).

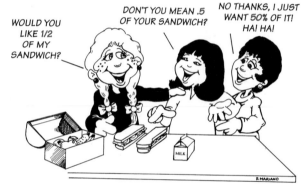

FIGURE 18-1 An easy way to remember how to convert decimals, percentages, and fractions is to think of this humorous cartoon.

Many health care workers use small calculators to assist them with calculations. During your health care studies, some instructors will allow the use of calculators, and others will not. It is always best to know how to do the basic functions by "long hand" (without a calculator). Calculators can quit working at any time during a test or at the workplace. In addition, some professional examinations required for licensure or certification do not allow the use of calculators.

WHOLE NUMBERS

Whole numbers are what we traditionally use to count (1, 2, 3, . . .). They do not contain fractions or decimals. For example, 30 is a whole number, while 30½ and 30.5 are not. Health care workers must be able to accurately add, subtract, multiply, and divide whole numbers.

Addition of Whole Numbers

Addition is adding two or more numbers together to find the *sum,* or total. A few examples of how addition is used in health care include:

♦ Counting and totaling supplies for an inventory

♦ Adding oral (by mouth) intake

♦ Adding intravenous or IV (into a vein) intake

♦ Measuring and totaling output from the body such as amounts of urine

♦ Completing statistical information such as the total number of patients diagnosed with lung cancer or the total number of surgeries performed in a hospital in a 1-year period

To add whole numbers together, the numbers are placed in a column and lined up on the right side of the column. The columns are then added together starting with the column on the right.

Example: A nurse assistant must encourage a patient to drink large amounts of fluid. For lunch, the patient drank 240 milliliters (mL) of milk, 120 mL of coffee, 45 mL of water, and 60 mL of juice. What is the total amount of fluids the patient drank?

$$\begin{array}{r} {}^{+1}2\,4\,0 \\ 1\,2\,0 \\ 4\,5 \\ +\ 6\,0 \\ \hline 4\,6\,5 \end{array}$$

Answer: The patient drank 465 mL of fluid.

Subtraction of Whole Numbers

Subtraction is the process of taking a number away from another number to find the *difference,* or *remainder,* between the numbers. A few examples of how subtraction is used in health care include:

♦ Determining weight loss or gain

♦ Maintaining an inventory of supplies

♦ Calculating a pulse deficit (difference between the number of times a heart beats and the actual pulse it creates)

♦ Performing laboratory tests

♦ Reporting statistical information such as number of deaths from a particular disease

To subtract whole numbers, the number to be subtracted is placed under the number from which it is to be subtracted. Both numbers must be lined up on the right-hand column. Starting at the right side, the bottom number is subtracted from the top number.

Example: A patient with a heart condition is on a weight-reduction plan. Last month, the patient weighed 214 pounds. This month, the patient weighs 195 pounds. How much weight did the patient lose?

$$\begin{array}{r} {}^{1}2\,{}^{0}1\,4 \\ -\ 1\,9\,5 \\ \hline 1\,9 \end{array}$$

Answer: The patient lost 19 pounds.

Multiplication of Whole Numbers

Multiplication is actually a simple method of addition. For example, if three *7s* are added together, the answer or sum is *21* $(7 + 7 + 7 = 21)$. If the number *7* is multiplied by *3,* the answer or product is *21* $(7 \times 3 = 21)$. A few examples of how multiplication is used in health care include:

♦ Maintaining payroll records including hours worked and salary earned

♦ Performing laboratory tests

♦ Determining the magnification power of a microscope

♦ Calculating prescription amounts such as the number of pills a patient should receive for a 30-day supply of medication

♦ Calculating caloric requirement based on body weight

To multiply whole numbers, write the number to be multiplied *(multiplicand)* first. If possible, use the largest number as the multiplicand. Under the multiplicand, write the number of times it is to be multiplied *(multiplier),* making sure the numbers are lined up on the right side. Then multiply every number in the multiplicand by every number in the multiplier. After all of the multipliers are used, the products obtained are added together to get the answer.

Example: A medical laboratory technician is preparing agar slant tubes. The tubes are used to grow microorganisms so the cause of a disease can be identified. The technician needs a total of 24 tubes. For each tube, 30 milliliters (mL) of broth and 15 mL of agar is needed (figure 18-2).

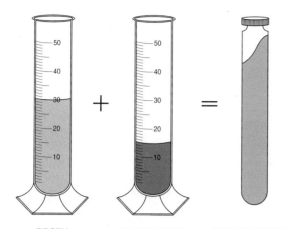

BROTH   BLOOD AGAR   AGAR SLANT TUBE

FIGURE 18-2 How much broth and agar is needed to fill 24 agar slant tubes?

What is the total amount of broth needed and the total amount of agar needed?

```
    30           15
 ×  24        ×  24
   120           60
 + 60         + 30
   720          360
```

Answer: The laboratory technician needs 720 mL of broth and 360 mL of agar to prepare 24 agar slant tubes.

Division of Whole Numbers

Division is a simple method used to determine how many times one number is present in another number. A few examples of how division is used in health care include:

♦ Calculating diets and amounts of nutrients allowed

♦ Determining cost per item while ordering bulk supplies or equipment

♦ Performing laboratory tests

♦ Compiling statistics on diseases and death rates

♦ Calculating budgets and salaries

Division involves the use of two numbers: a dividend and a divisor. The number to be divided is the *dividend*. The *divisor* is the number of times the dividend is to be divided. It is important to position these numbers correctly to obtain an answer, or *quotient*.

Example: A student doing research learns that statistics show 526,704 people die of cancer each year. On average, how many people die of cancer each month? (*Hint:* Remember that there are 12 months in a year.)

```
          43892
    12 √ 526704
       − 48
         46
       − 36
         107
        − 96
         110
       − 108
           24
         − 24
            0
```

Answer: On average, 43,892 people die of cancer each month.

DECIMALS

Decimals are one way of expressing parts of numbers or anything else that has been divided into parts. The parts are expressed in units of 10. That is, decimals represent the number of tenths, hundredths, thousandths, and so on that are available. For example, 0.7 represents 7 of the 10 parts into which something has been divided. When reading decimals verbally, it is necessary to know the placement values for the decimals (digits to the right of the decimal point) and that the decimal point is read as "and" (figure 18-3). For example:

♦ 0.5 is read "five tenths"

♦ 1.5 is read "one and five tenths"

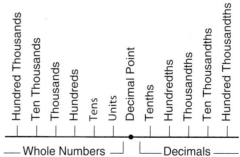

FIGURE 18-3 The position of the number to the left or the right of the decimal point is its place value. The value of each place *left* of the decimal point is *10 times* that of the place to its right. The value of each place *right* of the decimal point is *one-tenth* the value of the place to its left.

♦ 1.50 is read "one and fifty hundredths"

♦ 1.500 is read "one and five hundred thousandths"

♦ 1.5000 is read "one and five thousand ten thousandths"

Note that a zero is placed to the left of the decimal point if the number begins to the right of the point. This is necessary to prevent errors from occurring if the decimal point is not seen.

Decimals are added, subtracted, multiplied, and divided in the same way as whole numbers. The most common mistake is incorrect placement of the decimal point (table 18-1).

A few examples of how decimals are used in health care include:

♦ Determining medication dosages

♦ Performing laboratory tests

♦ Calculating dietary requirements or restrictions

♦ Measuring respiratory function

♦ Maintaining payroll records

♦ Billing charges on patient accounts

♦ Determining exposure to radiation

♦ Totaling the cost of supplies and equipment orders

Example: A dietitian is teaching teenagers about the high levels of fat in fast food. She notes that there are 44.51 grams (g) of fat in a bacon cheeseburger, 18.3 g in large serving of fries, and 13.83 g in a milkshake. How many grams of fat does this meal contain? (Remember to line up the decimal points to add the numbers together.)

$$\begin{array}{r} 44.51 \\ 18.3 \\ +\,13.83 \\ \hline 76.64 \end{array}$$

This meal contains 76.64 g of fat. If the recommended daily allowance for fat grams is 60 g in an 1,800-calorie diet, how many extra grams of fat are present in just this one meal? To solve this, subtract the recommended daily allowance from the total number of fat grams in the meal. Add

TABLE 18-1 Working with Decimals

FUNCTION	EXAMPLE	KEY POINTS
Add: (+)	1.5 + 2.25 3.75	1. Line up the decimal points. 2. Add the numbers. 3. Bring the decimal point straight down.
Subtract: (−)	3.75 − 1.25 2.50	1. Line up the decimal points. 2. Subtract the numbers. 3. Bring the decimal point straight down.
Multiply: (×)	2.5 × 2.5 125 + 50 6.25	1. Multiply the numbers. 2. Count the total number of digits to the right of the decimal points in the numbers you you are multiplying. 3. Count the same number of places in your answers. Start to the right of the last digit in your answer and move that number of places to the left. This is where the decimal point is placed.
Divide: (÷)	2.5)50.5 25.)505.0 20.2 25)505.0 50 5 0 50 50 0	1. Move the decimal point to the right in the number you are dividing by to make it a whole number. 2. Move the decimal point the same number of places to the right in the number being divided. Add zeros if necessary. 3. Divide the numbers. 4. Place the decimal point in the answer by moving it straight up from the number that was divided.

zeros to the right of the decimal point to make it easier to subtract the numbers.

$$
\begin{array}{r}
76.64 \\
-60.00 \\
\hline
16.64
\end{array}
$$

Answer: This fast-food meal contains 76.64 g of fat, which is 16.64 g more than is recommended for an entire day of meals.

FRACTIONS

Fractions are another way of expressing numbers that represent parts of a whole. A few examples of how fractions are used in health care include:

♦ Measuring solutions for laboratory tests

♦ Calculating height and weight

♦ Measuring head circumference on an infant

♦ Mixing solutions such as disinfectants for infection control

♦ Preparing dental materials and trimming dental models

♦ Mixing infant formulas or tube feedings

♦ Calculating dosages for certain medications

A fraction has a *numerator* (top number) and a *denominator* (bottom number). An example of a fraction is ³⁄₁₀, where 3 is the numerator and 10 is the denominator.

The 3 tells how many parts are present. The 10 tells how many parts make up the whole (figure 18-4). The fraction ³⁄₁₀ has been reduced to its lowest terms because no number can be divided evenly into both the numerator and denominator.

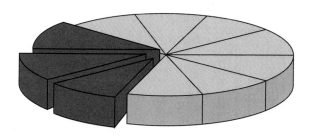

$$\frac{Part}{Whole} \quad \frac{3}{10}$$

FIGURE 18-4 A fraction is a comparison of parts (numerator) to a whole (denominator).

Some fractions must be *reduced* to their lowest terms. An example is 4/8. Both the numerator and denominator can be divided evenly by 4: 4 ÷ 4 = 1 and 8 ÷ 4 = 2. As a result, ⁴⁄₈ = ½.

Improper fractions have numerators that are larger than the denominators. To reduce these fractions, divide the denominator into the numerator. The result will be a whole number or a mixed number (whole number and a fraction). For example:

♦ The fraction ¹²⁄₄ would be reduced to the whole number 3 (12 ÷ 4 = 3)

♦ The fraction ¹¹⁄₄ would be reduced to the mixed number 2¾ (11 ÷ 4 = 2¾)

Performing calculations with fractions is not difficult, but it does require following a series of steps. These are described in table 18-2. When adding and subtracting fractions, it is necessary to change all the denominators to the same number to perform the calculations. This is known as *converting the fractions*. To do this, find a number that each denominator can divide into evenly. Then adjust the numerators to maintain an equivalent fraction. For example, to add ½ + ⅓, convert both fractions to sixths = ³⁄₆ + ²⁄₆ = ⁵⁄₆. The denominators 2 and 3 both divide into 6 evenly; then the numerator is multiplied by the number of times the old denominator divides into the new denominator (2 divides into 6 three times, so 1 × 3 then creates the new fraction of ³⁄₆; 3 divides into 6 two times, so 1 × 2 then creates the new fraction of ²⁄₆).

Multiplying fractions is straightforward. First multiply the two numerators and then the two denominators. For example, ½ × ½ is ¼ (1 × 1 = 1 and 2 × 2 = 4).

Dividing fractions requires the dividing fraction to be *inverted* (turned upside down). The new, upside-down fraction is called the **reciprocal.** The numerators and denominators are then multiplied to get the answer. For example, ½ ÷ ½ = ½ × ²⁄₁ = ²⁄₂ or 1.

Study the examples in table 18-2 to see how to add, subtract, multiply, and divide fractions. Then review these examples:

Example 1: A dental assistant has ½ ounce of disinfectant solution in one bottle and ⅔ ounce in a second bottle. Can the two bottles be combined in a 1½-ounce bottle? To solve this, add ½ and ⅔ together using the following steps:

First think of a number that both *2* and *3* divide into evenly. The answer is *6.*

TABLE 18-2 Working with Fractions

FUNCTION	EXAMPLE	KEY POINTS
Add: (+)	$\frac{1}{5} = \frac{6}{30}$ $+\frac{1}{6} = \frac{5}{30}$ $\frac{11}{30}$	1. If the denominators are not the same, find a number both denominators divide into evenly. 2. Multiply the numerators by the number of times the old denominators divide into the new denominator. 3. Add the numerators. 4. Place the new numerator over the denominator. 5. Reduce the fraction, if necessary.
Subtract: (−)	$\frac{1}{5} = \frac{6}{30}$ $-\frac{1}{6} = \frac{5}{30}$ $\frac{1}{30}$	1. If the denominators are not the same, find a number both denominators divide into evenly. 2. Multiply the numerators by the number of times the old denominators divide into the new denominator. 3. Subtract the numerators. 4. Place the new numerator over the denominator. 5. Reduce the fraction, if necessary.
Multiply: (×)	$\frac{1}{5} \times \frac{1}{6} = \frac{1}{30}$	1. Multiply numerators. 2. Multiply denominators. 3. Reduce the fraction, if necessary.
Divide: (÷)	$\frac{1}{5} \div \frac{1}{6} = \frac{1}{5} \times \frac{6}{1} = \frac{6}{5} = 1\frac{1}{5}$	1. Invert the dividing fraction. 2. Multiply numerators. 3. Multiply denominators. 4. Reduce the fraction, if necessary.

$$6 \div 2 = 3 \qquad 6 \div 3 = 2$$

Then multiply the numerator by the number of times the old denominator goes into 6.

$$1 \times 3 = 3 \qquad \frac{1}{2} = \frac{3}{6}$$
$$2 \times 2 = 4 \qquad \frac{2}{3} = \frac{4}{6}$$

Now add the two numerators together and place the answer over the common denominator.

$$\frac{3}{6} + \frac{4}{6} = \frac{7}{6}$$

The fraction $\frac{7}{6}$ is an improper fraction because the numerator is larger than the denominator. Divide the denominator into the numerator.

$$7 \div 6 = 1\frac{1}{6} \text{ ounces}$$

Will $1\frac{1}{6}$ ounces fit into a $1\frac{1}{2}$-ounce bottle? Change the $\frac{1}{2}$ to sixths.

$$6 \div 2 = 3 \qquad 3 \times 1 = 3 \qquad \frac{1}{2} = \frac{3}{6}$$

Answer: The bottle will hold $1\frac{3}{6}$ ounces, so $1\frac{1}{6}$ ounces will fit into the bottle.

Example 2: A pharmacist must prepare 24 ounces of a tube feeding for a patient. The mixture is $\frac{1}{3}$ formula and $\frac{2}{3}$ water. How much formula should she use? How much water?

To determine the amount of formula, multiply 24 (write as the fraction $\frac{24}{1}$) by $\frac{1}{3}$:

$$\frac{24}{1} \times \frac{1}{3} = ?$$

Multiply the numerators: $24 \times 1 = 24$.
Multiply the denominators: $1 \times 3 = 3$.
Put the new numerator over the new denominator: $\frac{24}{3}$.
Reduce the improper fraction by dividing the denominator into the numerator: $24 \div 3 = 8$.
Answer: The pharmacist will need 8 ounces of formula. To determine the amount of water, multiply 24 by $\frac{2}{3}$

$$\frac{24}{1} \times \frac{2}{3} = ?$$

Multiply the numerators: $24 \times 2 = 48$.
Multiply the denominators: $3 \times 1 = 3$.
Put the new numerator over the new denominator: $\frac{48}{3}$.
Reduce the improper fraction by dividing the denominator into the numerator: $48 \div 3 = 16$.
Answer: The pharmacist will need 16 ounces of water.

To check the answers, add 8 + 16 = 24. The answers are correct because 24 ounces is the total amount of tube feeding needed.

PERCENTAGES

Percentages are used to express either a whole or part of a whole. The whole is expressed as 100 percent (%). Refer to figure 18-4 and imagine this as a hot apple pie sliced into 10 equal pieces. The 10 slices together equal the whole, or 100%, of the pie. 100 divided by 10 equals 10. Therefore, each slice represents 10% of the pie. If each slice is 10%, then three slices represent 30% of the pie.

A few examples of how percentages are used in health care include:

◆ Recording statistics such as the percentage of people who die of lung cancer

◆ Preparing solutions for laboratory tests

◆ Mixing solutions for infection control such as a 10 percent bleach solution

◆ Calculating the amount of tax that must be subtracted from a salary check

◆ Determining dietary requirements or calculating special (therapeutic) diets

When working with percentages, it is easier to convert the percentage to a decimal and then perform the addition, subtraction, multiplication, and division. Converting percentages to decimals is explained in table 18-3. Look at the pie chart in figure 18-5 that shows emergency department admissions for a one-month period. Then use this information to find the answers to the following questions on percentages.

Example 1: What is the total percentage of people admitted due to heart attacks or respiratory problems?

The percentage admitted for heart attacks was 11.8%.

The percentage admitted for respiratory problems was 8.8%.

These two percentages can be added together by lining up the decimal points:

$$11.8\%$$
$$+\ \ 8.8\%$$
$$20.6\%$$

Answer: 20.6 percent of the people were admitted with heart attacks or respiratory problems.

Example 2: If a total of 364 patients were admitted to the emergency department during the one-month period, how many people were admitted because of an auto accident?

Check the pie chart: 26.1 percent of the admissions were for auto accidents.

First convert the 26.1 percent to decimals:

$$26.1\% = 26.1 \qquad 100 = 0.261$$

Now multiply the total number of patients, or 364, by 0.261:

$$
\begin{array}{r}
364 \\
\times\,0.261 \\
\hline
364 \\
2184 \\
728 \\
\hline
95004. = 95.004 = 95
\end{array}
$$

Starting at the right side, move the decimal point the same number of places to the left as it is in the multiplier. Because 0.261 has three decimal places, 95.004 is the correct answer.

Answer: A total of 95 people were admitted to the emergency department because of an auto accident. Note that the **4** at the end of the answer was ignored. When percentages are calculated, answers are often rounded to whole numbers.

RATIOS

Ratios show relationships between numbers or like values: how many of one number or value is present as compared with the other. For example, a bleach and water solution with a 1:2 ratio means that one part of bleach is added for every two parts of water. This relationship applies regardless of the units used:

◆ 1 cup of bleach and 2 cups of water

◆ 1 quart of bleach and 2 quarts of water

◆ ½ cup of bleach and 1 cup of water

◆ ¼ cup of bleach and ½ cup of water

The use of ratios to express the strength of a solution is commonly seen in health care. Solution strengths are also frequently expressed as percentages. A 50-percent bleach solution is the same as the 1:2 ratio. Conversions between ratios and percentages are explained in the next section.

TABLE 18-3 Converting Decimals, Fractions, and Percentages

CONVERTING	EXAMPLE	KEY POINTS
Decimals to fractions	$0.75 = 75/100$ $\dfrac{75}{100} = \dfrac{75}{100} \div \dfrac{25}{25} = \dfrac{3}{4}$	1. Drop the decimal point. 2. Position the number over its placement value (Figure 18-3). 3. If necessary, reduce the fraction.
Decimals to percentages	$5.275 = 5.275 \times 100 = 527.5$ 527.5%	1. Move the decimal point two places to the right because percentages are based on 100. This is the same as multiplying by 100. 2. Add the percentage sign.
Fractions to decimals	$3/5 = 3 \div 5 = 0.6$	1. Divide the numerator by the denominator.
Fractions to percentages	$7/8 = 7 \div 8 = 0.875$ $0.875 \times 100 = 87.5$ 87.5%	1. Divide the numerator by the denominator. 2. Move the decimal point two places to the right because percentages are based on 100. This is the same as multiplying by 100. 3. Add the percentage sign.
Percentages to decimals	$125.5\% = 125.5$ $125.5 \div 100 = 1.255$	1. Remove the percentage sign. 2. Move the decimal point two places to the left because percentages are based on 100. This is the same as dividing by 100.
Percentages to fractions	$5\% = 5$ $\dfrac{5}{100} = \dfrac{5 \div 5}{100 \div 5} = \dfrac{1}{20}$	1. Remove the percentage sign. 2. Place the number over 100. 3. If appropriate, simplify the fraction to its lowest terms.
Percentages to ratios	$75\% = 75$ 75:100	1. Remove the percentage sign. 2. Create a ratio using the former percentage and the number 100. 3. Insert a colon (:) between the numbers.
Ratios to percentages	$1:2 = 1 \div 2 = 0.5$ $0.5 \times 100 = 50$ $50 = 50\,\%$	1. Divide the number on the left of the colon by the number on the right of the ratio sign. 2. Move the decimal point two places to the right. Add zero(s) if necessary. This is the same as multiplying by 100. 3. Add the percentage sign.

EMERGENCY DEPARTMENT ADMISSIONS

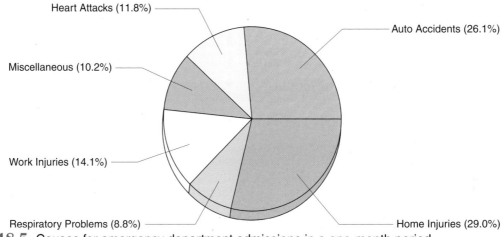

FIGURE 18-5 Causes for emergency department admissions in a one-month period.

CONVERTING DECIMALS, FRACTIONS, PERCENTAGES, AND RATIOS

Decimals, fractions, and percentages all express parts of a whole. The cartoon in figure 18-1 humorously portrayed how they are related: the fraction ½, the decimal 0.5, and the percentage 50% all represent the same amount of the sandwich. The steps used to convert between these numerical forms are shown in table 18-3.

ROUNDING NUMBERS

Rounding numbers means changing them to the nearest ten, hundred, thousand, and so on. Deciding which to use depends on the size of the original number and the degree of accuracy required. Deciding whether to round up or round down depends on the digits (numbers) located to the right of the value chosen for rounding. The following examples illustrate how these rules are applied:

Example 1: When rounding to the nearest 10: look at the digit to the right of the tens place (the ones place). If the number is 5 or greater, round up. If it is less than 5, round down.

88 rounds up to 90

83 rounds down to 80

Example 2: When rounding to the nearest 100: look at the digit to the right of the hundreds place (the tens place). If the number is 5 or greater, round up. If it is less than 5, round down.

67 rounds up to 100

133 rounds down to 100

668 rounds up to 700

621 rounds down to 600

Example 3: When rounding to the nearest 1,000, look at the digit to the right of the thousands place (the hundreds place). If the number is 5 or greater, round up. If it is less than 5, round down.

7777 rounds up to 8,000

7355 rounds down to 7,000

All numbers can be rounded. Review figure 18-3 and study the examples in table 18-4.

SOLVING PROBLEMS WITH PROPORTIONS

A **proportion** is a statement of equality between two ratios. For example, the proportion 2:6 = 3:9 means that 2 is related to 6 in the same way that 3

TABLE 18-4 Rounding Numbers

ROUND THE NUMBER 1234.5678 TO THE NEAREST:	RESULT	COMMENTS
Whole number	1234.5678 = 1235	The digit to the right of the whole number (1234) is 5, so you round up one number.
Tens	1234.5678 = 1230	The digit to the right of the tens place is 4, so you round down.
Hundreds	1234.5678 = 1200	The digit to the right of the hundreds place is 3, so you round down.
Thousands	1234.5678 = 1000	The digit to the right of the thousands place is 2, so you round down.
Tenths	1234.5678 = 1234.6	The digit to the right of the tenths place is 6, so you round up.
Hundredths	1234.5678 = 1234.57	The digit to the right of the hundredths place is 7, so you round up.
Thousandths	1234.5678 = 1234.568	The digit to the right of the thousandths place is 8, so you round up.
Ten thousandths	1234.56780 = 1234.5678	No change.

is related to 9. It is verbalized as "two is to six as three is to nine."

Proportions are used to solve many math problems in health care. Some common examples include:

♦ Calculating height to feet and inches

♦ Calculating weight to pounds and ounces

♦ Determining the proper dosage of a medicine

♦ Calculating a flow rate for IV (intravenous or into a vein) solutions

♦ Determining measurements to mix solutions

♦ Interpreting laboratory test results

Proportions are useful for converting from one unit to another when three of the terms in the proportion are known.
Example: You need $32.50 in quarters. How many quarters are needed? Three of the terms in the proportion are known:

♦ $32.50

♦ 4 (the number of quarters that are in $1.00)

♦ $1.00

The proportion is set up as follows:

$$\frac{4 \text{ quarters}}{x \text{ quarters}} = \frac{\$1.00}{\$32.50}$$

The purpose of the proportion is to answer the question: "If four quarters equal one dollar, how many quarters are there in thirty-two dollars and fifty cents?" Or put another way: "4 quarters is to $1.00 as x quarters are to $32.50." *Note that the two unit measurements on each side of the equation are the same* (quarters on the left and dollars on the right). The x stands for the number to be calculated.
To solve this problem, follow these steps:
Cross multiply:

$$\frac{4 \text{ quarters}}{x \text{ quarters}} = \frac{\$1.00}{\$32.50}$$

$$1 \times x = 4 \times 32.50 \qquad 1x = 130$$

Divide each side by the number in front of x (in this case, each number is divided by one and this does not alter the number)

$$1x \div 1 = x \text{ and } 130 \div 1 = 130$$
$$x = 130 \text{ quarters}$$

The completed proportion is:

$$\frac{4 \text{ quarters}}{130 \text{ quarters}} = \frac{\$1.00}{\$32.50}$$

Answer: 130 quarters are needed to make a payment of $32.50.

Converting units of measurement is another common application of proportions. When a patient's height is measured, the height bar on most medical scales provides the measurement in inches. This must be converted to feet and inches.
Example: A medical assistant measures the height of a small child at 36 inches. How many feet are in 36 inches? Three of the terms in the proportion are known:

♦ 29 inches

♦ 12 (the number of inches in 1 foot)

♦ 1 foot

The proportion is set up as follows:

$$\frac{1 \text{ foot}}{x \text{ feet}} = \frac{12 \text{ inches}}{36 \text{ inches}}$$

To solve this problem, follow these steps:
Cross multiply:

$$\frac{1 \text{ foot}}{x \text{ feet}} = \frac{12 \text{ inches}}{36 \text{ inches}}$$

$$12 \times x = 1 \times 36 \qquad 12x = 36$$

Divide each side by the number in front of x

$$12x \div 12 = x \text{ and } 36 \div 12 = 3$$
$$x = 3 \text{ feet}$$

The completed proportion is:

$$\frac{1 \text{ foot}}{3 \text{ feet}} = \frac{12 \text{ inches}}{36 \text{ inches}}$$

Answer: The small child is 3 feet tall.

A common application of proportions in health care is to find the value of an unknown when calculating the dosage of medications
Example: A physician orders a patient to have 50 g of a medication. When the nurse checks, she notes that the medication is only available in 12.5-g tablets. How many tablets should she give the patient?

Set up the proportion with the three known facts.

$$\frac{1 \text{ tablet}}{x \text{ tablets}} = \frac{12.5 \text{ g}}{50 \text{ g}}$$

Cross multiply:

$$\frac{1 \text{ tablet}}{x \text{ tablets}} = \frac{12.5 \text{ g}}{50 \text{ g}}$$

$$12.5 \times x = 1 \times 50 \qquad 12.5x = 50$$

Divide each side by the number in front of x

$$12.5x \div 12.5 = x \text{ and } 50 \div 12.5 = 4$$
$$x = 4 \text{ tablets}$$

The completed proportion is:

$$\frac{1 \text{ tablet}}{4 \text{ tablets}} = \frac{12.5 \text{ g}}{50 \text{ g}}$$

Answer: 4 tablets are needed to equal 50 g

18:2 INFORMATION

Estimating

Health care workers must work carefully and thoughtfully when performing calculations. An important skill to help check work is anticipating the results. This involves **estimating**— calculating the approximate answer—and judging if the calculated results seem reasonable. If calculations are performed without thought and answers simply accepted, errors can go unnoticed. It is easy for mistakes to occur when you're working in a hurry. Numbers can be placed in the wrong order, decimal points misplaced, or operations carried out incorrectly. Knowing when an answer "just doesn't look right" serves as an alert to double-check the results. Working on "automatic pilot" is not acceptable when using math in the workplace.

Learning to estimate and detect incorrect answers takes practice and thought. There are a few guidelines to make estimating useful. First, use rounding to get numbers that are easier to mentally compute. For example, when multiplying 47 times 83, round 47 up to 50 and 83 down to 80. 50 times 80 is much easier to mentally multiply than the original numbers. Second, watch place values carefully. In the 50 times 80 example, if 5 is multiplied times 8, two zeroes must be added to the quick result of 40. Third, look at the size of the answer. Does it make sense? For example, when multiplying whole numbers, the answer should be larger than either of the numbers in the problem. When dividing numbers, it should be smaller. Fourth, be careful about placing decimal points. Remember that everything to the right of the point is a fraction. Even 0.99999 does not equal 1.0.

18:3 INFORMATION

Roman Numerals

The traditional numbering system we use every day is referred to as Arabic numerals (1, 2, 3,. . .). In health care, it is necessary to know Roman numerals because they are used for some medications, solutions, and ordering systems. You may also see some files or materials organized using Roman numerals. When using **Roman numerals,** remember the following key points:

- All numbers can be expressed by using seven key numerals:
  I = 1
  V = 5
  X = 10
  L = 50
  C = 100
  D = 500
  M = 1000

- If a smaller numeral is placed in front of a larger numeral, the smaller numeral is *subtracted* from the larger numeral. For example: IV = 1 is placed before the 5, so it is subtracted (5 − 1 = 4)

- If a smaller numeral is placed after a larger numeral, the smaller numeral is *added* to the larger numeral. For example: VI = 1 is placed after the 5, so it is added (5 + 1 = 6)

- When the same numeral is placed next to itself it is added. For example:
  III = 1 + 1 + 1 = 3
  XX = 10 + 10 = 20
  IXX = this has two of the same numerals preceded by a smaller numeral, but the rules still apply (10 + 10 − 1 = 19 OR 10 − 1 = 9 + 10 = 19)

- The same numeral is *not* placed next to itself more than three times. For example:
  XXX = 30
  XL = 40 (XXXX is not correct)

- When Roman numerals are used with medication dosages, the lowercase (i, v, x, l, c, d, m) may be used rather than uppercase (capital letters). For example, ii = 2, iv = 4, ixx = 19.

Study table 18-5 to practice converting between Arabic and Roman numerals.

18:4 INFORMATION

Angles

Angles are used in health care when injecting medications, describing joint movement, and indicating bed positions. **Angles** are always defined by comparison to a **reference plane,** a

TABLE 18-5 Arabic and Roman Numeral Conversion Chart

ARABIC	ROMAN	ARABIC	ROMAN
1	I	23	XXIII
2	II	24	XXIV
3	III	25	XXV
4	IV	26	XXVI
5	V	27	XXVII
6	VI	28	XXVIII
7	VII	29	XXIX
8	VIII	30	XXX
9	IX	40	XL
10	X	50	L
20	XX	100	C
21	XXI	500	D
22	XXII	1000	M

real or imaginary flat surface from which the angle is measured. The distance between the plane and the line of the angle is measured in units called **degrees.** For example, if a flat stick is placed on a table (the reference plane), the angle is at 0 degrees. There is no distance between the plane and the stick. If the stick is lifted to stand straight up (perpendicular to the table), there is a 90-degree angle to the table. Moving the stick halfway between these two positions creates a 45-degree angle. Rotating the stick all the way around the arc and returning to the reference point creates a complete circle and represents 360 degrees (figure 18-6). The following examples illustrate how angles are used in health care:

Example 1: Angles for injecting needles vary, depending on the type of medication or proce-

dure being performed (figure 18-7). Note that in this case the reference plane is the surface of the skin.

Example 2: When describing the angle of extremities (arms and legs), the body in a full upright position is the reference plane (figure 18-8). Each joint (e.g., elbow, knee, hip) in the body has a normal range it is intended to move within. Physicians assess the range of a patient's joint compared with this normal range to chart loss of function or progress of recovery.

Example 3: After surgery on a joint (e.g., hip or knee replacement), the physician will order that the joint not be moved more than a certain number of degrees to prevent the new joint from "popping" out of place.

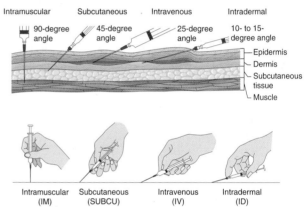

FIGURE 18-7 The correct angle must be used when inserting needles for administration of injections.

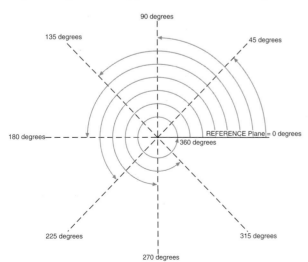

FIGURE 18-6 All angles are expressed in relation to a real or imaginary reference plane.

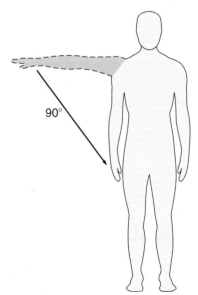

FIGURE 18-8 Body in full upright position with right arm lifted to 90-degree angle.

Example 4: Sometimes the physician will order to keep the head of the bed elevated by 30 to 45 degrees at all times. This is usually ordered to aid in respiration or to prevent aspiration (stomach contents entering the lungs). In this situation, the bed in the flat position is the reference plane.

18:5 INFORMATION

Systems of Measurement

Basic skills in calculation are applied when learning and using the various systems of measurement used in health care. Each system has its own terminology for designating distance (length), capacity (volume), and mass (weight). Converting between these systems requires the use of the skills presented in this chapter. The three systems used in health care are household, metric, and apothecary. Each system has its own **nomenclature** (method of naming).

HOUSEHOLD SYSTEM

The **household system** is probably the method of measurement most familiar to students who are educated in the United States (table 18-6). Note that "ounce" is used as both a measurement of capacity/volume and mass/weight. Health care workers use both. Liquids, such as an 8-ounce glass of water, are measured in terms of capacity

or volume. Determining mass or weight, such as with a 6-pound 12-ounce infant, is done by weighing with a scale. The various units of measurements in the household system relate to each other and can be converted among themselves. For example, volume/capacity is measured in drops, teaspoons, tablespoons, ounces, cups, pints, quarts, and gallons. Knowing the equivalencies of these units enables you to calculate each one in terms of the others (figure 18-9).

When the basic equivalents are known, unknown measurements can be determined using proportions. Suppose that 3 tablespoons of a liquid are needed, but the only measuring device available is a cup marked in ounces (oz). How many ounces are in 3 tablespoons (3 T)? Knowing that 2 T = 1 oz, the proportion would be set up as follows:

$$\frac{2\,T}{3\,T} = \frac{1\,oz}{x\,oz}$$
$$2x = 3\,oz$$
$$2x \div 2 = 3\,oz \div 2$$
$$x = 1.5\,oz$$

The next example involves measurement of height. If a patient is 63 inches tall and asks how many feet that is, the calculation would use the following proportion:

$$\frac{12\,inches}{63\,inches} = \frac{1\,foot}{x\,feet}$$
$$12x = 63$$
$$12x \div 12 = 63 \div 12$$
$$x = 5.25\,feet$$
$$x = 5.25\,feet$$

TABLE 18-6 Household Measurement System

TYPE OF MEASUREMENT	NOMENCLATURE	COMMON EQUIVALENTS
Distance/Length	inch (″ or in) foot (′ or ft) yard (yd) mile (mi)	12 in = 1 ft 3 ft = 1 yd 1760 yds = 1 mi
Capacity/Volume	drop (gtt) teaspoon (t or tsp) tablespoon (T or tbsp) ounce (oz) cup (C) pint (pt) quart (qt) gallon (gal)	60 gtts = 1 t 3 t = 1 T 2 T = 1 oz 8 oz = 1 C 2 C = 1 pt 2 pt = 1 qt 4 qt = 1 gal
Mass/Weight	ounce (oz) pound (lb)	16 oz = 1 lb

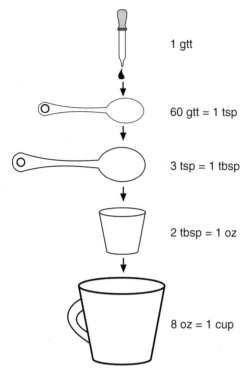

1 gtt

60 gtt = 1 tsp

3 tsp = 1 tbsp

2 tbsp = 1 oz

8 oz = 1 cup

FIGURE 18-9 Common household measurements used in health care.

Because most people do not say they are 5.25 feet tall, the decimal of 0.25 feet can be converted to inches. The following proportion can be used:

$$\frac{1 \text{ foot}}{0.25 \text{ ft}} = \frac{12 \text{ inches}}{x \text{ inches}}$$

Cross-multiply:

$$1 \times x = 1x \qquad 12 \times 0.25 = 3$$

Divide both by 1 to find the value of x

$$1x \div 1 = x \qquad 3 \div 1 = 3$$

The value of x is 3 inches. The patient is 5 feet 3 inches tall.

METRIC SYSTEM

The **metric system** is more accurate than the household system. Converting between numbers is easier because everything is based on a unit of 10. The nomenclature for the metric units is as follows:

♦ Distance/length: meter (m)

♦ Capacity/volume: liter (1 or L)

♦ Mass/weight: gram (g or gm)

The meter, liter, and gram are modified by adding the appropriate prefix to express larger or smaller units (table 18-7).

Because metric units are based on multiples of 10, conversions within the metric system are calculated by multiplying by 10, 100, 1,000, and so on:

♦ 1 *kilo*liter = 1,000 × 1 liter = 1,000 liters

♦ 1 *hecto*liter = 100 × 1 liter = 100 liters

♦ 1 *deca*liter = 10 × 1 liter = 10 liters

♦ 1 *deci*liter = 0.1 × 1 liter = 0.1 liter

♦ 1 *centi*liter = 0.01 × 1 liter = 0.01 liter

♦ 1 *milli*liter = 0.001 × 1 liter = 0.001 liter

A shortcut for performing these operations is to move the decimal point the number of places indicated by the prefix. Here are three examples:

TABLE 18-7 Common Prefixes of the Metric System

PREFIX	MEANING	EXAMPLES	MEANING OF EXAMPLES
kilo	1,000 times	kilogram kilometer kiloliter	1,000 grams 1,000 meters 1,000 liters
hecto	100 times	hectogram	100 grams
deca (also "deka")	10 times	decaliter	10 liters
meter, liter, gram	Whole units of measurement		
deci	1/10	decigram	1/10 of a gram
centi	1/100	centimeter	1/100 of a meter
milli	1/1,000	milliliter	1/1,000 of a liter
micro	1/1,000,000	microgram	1/1,000,000 of a gram

PREFIX	KILO-	HECTO-	DEKA-	BASE	DECI-	CENTI-	MILLI-	DECIMILLI-	CENTIMILLI-	MICROMILLI-
Common Units	kilogram			gram liter meter		centimeter	milligram milliliter millimeter			microgram
Value to Base	**1,000**	100	10	**1.0**	0.1	**0.01**	**0.001**	0.0001	0.00001	0.000001

FIGURE 18-10 Comparison of common metric units used in health care.

Example 1: Multiplying by 10 means moving the decimal point one place to the right. This may require adding one or more zeros. Multiplying 4.2 by 10 = 42.

Example 2: Multiplying by 100 means moving the decimal point two places to the right. This may require adding one or more zeros. Multiplying 4.2 by 100 = 420.

Example 3: Multiplying by 1,000 means moving the decimal point three places to the right. This may require adding one or more zeros. Multiplying 4.2 by 1,000 = 4,200.

Converting units within the metric system is accomplished by moving the decimal point. See figure 18-10 for a visual representation of decimal placement.

Example 1: A physician orders 2,000 milligrams (mg) of a medication. The medication is available in 1-g tablets. The 2,000 mg must be changed to grams. The conversion is made as follows:

♦ *Milli* is in the third place to the right of *gram*. Move the decimal point three spaces to the left toward gram: 2,000 = 2.000, or 2.

♦ Change unit name to grams: 2 g.

♦ The proper dose would be 2 g, or two 1-g tablets.

Example 2: A physical therapist measures a distance at 1,000 centimeters, but must know the distance in kilometers to check a patient's progress. The conversion is made as follows:

♦ *Centi* is five decimal places to the right of *kilo*, so move the decimal point five spaces to the left *toward* kilo. Add zeros as needed: 1,000 = 0.01.

♦ Change unit name to kilometers: 0.01 kilometer.

♦ 1,000 centimeters equals 0.01 kilometer.

In addition to moving the decimal point the correct number of places, it is critical that it be moved in the correct direction. This can be confusing. The easiest way is to determine whether the answer should be a larger or smaller number and then just move the decimal point accordingly:

♦ If converting from a larger to a smaller prefix (e.g., *kilo* to *milli*), the answer will be larger. It takes more smaller units to make up the larger unit.

♦ If converting from a smaller to a larger prefix (e.g., *milli* to *kilo*), the answer will be smaller. Many small units can be contained in a smaller number of large units.

A common health care application of the metric system is in the measurement of medications. Two units that represent the same amount are milliliters (mL) and cubic centimeters (cc). Both units measure volume and they are often interchanged when dispensing liquids. For example, 1 mL = 1 cc, 2 mL = 2 cc, and so forth. It is also worth noting that 1 mL or cc has a weight of 1 g (figure 18-11).

APOTHECARY SYSTEM

The **apothecary system** is the oldest and least used of the three systems of measurement presented. Some physicians still write orders using the apothecary system, so it is necessary to be familiar with these units of measurements (table 18-8). Health care workers must be able to con-

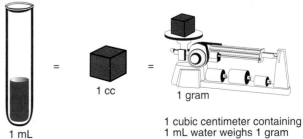

1 mL

1 cc

1 gram

1 cubic centimeter containing 1 mL water weighs 1 gram

FIGURE 18-11 The metric units that measure weight and volume are related.

TABLE 18-8 Apothecary Measurement System

TYPE OF MEASUREMENT	NOMENCLATURE	COMMON EQUIVALENTS
Distance/Length	N/A	N/A
Capacity/Volume	minim ♏ fluid dram (fl dr or f ʒ) fluid ounce (fl oz or f ʒ̄) pint (pt) quart (qt)	1 minim = 1 drop 60 minims = 1 fl dr 8 fl dr = 1 fl oz 16 fl oz = 1 pt 2 pt = 1 qt
Mass/Weight	grain (gr) dram (dr or ʒ) ounce (oz. or ʒ̄)	60 gr = 1 dr 480 gr = 1 oz

vert within the system as well as to convert to the metric system.

Roman numerals can be used in conjunction with the apothecary system, and may be seen in uppercase or lowercase. If lowercase is used, the Roman numeral for 1 is written with a line and a dot. For example, 2 would be written as ii. A commonly used abbreviation that originated with the apothecary system is s̄s̄, which means "half." For example, 2½ would be written as īīs̄s̄.

CONVERTING SYSTEMS OF MEASUREMENT

Health care work sometimes requires that units from one system of measurement are converted to those of another. This requires knowledge of the equivalencies between the units of the systems. There are frequently no exact equivalents, so when converting between systems, the answer is considered to be a close approximation (see table 18-9).

Using the appropriate equivalencies, a proportion is set up to identify and solve for the unknown quantity. The following steps are used for performing conversions:

♦ Identify an equivalent between the two systems.

♦ Set up a proportion so unit measurements on each side of the equation are the same.

♦ Use x for the unknown value being calculated.

♦ Cross-multiply.

♦ Solve for x.

♦ Verify that the answer is reasonable.

♦ If converting from a smaller unit to a larger unit, the answer will be smaller. For example, when converting 10 mL to teaspoons, the result will be smaller than 10 because a milliliter is a smaller unit than a teaspoon. Because there are 5 mL in 1 teaspoon, 10 mL = 2 teaspoons.

♦ If converting from a larger unit to a smaller unit, the answer will be larger. For example, when converting 2 grains to milligrams, the result will be a larger unit than 2 because a grain is a larger unit than a milligram. Because there are 60 mg in every grain, 2 grains = 120 mg.

The following examples illustrate how to perform conversions:

Example 1: Convert 19 inches to centimeters:

♦ Identify the equivalency: 1 inch = 2.5 centimeters

TABLE 18-9 Approximate Equivalents between Measuring Systems

DISTANCE/LENGTH	CAPACITY/VOLUME	MASS/WEIGHT
1 in = 2.5 cm	1 tsp = 5 mL = 5 cc	2.2 lb = 1 kg
39.4 in = 1 m	1 oz = 30 mL = 30 cc	1 grain = 60 milligrams
	1 qt = 1,000 mL = 1000 cc	15 grains = 1 gram

◆ Set up a proportion with the same units on each side of the equation. Use x for the unknown.
$$\frac{1 \text{ in}}{19 \text{ in}} = \frac{2.5 \text{ cm}}{x \text{ cm}}$$

◆ Cross-multiply:
$$1 \times x = 2.5 \times 19 \qquad 1x = 47.5 \text{ cm}$$

◆ Solve for x:
$$1x \div 1 = 47.5 \div 1$$
$$x = 47.5 \text{ cm}$$

◆ Verify that the answer is reasonable: It takes a larger number of centimeters (2½ times) to measure the same distance as 1 inch. Therefore, it makes sense that the answer is larger than 19.

Example 2: Convert 1.5 meters to inches:

◆ Identify the equivalency: 39.4 inches = 1 meter

◆ Set up a proportion with the same units on each side of equation. Use x for the unknown.
$$\frac{39.4 \text{ in}}{x \text{ in}} = \frac{1 \text{ m}}{1.5 \text{ m}}$$

◆ Cross-multiply:
$$1 \times x = 1.5 \times 39.4 \qquad 1x = 59.1 \text{ inches}$$

◆ Solve for x:
$$1x \div 1 = 59.1 \div 1$$
$$x = 59.1 \text{ inches}$$

◆ Verify that the answer is reasonable: It takes many inches to measure the distance designated by 1 meter. Therefore, the answer 59.1 makes sense.

Example 3: Convert 5 teaspoons to milliters:
$$\frac{1 \text{ tsp}}{5 \text{ tsp}} = \frac{5 \text{ mL}}{x \text{ mL}}$$
$$1 \times x = 5 \times 5 \qquad 1x = 25$$
$$x = 25 \text{ mL (25 cc)}$$

Example 4: Convert 75 mL to ounces:
$$\frac{1 \text{ oz}}{x \text{ oz}} = \frac{30 \text{ mL}}{75 \text{ mL}}$$
$$30x = 75 \text{ (Note that in solving for } x,$$
each side is divided by 30.)
$$x = 2.5 \text{ oz}$$

Example 5: Convert 120 pounds to kilograms:
$$\frac{2.2 \text{ lb}}{120 \text{ lb}} = \frac{1 \text{ kg}}{x \text{ kg}}$$
$$2.2x = 120 \text{ (Note that in solving for } x,$$
each side is divided by 2.2.)
$$x = 54.5 \text{ kg (rounded to nearest tenth)}$$

Example 6: Convert 15 gr to milligrams:
$$\frac{1 \text{ gr}}{15 \text{ gr}} = \frac{60 \text{ mg}}{x \text{ mg}}$$
$$x = 900 \text{ mg}$$

Example 7: Convert 2 g to grains:
$$\frac{15 \text{ gr}}{x \text{ gr}} = \frac{1 \text{ g}}{2 \text{ g}}$$
$$x = 30 \text{ gr}$$

Example 8: Convert 60 kg to ounces:
$$\frac{2.2 \text{ lb}}{x \text{ oz}} = \frac{1 \text{ kg}}{60 \text{ kg}}$$

This problem cannot be solved using this proportion, because the unit measurements on the left side of the equation are not the same size (pound and ounce). To solve this problem, pounds must first be converted to ounces. Refer back to the household system and table 18-6: 16 ounces = 1 pound.
$$\frac{16 \text{ oz}}{x} = \frac{1 \text{ lb}}{2.2 \text{ lb}}$$
$$x = 35.2 \text{ oz}$$

Knowing that 2.2 pounds = 35.2 ounces = 1 kilogram allows the appropriate proportion to be set up:
$$\frac{35.2 \text{ oz}}{x \text{ oz}} = \frac{1 \text{ kg}}{60 \text{ kg}}$$
$$x = 2,112 \text{ oz}$$

18:6 INFORMATION

Temperature Conversion

Thermometers using **Fahrenheit (F)** as the measuring unit are more familiar to people living in the United States. The **Celsius (C)** or **centigrade (C)** system of measurement, however, is frequently seen in medical practice. One way to start understanding the difference between the two systems is to compare how each one expresses the boiling and freezing points of water.

Boiling points: 212°F = 100°C
Freezing points: 32°F = 0°C

See figure 18-12 for a comparison of Fahrenheit (F) and Centigrade (C) thermometers and table 18-10 for a conversion chart. Health care workers may have to convert between the Fahrenheit and Celsius systems when a conversion chart is not available. Table 18-11 contains the formulas for conversion. There is a fraction and a decimal approach that give the same results. Deciding which to use depends on whether you have stronger skills working with fractions or decimals. All the formulas include parentheses. These are used to indicate that the enclosed calculation must be performed first. For example,

TABLE 18-10 Fahrenheit–Centigrade Conversion Chart

FAHRENHEIT	CENTIGRADE
32 (freezing point)	0 (freezing point)
95	35
96	35.6
97	36.1
97.4	36.3
98	36.7
98.6	37
99	37.2
99.4	37.4
100	37.8
101	38.3
102	38.9
103	39.4
104	40
212 (boiling point)	100 (boiling point)

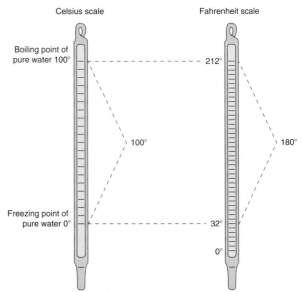

FIGURE 18-12 Comparison of Fahrenheit and Centigrade temperature scales.

the steps to solve the formula (°F − 32) × ⅝ = °C are to first subtract 32 from the value for °F and *then* multiply that value by ⅝.

18:7 INFORMATION

Military Time

Military time is frequently used in health care to avoid the confusion created by the AM and PM used in the traditional system to designate the correct time. The problem with the traditional system is that if the AM or PM is omitted or misread, an error of 12 hours is made. Errors in recording times are unacceptable in health care. For example, accuracy is critical when entering data on a patient chart, reporting when medications are given, or signing off on physician orders.

When **military time** is the standard used, all time designations are made with the 24-hour clock. The 12th hour is at 12 noon and the 24th hour is at 12 midnight.

See figure 18-13. When using the 24-hour clock, remember the following key points:

♦ Time is always expressed using four digits (e.g., 0030, 0200, 1200, 1700)

♦ AM hours are expressed with the same numbers as the traditional clock:

1 AM: 0100

TABLE 18-11 Temperature Scale Conversion Formulas

CONVERT FROM:	FRACTION FORMULA	DECIMAL FORMULA
Celsius to Fahrenheit	(°C × 9/5) + 32 = °F Example: 37°C (37 × 9/5) + 32 = °F 333/5 + 32 = °F 66.6 + 32 = 98.6°F	(°C × 1.8) + 32 = °F Example: 37°C (37 × 1.8) + 32 = °F 66.6 + 32 = 98.6°F
Fahrenheit to Celsius	(°F − 32) × 5/9 = °C Example: 101°F (101 − 32) × 5/9 = °C 69 × 5/9 = °C 345/9 = 38.3°C (rounded to nearest tenth)	(°F − 32) ÷ 1.8 = °C Example: 101°F (101 − 32) ÷ 1.8 = °C 69 ÷ 1.8 = 38.3°C (rounded to nearest tenth)

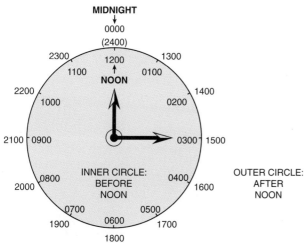

FIGURE 18-13 The military clock is based on a 24-hour day.

5:30 AM: 0530

10 AM: 1000

♦ An easy way to convert the PM hours is to add the time to 1200. Example:

1 PM: 1200 + 0100 (1:00 PM expressed in four digits) = 1300

5:30 PM: 1200 + 0530 (5:30 PM expressed in four digits) = 1730

10 PM: 1200 + 1000 (10:00 PM expressed in four digits) = 2200

♦ When times are verbalized, there is a specific way in which it is expressed:

1300 = thirteen hundred hours

1301 = thirteen oh one

1730 = seventeen thirty hours

2200 = twenty-two hundred hours

Study table 18-12 to practice converting between traditional and military times.

STUDENT: *Go to the workbook and complete the assignment sheet for Chapter 18, Medical Math.*

CHAPTER 18 SUMMARY

Work in health care requires the use of math skills to measure and perform various types of calculations. To work safely in health care, it is essential to be able to add, subtract, multiply, and divide whole numbers, decimals, fractions, and percentages. An understanding of equivalents when using decimals, fractions, and percentages is also needed.

TABLE 18-12 Military (24-Hour Clock) and Traditional Time Conversion Chart

TRADITIONAL	24-HOUR TIME	TRADITIONAL	24-HOUR TIME
12:01 AM	0001	12:01 PM	1201
12:30 AM	0030	12:30 PM	1230
1:00 AM	0100	1:00 PM	1300
2:00 AM	0200	2:00 PM	1400
3:00 AM	0300	3:00 PM	1500
4:00 AM	0400	4:00 PM	1600
5:00 AM	0500	5:00 PM	1700
6:00 AM	0600	6:00 PM	1800
7:00 AM	0700	7:00 PM	1900
8:00 AM	0800	8:00 PM	2000
9:00 AM	0900	9:00 PM	2100
10:00 AM	1000	10:00 PM	2200
11:00 AM	1100	11:00 PM	2300
12:00 noon	1200	12:00 midnight	2400

TODAY'S RESEARCH: TOMORROW'S HEALTH CARE

Scorpions and snakes to cure cancer?

Twenty thousand people each year experience development of a glioma, a cancerous brain tumor. Gliomas grow at a rapid rate and can kill a person in a matter of weeks. In most cases, surgical removal of the tumors will destroy too much brain tissue, so treatment is extremely limited. Few patients live more than 6 to 8 months after the tumor is diagnosed.

Now there is hope for people with gliomas. Dr. Harald Sontheimer is working with a research team at the University of Alabama at Birmingham. He discovered that a giant Israeli golden scorpion secretes a venom that is safe to humans but paralyzes muscles of a cockroach. The toxic molecules of the venom target a specific protein on the muscles of the cockroach, killing the cockroach. Through research, Sonteheimer found that the same protein is present on the cancerous glioma cells. When the venom seeks out the tumor cells, it kills the cells and stops the growth of the glioma without harming the healthy cells in the brain. Currently, clinical trials are being conducted on more than 60 people with gliomas. If the trials are successful, the Food and Drug Administration may approve this venom-derived drug as an accepted form of treatment.

Many other researchers are working with snake venom. They are trying to use snake venom to destroy the blood vessels that supply cancerous tumors with nourishment and fluid. If access to nourishment is restricted, tumors will not be able to grow. Another group of researchers is trying to use the venom from bees to kill malignant cells and destroy cancerous tumors. One of the leading causes of death will be eliminated if research finds that readily available venom from scorpions, snakes, and bees cures a cancerous tumor.

An important skill to help check work is anticipating the results. Learning to estimate and detect incorrect answers takes practice and thought.

Roman numerals are used in health care for some medications, solutions, and ordering systems. Angles are used when injecting medications, describing joint movement, and indicating bed positions.

The three systems of measurement used in health care are household, metric, and apothecary. Health care work sometimes requires that units from one system of measurement be converted to those of another. This requires knowledge of the equivalencies between the units of the systems. Health care workers may have to convert between the Fahrenheit and Celsius systems of temperature measurement, because the Celsius or centigrade system of measurement is frequently seen in medical practice.

Military time is frequently used in health care to avoid the confusion created by the AM and PM used in the traditional system. Errors in recording times are unacceptable in health care.

Accuracy is critical such as when entering data on a patient chart, reporting when medications are given, or signing off on physicians orders.

Health care workers must work carefully and thoughtfully when performing calculations. Errors in math can have serious effects on the patient; therefore, health care workers must strive for 100 percent accuracy.

INTERNET SEARCHES

Use the suggested search engines in Chapter 17:4 of this textbook to search the Internet for additional information on the following topics:

1. *Math:* search words such as math, basic math, basic calculations, fractions, and percentages

2. *Roman numerals:* search for additional information on using Roman numerals

3. *Measurement:* search words such as measurement, mass/weight, volume, converting measures, metric system, and equivalents

4. *Temperature:* search for information on Fahrenheit, centigrade, Celsius, and converting temperatures

5. *Military time:* search words such as time, military time, and 24-hour clock

REVIEW QUESTIONS

1. A patient's oral intake is being measured. For breakfast, he drinks 240 milliliters (mL) of coffee, 120 mL of juice, and 60 mL of water. What is the total fluid intake?

2. A patient is on a diet to lose weight. Last month, she weighed 172 pounds. This month, she weighs 159 pounds. How much weight did she lose?

3. A physical therapist is buying elastic bandages. Each roll costs $3.25. How much would 30 rolls cost?

4. A central supply worker orders 12 new stethoscopes for a total cost of $108.48. How much does each stethoscope cost?

5. A surgical nurse works $1\frac{1}{4}$ hours in preoperative (before surgery) care, $2\frac{1}{2}$ hours in the operating room, and $3\frac{3}{4}$ hours in the recovery room. What is the total number of hours worked?

6. An electrocardiograph technician knows that one small block on electrocardiographic paper represents $\frac{1}{25}$ of a second. How many seconds are represented by 150 small blocks?

7. A laboratory technician counts 7,742 leukocytes (white blood cells). If 36% of the leukocytes are lymphocytes, how many lymphocytes are present?

8. A doctor orders 500 mg of sumycin for a patient. Sumycin, an antibiotic, is available in 250-mg capsules. How many capsules should be given to the patient?

9. A medical assistant orders MM pairs of gloves. How many gloves were ordered?

10. How many liters are in 2.5 kiloliters?

11. A patient drinks 90 mL of water. How many ounces did the patient drink?

12. A doctor orders a saline irrigation with 2,000 mL. How many quarts of solution must be used?

13. An emergency medical technician must report to work at 1830. What does this mean in traditional time?

14. Convert 70 degrees Fahrenheit to Celsius.

Source: Mitchell, Joyce & Haroun, Lee. *Introduction to Health Care, 2/E*, Cengage Learning, 2007.

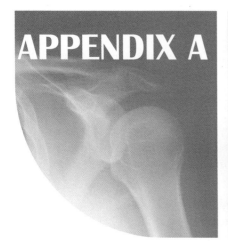

APPENDIX A

Career and Technical Student Organizations (CTSOs)

Career and technical student organizations provide both secondary (high school) and post-secondary (after high school) career/technical students with the opportunity to associate with other students enrolled in the same programs or career areas. Some purposes of these organizations are to:

♦ Develop leadership abilities, citizenship skills, social competencies, and a wholesome attitude about life and work

♦ Strengthen creativity, thinking skills, decision-making abilities, and self-confidence

♦ Enhance the quality and relevance of education by developing the knowledge, skills, and attitudes that lead to successful employment and continuing education

♦ Promote quality of work and pride in occupational excellence through competitive activities

♦ Obtain scholarships for post-secondary education from corporations that recognize the importance of these organizations

The United States Department of Education recognizes and supports the following eight career and technical student organizations:

♦ Business Professionals of America (BPA)

♦ Distributive Education Clubs of America (DECA)

♦ Future Business Leaders of America (FBLA)

♦ National FFA Organization (Agriculture Science Education)

♦ Family, Career, and Community Leaders of America (FCCLA)

♦ HOSA (Health Occupations Students of America)

♦ Technology Students Association (TSA)

♦ SkillsUSA

Two organizations that supplement health-science technology education are discussed: HOSA and SkillsUSA.

HOSA

HOSA (pronounced *Ho'sa*) is the national organization for secondary and post-secondary/collegiate students enrolled in health science technology education (HSTE) programs. HOSA is endorsed by the U.S. Department of Education and the Health Science Technology Education Division of the Association for Career and Technical Education (ACTE). Membership begins at the local level, where students who are enrolled in an HSTE program join together under the supervision of their classroom instructor, who serves as the HOSA local chapter advisor. Local chapters associate with the HOSA state association and the HOSA national organization.

Members of HOSA are involved in community-oriented, career-related, team-building, and leadership-development activities. All HOSA activities relate to the classroom instructional program and the health care delivery system. Furthermore, HOSA is an integral part of the HSTE program, meaning that HOSA activities motivate students and enhance what the students learn in the classroom and on the job.

The mission of HOSA is "to enhance the delivery of compassionate, quality health care by providing opportunities for knowledge, skills, and leadership development of all HSTE students, therefore helping the student meet the needs of the health care community." The HOSA motto is "The hands of HOSA mold the health of tomorrow." The HOSA slogan is "Health Science and HOSA: A Healthy Partnership." Goals that HOSA believes are vital for each member are:

♦ To promote physical, mental, and social well-being

♦ To develop effective leadership qualities and skills

♦ To develop the ability to communicate more effectively with people

♦ To develop character

♦ To develop responsible citizenship traits

♦ To understand the importance of pleasing oneself as well as being of service to others

♦ To build self-confidence and pride in one's work

♦ To make realistic career choices and seek successful employment in the health care field

♦ To develop an understanding of the importance of interacting and cooperating with other students and organizations

♦ To encourage individual and group achievement

♦ To develop an understanding of current health care issues, environmental concerns, and survival needs of the community, the nation, and the world

♦ To encourage involvement in local, state, and national health care and education projects

♦ To support HSTE instructional objectives

♦ To promote career opportunities in health care

In addition to providing activities that allow members to develop occupational skills, leadership qualities, and fellowship through social and recreational activities, HOSA also encourages skill development and a healthy competitive spirit through participation in the National Competitive Events Program. Competition is held at the local, district/regional, state, and national levels. Some of the competitive events include contests in prepared and extemporaneous speaking, job-seeking skills, CPR/first aid, dental assisting, dental laboratory technology, emergency

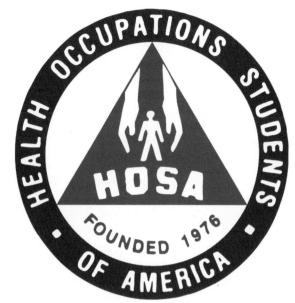

FIGURE A-1 The HOSA emblem. *(Reprinted with permission of HOSA)*

medical technician, clinical and administrative medical assisting, medical laboratory assisting, nursing assisting, practical nursing, physical therapy aide, veterinary assisting, dental spelling and terminology, medical spelling and terminology, extemporaneous health poster, community awareness project (of health-related issues), creative problem solving, biomedical debate, parliamentary procedure, and the HOSA Bowl.

HOSA has an official emblem (figure A-1). The circle represents the continuity of health care; the triangle represents the three aspects of human well-being: social, physical, and mental; and the hands signify the caring of each HOSA member. The colors of HOSA—maroon, medical white, and navy blue—are represented in the emblem. Navy blue represents loyalty to the health care profession. Medical white represents purity of purpose. Maroon represents the compassion of HOSA members.

The HOSA handbook provides detailed information about the structure, purposes, competitive events, and activities of HOSA. Students interested in further details should refer to this handbook or obtain additional information from the Internet by contacting HOSA at *www.hosa.org*.

SkillsUSA

Students in HSTE programs can also participate in SkillsUSA. SkillsUSA is a partnership of students, teachers, and industry working together to ensure America has a skilled workforce. It is a national organization for secondary and post-secondary/collegiate students enrolled in training programs in technical, skilled, and service occupations, including health careers. Examples of these programs include auto services, cosmetology, carpentry, collision repair, computer-aided drafting, electronics, masonry, precision machining, welding, and health occupations. Membership begins with local chapters that affiliate with a state association and then the national organization.

A national program of work sets the pace for SkillsUSA chapters. All SkillsUSA programs are in some way related to these seven major goals: professional development, community service, employment, ways and means, championships, public relations, and social activities.

The SkillsUSA motto is "Preparing for leadership in the world of work." Some of the purposes include:

♦ To unite in a common bond all students enrolled in trade, industrial, technical, and HSTE

♦ To develop leadership abilities through participation in educational, technical, civic, recreational, and social activities

♦ To foster a deep respect for the dignity of work

♦ To assist students in establishing realistic goals

♦ To help students attain purposeful lives

♦ To create enthusiasm for learning

♦ To promote high standards in trade ethics, workmanship, scholarship, and safety

♦ To develop the ability of students to plan together, organize, and carry out worthy activities and projects through the use of the democratic process

♦ To develop patriotism through a knowledge of our nation's heritage and the practice of democracy

To achieve these purposes, SkillsUSA offers a *Professional Development Program (PDP)*, and SkillsUSA Championships. The PDP is a self-paced curriculum for students to obtain skills in areas such as effective communication, management, teamwork, networking, workplace ethics, and job interviewing. The PDP is designed to help students develop the skills they need to make a smooth transition to the workforce or higher education.

SkillsUSA Championships offer skill competition in both leadership and occupational areas. Competition is held at the local, district/ regional, state, and national levels. Examples of leadership contests include prepared and extemporaneous speech, SkillsUSA opening and closing ceremonies, chapter business procedure, action skills, job interview, and safety promotion. Examples of career contests for HSTE students include medical assisting, dental assisting, nurse assisting, practical nursing, basic health care skills, first aid and CPR, health occupations professional portfolio, and a health knowledge bowl.

The ceremonial emblem of SkillsUSA is shown in figure A-2. The shield represents patriotism, or a belief in democracy, liberty, and the American way of life. The torch represents knowledge. The orbital circles represent technology and the training needed to master new technical frontiers along with the need for continuous education. The gear represents the industrial society and the cooperation of the individual working with labor and management for the betterment of humankind. The hands represent the individual and portray a search for knowledge along with the desire to acquire a skill.

The colors of the SkillsUSA organization are red, white, blue, and gold. Red and white represent the individual states and chapters. Blue represents the common union of the states and

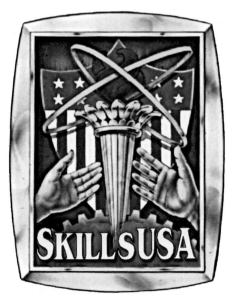

FIGURE A-2 The SkillsUSA emblem. *(Reprinted with permission of SkillsUSA)*

chapters. Gold represents the individual, the most important element of the organization.

The SkillsUSA Leadership Handbook and other SkillsUSA publications provide more information on the various activities and programs. Students interested in further details should refer to these sources of information or obtain additional information from the Internet by contacting SkillsUSA at *www.skillsusa.org*.

OTHER SOURCES OF INFORMATION

♦ National HOSA
6021 Morris Rd., Suite 111
Flower Mound, TX 75028
800-321-HOSA
Internet address: *www.hosa.org*

♦ SkillsUSA
P.O. Box 3000
Leesburg, Virginia 20177-0300
703-777-8810
Internet address: *www.skillsusa.org*

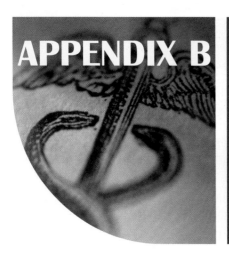

APPENDIX B

Correlation to National Health Care Skill Standards

Introduction to Health Science Technology Chapter	Health Care Core Standards	Therapeutic Services	Diagnostic Services	Health Informatics	Support Services	Biotechnology Research and Development
1. History and Trends of Health Care	X	X	X	X	X	X
2. Health Care Systems	X	X	X	X	X	X
3. Careers in Health Care	X	X	X	X	X	X
4. Personal and Professional Qualities of a Health Care Worker	X	X	X	X	X	X
5. Legal and Ethical Responsibilities	X	X	X	X	X	X
6. Medical Terminology	X	X	X	X	X	X
7. Anatomy and Physiology	X	X	X	X	X	X
8. Human Growth and Development	X	X	X	X	X	X
9. Nutrition and Diets	X	X	X	X	X	X
10. Cultural Diversity	X	X	X	X	X	X
11. Geriatric Care	X	X	X	X	X	X
12. Promotion of Safety	X	X	X	X	X	X
13. Infection Control	X	X	X	X	X	X
14. Vital Signs		X	X	X	X	X
15. First Aid	X	X	X	X	X	X
16. Preparing for the World of Work	X	X	X	X	X	X
17. Computer Technology in Health Care	X	X	X	X	X	X
18. Medical Math	X	X	X	X	X	X

Glossary

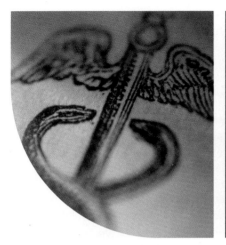

A

abbreviation—A shortened form of a word, usually just letters.

abdominal—Pertaining to the cavity or area in the front of the body and containing the stomach, the small intestine, part of the large intestine, the liver, the gallbladder, the pancreas, and the spleen.

abduction—Movement away from the midline.

abrasion—Injury caused by rubbing or scraping the skin.

absorption—Act or process of sucking up or in; taking in of nutrients.

abuse—Any care that results in physical harm or pain, or mental anguish.

acceptance—The process of receiving or taking; approval; belief.

accreditation—Process where an educational program is recognized and/or approved for meeting and maintaining standards that qualify its graduates for professional practice.

acculturation—Process of learning the beliefs and behaviors of a dominant culture and assuming some of the characteristics.

acidosis—A pathological condition resulting from a disturbance in the acid–base balance in the blood and body tissues.

activities of daily living (ADL)—Daily activities necessary to meet basic human needs, for example, feeding, dressing, and elimination.

acupuncture—Puncturing the skin at specific points with thin needles to relieve pain and/or treat disease.

acute—Lasting a short period of time but relatively severe (for example, an acute illness).

addiction—State of being controlled by a habit, as can happen with alcohol and drugs.

adduction—Movement toward the midline.

adipose—Fatty tissue; fat.

adolescence—Period of development from 12 to 18 years of age; teenage years.

adrenal—One of two endocrine glands located one above each kidney.

advance directive—A legal document designed to indicate a person's wishes regarding care in case of a terminal illness or during the dying process.

aerobic—Requiring oxygen to live and grow.

afebrile—Without a fever.

agent—Someone who has the power or authority to act as the representative of another.

agnostic—Person who believes that the existence of God cannot be proved or disproved.

alimentary canal—The digestive tract from the esophagus to the rectum.

alternative therapy—Method of treatment used in place of biomedical therapies.

alveoli—Microscopic air sacs in the lungs.

Alzheimer's disease—Progressive, irreversible disease involving memory loss, disorientation, deterioration of intellectual function, and speech and gait disturbances.

amino acid—The basic component of proteins.

amputation—The cutting off or separation of a body part from the body.

anaerobic—Not requiring oxygen to live and grow; able to thrive in the absence of oxygen.

anaphylactic shock—An extreme, sometimes fatal, allergic reaction or sensitivity to a specific antigen, such as a medication, insect sting, or specific food.

anatomy—The study of the structure of an organism.

anemia—Disease caused by lack of blood or an insufficient number of red blood cells.

anger—Feeling of displeasure or hostility; mad.

angles—Figures formed by two lines diverging from a common point.

anorexia—Loss of appetite.

anorexia nervosa—Psychological disorder involving loss of appetite and excessive weight loss not caused by a physical disease.

anoxia—Without oxygen; synonymous with suffocation.

antecubital—The space located on the inner part of the arm and near the elbow.

anterior—Before or in front of.

antioxidants—Enzymes or organic molecules; help protect the body from harmful chemicals called *free radicals*.

antisepsis—Aseptic control that inhibits, retards growth of, or kills pathogenic organisms; not effective against spores and viruses.

anuria—Without urine; producing no urine.

anus—External opening of the anal canal, or rectum.

aorta—Largest artery in the body; carries blood away from the heart.

aortic valve—Flap or cusp located between the left ventricle of the heart and the aorta.

aphasia—Language impairment; loss of ability to comprehend or speak normally.

apical pulse—Pulse taken with a stethoscope and near the apex of the heart.

apnea—Absence of respirations; temporary cessation of respirations.

apoplexy—A stroke; *see* **cerebrovascular accident.**

Apothecary system—Older system of measurement used for some medications.

appendicular skeleton—The bones that form the limbs or extremities of the body.

application form—A form or record completed when applying for a job.

aqueous humor—Watery liquid that circulates in the anterior chamber of the eye.

aromatherapy—Use of natural scents and smells to promote health and well-being.

arrhythmia—Irregular or abnormal rhythm, usually referring to the heart rhythm.

arterial—Pertaining to an artery.

arteriole—Smallest branch of an artery; vessel that connects arteries to capillaries.

arteriosclerosis—Hardening and/or narrowing of the walls of arteries.

artery—Blood vessel that carries blood away from the heart.

asepsis—Being free from infection.

assault—Physical or verbal attack on another person; treatment or care given to a person without obtaining proper consent.

assistant—Level of occupational proficiency where an individual can work in an occupation after a period of education or on-the-job training.

associate degree—Degree awarded by a vocational–technical school or community college after successful completion of a two-year course of study or its equivalent.

atheist—Person who does not believe in any deity.

atherosclerosis—Form of arteriosclerosis characterized by accumulation of fats or mineral deposits on the inner walls of the arteries.

atrium—Also called an *auricle*; an upper chamber of the heart.

audiologist—Individual specializing in diagnosis and treatment of hearing disorders.

aural temperature—Measurement of body temperature at the tympanic membrane in the ear.

auricle—Also called the *pinna*; external part of the ear.

autoclave—Piece of equipment used to sterilize articles by way of steam under pressure and/or dry heat.

autocratic leader—A dictator type of leader who maintains total control and makes all the decisions.

automated external defibrillator (AED)—Machine used to assess the heart rhythm and provide an electric shock to restore normal heart rhythm.

autonomic nervous system—That division of the nervous system concerned with reflex, or involuntary, activities of the body.

autopsy—Examination of the body after death to determine the cause of death.

avulsion—A wound that occurs when tissue is separated from the body.

axial skeleton—The bones of the skull, rib cage, and spinal column; the bones that form the trunk of the body.

axilla—Armpit; that area of the body under the arm.

B

bachelor's degree—Degree awarded by a college or university after a person has completed a four-year course of study or its equivalent.

backup—Copying or saving data in a secure location to prevent loss in the event of computer failure or a disaster.

bacteria—One-celled microorganisms, some of which are beneficial and some of which cause disease.

bandage—Material used to hold dressings in place, secure splints, and support and protect body parts.

bargaining—Process of negotiating an agreement, sale, or exchange.

Bartholin's glands—Two small mucous glands near the vaginal opening.

basal metabolism—The amount of energy needed to maintain life when the subject is at complete rest.

base of support—Standing with feet 8–10 inches apart to provide better balance.

battery—Unlawfully touching another person without that person's consent.

benign—Not malignant or cancerous.

bias—A preference that inhibits impartial judgment.

bile—Liver secretion that is concentrated and stored in the gallbladder; aids in the emulsification of fats during digestion.

bioethics—Branch of medicine concerned with moral issues resulting from technologic advances and medical research.

biohazardous—Contaminated with blood or body fluid and having the potential to transmit disease.

bioterrorism—The use of biological agents, such as pathogens, for terrorist purposes.

bladder—Membranous sac or storage area for a secretion (gallbladder); also, the vesicle that acts as the reservoir for urine.

bland diet—Diet containing only mild-flavored foods with soft textures.

blood—Fluid that circulates through the vessels in the body to carry substances to all body parts.

blood pressure—Measurement of the force exerted by the heart against the arterial walls when the heart contracts (beats) and relaxes.

bloodborne—An infectious disease or pathogenic organism that is transmitted through blood.

body mechanics—The way in which the body moves and maintains balance; proper body mechanics involves the most efficient use of all body parts.

bowel—The intestines.

Bowman's capsule—Part of the renal corpuscle in the kidney; picks up substances filtered from the blood by the glomerulus.

brachial—Pertaining to the brachial artery in the arm, which is used to measure blood pressure.

bradycardia—Slow heart rate, usually below 60 beats per minute.

bradypnea—Slow respiratory rate, usually below 10 respirations per minute.

brain—Soft mass of nerve tissue inside the cranium.

breast—Mammary, or milk, gland located on the upper part of the front surface of the body.

bronchi—Two main branches of the trachea; air tubes to and from the lungs.

bronchioles—Small branches of the bronchi; carry air in the lungs.

browser—Special software that allows an individual to view information on the Internet.

budget—An itemized list of income and expected expenditures for a period of time.

bulimarexia—Psychological condition in which a person eats excessively and then uses laxatives or vomits to get rid of the food.

bulimia—Psychological condition in which a person alternately eats excessively and then fasts or refuses to eat.

burn—Injury to body tissue caused by heat, caustics, radiation, and/or electricity.

C

calorie—Unit of measurement of the fuel value of food.

cancer—A group of diseases caused by abnormal cell division and/or growth.

capillary—Tiny blood vessel that connects arterioles and venules and allows for exchange of nutrients and gases between the blood and the body cells.

carbohydrate-controlled diet—Diet in which the number and types of carbohydrates are restricted or limited.

carbohydrates—Group of chemical substances including sugars, cellulose, and starches; nutrients that provide the greatest amount of energy in the average diet.

carcinogen—Any cancer-causing substance.

carcinoma—Malignant (cancerous) tumor of connective tissue.

cardiac—Pertaining to the heart.

cardiac arrest—Sudden and unexpected stoppage of heart action.

cardiopulmonary—Pertaining to the heart and lungs.

cardiopulmonary resuscitation (CPR)—Procedure of providing oxygen and chest compressions to a victim whose heart has stopped beating.

cardiovascular—Pertaining to the heart and blood vessels.

carpal—Bone of the wrist.

cataract—Condition of the eye where the lens becomes cloudy or opaque, leading to blindness.

caudal—Pertaining to any tail or tail-like structure.

cavitation—The cleaning process employed in an ultrasonic unit; bubbles explode to drive cleaning solution onto article being cleaned.

cavity—A hollow space, such as a body cavity (which contains organs) or a hole in a tooth.

cell—Mass of protoplasm; the basic unit of structure of all animals and plants.

cell membrane—Outer, protective, semipermeable covering of a cell.

cellulose—Fibrous form of carbohydrate.

Centigrade—Temperature scale that registers the freezing point of water as 0° and the boiling point as 100°.

central nervous system—The division of the nervous system consisting of the brain and spinal cord.

central processing unit (CPU)—Unit that controls all of the work of a computer; frequently called the "brains" of the computer.

centrosome—That area of cell cytoplasm that contains two centrioles; important in reproduction of the cell.

cerebellum—The section of the brain that is dorsal to the pons and medulla oblongata; maintains balance and equilibrium.

cerebrospinal fluid—Watery, clear fluid that surrounds the brain and spinal cord.

cerebrovascular accident—Also called a *stroke* or *apoplexy*; an interrupted supply of blood to the brain, caused by formation of a clot, blockage of an artery, or rupture of a blood vessel.

cerebrum—Largest section of brain; involved in sensory interpretation and voluntary muscle activity.

certification—The issuing of a statement or certificate by a professional organization to a person who has met the requirements of education and/or experience and who meets the standards set by the organization.

cervical—Pertaining to the neck portion of the spinal column or to the lower part of the uterus.

cervix—Anatomical part of a tooth where the crown joins with the root; entrance to or lower part of the uterus.

chain of infection—Factors that lead to the transmission or spread of disease.

character—The quality of respirations (for example, deep, shallow, or labored).

chemical—The method of aseptic control in which substances or solutions are used to disinfect articles; does not always kill spores and viruses.

chemical abuse—Use of chemical substances without regard for accepted practice; dependence on alcohol or drugs.

chemotherapy—Treatment of a disease by way of chemical agents.

Cheyne–Stokes respirations—Periods of difficult breathing (dyspnea) followed by periods of no respirations (apnea).

chiropractic—System of treatment based on manipulation of the spinal column and other body structures.

cholesterol—Fatlike substance synthesized in the liver and found in body cells and animal fats.

choroid—Middle or vascular layer of the eye, between the sclera and retina.

chromatin network—That structure in the nucleus of a cell that contains chromosomes with genes, which carry inherited characteristics.

chronic—Lasting a long period of time; reoccurring.

cilia—Hairlike projections.

circumduction—Moving in a circle at a joint, or moving one end of a body part in a circle while the other end remains stationary.

clavicle—Collarbone.

clean—Free from organisms causing disease.

clear-liquid diet—Diet containing only water-based liquids; nutritionally inadequate.

client—Person receiving service or care; a patient in health care.

clinic—Institution that provides care for outpatients; a group of specialists working in cooperation.

coccyx—The tailbone; lowest bones of the vertebral column.

cochlea—Snail-shaped section of the inner ear; contains the organ of Corti for hearing.

colon—The large intestine.

communicable disease—Disease that is transmitted from one individual to another.

communication—Process of transmission; exchange of thoughts or information.

compensation—Something given or received as an equivalent for a loss, service, or debt; defense mechanism involving substitution of one goal for another goal to achieve success.

competent—Able, capable.

complementary therapy—Method of treatment used in conjunction with biomedical therapies.

computer-assisted instruction (CAI)—Teaching method in which a computer and computer programs are used to control the learning process and deliver the instructional material to the learner.

computerized tomography (CT)—A scanning and detection system that uses a minicomputer and display screen to visualize an internal portion of the human body; formerly known as *CAT (computerized axial tomography)*.

confidential—Not to be shared or told; to be held in confidence, or kept to oneself.

congenital—Present at birth (as in a congenital defect).

conjunctiva—Mucous membrane that lines the eyelids and covers the anterior part of the sclera of the eye.

connective tissue—Body tissue that connects, supports, or binds body organs.

contagious—Easily spread; communicable.

contamination—Containing infection or infectious organisms or germs.

contract—To shorten, decrease in size, or draw together; an agreement between two or more persons.

contracture—Tightening or shortening of a muscle.

contusion—An injury that results in a hemorrhage (bleeding) beneath intact skin; a bruise.

convulsion—Also called a *seizure*; a violent, involuntary contraction of muscles.

cornea—The transparent section of the sclera; allows light rays to enter the eye.

cost containment—Procedures used to control costs or expenses.

Cowper's glands—The pair of small mucous glands near the male urethra.

cranial—Pertaining to the skull or cranium.

cranium—Part of the skull; the eight bones of the head that enclose the brain.

crust—A scab; outer covering or coat.

cultural assimilation—Absorption of a culturally distinct group into a dominant or prevailing culture.

cultural diversity—Differences among individuals based on cultural, ethnic, and racial factors.

culture—Values, beliefs, ideas, customs, and characteristics passed from one generation to the next.

cyanosis—Bluish color of the skin, nail beds, and/or lips due to an insufficient amount of oxygen in the blood.

cytoplasm—The fluid inside a cell; contains water, proteins, lipids, carbohydrates, minerals, and salts.

D

database—Organized collection of information.

daydreaming—Defense mechanism of escape; dreamlike musing while awake.

decimal—A part of a number expressed as a unit of 10.

deduction—Something subtracted or taken out (for example, monies taken out of a paycheck for various purposes).

defamation—Slander or libel; a false statement that causes ridicule or damage to a reputation.

defense mechanism—Physical or psychological reaction of an organism used in self-defense or to protect self-image.

defibrillate—Use of an electric shock to restore normal heart rhythm.

degrees—Units of measurement for temperature and angles.

dehydration—Insufficient amounts of fluid in the tissues.

delirium—Acute, reversible mental confusion caused by illness, medical problems, and/or medications.

delusion—A false belief.

dementia—Loss of mental ability characterized by decrease in intellectual ability, loss of memory, impaired judgment, and disorientation.

democratic leader—A leader who encourages the participation of all individuals in a group.

dental hygienist—A licensed individual who works with a dentist to provide care and treatment for the teeth and gums.

dentist—A doctor who specializes in diagnosis, prevention, and treatment of diseases of the teeth and gums.

dentition—The number, type, and arrangement of teeth in the mouth.

dependable—Capable of being relied on; trustworthy.

dermis—The skin.

diabetes mellitus—Metabolic disease caused by an insufficient secretion or utilization of insulin and leading to an increased amount of glucose (sugar) in the blood and urine.

diabetic coma—An unconscious condition caused by an increased level of glucose (sugar) and ketones in the bloodstream of a person with diabetes mellitus.

diagnosis—Determination of the nature of a person's disease.

diaphysis—The shaft, or middle section, of a long bone.

diastole—Period of relaxation of the heart.

diastolic pressure—Measurement of blood pressure taken when the heart is at rest; measurement of the constant pressure in arteries.

diencephalon—The section of the brain between the cerebrum and midbrain; contains the thalamus and hypothalamus.

dietitian—An individual who specializes in the science of diet and nutrition.

digestion—Physical and chemical breakdown of food by the body in preparation for absorption.

disability—A physical or mental handicap that interferes with normal function; incapacitated, incapable.

discretion—Ability to use good judgment and self-restraint in speech or behavior.

disease—Any condition that interferes with the normal function of the body.

disinfection—Aseptic-control method that destroys pathogens but does not usually kill spores and viruses.

dislocation—Displacement of a bone at a joint.

disorientation—Confusion with regard to the identity of time, place, or person.

displacement—Defense mechanism in which feelings about one person are transferred to someone else.

distal—Most distant or farthest from the trunk; center or midline.

doctorate—Degree awarded by a college or university after completion of a prescribed course of study beyond a bachelor's or master's degree.

dorsal—Pertaining to the back; in back of.

dressing—Covering placed over a wound or injured part.

duodenum—First part of the small intestine; connects the pylorus of the stomach and the jejunum.

dysphagia—Difficulty in swallowing.

dyspnea—Difficult or labored breathing.

dysrhythmia—An abnormal rhythm in the electrical activity of the brain or heart.

dysuria—Difficult or painful urination.

E

early adulthood—Period of development from 19 to 40 years of age.

early childhood—Period of development from 1 to 6 years of age.

echocardiography—A diagnostic test that uses ultra-high-frequency sound waves to evaluate the structure and function of the heart.

edema—Swelling; excess amount of fluid in the tissues.

ejaculatory duct—In the male, duct or tube from the seminal vesicle to the urethra.

electrocardiogram (ECG)—Graphic tracing of the electrical activity of the heart.

electroencephalogram (EEG)—Graphic recording of the brain waves or electrical activity in the brain.

electronic mail (e-mail)—Form of communication that is sent, received, and forwarded online from one computer to another by means of a modem.

embolus—A blood clot or mass of material circulating in the blood vessels.

emotional—Pertaining to feelings or psychological states.

empathy—Identifying with another's feelings but being unable to change or solve the situation.

endocardium—Serous membrane lining of the heart.

endocrine—Ductless gland that produces an internal secretion discharged into the blood or lymph.

endodontics—Branch of dentistry involving treatment of the pulp chamber and root canals of the teeth; root canal treatment.

endogenous—Infection or disease originating within the body.

endoplasmic reticulum—Fine network of tubular structures in the cytoplasm of a cell; allows for the transport of materials in and out of the nucleus and aids in the synthesis and storage of protein.

entrepreneur—Individual who organizes, manages, and assumes the risk of a business.

epidemic—An infectious disease that affects a large number of people within a population, community, or region at the same time.

epidemiology—The study of the history, cause, and spread of an infectious disease.

epidermis—The outer layer of the skin.

epididymis—Tightly coiled tube in the scrotal sac; connects the testes with the vas or ductus deferens.

epigastric—Pertaining to the area of the abdomen above the stomach.

epiglottis—Leaf-shaped structure that closes over the larynx during swallowing.

epilepsy—A chronic disease of the nervous system characterized by motor and sensory dysfunction, sometimes accompanied by convulsions and unconsciousness.

epiphysis—The end or head at the extremity of a long bone.

epistaxis—Nosebleed.

epithelial tissue—Tissue that forms the skin and parts of the secreting glands, and that lines the body cavities.

ergonomics—An applied science used to promote the safety and well-being of a person by adapting the environment and using techniques to prevent injuries.

erythema—Redness of the skin.

erythrocyte—Red blood cell (RBC).

esophagus—Tube that extends from the pharynx to the stomach.

essential nutrients—Those elements in food required by the body for proper function.

estimate—Calculate an approximate answer.

ethics—Principles of right or good conduct.

ethnicity—Classification of people based on national origin and/or culture.

ethnocentric—Belief in the superiority of one's own ethnic group.

etiology—The study of the cause of a disease.

eustachian tube—Tube that connects the middle ear and the pharynx, or throat.

exocrine—Gland with a duct that produces a secretion.

exogenous—Infection or disease originating outside of or external to the body.

expiration—The expulsion of air from the lungs; breathing out air.

extension—Increasing the angle between two parts; straightening a limb.

external auditory canal—Passageway or tube extending from the auricle of the ear to the tympanic membrane.

F

facsimile—Machine that utilizes telephone lines to send messages and/or documents from one location to another location; a fax.

Fahrenheit—Temperature scale that registers the freezing point of water as 32° and the boiling point as 212°.

fainting—Partial or complete loss of consciousness caused by a temporary reduction in the supply of blood to the brain.

Fallopian tubes—Oviducts; in the female, passageway for the ova (egg) from the ovary to uterus.

false imprisonment—Restraining an individual or restricting an individual's freedom.

fascia—Fibrous membrane covering, supporting, and separating muscles.

fat—Also called a *lipid*; nutrient that provides the most concentrated form of energy; highest-calorie energy nutrient; overweight.

fat-restricted diet—Diet with limited amounts of fats, or lipids.

fax—*See* **facsimile**.

febrile—Pertaining to a fever, or elevated body temperature.

femur—Thigh bone of the leg; the longest and strongest bone in the body.

fever—Elevated body temperature, usually above 101°F, or 38.3°C, rectally.

fibula—Outer and smaller bone of the lower leg.

field—A specific data category within a computer database, for example, the entry of an address in a patient information database.

file—A group of related records in a computerized system.

fire extinguisher—A device that can be used to put out fires.

firewall—A software program or hardware device designed to prevent unauthorized access to a computer system.

first aid—Immediate care given to a victim of an injury or illness to minimize the effects of the injury or illness.

fixed expenses—Those items in a budget that are set and usually do not change (for example, rent and car payments).

flexion—Decreasing the angle between two parts; bending a limb.

fomite—Any substance or object that adheres to and transmits infectious material.

foramina—A passage or opening; a hole in a bone through which blood vessels or nerves pass.

fractions—Numbers that represent parts of a whole expressed with a numerator (top number) and denominator (bottom number).

fracture—A break (usually, a break in a bone or tooth).

frontal (coronal) plane—Imaginary line that separates the body into a front section and a back section.

frostbite—Actual freezing of tissue fluid resulting in damage to the skin and underlying tissue.

full liquid diet—Diet consisting of liquids and foods that are liquid at body temperature.

fungi—Group of simple, plantlike animals that live on dead organic matter (for example, yeast and molds).

G

gallbladder—Small sac near the liver; concentrates and stores bile.

geriatrics, gerontology—The study of the aged or old age and treatment of related diseases and conditions.

glaucoma—Eye disease characterized by increased intraocular pressure.

glomerulus—Microscopic cluster of capillaries in Bowman's capsule of the nephron in the kidney.

glucose—The most common type of sugar in the body.

glycosuria—Presence of sugar in the urine.

goal—Desired result or purpose toward which one is working.

Golgi apparatus—That structure in the cytoplasm of a cell that produces, stores, and packages secretions for discharge from the cell.

gonads—Sex glands, ovaries in the female and testes in the male.

gross income—Amount of pay earned before deductions are taken out.

gynecology—The study of diseases of women, especially those affecting the reproductive organs.

H

hantavirus—A virus spread by contact with rodents (rats and mice) or their excretions.

hard copy—Computer term for a printed copy of information.

hard palate—Bony structure that forms the roof of the mouth.

hardware—Machine or physical components of a computer system (usually, the parts of the computer and the peripherals).

Health Insurance Portability and Accountability Act (HIPAA)—Set of federal regulations adopted to protect the confidentiality of patient information and the ability to retain health insurance coverage.

heart attack—*See* **myocardial infarction**.

heat cramp—Muscle pain and spasm resulting from exposure to heat and inadequate fluid and salt intake.

heat exhaustion—Condition resulting from exposure to heat and excessive loss of fluid through sweating.

heat stroke—Medical emergency caused by prolonged exposure to heat, resulting in high body temperature and failure of sweat glands.

hemiplegia—Paralysis on one side of the body.

hemoglobin—The iron-containing protein of the red blood cells; serves to carry oxygen from the lungs to the tissues.

hemorrhage—Excessive loss of blood; bleeding.

heparin—A substance formed in the liver to prevent the clotting of blood; an anticoagulant.

hepatitis—Inflammation of the liver.

high-fiber diet—Diet containing large amounts of fiber, or indigestible food.

high-protein diet—Diet containing large amounts of protein-rich foods.

HIPAA—*See* **Health Insurance Portability and Accountability Act**.

histology—Study of tissue.

holistic health care—Care that promotes physical, emotional, social, intellectual, and spiritual well-being.

home health care—Any type of health care provided in a patient's home environment.

homeostasis—A constant state of natural balance within the body.

honesty—Truthfulness; integrity.

hormone—Chemical substance secreted by an organ or gland.

HOSA—Health Occupations Students of America, a national organization for students enrolled in health occupations programs.

hospice—Program designed to provide care for the terminally ill while allowing them to die with dignity.

hospital—Institution that provides medical or surgical care and treatment for the sick or injured.

humerus—Long bone of the upper arm.

hyperglycemia—Presence of sugar in the blood; high blood sugar.

hyperopia—Farsightedness; defect in near vision.

hyperpnea—An increased respiratory rate.

hypertension—High blood pressure.

hyperthermia—Condition that occurs when body temperature exceeds 104°F, or 40°C, rectally.

hypoglycemia—Low blood sugar.

hypotension—Low blood pressure.

hypothalamus—That structure in the diencephalon of the brain that regulates and controls many body functions.

hypothermia—Condition in which body temperature is below normal, usually below 95°F (35°C) and often in the range of 78–95°F (26–35°C).

hypoxia—Without oxygen; a deficiency of oxygen.

I

idiopathic—Without recognizable cause; condition that is self-originating.

ileum—Final section of small intestine; connects the jejunum and large intestine.

immunity—Condition of being protected against a particular disease.

improper fraction—A fraction in which the numerator is larger than the denominator.

incision—Cut or wound of body tissue caused by a sharp object; a surgical cut.

income—Total amount of money received in a given period (usually a year); salary is usually the main source.

infancy—Period of development from birth to 1 year of age.

infection—Invasion by organisms; contamination by disease-producing organisms, or pathogens.

inferior—Below; under.

inflammation—Tissue reaction to injury characterized by heat, redness, swelling, and pain.

informed consent—Permission granted voluntarily by a person who is of sound mind and aware of all factors involved.

ingestion—Taking food, fluids, or medications into the body through the mouth.

inhalation—Breathing in.

initiative—Ability to begin or follow through with a plan or task; determination.

input—Computer term for information that is entered into a computer.

inspiration—Breathing in; taking air into the lungs.

insulin—A hormone secreted by the islets of Langerhans in the pancreas; essential for the metabolism of glucose.

insulin shock—Condition that occurs in individuals with diabetes when there is an excess amount of insulin and a low level of glucose (sugar) in the blood.

integumentary—Pertaining to the skin or a covering.

interactive video—The color, sound, and motion of video technology integrated with computer-assisted instruction to create a new technology.

intercostal—Pertaining to the space between the ribs (costae).

Internet—Worldwide computer network.

intestine—That portion of the alimentary canal from the stomach to the rectum and anus.

intradermal—Inserted or put into the skin.

intramuscular—Injected or put into a muscle.

intravenous—Injected or put into a vein.

invasion of privacy—Revealing personal information about an individual without his or her consent.

invasive—Pertains to a test or procedure that involves penetrating or entering the body.

involuntary—Independent action not controlled by choice or desire.

iris—Colored portion of the eye; composed of muscular, or contractile, tissue that regulates the size of the pupil.

isolation—Method or technique of caring for persons who have communicable diseases.

J

jaundice—Yellow discoloration of the skin and eyes, frequently caused by liver or gallbladder disease.

jejunum—The middle section of the small intestine; connects the duodenum and ileum.

job interview—A face-to-face meeting or conversation between an employer and an applicant for a job.

joint—An articulation, or area where two bones meet or join.

K

kcal-controlled diet—Diet containing low-calorie foods; frequently prescribed for weight loss.

kidney—Bean-shaped organ that excretes urine; located high and in back of the abdominal cavity.

kilocalorie—Unit used to measure the energy value of food.

kilojoule—Metric unit used to measure the energy value of food.

L

labia majora—Two large folds of adipose tissue lying on each side of the vulva in the female; hairy outer lips.

labia minora—Two folds of membrane lying inside the labia majora; hairless inner lips.

laboratory—A room or building where scientific tests, research, experiments, or learning takes place.

laceration—Wound or injury with jagged, irregular edges.

lacrimal—Pertaining to tears; glands that secrete and expel tears.

lacteal—Specialized lymphatic capillary that picks up digested fats or lipids in the small intestine and transports them to the thoracic duct.

laissez-faire leader—An informal type of leader who believes in noninterference in the affairs of others.

larynx—Voice box, located between the pharynx and trachea.

late adulthood—Period of development beginning at 65 years of age and ending at death.

late childhood—Period of development from 6 to 12 years of age.

leadership—Ability to lead, guide, and direct others.

legal—Authorized or based on law.

legal disability—A condition in which a person does not have legal capacity and is therefore unable to enter into a legal agreement (for example, as is the case with a minor).

lens—Crystalline structure suspended behind the pupil of the eye; refracts or bends light rays onto the retina; also, the magnifying glass in a microscope.

leukocyte—White blood cell (WBC).

liability—A legal or financial responsibility.

libel—False written statement that causes a person ridicule or contempt or causes damage to the person's reputation.

licensure—Process by which a government agency authorizes individuals to work in a given occupation.

life stages—Stages of growth and development experienced by an individual from birth to death.

ligament—Fibrous tissue that connects bone to bone.

light diet—Also called a *convalescent diet*; diet that contains easy-to-digest foods.

listen—To pay attention, make an effort to hear.

liver—Largest gland in the body; located in the upper right quadrant of the abdomen; two of its main functions are excreting bile and storing glycogen.

living will—A legal document stating a person's desires on what measures should or should not be taken to prolong life when his or her condition is terminal.

low-cholesterol diet—Diet that restricts foods high in saturated fat.

low-protein diet—Diet that limits foods high in protein.

low-residue diet—Diet that limits foods containing large amounts of residue, or indigestibles.

lung—Organ of respiration located in the thoracic cavity.

lymph—Fluid formed in body tissues and circulated in the lymphatic vessels.

lymph node—A round body of lymph tissue that filters lymph.

lymphatic duct—Short tube that drains purified lymph from the right sides of the head and neck and the right arm.

lymphatic vessels—Thin-walled vessels that carry lymph from tissues.

lysosomes—Those structures in the cytoplasm of a cell that contain digestive enzymes to digest and destroy old cells, bacteria, and foreign matter.

M

macule—A discolored but neither raised nor depressed spot or area on the skin.

magnetic resonance imaging (MRI)—Process that uses a computer and magnetic forces, instead of X-rays, to visualize internal organs.

mainframe computer—Largest type of computer; many users can access this computer at the same time.

malignant—Harmful or dangerous; likely to spread and cause destruction and death (for example, cancer).

malnutrition—Poor nutrition; without adequate food and nutrients.

malpractice—Providing improper or unprofessional treatment or care that results in injury to another person.

managed care—A health care delivery system designed to reduce the cost of health care while providing access to care through designated providers.

master's degree—Degree awarded by a college or university after completion of one or more years of prescribed study beyond a bachelor's degree.

Material Safety Data Sheets (MSDSs)—Information sheets that must be provided by the manufacturer for all hazardous products.

matriarchal—Social organization in which the mother or oldest woman is the authority figure.

medial—Pertaining to the middle or midline.

Medicaid—Government program that provides medical care for people whose incomes are below a certain level.

medical record—Also called a *patient chart*; written record of a patient's diagnosis, care, treatment, test results, and prognosis.

Medicare—Government program that provides medical care for elderly and/or disabled individuals.

medication—Drug used to treat a disease or condition.

Medigap policy—An insurance plan that serves as supplemental insurance to Medicare; usually pays deductible for Medicare and co-payments of care.

medulla oblongata—The lower part of the brainstem; controls vital processes such as respiration and heartbeat.

medullary canal—Inner, or central, portion of a long bone.

meiosis—The process of cell division that occurs in gametes, or sex cells (ovum and spermatozoa).

melanin—Brownish black pigment found in the skin, hair, and eyes.

meninges—Membranes that cover the brain and spinal cord.

menopause—Permanent cessation of menstruation.

mental—Pertaining to the mind.

metabolism—The use of food nutrients by the body to produce energy.

metacarpal—Bone of the hand between the wrist and each finger.

metastasis—The spread of tumor or cancer cells from the site of origin.

metatarsal—Bone of the foot between the instep and each toe.

microcomputer—Desktop or personal computer found in the home or office.

microorganism—Small, living plant or animal not visible to the naked eye; a microbe.

midbrain—That portion of the brain that connects the pons and cerebellum; relay center for impulses.

middle adulthood—Period of development from 40–65 years of age.

midsagittal—An imaginary line drawn down the midline of the body to divide the body into a right side and a left side.

military time—System of time that expresses time in four digits ranging from 0001 (one minute after midnight) to 2400 (12 midnight).

minerals—Inorganic substances essential to life.

mitochondria—Those structures in a cell that provide energy and are involved in the metabolism of the cell.

mitosis—Process of asexual reproduction by which cells divide into two identical cells.

modem—Device that converts outgoing messages from a computer into a form than can be sent over telephone lines.

mouth—Oral cavity; opening to the digestive tract, or alimentary canal.

muscle tissue—Body tissue composed of fibers that produce movement.

muscle tone—State of partial muscle contraction providing a state of readiness to act.

myocardial infarction—Heart attack; a reduction in the supply of blood to the heart resulting in damage to the muscle of the heart.

myocardium—Muscle layer of the heart.

myopia—Nearsightedness; defect in distant vision.

myth—A false belief; an established belief with no basis.

N

nasal cavity—Space between the cranium and the roof of the mouth.

nasal septum—Bony and cartilaginous partition that separates the nasal cavity into two sections.

need—Lack of something required or desired; urgent want or desire.

negligence—Failure to give care that is normally expected, resulting in injury to another person.

nephron—Structural and functional unit of the kidney.

nerve—Group of nerve tissues that conducts impulses.

nerve tissue—Body tissue that conducts or transmits impulses throughout the body.

net income—Amount of pay received for hours worked after all deductions have been taken out; take-home pay.

network—Connection of two or more computers to share data and hardware.

neurology—The study of the nervous system.

neuron—Nerve cell.

nocturia—Excessive urination at night.

noninvasive—Pertaining to a test or procedure that does not require penetration or entrance into the body.

nonpathogen—A microorganism that is not capable of causing a disease.

nonverbal—Without words or speech.

nose—The projection in the center of the face; the organ for smelling and breathing.

nosocomial—Pertaining to or originating in a health care facility such as a hospital.

nucleolus—The spherical body in the nucleus of a cell that is important in reproduction of the cell.

nucleus—The structure in a cell that controls cell activities such as growth, metabolism, and reproduction.

nutrition—All body processes related to food; the body's use of food for growth, development, and health.

nutritional status—The state of one's nutrition.

O

obstetrics—The branch of medicine dealing with pregnancy and childbirth.

occupational therapy—Treatment directed at preparing a person requiring rehabilitation for a trade or for return to the activities of daily living.

olfactory—Pertaining to the sense of smell.

oliguria—Decreased or less-than-normal amounts of urine secretion.

ombudsman—Specially trained individual who acts as an advocate for others to improve care or conditions.

Omnibus Budget Reconciliation Act (OBRA)—Federal law that regulates the education and testing of nursing assistants.

oncology—The branch of medicine dealing with tumors or abnormal growths (for example, cancer).

ophthalmologist—A medical doctor who specializes in diseases of the eye.

ophthalmology—The study of the eye and diseases and disorders affecting the eye.

opportunistic infection—An infection that occurs when the body's immune system cannot defend itself from pathogens normally found in the environment.

optician—An individual who makes or sells lenses, eyeglasses, and other optical supplies.

optometrist—A licensed, nonmedical practitioner who specializes in the diagnosis and treatment of vision defects.

oral cavity—The mouth.

organ—Body part made of tissues that have joined together to perform a special function.

organ of Corti—Structure in the cochlea of the ear; organ of hearing.

organelles—Structures in the cytoplasm of a cell, including the nucleus, mitochondria, ribosomes, lysosomes, and Golgi apparatus.

orthodontics—The branch of dentistry dealing with prevention and correction of irregularities of the alignment of teeth.

orthopedics—The branch of medicine/surgery dealing with the treatment of diseases and deformities of the bones, muscles, and joints.

orthopnea—Severe dyspnea in which breathing is very difficult in any position other than sitting erect or standing.

os coxae—The hipbone; formed by the union of the ilium, ischium, and pubis.

ossicles—Small bones, especially the three bones of the middle ear that amplify and transmit sound waves.

osteopathy—A field of medicine and treatment based on manipulation, especially of the bones, to treat disease.

osteoporosis—Condition in which bones become porous and brittle because of lack or loss of calcium, phosphorus, and other minerals.

output—Computer term for processed information, or the final product obtained from the computer; also, total amount of liquid expelled from the body.

ovary—Endocrine gland or gonad that produces hormones and the female sex cell, or ovum.

P

palate—Structure that separates the oral and nasal cavities; roof of the mouth.

palliative—Measures taken to treat symptoms and/or pain even though it will not cure a disease; comfort measures.

pallor—Paleness; lack of color.

pancreas—Gland that is dorsal to the stomach; secretes insulin and digestive juices.

pandemic—An infectious disease that affects many people over a wide geographic area; a worldwide epidemic.

papule—Solid, elevated spot or area on the skin.

paralysis—Loss or impairment of the ability to feel or move parts of the body.

paraplegia—Paralysis of the lower half of the body.

parasite—Organism that lives on or within another living organism.

parasympathetic—A division of the autonomic nervous system.

parathyroid—One of four small glands located on the thyroid gland; regulates calcium and phosphorus metabolism.

patella—The kneecap.

pathogen—Disease-producing organisms.

pathology—The study of the cause or nature of a disease.

pathophysiology—Study of how disease occurs and the responses of living organisms to disease processes.

patience—Ability to wait, persevere; capacity for calm endurance.

patients' rights—Factors of care that all patients can expect to receive.

patriarchal—Social organization in which the father or oldest male is the authority figure.

pediatrics—The branch of medicine dealing with care and treatment of diseases and disorders of children.

pedodontics—The branch of dentistry dealing with treatment of teeth and oral conditions of children.

penis—External sex organ of the male.

percentage—A proportion or share in relation to a whole, with the whole represented as 100.

pericardium—Membrane sac that covers the outside of the heart.

perineum—Region between the vagina and anus in the female and between the scrotum and anus in the male.

periodontics—The branch of dentistry dealing with the treatment of the gingiva (gum) and periodontium (supporting tissues) surrounding the teeth.

periosteum—Fibrous membrane that covers the bones except at joint areas.

peripheral—That part of the nervous system apart from the brain and spinal cord; also, a device connected to a computer.

peristalsis—Rhythmic, wavelike motion of involuntary muscles.

peritoneal—Pertaining to the body cavity containing the liver, stomach, intestines, urinary bladder, and internal reproductive organs.

personal protective equipment (PPE)—Protective barriers such as a mask, gown, gloves, and protective eyewear that help protect a person from contact with infectious material.

perspiration—The secretion of sweat.

phalanges—Bones of the fingers and toes.

pharmacology—The study of drugs.

pharynx—The throat.

phlebotomist—Also called a *venipuncture technician*; individual who collects blood and prepares it for tests.

physiatrist—Medical doctor specializing in rehabilitation.

physical therapy—Treatment by physical means, such as heat, cold, water, massage, or electricity.

physiological needs—Basic physical or biological needs required by every human being to sustain life.

physiology—The study of the processes or functions of living organisms.

pineal—Glandlike structure in the brain.

pinna—Also called the *auricle*; external portion of the ear.

pituitary—Small, rounded endocrine gland at the base of the brain; regulates function of other endocrine glands and body processes.

placenta—Temporary endocrine gland created during pregnancy to provide nourishment for the fetus; the afterbirth.

plane—Flat or relatively smooth surface; an imaginary line drawn through the body at various parts to separate the body into sections.

plasma—Liquid portion of the blood.

platelet—*See* **thrombocyte**.

pleura—A serous membrane that covers the lungs and lines the thoracic cavity.

podiatrist—An individual who specializes in the diagnosis and treatment of diseases and disorders of the feet.

poisoning—Condition that occurs when contact is made with any chemical substance that causes injury, illness, or death.

polycythemia—Excess number of red blood cells.

polydipsia—Excessive thirst.

polyuria—Increased production and discharge of urine; excessive urination.

pons—That portion of the brainstem that connects the medulla oblongata and cerebellum to the upper portions of the brain.

positron emission tomography (PET)—Computerized body scanning technique in which the computer detects a radioactive substance injected into a patient.

posterior—Toward the back; behind.

Power of Attorney (POA)—A legal document authorizing a person to act as another person's legal representative or agent.

prefix—An affix attached to the beginning of a word.

prejudice—Strong feeling or belief about a person or subject that is formed without reviewing facts or information.

privileged communications—All personal information given to health personnel by a patient; must be kept confidential.

prognosis—Prediction regarding the probable outcome of a disease.

projection—Defense mechanism in which an individual places the blame for his or her actions on someone else or circumstances.

prostate gland—In the male, gland near the urethra; contracts during ejaculation to prevent urine from leaving the bladder.

prosthodontics—The branch of dentistry dealing with the construction of artificial appliances for the mouth.

protective isolation—*See* **reverse isolation**.

protein—One of six essential nutrients needed for growth and repair of tissues.

protoplasm—Thick, viscous substance that is the physical basis of all living things.

protozoa—Microscopic, one-celled animals often found in decayed materials and contaminated water.

proximal—Closest to the point of attachment or area of reference.

psychiatry—The branch of medicine dealing with the diagnosis, treatment, and prevention of mental illness.

psychology—The study of mental processes and their effects on behavior.

psychosomatic—Pertaining to the relationship between the mind or emotions and the body.

puberty—Period of growth and development during which secondary sexual characteristics begin to develop.

pulse—Pressure of the blood felt against the wall of an artery as the heart contracts or beats.

pulse deficit—The difference between the rate of an apical pulse and the rate of a radial pulse.

pulse pressure—The difference between systolic and diastolic blood pressure.

puncture wound—Injury caused by a pointed object such as a needle or nail.

pupil—Opening or hole in the center of the iris of the eye; allows light to enter the eye.

pustule—Small, elevated, pus- or lymph-filled area of the skin.

pyrexia—Fever.

pyuria—Pus in the urine.

Q

quadriplegia—Paralysis below the neck; paralysis of arms and legs.

R

race—Classification of people based on physical or biological characteristics.

radiology—The branch of medicine dealing with X-rays and radioactive substances.

radius—Long bone of the forearm, between the wrist and elbow.

rale—Bubbling or noisy sound caused by fluid or mucus in the air passages.

random access memory (RAM)—Form of computer memory known as read/write memory because data can be stored or retrieved from it.

range of motion (ROM)—The full range of movement of a muscle or joint; exercises designed to move each joint and muscle through its full range of movement.

rate—Number per minute, as with pulse and respiration counts.

ratio—Relationship between numbers; shows how many of one number is present as compared with another number.

rationalization—Defense mechanism involving the use of a reasonable or acceptable excuse as explanation for behavior.

read only memory (ROM)—Nonerasable, permanent form of computer memory built into a computer to control many of the computer's internal operations.

reality orientation—Activities to help promote awareness of time, place, and person.

record—A collection of related data in a computer.

rectal, rectum—Pertaining to or the lower part of the large intestine, the temporary storage area for indigestibles.

red marrow—Soft tissue in the epiphyses of long bones.

reference plane—Real or imaginary flat surface from which an angle is measured.

registration—Process whereby a regulatory body in a given health care area administers examinations and/or maintains a list of qualified personnel.

rehabilitation—The restoration to useful life through therapy and education.

religion—Spiritual beliefs and practices of an individual.

repression—Defense mechanism involving the transfer of painful or unacceptable ideas, feelings, or thoughts into the subconscious.

resident—An individual who lives in a long-term care facility.

resistant—Able to oppose; organisms that remain unaffected by harmful substances in the environment.

respiration—The process of taking in oxygen (inspiration) and expelling carbon dioxide (expiration) by way of the lungs and air passages.

responsibility—Being held accountable for actions or behaviors; willing to meet obligations.

résumé—A summary of a person's work history and experience, submitted when applying for a job.

retina—The sensory membrane that lines the eye and is the immediate instrument of vision.

reverse isolation—Technique used to provide care to patients requiring protection from organisms in the environment.

rhythm—Referring to regularity; regular or irregular.

ribs—Also called *costae*; 12 pairs of narrow, curved bones that surround the thoracic cavity.

rickettsiae—Parasitic microorganisms that live on other living organisms.

Roman numerals—Older system of numbering that uses symbols (I, V, X, L, C, D, M) and a combination of symbols to express an amount.

rotation—Movement around a central axis; a turning.

S

safety standards—Set of rules designed to protect both the patient and the health care worker.

salivary glands—Glands of the mouth that produce saliva, a digestive secretion.

scapula—Shoulder blade or bone.

sclera—White outer coat of the eye.

scrotum—Double pouch containing the testes and epididymis in the male individual.

search engine—Computer program designed to locate specific information on the Internet.

sebaceous gland—Oil-secreting gland of the skin.

seizure—A convulsion; involuntary contraction of muscles.

self-actualization—Achieving one's full potential.

self-esteem—Satisfaction with oneself.

self-motivation—Ability to begin or to follow through with a task without the assistance of others.

semicircular canals—Structures of the inner ear that are involved in maintaining balance and equilibrium.

seminal vesicle—One of two saclike structures behind the bladder and connected to the vas deferens in the male individual; secretes thick, viscous fluid for semen.

senile lentigines—Dark-yellow or brown spots that develop on the skin as aging occurs.

senility—Feebleness of body or mind caused by aging.

sensitive—Susceptible to a substance; organisms that are affected by an antibiotic in a culture and sensitivity study.

sensitivity—Ability to recognize and appreciate the personal characteristics of others.

septum—Membranous wall that divides two cavities.

sharps container—A puncture-resistant container for disposal of needles, syringes, and other sharp objects contaminated by blood or body fluids.

shock—Clinical condition characterized by various symptoms and resulting in an inadequate supply of blood and oxygen to body organs, especially the brain and heart.

sign—Objective evidence of disease; something that is seen.

sinus—Cavity or air space in a bone.

skeleton—The bony structure of the body.

SkillsUSA—An organization for students enrolled in career and technical programs.

slander—Spoken comment that causes a person ridicule or contempt or damages the person's reputation.

small intestine—That section of the intestine that is between the stomach and large intestine; site of most absorption of nutrients.

sodium-restricted diet—Special diet containing low or limited amounts of sodium (salt).

soft diet—Special diet containing only foods that are soft in texture.

soft palate—Tissue at the back of the roof of the mouth; separates the mouth from the nasopharynx.

software—Programs or instructions that allow computer hardware to function intelligently.

sphygmomanometer—Instrument calibrated for measuring blood pressure in millimeters of mercury (mm Hg).

spinal cord—A column of nervous tissue extending from the medulla oblongata of the brain to the second lumbar vertebra in the vertebral column.

spirituality—Individualized and personal set of beliefs and practices that evolve and change throughout an individual's life.

spleen—Ductless gland below the diaphragm and in the upper-left quadrant of the abdomen; serves to form, store, and filter blood.

sprain—Injury to a joint accompanied by stretching or tearing of the ligaments.

spreadsheet—Worksheet created by using a computer's ability to perform high-speed mathematical calculations; used for budgets, accounts, financial records.

standard precautions—Recommendations that must be followed to prevent transmission of pathogenic organisms by way of blood and body fluids.

stereotyping—Process of assuming that everyone in a particular group is the same.

sterile—Free of all organisms, including spores and viruses.

sterilization—Process that results in total destruction of all microorganisms; also, surgical procedure that prevents conception of a child.

sternum—Breastbone.

stethoscope—Instrument used for listening to internal body sounds.

stomach—Enlarged section of the alimentary canal, between the esophagus and the small intestine; serves as an organ of digestion.

strain—Injury caused by excessive stretching, overuse, or misuse of a muscle.

stress—Body's reaction to any stimulus that requires a person to adjust to a changing environment.

stroke—*See* **cerebrovascular accident**.

subcutaneous fascia (hypodermis)—Layer of tissue that is under the skin and connects the skin to muscles and underlying tissues.

sublingual—Under the tongue.

sudoriferous gland—Sweat-secreting gland of the skin.

suffix—An affix attached to the end of a word.

suicide—Killing oneself.

superior—Above, on top of, or higher than.

suppression—Defense mechanism used by an individual who is aware of unacceptable feelings or thoughts but refuses to deal with them.

surgery—The branch of medicine dealing with operative procedures to correct deformities, repair injuries, or treat disease.

sympathetic—That division of the autonomic nervous system that allows the body to respond to emergencies and stress; also, to understand and attempt to solve the problems of another.

symptom—A subjective indication of disease that is felt by the patient.

syncope—Fainting; temporary period of unconsciousness.

system—A group of organs and other parts that work together to perform a certain function.

systemic—Pertaining to the whole body.

systole—Period of work, or contraction, of the heart.

systolic pressure—Measurement of blood pressure taken when the heart is contracting and forcing blood into the arteries.

T

tachycardia—Fast, or rapid, heartbeat (usually more than 100 beats per minute in an adult).

tachypnea—Respiratory rate above 25 respirations per minute.

tactful—Able to do or say the correct thing; thoughtful.

tarsal—One of seven bones that forms the instep of the foot.

teamwork—Cooperative effort by the members of a group to achieve a common goal.

technician—A level of proficiency usually requiring a 2-year associate's degree or 3 to 4 years of on-the-job training.

technologist—A class of expertise in a health career field, usually requiring at least 3 to 4 years of college plus work experience.

teeth—Structures in the mouth that physically break down food by chewing and grinding.

temperature—The measurement of the balance between heat lost and heat produced by the body.

temporal temperature—Measurement of body temperature at the temporal artery on the forehead.

tendon—Fibrous connective tissue that connects muscles to bones.

tension—Uncomfortable inner sensation, discomfort, strain, or stress that affects the mind.

terminal illness—An illness that will result in death.

testes—Gonads or endocrine glands that are located in the scrotum of the male and that produce sperm and male hormones.

thalamus—That structure in the diencephalon of the brain that acts as a relay center to direct sensory impulses to the cerebrum.

therapeutic diet—Diet used in the treatment of disease.

therapy—Remedial treatment of a disease or disorder.

thermometer—Instrument used to measure temperature.

thoracic duct—Main lymph duct of the body; drains lymph from the lymphatic vessels into the left subclavian vein.

thrombocyte—Also called a *platelet*; blood cell required for clotting of the blood.

thymus—Organ in the upper part of the chest, lymphatic tissue and endocrine gland that atrophies at puberty.

thyroid—Endocrine gland that is located in the neck and regulates body metabolism.

tibia—Inner and larger bone of the lower leg, between the knee and ankle.

time management—System of practical skills that allows an individual to use time in the most effective and productive way.

tissue—A group of similar cells that join together to perform a particular function.

tongue—Muscular organ of the mouth; aids in speech, swallowing, and taste.

tonsil—Mass of lymphatic tissue found in the pharynx (throat) and mouth.

tort—A wrongful or illegal act of civil law not involving a contract.

trachea—Windpipe; air tube from the larynx to the bronchi.

transverse plane—Imaginary line drawn through the body to separate the body into a top half and a bottom half.

triage—A method of prioritizing treatment.

tricuspid valve—Flap or cusp between the right atrium and right ventricle in the heart.

tympanic membrane—The eardrum.

U

ulcer—An open lesion on the skin or mucous membrane.

ulna—Long bone in the forearm, between the wrist and elbow.

ultrasonic unit—Piece of equipment that cleans with sound waves.

ultrasonography—Noninvasive, computerized scanning technique that uses high-frequency sound waves to create pictures of body parts.

uremia—Excessive amounts of urea (a waste product) in the blood.

ureter—Tube that carries urine from the kidney to the urinary bladder.

urethra—Tube that carries urine from the urinary bladder to outside the body.

urinary meatus—External opening of the urethra.

urinate—To expel urine from the bladder.

urine—The fluid excreted by the kidney.

urology—The branch of medicine dealing with urine and diseases of the urinary tract.

urticaria—Hives.

uterus—Muscular, hollow organ that serves as the organ of menstruation and the area for development of the fetus in the female body.

V

vaccine—Substance given to an individual to produce immunity to a disease.

vagina—Tube from the uterus to outside the body in a female individual.

variable expense—In a budget, an expense that can change or be adjusted (for example, expenses for clothing and entertainment).

vas deferens—Also called the *ductus deferens*; the tube that carries sperm and semen from the epididymis to the ejaculatory duct in the male body.

vascular—Pertaining to blood vessels.

vasoconstriction—Constriction (decrease in diameter) of the blood vessels.

vasodilation—Dilation (increase in diameter) of the blood vessels.

vector—A carrier of disease; an insect, rodent, or small animal that transmits disease.

vein—Blood vessel that carries blood back to the heart.

ventilation—Process of breathing.

ventral—Pertaining to the front, or anterior, part of the body; in front of.

ventricle—One of two lower chambers of the heart; also, a cavity in the brain.

venule—The smallest type of vein; connects capillaries and veins.

vertebrae—Bones of the spinal column.

vesicle—Blister; a sac full of water or tissue fluid.

vestibule—Small space or cavity at the beginning of a canal.

veterinary—Pertaining to the medical treatment of animals.

villi—Tiny projections from a surface; in the small intestine, projections that aid in the absorption of nutrients.

virtual communities—Individuals who use the Internet to communicate and share information.

virus—One of a large group of very small microorganisms, many of which cause disease.

vital signs—Determinations that provide information about body conditions; include temperature, pulse, respirations, and blood pressure.

vitamins—Organic substances necessary for body processes and life.

vitreous humor—Jelly-like mass that fills the cavity of the eyeball, behind the lens.

volume—The degree of strength of a pulse (for example, strong or weak).

vulva—External female genitalia; includes the labia majora, labia minora, and clitoris.

W

wellness—State of being in good health; well.

wheezing—Difficult breathing with a high-pitched whistling or sighing sound during expiration.

whole numbers—Numbers that do not contain fractions or decimals

withdrawal—Defense mechanism in which an individual either ceases to communicate or physically removes self from a situation.

word root—Main word or part of word to which prefixes and suffixes can be added.

Workers' Compensation—Payment and care provided to an individual who is injured on the job.

wound—An injury to tissues.

X

xiphoid process—The small, bony projection at the lower end of the sternum (breastbone).

Y

yellow marrow—Soft tissue in the diaphyses of long bones.

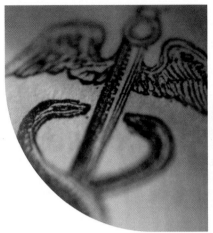
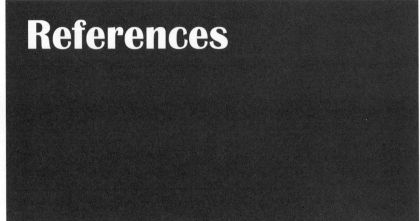

References

Acello, B. (2002). *The OBRA guidelines for quality improvement* (4th ed.). Clifton Park, NY: Delmar Learning.

Acello, B. (2002). *The OSHA handbook: Guidelines for compliance in health care facilities* (3rd ed.). Clifton Park, NY: Delmar Learning.

Acello, B. (2005). *Nursing assisting: Essentials for long-term care* (2nd ed.). Clifton Park, NY: Delmar Learning.

Acello, B. (2005). *Nutrition assistant essentials.* Clifton Park, NY: Delmar Learning.

Aehlert, B. (2007). *ACLS (Advanced Cardiac Life Support) review* (3rd ed.). St. Louis, MO: Mosby.

Agency for Instructional Technology. (2002). *Communicating with your team* (2nd ed.). Cincinnati, OH: South-Western.

Agency for Instructional Technology. (2002). *Communication and diversity* (2nd ed.). Cincinnati, OH: South-Western.

Agency for Instructional Technology. (2002). *Communication 2000: Resolving problems and conflicts* (2nd ed.). Cincinnati, OH: South-Western.

Aiken, T. D. (2003). *Legal and ethical issues in health occupations.* Philadelphia: W. B. Saunders.

Allen, E., & Marotz, L. (2007). *Developmental profiles: Pre-birth to eight* (5th ed.). Clifton Park, NY: Delmar Learning.

Alternative Link Systems, Inc. (2001). *The state legal guide to complementary and alternative medicine and nursing.* Clifton Park, NY: Delmar Learning.

Altman, G. (2004). *Delmar's fundamental and advanced nursing skills* (2nd ed.). Clifton Park, NY: Delmar Learning.

American Heart Association. (2004). *Recommendations for blood pressure measurements in humans.* Dallas, TX: American Heart Association.

American Heart Association. (2005). *American Heart Association to your health: A guide to health smart living.* Dallas, TX: American Heart Association.

American Heart Association. (2006). *BLS for healthcare providers.* Dallas, TX: American Heart Association.

American Heart Association. (2006). *Handbook of emergency cardiovascular care for healthcare providers.* Dallas, TX: American Heart Association.

American Heart Association. (2006). *Heart diseases and stroke statistics.* Dallas, TX: American Heart Association.

American Heart Association. (2006). *Know the facts: Get the stats.* Dallas, TX: American Heart Association.

American Heart Association. (2006). *Stroke facts 2006: All Americans.* Dallas, TX: American Heart Association.

American Heart Association. (2007). *Heartsaver® AED.* Dallas, TX: American Heart Association.

American Heart Association. (2007). *Heartsaver® CPR.* Dallas, TX: American Heart Association.

American Heart Association. (2007). *Heartsaver® first aid.* Dallas, TX: American Heart Association.

American Medical Association. (2009). *Health professions career and education directory.* Chicago: American Medical Association.

American Red Cross. (2005). *Bloodborne pathogens training: Preventing disease transmission.* Boston: StayWell.

American Red Cross. (2005). *Disaster preparedness guide.* Washington, DC: American Red Cross.

American Red Cross. (2005). *First aid fast.* Boston: StayWell.

American Red Cross. (2006). *CPR/AED for the professional rescuer.* Boston: StayWell.

American Red Cross. (2006). *General first aid/CPR/AED.* Boston: StayWell.

American Red Cross. (2006). *Responding to emergencies.* Boston: StayWell.

Andrews, M., & Boyle, J. (2002). *Transcultural concepts in nursing care* (4th ed.). Philadelphia: Lippincott Williams & Wilkins.

Anspaugh, D., Hamrick, M., & Rosato, F. (2006). *Wellness: Concepts and applications* (6th ed.). New York: McGraw-Hill.

Bailey, L. (2007). *Working* (4th ed.). Cincinnati, OH: South-Western.

Beck, M. (2006). *Theory and practice of therapeutic massage* (4th ed.). Clifton Park, NY: Delmar Learning.

Beebe, R., & Funk, D. (2005). *Fundamentals of emergency care* (2nd ed.). Clifton Park, NY: Delmar Learning.

Beers, M., & Berkow, R. (2006). *The Merck manual of diagnosis and therapy* (18th ed.). Whitehouse Station, NJ: Merck and Company.

Beers, M., & Jones, T. V. (2005). *The Merck manual of geriatrics* (3rd ed.). Whitehouse Station, NJ: Merck and Company.

Beers, M., & Jones, T. V. (2005). *The Merck manual of health and aging.* Whitehouse Station, NJ: Merck and Company.

Bonewit-West, K., Fulcher, E., & Burton, B. (2006). *Clinical procedures for medical assistants* (6th ed.). Philadelphia: W. B. Saunders.

Bos, T. J., & Somers, K. D. (2006). *Microbiology and infectious diseases.* New York: McGraw-Hill.

Bowman, M., & Lawlis, G. F. (2003). *Complementary and alternative medicine management.* Clifton Park, NY: Delmar Learning.

Brannigan, M. (2005). *Ethics across cultures.* New York: McGraw-Hill.

Buck, G. (2002). *Preparing for biological terrorism: An emergency services guide.* Clifton Park, NY: Delmar Learning.

Buck, G., Buck, L., & McGill, B. (2003). *Preparing for terrorism: The public safety communicator's guide.* Clifton Park, NY: Delmar Learning.

Buckley, W., & Okrent, K. (2004). *Torts and personal injury law* (3rd ed.). Clifton Park, NY: Delmar Learning.

Burke, L., & Weill, B. (2005). *Information technology for the health professions* (2nd ed.). Upper Saddle River, NJ: Prentice Hall.

Burkhardt, M., & Nathaniel, A. (2002). *Ethics and issues in contemporary nursing* (2nd ed.). Clifton Park, NY: Delmar Learning.

Burkhardt, M. A., & Naqai-Jacobson, M. G. (2002). *Spirituality: Living our connectedness.* Clifton Park, NY: Delmar Learning.

Burton, G. R., & Engelkirk, P. G. (2006). *Microbiology for the health sciences* (8th ed.). Philadelphia: Lippincott Williams & Wilkins.

Capellini, S. (2006). *Massage therapy career guide for hands-on success* (2nd ed.). Clifton Park, NY: Delmar Learning.

Carlton, R. R., & McKenna Adler, A. (2006). *Principles of radiographic imaging* (4th ed.). Clifton Park, NY: Delmar Learning.

Charlesworth, R. (2004). *Understanding child development* (6th ed.). Clifton Park, NY: Delmar Learning.

Cohen, B. (2005). *Memmler's structure and function of the human body* (8th ed.). Philadelphia: Lippincott Williams & Wilkins.

Cohen, B. (2005). *Memmler's the human body in health and disease* (10th ed.). Philadelphia: Lippincott Williams & Wilkins.

Coker Group. (2005). *Handbook of medical office communications: Effective letters, memos, and e-mails.* Chicago: American Medical Association.

Colbert, B. J. (2006). *Workplace readiness for health occupations.* (2nd ed.). Clifton Park, NY: Delmar Learning.

Comer, S. R. (2005). *Delmar's geriatric nursing care plans.* Clifton Park, NY: Delmar Learning.

Conklin, W. A., White, G., Cothren, C., Williams, D., & Davis, R. (2005). *Principles of computer security.* New York: McGraw-Hill.

Correa, C. (2005). *Getting started in the computerized medical office: Fundamentals and practice.* Clifton Park, NY: Delmar Learning.

Course Technology. (2005). *Guide to the Internet* (3rd ed.). Cincinnati, OH: South-Western.

Cowan, M., & Park Talaro, K. (2006). *Microbiology.* New York: McGraw-Hill.

Cronin, A., & Mandich, M. B. (2005). *Human development and performance throughout the lifespan.* Clifton Park, NY: Delmar Learning.

Cumming, A., Simpson, K., & Brown, D. (2007). *Complementary and alternative medicine.* New York: Churchill Livingstone.

Dalton, M., Hoyle, D. G., & Watts, M. W. (2006). *Human relations* (3rd ed.). Cincinnati, OH: South-Western.

Damjanov, I. (2006). *Pathology for the health professions* (3rd ed.). Philadelphia: W. B. Saunders.

D'Avanzo, C., & Geissler, E. (2003). *Pocket guide to cultural assessment* (3rd ed.). St. Louis, MO: Mosby.

Davies, J. (2002). *Essentials of medical terminology* (2nd ed.). Clifton Park, NY: Delmar Learning.

Davies, J. J. (2007). *Illustrated guide to medical terminology.* Clifton Park, NY: Delmar Learning.

Davis, B. K. (2002). *Phlebotomy: A customer service approach.* Clifton Park, NY: Delmar Learning.

Deem, S., & Deem, J. (2000). *Health care exploration.* Clifton Park, NY: Delmar Learning.

Delmar's medical terminology Flash! Computerized flashcards. (2002). Clifton Park, NY: Delmar Learning.

Dennerll, J. T. (2007). *Medical terminology made easy* (4th ed.). Clifton Park, NY: Delmar Learning.

Dennerll, J. T., & Davis, P. (2005). *Medical terminology: A programmed systems approach* (9th ed.). Clifton Park, NY: Delmar Learning.

DesJardins, T. (2002). *Cardiopulmonary anatomy and physiology* (4th ed.). Clifton Park, NY: Delmar Learning.

Dietz-Bourquignon, E. (2002). *Safety standards and infection control for dental assistants.* Clifton Park, NY: Delmar Learning.

Dikel, M., & Roehm, F. (2007). *Guide to Internet job searching.* Indianapolis, IN: Jist Works.

Diller, J., & Moule, J. (2005). *Cultural competence.* Pacific Grove, CA: Brooks/Cole.

Diller, J. (2007). *Cultural diversity: A primer for the human services* (3rd ed.). Pacific Grove, CA: Brooks/Cole.

Dorland's illustrated medical dictionary (31st ed.). (2007). Philadelphia: W. B. Saunders.

Doscher, M. (2005). *HIPAA: A short- and long-term perspective for health care.* Chicago: American Medical Association.

Edge, R., & Groves, J. (2006). *Ethics of health care: A guide for clinical practice* (3rd ed.). Clifton Park, NY: Delmar Learning.

Eggland, S. A., & WIlliams, J. W. (2005). *Human relations for career success* (6th ed.). Cincinnati, OH: South-Western.

Ehrlich, A., & Schroeder, C. L. (2005). *Medical terminology for health professions* (5th ed.). Clifton Park, NY: Delmar Learning.

Elahi, A. (2006). *Data, network, and Internet communications technology*. Clifton Park, NY: Delmar Learning.

Elling, Bob. (2003). *Principles of patient assessment in EMS*. Clifton Park, NY: Delmar Learning.

Engelkirk, P., & Burton, G. (2007). *Burton's microbiology for the health sciences* (8th ed.). Philadelphia: Lippincott Williams & Wilkins.

Estes, M. E. Z. (2006). *Health assessment* (3rd ed.). Clifton Park, NY: Delmar Learning.

Evashwick, C. (2005). *The continuum of long-term care* (3rd ed.). Clifton Park, NY: Delmar Learning.

Farr, M. (2006). *Job searching fast and easy*. Clifton Park, NY: Delmar Learning.

Farr, M. (2006). *Landing your dream job*. Clifton Park, NY: Delmar Learning.

Farr, M. (2006). *Seven step job search* (2nd ed.). Indianapolis, IN: Jist Works.

Feldstein, P. J. (2005). *Health care economics* (6th ed.). Clifton Park, NY: Delmar Learning.

Fetrow, C., & Avila, J. R. (2003). *Professional's handbook of complementary and alternative medicine* (3rd ed.). Philadelphia: Lippincott Williams & Wilkins.

Flight, M. R. (2004). *Law, liability, and ethics for the medical office professional* (4th ed.). Clifton Park, NY: Delmar Learning.

Fordney, M., French, L., & Follis, J. (2004). *Administrative medical assisting* (5th ed.). Clifton Park, NY: Delmar Learning.

Frazier, M. S., & Drzymkowski, J. (2004). *Essentials of human disease and conditions* (3rd ed.). Philadelphia: W. B. Saunders.

Fremgen, B. F. (2005). *Medical law and ethics* (2nd ed.). Upper Saddle River, NJ: Prentice Hall.

Frey, K., & Price, P. (2005). *Surgical anatomy and physiology for surgical technologists*. Clifton Park, NY: Delmar Learning.

Fry, R. (2003). *101 great resumes* (2nd ed.). Clifton Park, NY: Delmar Learning.

Fry, R. (2005). *Get organized* (3rd ed.). Clifton Park, NY: Delmar Learning.

Fry, R. (2005). *How to study* (6th ed.). Clifton Park, NY: Delmar Learning.

Fry, R. (2007). *101 great answers to the toughest interview questions* (5th ed.). Clifton Park, NY: Delmar Learning.

Fry, R. (2007). *101 smart questions to ask on your interview* (2nd ed.). Clifton Park, NY: Delmar Learning.

Garwood-Growers, A., Tingle, J., & Wheat, K. (2005). *Contemporary issues in healthcare law and ethics*. Philadelphia: W. B. Saunders.

Gaviola, S. (2005). *My pocket mentor, a health care professional's guide to success*. Clifton Park, NY: Delmar Learning.

Giger, J. N., & Davidhizar, R. E. (2004). *Transcultural nursing: Assessment and intervention* (4th ed.). St. Louis, MO: Mosby.

Gould, B. (2006). *Pathophysiology for the health related professions* (3rd ed.). Philadelphia: W. B. Saunders.

Green, M., & Bowie, M. J. (2005). *Essentials of health information management: Principles and practices*. Clifton Park, NY: Delmar Learning.

Grover-Lakomia, L., & Fong, E. (2000). *Microbiology for health careers* (6th ed.). Clifton Park, NY: Delmar Learning.

Haroun, L. (2006). *Career development for health professionals* (2nd ed.). Philadelphia: Saunders.

Haroun, L., & Royce, S. (2004). *Delmar's teaching ideas and classroom activities for health occupations*. Clifton Park, NY: Delmar Learning.

Hegner, B., & Acello, B. (2004). *On the job: The essentials of nursing assisting*. Clifton Park, NY: Delmar Learning.

Hegner, B., Acello, B., & Caldwell, E. (2004). *Nursing assistant: A nursing process approach* (9th ed.). Clifton Park, NY: Delmar Learning.

Hegner, B., Needham, J., & Gerlach, M. J. (2007). *Assisting in long-term care* (5th ed.). Clifton Park, NY: Delmar Learning.

Heller, M., & Veach, L. (2007). *Clinical medical assisting*. Clifton Park, NY: Delmar Learning.

Henderson, D. A., O'Toole, T., & Inglesly, T. V. (2005). *Bioterrorism: A guideline for medical and public health management*. Chicago: American Medical Association.

Hernandez, L. de. (2002). *Emergencia: Emergency translation manual*. Clifton Park, NY: Delmar Learning.

Hirsch, A. (2005). *Job search and career checklist*. Indianapolis, IN: Jist Works.

Hoffman, S. M. (2006). *Child care in action: Infants and toddlers*. Clifton Park, NY: Delmar Learning.

Hogan, M. (2003). *Four skills of cultural diversity: A process for understanding and practice* (2nd ed.). Pacific Grove, CA: Brooks/Cole.

Hogstel, M. (2001). *Nursing care of the older adult*. Clifton Park, NY: Delmar Learning.

Hosley, J., & Molle-Matthews, E. (2006). *A practical guide to therapeutic communication for health professionals*. Philadelphia: W. B. Saunders.

Hover-Kramer, D. (2002). *Healing touch: A guide book for practitioners* (2nd ed.). Clifton Park, NY: Delmar Learning.

Humphrey, D., & Sigler, K. (2004). *Contemporary medical office procedures* (3rd ed.). Clifton Park, NY: Delmar Learning.

Jonas, W. (2005). *Mosby's dictionary of complementary and alternative medicine*. St. Louis, MO: Mosby.

Jones, B. D., & Davies, J. J. (2006). *Delmar's comprehensive medical terminology* (2nd ed.). Clifton Park, NY: Delmar Learning.

Keegan, L. (2001). *Healing with complementary and alternative therapies.* Clifton Park, NY: Delmar Learning.

Keegan, L. (2002). *Healing nutrition* (2nd ed.). Clifton Park, NY: Delmar Learning.

Keir, L., Krebs, C., & Wise, B. A. (2006). *Medical assisting: Administrative and clinical competencies 2006 update* (5th ed.). Clifton Park, NY: Delmar Learning.

Kelz, R. (1999). *Conversational Spanish for health professions.* Clifton Park, NY: Delmar Learning.

Kennamer, M. (2005). *Math for health care professionals.* Clifton Park, NY: Delmar Learning.

Kennamer, M. (2007). *Basic infection control for the health care professional* (2nd ed.). Clifton Park, NY: Delmar Learning.

Klinoff, R. (2007). *Introduction to fire protection* (3rd ed.). Clifton Park, NY: Delmar Learning.

Krager, D., & Krager, C. (2005). *HIPAA for medical office personnel.* Clifton Park, NY: Delmar Learning.

Kramer, C. (2002). *Success in on-line learning.* Clifton Park, NY: Delmar Learning.

Krantman, S. (2001). *The resume writer's workbook* (2nd ed.). Clifton Park, NY: Delmar Learning.

Kubler-Ross, E. (1975). *Death: The final stage of growth.* Englewood Cliffs, NJ: Prentice-Hall.

Lafferty, S., & Baird, M. (2001). *Tele-nurse: Telephone triage protocols.* Clifton Park, NY: Delmar Learning.

Layman, D. (2006). *Medical terminology demystified.* New York: McGraw-Hill.

Leininger, M., & McFarland, M. R. (2002). *Transcultural nursing.* New York: McGraw-Hill.

Leonard, P. C. (2007). *Quick and easy medical terminology* (5th ed.). Philadelphia: W. B. Saunders.

Lesmeister, M. B. (2005). *Math basics for the health care professional* (2nd ed.). Upper Saddle River, NJ: Prentice Hall.

Lesmeister, M. B. (2007). *Writing basics for the health care professional* (2nd ed.). Upper Saddle River, NJ: Prentice Hall.

Libster, M. (2002). *Delmar's integrative herb guide for nurses.* Clifton Park, NY: Delmar Learning.

Limmer, D., O'Keefe, M., Dickinson, E., Grant, H., Murray, B., & Bergeron, J. D. (2005). *Emergency care* (10th ed.). Upper Saddle River, NJ: Brady/Prentice Hall.

Lindh, W. (2002). *Therapeutic communications for health professionals* (2nd ed.). Clifton Park, NY: Delmar Learning.

Lindh, W., Pooler, M., Tamparo, C., & Dahl, B. (2006). *Thomson Delmar learning's comprehensive medical assisting: Administrative and clinical competencies* (3rd ed.). Clifton Park, NY: Delmar Learning.

Makely, S. (1999). *Multiskilling: Team building for the health care provider.* Clifton Park, NY: Delmar Learning.

Mandleco, B. (2004). *Growth and development handbook: Newborn through adolescent.* Clifton Park, NY: Delmar Learning.

Mappes, T., & DeGrazia, D. (2006). *Biomedical ethics* (6th ed.). New York: McGraw-Hill.

Marotz, L., Cross, M. Z., Rush, J. (2005). *Health, safety, and nutrition for the young child* (6th ed.). Clifton Park, NY: Delmar Learning.

McArdle, W., Katch, F., & Katch, V. (2006). *Exercise physiology: Energy, nutrition, and human performance* (6th ed.). Philadelphia: Lippincott Williams & Wilkins.

McCutcheon, M., & Phillips, M. (2006). *Exploring health careers* (3rd ed.). Clifton Park, NY: Delmar Learning.

McElroy, O. H., & Grabb, L. L. (2006). *Spanish-English English-Spanish medical dictionary* (3rd ed.). Philadelphia: Lippincott Williams & Wilkins.

Merriam-Webster's medical desk dictionary (3rd ed.). (2006). Clifton Park, NY: Delmar Learning.

Milliken, M. E. (2004). *Understanding human behavior* (7th ed.). Clifton Park, NY: Delmar Learning.

Mitchell, J., & Haroun, L. (2007). *Introduction to health care* (2nd ed.). Clifton Park, NY: Delmar Learning.

Mitchell, M. K. (2003). *Nutrition across the life span* (2nd ed.). Philadelphia: W. B. Saunders.

Mosby's dictionary of medicine, nursing, and health professions (7th ed.). (2006). St. Louis, MO: Mosby.

Moisio, M. (2002). *Medical terminology: A student centered approach.* Clifton Park, NY: Delmar Learning.

Mullins, D. F. (2006). *501 human diseases.* Clifton Park, NY: Delmar Learning.

Mulvihill, M. L., Zelman, M., Holdaway, P., Tompary, E., & Raymond, J. (2006). *Human diseases: A systemic approach* (6th ed.). Upper Saddle River, NJ: Prentice Hall.

Munoz, C., & Luckmann, J. (2005). *Transcultural communication in nursing* (2nd ed.). Clifton Park, NY: Delmar Learning.

Myers, J., Neighbors, M., & Tannehill-Jones, R. (2002). *Principles of pathophysiology and emergency medical care.* Clifton Park, NY: Delmar Learning.

Nasso, J., & Celia, L. (2007). *Dementia care.* Clifton Park, NY: Delmar Learning.

National Health Council. (2002). *300 ways to put your talent to work in the health field.* New York: National Health Council.

National Health Council. (2008). *Guide to voluntary health agencies.* New York: National Health Council.

National Safety Council. (2007). *Standard first aid, CPR, and AED* (2nd ed.). New York: McGraw-Hill.

Neighbors, M., & Tannehill-Jones, R. (2006). *Human diseases* (2nd ed.). Clifton Park, NY: Delmar Learning.

Nicoll, L. (2009). *CIN: Computers, informatics, nursing.* Philadelphia: Lippincott Williams & Wilkins.

Nielsen, R. (2000). *OSHA regulations and guidelines: A guide for health care providers.* Clifton Park, NY: Delmar Learning.

Nix, S. (2005). *Williams' basic nutrition and diet therapy* (12th ed.). St. Louis, MO: Mosby.

Nowak, T. J., & Handford, A. G. (2004). *Pathophysiology concepts and applications for health care professionals* (3rd ed.). New York: McGraw-Hill.

O'Donnell, M. (2002). *Health promotion in the workplace* (3rd ed.). Clifton Park, NY: Delmar Learning.

Olson, M. (2002). *Healing the dying* (2nd ed.). Clifton Park, NY: Delmar Learning.

Papalia, D. E., Sterns, H., Feldman, R., & Camp, C. (2007). *Adult development and aging* (3rd ed.). New York: McGraw-Hill.

Papalia, D. E., Wendkos Olds, S., & Duskin Feldman, R. (2006). *A child's world: Infancy through adolescence* (10th ed.). New York: McGraw-Hill.

Parry, J., & Ryan, A. (2003). *A cross-cultural look at death, dying, and religion.* New York: McGraw-Hill.

Payne, R. A. (2005). *Relaxation techniques: A practical handbook for the health care professional* (3rd ed.). New York: Churchill Livingston.

Physicians' desk reference. (2009). Montvale, NJ: Thomson Healthcare.

Pigford, L. (2001). *The successful interview and beyond.* Clifton Park, NY: Delmar Learning.

Price, P., & Frey, K. (2003). *Microbiology for surgical technologists.* Clifton Park, NY: Delmar Learning.

Quill, T. (1993). *Death and dignity.* New York: W. W. Norton and Company.

Quill, T., & Battin, M. P. (2004). *Physician-assisted dying: The case for palliative care and patient choice.* Baltimore, MD: Johns Hopkins University Press.

Raffel, M. W., & Barsukiewicz, C. K. (2002). *The US health system origins and functions* (5th ed.). Clifton Park, NY: Delmar Learning.

Rasberry, R. (2004). *Employment strategies for career success.* Cincinnati, OH: South-Western.

Reichman, E. F. (2007). *Pocket atlas of emergency procedures.* New York: McGraw-Hill.

Rios, J., & Fernandez, J. (2005). *Spanish for health care providers.* New York: McGraw-Hill.

Rizzo, D. (2006). *Delmar's fundamentals of anatomy and physiology* (2nd ed.). Clifton Park, NY: Delmar Learning.

Robertson, C. (2007). *Safety, health, and nutrition in early education* (3rd ed.). Clifton Park, NY: Delmar Learning.

Robinson, J., & McCormick, D. J. (2005). *Essentials of health and wellness.* Clifton Park, NY: Delmar Learning.

Roth, R. A., & Townsend, C. E. (2007). *Nutrition and diet therapy* (9th ed.). Clifton Park, NY: Delmar Learning.

Ryan, J. S. (2006). *Managing your personal finances* (5th ed.). Cincinnati, OH: South-Western.

Saba, V., & McCormick, K. (2006). *Essentials of computers: Nursing informatics* (4th ed.). New York: McGraw-Hill.

Schultheis, R., & Kaczmarski, R. (2006). *Business math* (16th ed.). Cincinnati, OH: South-Western.

Scott, A., & Fong, E. (2004). *Body structures and functions* (10th ed.). Clifton Park, NY: Delmar Learning.

Scott, A., Fong, E., & Beebee, R. (2002). *Functional anatomy for emergency medical services.* Clifton Park, NY: Delmar Learning.

Segen, J. (2006). *Concise dictionary of modern medicine.* New York: McGraw-Hill.

Shortell, S., & Kaluzny, A. (2006). *Health care management, organization, design, and behavior* (5th ed.). Clifton Park, NY: Delmar Learning.

Simmers, L. (2005). *Practical problems in mathematics for health occupations* (2nd ed.). Clifton Park, NY: Delmar Learning.

Slaven, E. M., Stone, S. C., & Lopez, A. A. (2006). *Infectious diseases.* New York: McGraw-Hill.

Sormunen, C. (2003). *Terminology for allied health professionals* (5th ed.). Clifton Park, NY: Delmar Learning.

Sorrentino, S. (2006). *Mosby's essentials for nursing assistants* (3rd ed.). St. Louis, MO: Mosby.

Spatz, A., & Balduzzi, S. (2005). *Homemaker/home health aide* (6th ed.). Clifton Park, NY: Delmar Learning.

Stedman, T. L. (2005). *Stedman's alternative and complementary medicine words* (2nd ed.). Philadelphia: Lippincott Williams & Wilkins.

Stedman's medical dictionary for the health professions and nursing (5th ed.). (2005). Philadelphia: Lippincott Williams & Wilkins.

Stoy, W., Platt, T., & Lejeune, D. A. (2005). *Mosby's EMT-basic textbook* (2nd ed.). St. Louis, MO: Mosby.

Terryberry, K. (2005). *Writing for the health professions.* Clifton Park, NY: Delmar Learning.

Thibodeau, G., & Patton, K. (2004). *Structure and function of the body* (12th ed.). St. Louis, MO: Mosby.

Thibodeau, G., & Patton, K. (2005). *Human body in health and disease* (4th ed.). St. Louis, MO: Mosby.

Thibodeau, G., & Patton, K. (2007). *Anatomy and physiology* (6th ed.). St. Louis, MO: Mosby.

Thomson Delmar Learning. (2005). *Delmar learning's quick reference for health care providers.* Clifton Park, NY: Delmar Learning.

Thomson Delmar Learning. (2005). *Health care career exploration CD-ROM.* Clifton Park, NY: Delmar Learning.

Thomson Delmar Learning. (2006). *Vital signs for medical assistants interactive CD.* Clifton Park, NY: Delmar Learning.

Throop, R. K., & Castellucci, M. (2006). *Personal excellence.* Clifton Park, NY: Delmar Learning.

Tideiksaar, R. (2006). *Avoiding falls: A guideline for certified nursing assistants.* Clifton Park, NY: Delmar Learning.

U.S. Department of Agriculture. (2005). *Dietary guidelines for Americans.* Washington, DC: U.S. Government Printing Office.

U.S. Department of Agriculture. (2005). *Finding your way to a healthier you.* Washington, DC: U.S. Government Printing Office.

U.S. Department of Health and Human Services. (2007) *Guidelines for isolation precautions in hospitals.* Retrieved from http://www.cdc.gov/incidod/dhqp/gl_isolation.html

U.S. Department of Labor. (2009). *Occupational outlook handbook.* Washington, DC: U.S. Government Printing Office.

Villemarie, L., & Villemarie, D. (2006). *Grammar and writing skills for the health care professional* (2nd ed.). Clifton Park, NY: Delmar Learning.

Wallace, H. R., & Masters, A. (2006). *Personal development for life and work* (9th ed.). Cincinnati, OH: South-Western.

Walter, A., Rutledge, M., Edgar, C., & Davis, R. (2004). *First responder handbook*. Clifton Park, NY: Delmar Learning.

Walz, B. J. (2002). *Introduction to EMS systems*. Clifton Park, NY: Delmar Learning.

Waughfield, C. (2002). *Mental health concepts*. Clifton Park, NY: Delmar Learning.

Wendleton, K. (2006). *Launching the right career*. Clifton Park, NY: Delmar Learning.

Wendleton, K. (2006). *Mastering the job interview and winning the money game*. Clifton Park, NY: Delmar Learning.

Wendleton, K. (2006). *Packaging yourself: The targeted resume*. Clifton Park, NY: Delmar Learning.

Wendleton, K. (2007). *The five o'clock club job search workbook*. Clifton Park, NY: Delmar Learning.

Wertz, E. (2002). *Emergency care for children*. Clifton Park, NY: Delmar Learning.

Wheeler, S. Q. (2002). *Telephone triage protocols* (2nd ed.). Clifton Park, NY: Delmar Learning.

White, L. (2005). *Foundations of basic nursing* (2nd ed.). Clifton Park, NY: Delmar Learning.

Whittle, J. (2001). *911 responding for life: Case studies in emergency care*. Clifton Park, NY: Delmar Learning.

Williams, S. J. (2005). *Essentials of health services* (3rd ed.). Clifton Park, NY: Delmar Learning.

Williams, S. J., & Torrens, P. (2002). *Introduction to health services* (6th ed.). Clifton Park, NY: Delmar Learning.

Williams, S., & Schlenker, E. (2007). *Essentials of nutrition and diet therapy* (9th ed.). St. Louis, MO: Mosby.

Wischnitzer, S., & Wischnitzer, E. (2005). *Top 100 healthcare careers* (2nd ed.). Indianapolis, IN: Jist Works.

Wolfinger, A. (2007). *Best career and education Web sites* (5th ed.). Indianapolis, IN: Jist Works.

Wright, P., & Field, B. (2000). *Better job search in 3 easy steps*. Clifton Park, NY: Delmar Learning.

Wright, P., & Field, B. (2000). *Better job skills in 3 easy steps*. Clifton Park, NY: Delmar Learning.

Wright, P., & Field, B. (2000). *Better resumes in 3 easy steps*. Clifton Park, NY: Delmar Learning.

Zalenski, R., & Stone, S. C. (2008). *Emergency palliative care*. St. Louis, MO: McGraw-Hill.

Zedlitz, R. H. (2003). *How to get a job in health care*. Clifton Park, NY: Delmar Learning.

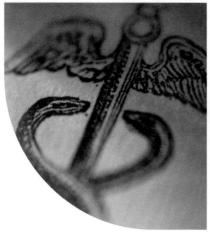

INDEX

IMPORTANT! READ CAREFULLY: This End User License Agreement ("Agreement") sets forth the conditions by which Delmar Cengage Learning will make electr access to the Delmar Cengage Learning-owned licensed content and associated media, software, documentation, printed materials, and electronic documenta contained in this package and/or made available to you via this product (the "Licensed Content"), available to you (the "End User"). BY CLICKING THE "I ACCE BUTTON AND/OR OPENING THIS PACKAGE, YOU ACKNOWLEDGE THAT YOU HAVE READ ALL OF THE TERMS AND CONDITIONS, AND THAT YOU AGREE BE BOUND BY ITS TERMS, CONDITIONS, AND ALL APPLICABLE LAWS AND REGULATIONS GOVERNING THE USE OF THE LICENSED CONTENT.

1.0 SCOPE OF LICENSE

1.1 <u>Licensed Content.</u> The Licensed Content may contain portions of modifiable content ("Modifiable Content") and content which may not be modifie otherwise altered by the End User ("Non-Modifiable Content"). For purposes of this Agreement, Modifiable Content and Non-Modifiable Content ma collectively referred to herein as the "Licensed Content." All Licensed Content shall be considered Non-Modifiable Content, unless such Licensed Conte presented to the End User in a modifiable format and it is clearly indicated that modification of the Licensed Content is permitted.

1.2 Subject to the End User's compliance with the terms and conditions of this Agreement, Delmar Cengage Learning hereby grants the End User, a nontran able, nonexclusive, limited right to access and view a single copy of the Licensed Content on a single personal computer system for noncommercial, inte personal use only. The End User shall not (i) reproduce, copy, modify (except in the case of Modifiable Content), distribute, display, transfer, sublicense, pare derivative work(s) based on, sell, exchange, barter or transfer, rent, lease, loan, resell, or in any other manner exploit the Licensed Content; (ii) rem obscure, or alter any notice of Delmar Cengage Learning's intellectual property rights present on or in the Licensed Content, including, but not limite copyright, trademark, and/or patent notices; or (iii) disassemble, decompile, translate, reverse engineer, or otherwise reduce the Licensed Content.

2.0 TERMINATION

2.1 Delmar Cengage Learning may at any time (without prejudice to its other rights or remedies) immediately terminate this Agreement and/or suspend acce some or all of the Licensed Content, in the event that the End User does not comply with any of the terms and conditions of this Agreement. In the event of termination by Delmar Cengage Learning, the End User shall immediately return any and all copies of the Licensed Content to Delmar Cengage Learning.

3.0 PROPRIETARY RIGHTS

3.1 The End User acknowledges that Delmar Cengage Learning owns all rights, title and interest, including, but not limited to, all copyright rights therein, in to the Licensed Content, and that the End User shall not take any action inconsistent with such ownership. The Licensed Content is protected by U.S. nadian and other applicable copyright laws and by international treaties, including the Berne Convention and the Universal Copyright Convention. Not contained in this Agreement shall be construed as granting the End User any ownership rights in or to the Licensed Content.

3.2 Delmar Cengage Learning reserves the right at any time to withdraw from the Licensed Content any item or part of an item for which it no longer retains right to publish, or which it has reasonable grounds to believe infringes copyright or is defamatory, unlawful, or otherwise objectionable.

4.0 PROTECTION AND SECURITY

4.1 The End User shall use its best efforts and take all reasonable steps to safeguard its copy of the Licensed Content to ensure that no unauthorized repro tion, publication, disclosure, modification, or distribution of the Licensed Content, in whole or in part, is made. To the extent that the End User beco aware of any such unauthorized use of the Licensed Content, the End User shall immediately notify Delmar Cengage Learning. Notification of such v tions may be made by sending an e-mail to delmarhelp@cengage.com.

5.0 MISUSE OF THE LICENSED PRODUCT

5.1 In the event that the End User uses the Licensed Content in violation of this Agreement, Delmar Cengage Learning shall have the option of electing liquid damages, which shall include all profits generated by the End User's use of the Licensed Content plus interest computed at the maximum rate permitte law and all legal fees and other expenses incurred by Delmar Cengage Learning in enforcing its rights, plus penalties.

6.0 FEDERAL GOVERNMENT CLIENTS

6.1 Except as expressly authorized by Delmar Cengage Learning, Federal Government clients obtain only the rights specified in this Agreement and no rights. The Government acknowledges that (i) all software and related documentation incorporated in the Licensed Content is existing commercial c puter software within the meaning of FAR 27.405(b)(2); and (2) all other data, delivered in whatever form, is limited rights data within the meaning of 27.401. The restrictions in this section are acceptable as consistent with the Government's need for software and other data under this Agreement.

7.0 DISCLAIMER OF WARRANTIES AND LIABILITIES

7.1 Although Delmar Cengage Learning believes the Licensed Content to be reliable, Delmar Cengage Learning does not guarantee or warrant (i) any info tion or materials contained in or produced by the Licensed Content, (ii) the accuracy, completeness or reliability of the Licensed Content, or (iii) tha Licensed Content is free from errors or other material defects. THE LICENSED PRODUCT IS PROVIDED "AS IS," WITHOUT ANY WARRANTY OF ANY K AND DELMAR CENGAGE LEARNING DISCLAIMS ANY AND ALL WARRANTIES, EXPRESSED OR IMPLIED, INCLUDING, WITHOUT LIMITATION, V RANTIES OF MERCHANTABILITY OR FITNESS FOR A PARTICULAR PURPOSE. IN NO EVENT SHALL DELMAR CENGAGE LEARNING BE LIABLE INDIRECT, SPECIAL, PUNITIVE OR CONSEQUENTIAL DAMAGES INCLUDING FOR LOST PROFITS, LOST DATA, OR OTHERWISE. IN NO EVENT SH DELMAR CENGAGE LEARNING'S AGGREGATE LIABILITY HEREUNDER, WHETHER ARISING IN CONTRACT, TORT, STRICT LIABILITY OR OTHERW EXCEED THE AMOUNT OF FEES PAID BY THE END USER HEREUNDER FOR THE LICENSE OF THE LICENSED CONTENT.

8.0 GENERAL

8.1 <u>Entire Agreement.</u> This Agreement shall constitute the entire Agreement between the Parties and supercedes all prior Agreements and understanding or written relating to the subject matter hereof.

8.2 <u>Enhancements/Modifications of Licensed Content.</u> From time to time, and in Delmar Cengage Learning's sole discretion, Delmar Cengage Learning advise the End User of updates, upgrades, enhancements and/or improvements to the Licensed Content, and may permit the End User to access and subject to the terms and conditions of this Agreement, such modifications, upon payment of prices as may be established by Delmar Cengage Learning

8.3 <u>No Export.</u> The End User shall use the Licensed Content solely in the United States and shall not transfer or export, directly or indirectly, the Licensed Con outside the United States.

8.4 <u>Severability.</u> If any provision of this Agreement is invalid, illegal, or unenforceable under any applicable statute or rule of law, the provision shall be dee omitted to the extent that it is invalid, illegal, or unenforceable. In such a case, the remainder of the Agreement shall be construed in a manner as to greatest effect to the original intention of the parties hereto.

8.5 <u>Waiver.</u> The waiver of any right or failure of either party to exercise in any respect any right provided in this Agreement in any instance shall not be dee to be a waiver of such right in the future or a waiver of any other right under this Agreement.

8.6 <u>Choice of Law/Venue.</u> This Agreement shall be interpreted, construed, and governed by and in accordance with the laws of the State of New York, applie to contracts executed and to be wholly preformed therein, without regard to its principles governing conflicts of law. Each party agrees that any procee arising out of or relating to this Agreement or the breach or threatened breach of this Agreement may be commenced and prosecuted in a court in the and County of New York. Each party consents and submits to the nonexclusive personal jurisdiction of any court in the State and County of New Yo respect of any such proceeding.

8.7 <u>Acknowledgment.</u> By opening this package and/or by accessing the Licensed Content on this Web site, THE END USER ACKNOWLEDGES THAT IT HAS THIS AGREEMENT, UNDERSTANDS IT, AND AGREES TO BE BOUND BY ITS TERMS AND CONDITIONS. IF YOU DO NOT ACCEPT THESE TERMS AND DITIONS, YOU MUST NOT ACCESS THE LICENSED CONTENT AND RETURN THE LICENSED PRODUCT TO DELMAR CENGAGE LEARNING (WITH CALENDAR DAYS OF THE END USER'S PURCHASE) WITH PROOF OF PAYMENT ACCEPTABLE TO DELMAR CENGAGE LEARNING, FOR A CREDIT OR A FUND. Should the End User have any questions/comments regarding this Agreement, please contact Delmar Cengage Learning at delmarhelp@cengage.